NURSE'S POCKET DRUG GUIDE 2009

EDITOR
Judith A. Barberio, PhD, APN,C, ANP, FNP, GNP

CONSULTING EDITOR
Leonard G. Gomella, MD, FACS

ASSOCIATE EDITORS
Steven A. Haist, MD, MS, FACP
Aimee Gelhot Adams, PharmD
Kelly M. Smith, PharmD, FASHP

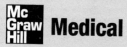

McGraw Hill Medical

New York Chicago San Francisco Lisbon
London Madrid Mexico City Milan New Delhi
San Juan Seoul Singapore Sydney Toronto

The McGraw·Hill Companies

Nurse's Pocket Drug Guide 2009

Copyright © 2009 by Judith A. Barberio. Based on *Clinician's Pocket Drug Reference 2008*. Copyright © 2008 by Leonard G. Gomella. Published by The McGraw-Hill Companies, Inc. All rights reserved. Printed in Canada. Except as permitted under the United States Copyright Act of 1976, no part of this publication may be reproduced or distributed in any form or by any means, or stored in a data base or retrieval system, without the prior written permission of the publisher.

ISBN 978-0-07-154970-7
MHID 0-07-154970-6
ISSN 1550-2554

The book was set in Times by International Typesetting and Composition
The editors were Quincy McDonald and Karen Davis.
The senior production supervisor was Sherri Souffrance.
The text designer was Marsha Cohen/Parallelogram Graphics.
The production manager was Preeti Longia Sinha, International Typesetting and Composition.
Transcontinental Gagne was printer and binder.

This book is printed on acid-free paper.

CONTENTS

Kelly M. Smith, PharmD, FASHP
Associate Professor
Department of Pharmacy Practice and Science
University of Kentucky College of Pharmacy
Clinical Specialist, Medical Use Policy
University of Kentucky Medical Center
Lexington, Kentucky

PREFACE

WE ARE PLEASED TO PRESENT THE FIFTH EDITION OF THE *NURSE'S POCKET DRUG GUIDE*. Our goal is to identify the most frequently used and clinically important medications, including branded, generic, and OTC products. The book includes over 1000 generic medications and is designed to represent a cross section of commonly used products in health care practices across the country.

The style of drug presentation includes key "must know" facts of commonly used medications and herbs, essential information for the student, practicing nurse, and health care provider. The inclusion of common uses of medications rather than just the official FDA-labeled indications are based on the uses of the medication and herbs supported by publications and community standards of care. All uses have been reviewed by our editorial board.

It is essential that students, registered nurses, and advanced-practice nurses learn more than the name and dose of the medications they administer and prescribe. Certain common side effects and significant contraindications are associated with most prescription medications. Although nurses and other health care practitioners should ideally be completely familiar with the entire package insert of any medication prescribed, such a requirement is unreasonable. References such as the *Physicians' Desk Reference* and the drug manufacturer's Web site make package inserts readily available for many medications, but may not highlight clinically significant facts or key data for generic drugs and those available over the counter.

The limitations of difficult-to-read package inserts were acknowledged by the Food and Drug Administration in early 2001, when it noted that health care providers do not have time to read the many pages of small print in the typical package insert. Newer drugs are producing more user-friendly package insert summaries that will highlight important drug information for easier nursing reference. Although useful, these summaries do not commingle with similarly approved generic or "competing" similar products.

The editorial board has analyzed the information on both brand and generic medications and has made this key prescribing information available in this pocket-sized book. Information in this book is meant for use by health care professionals who are familiar with these commonly prescribed medications.

This 2009 edition has been completely reviewed and updated by our editorial board. Over 55 new drugs and herbs have been added, and changes in other medications based on FDA actions have been incorporated, including deletions of discontinued brand names and compounds. New to this edition are the therapeutic and pharmacologic classifications for each drug and a section on commonly used vitamin combinations.

Where appropriate, emergency cardiac care (ECC) guidelines are provided based on the latest recommendations for the American Heart Association (Circulation, Volume 112, Issue 24 Supplement; December 13, 2005).

We express special thanks to our families for their long-term support of this book. The contributions of the members of the editorial board are deeply appreciated. The assistance of Quincy McDonald, and the team at McGraw-Hill are also to be thanked for their support in our goal of creating a pocket drug guide for nursing professionals.

Your comments and suggestions are always welcome and encouraged because improvements to this book would be impossible without the interest and feedback of our readers. We hope this book will help you learn some of the key elements in prescribing medications and allow you to care for your patients in the best way possible.

Judith A. Barberio, PhD, APN,C, ANP, FNP, GNP
Newark, New Jersey
JABPHD83@aol.com

Leonard G. Gomella, MD, FACS
Philadelphia, Pennsylvania
Leonard.Gomella@jefferson.edu

MEDICATION KEY

Medications are listed by prescribing class, and the individual medications are then listed in alphabetical order by generic name. Some of the more commonly recognized trade names are listed for each medication (in parentheses after the generic name) or if available without prescription, noted as OTC (over the counter).

> **Generic Drug Name (Selected Common Brand Names [Controlled Substance])** **WARNING:** Summarized version of the "Black Box" precautions deemed necessary by the FDA. These are significant precautions and contraindications concerning the individual medication. **Therapeutic and/or Pharmacologic Class:** Class is presented in brackets immediately following the brand name drug. The therapeutic drug class appears first and describes the disease state that the drug treats. The pharmacologic drug class follows and is based on the drug's mechanism of action. **Uses:** This includes both FDA labeled indications bracketed by * and other "off label" uses of the medication. Because many medications are used to treat various conditions based on the medical literature and not listed in their package insert, we list common uses of the medication rather than the official "labeled indications" (FDA approved) based on input from our editorial board **Action:** How the drug works. This information is helpful in comparing classes of drugs and understanding side effects and contraindications. *Spectrum:* Specifies activity against selected microbes **Dose:** *Adults.* Where no specific pediatric dose is given, the implication is that this drug is not commonly used or indicated in that age group. At the end of the dosing line, important dosing modifications may be noted (ie, take with food, avoid antacids, etc) **Caution:** [pregnancy/fetal risk categories, breast-feeding (as noted above)] cautions concerning the use of the drug in specific settings **Contra:** Contraindications **Disp:** Common dosing forms **SE:** Common or significant side effects **Notes:** Other key information about the drug **Interactions:** Common drug—drug, drug—herb, and drug—food interactions that may change the drug response **Labs:** Common laboratory test results that are changed by the drug or significant lab monitoring requirements **NIPE:** (Nursing Indications and/or Patient Education) Significant information that the nurse must be aware of with administration of the drug or information that should be given to any patient taking the drug.

CONTROLLED SUBSTANCE CLASSIFICATION

Medications under the control of the US Drug Enforcement Agency (Schedule I–V controlled substances) are indicated by the symbol [C]. Most medications are "uncontrolled" and do not require a DEA prescriber number on the prescription. The following is a general description for the schedules of DEA controlled substances:

Schedule (C–I) I: All nonresearch use forbidden (eg, heroin, LSD, mescaline, etc.).

Schedule (C–II) II: High addictive potential; medical use accepted. No telephone call-in prescriptions; no refills. Some states require special prescription form (eg, cocaine, morphine, methadone).

Schedule (C–III) III: Low to moderate risk of physical dependence, high risk of psychologic dependence; prescription must be rewritten after 6 months or five refills (eg, acetaminophen plus codeine).

Schedule (C–IV) IV: Limited potential for dependence; prescription rules same as for schedule III (eg, benzodiazepines, propoxyphene).

Schedule (C–V) V: Very limited abuse potential; prescribing regulations often same as for uncontrolled medications; some states have additional restrictions.

FDA FETAL RISK CATEGORIES

Category A: Adequate studies in pregnant women have not demonstrated a risk to the fetus in the first trimester of pregnancy; there is no evidence of risk in the last two trimesters.

Category B: Animal studies have not demonstrated a risk to the fetus, but no adequate studies have been done in pregnant women.

or

Animal studies have shown an adverse effect, but adequate studies in pregnant women have not demonstrated a risk to the fetus during the first trimester of pregnancy and there is no evidence of risk in the last two trimesters.

Category C: Animal studies have shown an adverse effect on the fetus, but no adequate studies have been done in humans. The benefits from the use of the drug in pregnant women may be acceptable despite its potential risks.

or

No animal reproduction studies and no adequate studies in humans have been done.

Category D: There is evidence of human fetal risk, but the potential benefits from the use of the drug in pregnant women may be acceptable despite its potential risks.

Category X: Studies in animals or humans or adverse reaction reports, or both, have demonstrated fetal abnormalities. The risk of use in pregnant women clearly outweighs any possible benefit.

Category ?: No data available (not a formal FDA classification; included to provide complete data set).

BREAST-FEEDING

No formally recognized classification exists for drugs and breast-feeding. This shorthand was developed for the *Nurse's Pocket Drug Guide*.

+	Compatible with breast-feeding
M	Monitor patient or use with caution
±	Excreted, or likely excreted, with unknown effects or at unknown concentrations
?/–	Unknown excretion, but effects likely to be of concern
–	Contraindicated in breast-feeding
?	No data available

ABBREVIATIONS

v: check or monitor
Ab: Antibody
ABMT: autologous bone marrow transplantation
Ac: before meals
ACE: angiotensin-converting enzyme
ACEI: angiotensin-converting enzyme inhibitor
ACLS: advanced cardiac life support
ACS: acute coronary syndrome, American Cancer Society, American College of Surgeons
ADH: antidiuretic hormone
ADHD: attention-deficit hyperactivity disorder
ADR: adverse drug reaction
AF: atrial fibrillation
Al: aluminum
ALL: acute lymphocytic leukemia
ALT: alanine aminotransferase
AMI: acute myocardial infarction
AML: acute myelogenous leukemia
Amp: ampule
ANC: absolute neutrophil count
APAP: acetaminophen: [*N*-acetyl-*p*-aminophenol]
aPTT: activated partial thromboplastin time
ARB: angiotensin II receptor blocker
ARDS: adult respiratory distress syndrome
ASA: aspirin (acetylsalicylic acid)

AUC: area under the curve
AV: atrioventricular
AVM: arteriovenous malformation
BCL: B-cell lymphoma
BM: bone marrow; bowel movement
↓ BM: hypotension
↓BM: bone marrow suppression, myelosuppression
BMT: bone marrow transplantation
BOO: bladder outlet obstruction
BP: blood pressure
BSA: body surface area
BUN: blood urea nitrogen
Ca: calcium
CA: cancer
CAD: coronary artery disease
CAP: community acquired pneumonia
CBC: complete blood count
CCB: calcium channel blocker
CF: cystic fibrosis
CHF: congestive heart failure
CLA: Cis-linoleic acid
CLL: chronic lymphocytic leukemia
CML: chronic myelogenous leukemia
CMV: cytomegalovirus
CNS: central nervous system
COMT: catechol-O-methyltransferase
Contra: contraindicated
COPD: chronic obstructive pulmonary disease
CP: chest pain

CPK: creatine phosphokinase
CPP: central precocious puberty
CR: controlled release
CrCl: creatinine clearance
CRF: chronic renal failure
CV: cardiovascular
CVA: cerebrovascular accident, costovertebral angle
CVH: common variable hypergammaglobulinemia
D: diarrhea
D5LR: 5% dextrose in lactated Ringer's solution
D5NS: 5% dextrose in normal saline
D5W: 5% dextrose in water
D/C: discontinue
DI: diabetes insipidus
Disp: dispensed as, how the drug is supplied
DKA: diabetic ketoacidosis
dL: deciliter
DM: diabetes mellitus
DMARD: Disease-modifying antirheumatic drug; drugs defined in randomized trials to decrease erosions and joint space narrowing in rheumatoid arthritis (eg, D-penicillamine, methotrexate, azathioprine)
DN: diabetic nephropathy
dppr: dropper
DOT: directly observed therapy
d/t: due to
DVT: deep venous thrombosis
Dz: disease
EC: enteric-coated
ECC: emergency cardiac care
ECG: electrocardiogram
ED: erectile dysfunction
EGFR: epidermal growth factor receptor

ELISA: enzyme-linked immunosorbent assay
EMIT: enzyme-multiplied immunoassay text
EPS: extrapyramidal symptoms (tardive dyskinesia, tremors and rigidity, restlessness [akathisia], muscle contractions [dystonia], changes in breathing and heart rate)
ER: extended release
ESRD: end-stage renal disease
ET: endotracheal
EtOH: ethanol
FSH: follicle-stimulating hormone
5-FU: fluorouracil
Fxn: function
g: gram
GABA: gama-aminobutyric acid
G-CSF: granulocyte colony-stimulating factor
gen: generation
GERD: gastroesophageal reflux disease
GF: growth factor
GFR: glomerular filtration rate
GH: growth hormone
GI: gastrointestinal
GIST: Gastrointestinal stromal tumor
GLA: Gamma-linoleic Acid
GM-CSF: granulocyte-macrophage colony-stimulating factor
GnRH: gonadotropin-releasing hormone
gt, gtt: drop, drops (*gutta*)
GTT: Glucose Tolerance Test
GUHD: Graft URS Host Disease
HA: headache
HCG: human chorionic gonadotropin
HCL: hairy cell leukemia
Hct: hematocrit

HCTZ: hydrochlorothiazide
HD: hemodialysis
HF: heart failure
Hgb: hemoglobin
HIT: heparin-induced
 thrombocytopenia
HIV: human immunodeficiency virus
HMG-CoA: hydroxymethylglutaryl
 coenzyme A
h/o: history of
HR: heart rate
↑ HR: increased heart rate
 (tachycardia)
hs: at bedtime (*hora somni*)
HSV: herpes simplex virus
5-HT: 5-hydroxytryptamine
HTN: hypertension
Hx: History of
I: Iodine
IBD: irritable bowel disease
IBS: irritable bowel syndrome
ICP: intracranial pressure
IFIS: Intraoperative Floppy Iris
 Syndrome
Ig: immunoglobulin
IM: intramuscular
Inf: infusion
Infxn: infection
Inh: inhalation
INH: isoniazid
INR: international normalized ratio
Insuff: insufficiency
Intravag: intravaginal
I&O: intake & output
IOP: intraocular pressure
ISA: intrinsic sympathomimetic
 activity
IT: intrathecal
ITP: idiopathic thrombocytopenic
 purpura
IV: intravenous

K/K⁺: potassium
LA: long acting
L/d: liters per day
LDL: low-density lipoprotein
LFT: liver function test
LH: luteinizing hormone
LHRH: luteinizing hormone-
 releasing hormone
Li: lithium
Liq: liquid
LMW: low molecular weight
LVD: left ventricular dysfunction
LVEF: left ventricular ejection
 fraction
LVSD: left ventricular systolic
 dysfunction
MAC: *Mycobacterium avium*
 complex
MAO/MAOI: monoamine
 oxidase/inhibitor
MDI: multidose inhaler
mEq: milliequivalent
Mg/Mg⁺²: magnesium
MI: myocardial infarction, mitral
 insufficiency
mL: milliliter
MoAb: monoclonal antibody
MRSA: methicillin-resistant
 Staphylococcus aureus
MS: multiple sclerosis
MSSA: methicillin-sensitive
 Staphylococcus aureus
MTT: monotetrazolium
MTX: methotrexate
MyG: myasthenia gravis
N: nausea
na: sodium
NA: narrow angle
NAG: narrow angle glaucoma
ng: nanogram
NG: nasogastric

NHL: non-Hodgkin's lymphoma
NIDDM: non-insulin-dependent diabetes mellitus
nl: normal
NMDA: N-Methyl-D-Aspartate
NNRTI: nonnucleoside reverse transcriptase inhibitor
NO: nitric oxide
NPO: nothing by mouth (*nil per os*)
NRTI: nucleoside reverse transcriptase inhibitor
NS: normal saline
NSAID: nonsteroidal anti-inflammatory drug
NSCLC: non-small-cell lung cancer
N/V: nausea and vomiting
N/V/D: nausea, vomiting, diarrhea
OAB: overactive bladder
OCP: oral contraceptive pill
OD: overdose
ODT: orally disintegrating tablets
OK: recommended
OTC: over the counter
P: phosphorus
PABA: para-amino benzoic acid
PAT: paroxysmal atrial tachycardia
pc: after eating (*post cibum*)
PCa: cancer of the prostate
PCN: penicillin
PCP: *Pneumocystis jiroveci* (formerly *carinii*) pneumonia
PCWP: pulmonary capillary wedge pressure
PDE5: phosphodiesterase type 5
PDGF: platelet-derived growth factor
PE: pulmonary embolus, physical examination, pleural effusion
PFT: pulmonary function test
pg: picogram
PID: pelvic inflammatory disease
plt: platelet

↓ plt; decreased platelets (thrombocytopenia)
PMDD: premenstrual dysphoric disorder
PO: by mouth (*per os*)
PPD: purified protein derivative
PR: by rectum
Prep: preparation
PRG: pregnancy
PRN: as often as needed (*pro re nata*)
PSVT: paroxysmal supraventricular tachycardia
pt: patient
PT: prothrombin time
PTCA: percutaneous transluminal coronary angioplasty
PTH: parathyroid hormone
PTT: partial thromboplastin time
PUD: peptic ulcer disease
PVC: premature ventricular contraction
PVD: peripheral vascular disease
PWP: pulmonary wedge pressure
Px: prevention
q: every (*quaque*)
qd: every day
qh: every hour
q_h: every _ hours
qhs: every hour of sleep (before bedtime)
qid: four times a day (*quater in die*)
qod: every other day
RA: rheumatoid arthritis
RCC: renal cell carcinoma
RDA: recommended dietary allowance
RDS: respiratory distress syndrome
resp: respiratory
RSV: respiratory syncytial virus
RT: reverse transcriptase
RTA: renal tubular acidosis
Rx: prescription or therapy

Rxn: reaction
SCr: serum creatinine
SDV: Single Dose Vial
SIADH: syndrome of inappropriate
   antidiuretic hormone
SL: sublingual
SLE: systemic lupus erythematosus
Sol/soln: solution
Sp: species
SPAG: small particle aerosol
   generator
SNRIs: serotonin-norepinephrine
   reuptake inhibitors
SQ: subcutaneous
SR: sustained release
SSRI: selective serotonin reuptake
   inhibitor
SSS: sick sinus syndrome
S/Sys: signs & symptoms
stat: immediately (*statim*)
supl: supplement
supp: suppository
SVT: supraventricular tachycardia
Sx: symptom
Sz: seizure
tab/tabs: tablet/tablets
TB: tuberculosis
TCA: tricyclic antidepressant
TFT: thyroid function test
TIA: transient ischemic attack
tid: three times a day (*ter in die*)
tinc: tincture
TMP: trimethoprim
TMP–SMX:
   trimethoprim–sulfamethoxazole

TNF: tumor necrosis factor
tox: toxicity
TPA: tissue plasminogen activator
tri: trimester
TSH thyroid stimulating hormone
Tsp: teaspoon
TTP: thrombotic thrombocytopenic
   purpura
TTS: transdermal therapeutic system
Tx: treatment
uln: upper limits of normal
UPA: pyrrolizidine alkaloids
URI: upper respiratory infection
UTI: urinary tract infection
Vag: vaginal
VF: ventricular fibrillation
VRE: vancomycin-resistant
   Enterococcus
VT: ventricular tachycardia
W/: with
WHI: Women's Health Initiative
W/in: within
Wk: week
WNL: within normal limits
w/o: without
WPW: Wolff–Parkinson–White
   syndrome
Wt: weight
XR: extended release
ZE: Zollinger–Ellison (syndrome)
>: greater than; older than
↑: increase
↓: decrease
∅: not recommended; do not take
÷/%: divided dose

CLASSIFICATION (Generic and common brand names)

ALLERGY

Antihistamines

Azelastine (Astelin, Optivar)
Cetirizine (Zyrtec, Zyrtec D)
Chlorpheniramine (Chlor-Trimeton)

Clemastine Fumarate (Tavist)
Cyproheptadine (Periactin)
Desloratadine (Clarinex)
Diphenhydramine (Benadryl)

Fexofenadine (Allegra)
Hydroxyzine (Atarax, Vistaril)
Loratadine (Claritin, Alavert)

Miscellaneous Antiallergy Agents

Budesonide (Rhinocort, Pulmicort)

Cromolyn Sodium (Intal, NasalCrom, Opticrom)

Montelukast (Singulair)

ANTIDOTES

Acetylcysteine (Aceta-dote, Mucomyst)
Activated Charcoal (SuperChar, Actidose, Liqui-Char)
Amifostine (Ethyol)
Atropine (AtroPen)
Deferasirox (Exjade)

Dexrazoxane (Zinecard)
Digoxin Immune Fab (Digibind, DigiFab)
Flumazenil (Romazicon)
Hydroxocobalamin (Cyanokit)
Ipecac Syrup, an over-the-counter (OTC) syrup

Mesna (Mesnex)
Naloxone (Narcan, Nalone, Narcanti)
Physostigmine (Antilirium)
Succimer (Chemet)

ANTIMICROBIAL AGENTS

Antibiotics

AMINOGLYCOSIDES

Amikacin (Amikin)
Gentamicin (Garamycin, G-Mycitin)

Neomycin
Streptomycin

Tobramycin (Nebcin)

CARBAPENEMS

Ertapenem (Invanz)   Imipenem-Cilastatin   Meropenem (Merrem)
                              (Primaxin)

CEPHALOSPORINS, FIRST GENERATION

Cefadroxil (Duricef,   Cephalexin (Keflex)   Cephradine (Velosef)
  Ultracef)
Cefazolin (Ancef, Kefzol)

CEPHALOSPORINS, SECOND GENERATION

Cefaclor (Ceclor)   Cefprozil (Cefzil)   Loracarbef (Lorabid)
Cefonicid (Monocid)   Cefuroxime (Ceftin
Cefotetan (Cefotan)   [oral], Zinacef
Cefoxitin (Mefoxin)   [parenteral])

CEPHALOSPORINS, THIRD GENERATION

Cefdinir (Omnicef)   Cefpodoxime (Vantin)   Ceftibuten (Cedax)
Cefditoren (Spectracef)   Ceftazidime (Fortaz,   Ceftizoxime (Cefizox)
Cefixime (Suprax)   Tazicef)   Ceftriaxone (Rocephin)
Cefoperazone (Cefobid)
Cefotaxime (Claforan)

CEPHALOSPORINS, FOURTH GENERATION

Cefepime (Maxipime)

FLUOROQUINOLONES

Ciprofloxacin (Cipro)   Lomefloxacin   Norfloxacin Ophthalmic
Gemifloxacin (Factive)   (Maxaquin)   (Noroxin, Chibroxin)
Levofloxacin (Levaquin,   Moxifloxacin   Ofloxacin Ophthalmic
  Quixin Ophthalmic)   (Avelox)   (Floxin, Ocuflox)

KETOLIDE

Telithromycin (Ketek)

MACROLIDES

Azithromycin   Dirithromycin (Dynabac)   Erythromycin &
  (Zithromax)   Erythromycin (E-Mycin,   Sulfisoxazole (Eryzole,
Clarithromycin   E.E.S., Ery-Tab)   Pediazole)
  (Biaxin)

PENICILLINS

Amoxicillin (Amoxil, Polymox)
Amoxicillin & Clavulanic Acid (Augmentin)
Ampicillin (Amcill, Omnipen)
Ampicillin-Sulbactam (Unasyn)
Dicloxacillin (Dynapen, Dycill)

Nafcillin (Nallpen)
Oxacillin (Bactocill, Prostaphlin)
Penicillin G, Aqueous (Potassium or Sodium) (Pfizerpen, Pentids)
Penicillin G Benzathine (Bicillin)
Penicillin G Procaine (Wycillin)

Penicillin V (Pen-Vee K, Veetids)
Piperacillin (Pipracil)
Piperacillin-Tazobactam (Zosyn)
Ticarcillin (Ticar)
Ticarcillin/Potassium Clavulanate (Timentin)

TETRACYCLINES

Doxycycline (Adoxa, Periostat, Oracea, Vibramycin, Vibra-Tabs)

Tetracycline (Achromycin V, Sumycin)

Tigecycline (Tygacil)

Miscellaneous Antibiotic Agents

Aztreonam (Azactam)
Clindamycin (Cleocin, Cleocin-T)
Fosfomycin (Monurol)
Linezolid (Zyvox)

Metronidazole (Flagyl, MetroGel)
Quinupristin-Dalfopristin (Synercid)
Rifaximin (Xifaxan)
Trimethoprim

Trimethoprim Sulfamethoxazole [Cotrimoxazole] (Bactrim, Septra)
Vancomycin (Vancocin, Vancoled)

ANTIFUNGALS

Amphotericin B (Fungizone)
Amphotericin B Cholesteryl (Amphotec)
Amphotericin B Lipid Complex (Abelcet)
Amphotericin B Liposomal (AmBisome)

Anidulafungin (Eraxis)
Caspofungin (Cancidas)
Clotrimazole (Lotrimin, Mycelex)
Clotrimazole & Betamethasone (Lotrisone)
Econazole (Spectazole)
Fluconazole (Diflucan)
Itraconazole (Sporanox)

Ketoconazole (Nizoral)
Miconazole (Monistat)
Nystatin (Mycostatin)
Oxiconazole (Oxistat)
Posaconazole (Noxafil)
Sertaconazole (Ertaczo)
Terbinafine (Lamisil)
Triamcinolone & Nystatin (Mycolog-II)
Voriconazole (VFEND)

Antimycobacterials

Dapsone, Oral
Ethambutol (Myambutol)
Isoniazid (INH)

Pyrazinamide
Rifabutin (Mycobutin)
Rifampin (Rifadin)

Rifapentine (Priftin)
Streptomycin

Antiprotozoals

Nitazoxanide (Alinia)

Tinidazole (Tindamax)

ANTINEOPLASTIC AGENTS

Alkylating Agents

Altretamine (Hexalen)
Busulfan (Myleran,
   Busulfex)

Carboplatin (Paraplatin)
Cisplatin (Platinol)
Oxaliplatin (Eloxatin)

Procarbazine (Matulane)
Triethylenethiophospho-
   ramide (Thiotepa)

NITROGEN MUSTARDS

Chlorambucil
   (Leukeran)
Cyclophosphamide
   (Cytoxan, Neosar)

Ifosfamide (Ifex,
   Holoxan)
Mechlorethamine
   (Mustargen)

Melphalan [L-PAM]
   (Alkeran)

NITROSOUREAS

Carmustine [BCNU]
   (BiCNU, Gliadel)

Streptozocin (Zanosar)

Antibiotics

Bleomycin Sulfate
   (Blenoxane)
Dactinomycin
   (Cosmegen)

Daunorubicin (Dauno-
   mycin, Cerubidine)
Doxorubicin
   (Adriamycin, Rubex)

Epirubicin (Ellence)
Idarubicin (Idamycin)
Mitomycin (Mutamycin)

Antimetabolites

Clofarabine (Clolar)
Cytarabine [ARA-C]
   (Cytosar-U)
Cytarabine Liposome
   (DepoCyt)
Floxuridine
   (FUDR)

Fludarabine Phosphate
   (Flamp, Fludara)
Fluorouracil [5-FU]
   (Adrucil)
Gemcitabine (Gemzar)
Mercaptopurine [6-MP]
   (Purinethol)

Methotrexate
   (Rheumatrex)
Nelarabine (Arranon)
Pemetrexed (Alimta)
6-Thioguanine [6-TG]

Hormones

Anastrozole (Arimidex)
Bicalutamide (Casodex)
Estramustine Phosphate (Estracyt, Emcyt)
Exemestane (Aromasin)
Fluoxymesterone (Halotestin, Androxy)
Flutamide (Eulexin)

Fulvestrant (Faslodex)
Goserelin (Zoladex)
Leuprolide (Lupron, Viadur, Eligard)
Levamisole (Ergamisol)

Megestrol Acetate (Megace)
Nilutamide (Nilandron)
Tamoxifen
Triptorelin (Trelstar Depot, Trelstar LA)

Mitotic Inhibitors

Etoposide [VP-16] (VePesid)
Vinblastine (Velban, Velbe)

Vincristine (Oncovin, Vincasar PFS)

Vinorelbine (Navelbine)

Monoclonal Antibodies

Cetuximab (Erbitux)
Erlotinib (Tarceva)

Panitumumab (Vectibix)

Trastuzumab (Herceptin)

Miscellaneous Antineoplastic Agents

Aldesleukin [Interleukin-2, IL-2] (Proleukin)
Aminoglutethimide (Cytadren)
L-Asparaginase (Elspar, Oncaspar)
BCG [Bacillus Calmette-Guérin] (TheraCys, Tice BCG)
Bevacizumab (Avastin)
Bortezomib (Velcade)
Cladribine (Leustatin)
Dacarbazine (DTIC)
Docetaxel (Taxotere)

Gefitinib (Iressa)
Gemtuzumab Ozogamicin (Mylotarg)
Hydroxyurea (Hydrea, Droxia)
Imatinib (Gleevec)
Irinotecan (Camptosar)
Letrozole (Femara)
Leucovorin (Wellcovorin)
Mitoxantrone (Novantrone)
Paclitaxel (Taxol, Abraxane)
Panitumumab (Vectibix)

Pemetrexed (Alimta)
Rasburicase (Elitek)
Sorafenib (Nexavar)
Sunitinib (Sutent)
Temsirolimus (Torisel Kit)
Thalidomide (Thalomid)
Topotecan (Hycamtin)
Tretinoin, Topical [Retinoic Acid] (Retin-A, Avita, Renova, Retin-A Micro)

ANTIRETROVIRALS

Abacavir (Ziagen)
Amprenavir (Agenerase)
Delavirdine (Rescriptor)
Didanosine [ddI] (Videx)
Efavirenz (Sustiva)
Efavirenz/Emtricitabine/
  Tenofovir (Atripla)
Fosamprenavir (Lexiva)
Indinavir (Crixivan)

Lamivudine (Epivir,
  Epivir-HBV)
Lopinavir/Ritonavir
  (Kaletra)
Nelfinavir (Viracept)
Nevirapine (Viramune)
Ritonavir (Norvir)
Saquinavir (Fortovase)
Stavudine (Zerit)

Telbivudine (Tyzeka)
Tenofovir (Viread)
Tenofovir/Emtricitabine
  (Truvada)
Tipranavir (Aptivus)
Zidovudine (Retrovir)
Zidovudine & Lamivudine
  (Combivir)

Antivirals

Acyclovir (Zovirax)
Adefovir (Hepsera)
Amantadine
  (Symmetrel)
Atazanavir (Reyataz)
Cidofovir (Vistide)
Emtricitabine
  (Emtriva)
Enfuvirtide (Fuzeon)
Famciclovir (Famvir)

Foscarnet (Foscavir)
Ganciclovir (Cytovene,
  Vitrasert)
Interferon Alfa-2b &
  Ribavirin Combo
  (Rebetron)
Oseltamivir (Tamiflu)
Palivizumab (Synagis)
Peginterferon Alfa-2a
  (Pegasys)

Peginterferon Alfa 2b
  (PEG-Intron)
Penciclovir (Denavir)
Ribavirin (Virazole)
Rimantadine (Flumadine)
Telbivudine (Tyzeka)
Valacyclovir (Valtrex)
Valganciclovir (Valcyte)
Zanamivir (Relenza)

Miscellaneous Antiviral Agents

Atovaquone (Mepron)
Atovaquone/Proguanil
  (Malarone)

Daptomycin (Cubicin)
Pentamidine (Pentam
  300, NebuPent)

Retapamulin (Altabax)
Trimetrexate (Neutrexin)

CARDIOVASCULAR (CV) AGENTS

ALDOSTERONE ANTAGONIST

Eplerenone (Inspra)

Alpha₁-Adrenergic Blocker

Doxazosin (Cardura)   Prazosin (Minipress)   Terazosin (Hytrin)

Angiotensin-Converting Enzyme (ACE) Inhibitors

Benazepril (Lotensin)
Captopril (Capoten)
Enalapril (Vasotec)
Fosinopril (Monopril)

Lisinopril (Prinivil, Zestril)
Moexipril (Univasc)
Perindopril Erbumine
  (Aceon)

Quinapril (Accupril)
Ramipril (Altace)
Trandolapril (Mavik)

Angiotensin II Receptor Antagonists

Candesartan (Atacand)
Eprosartan (Teveten)

Irbesartan (Avapro)
Losartan (Cozaar)

Telmisartan (Micardis)
Valsartan (Diovan)

Antiarrhythmic Agents

Adenosine (Adenocard)
Amiodarone (Cordarone, Pacerone)
Atropine
Digoxin (Digitek, Lanoxin, Lanoxicaps)
Disopyramide (NAPamide, Norpace, Norpace CR, Rhythmodan)

Dofetilide (Tikosyn)
Esmolol (Brevibloc)
Flecainide (Tambocor)
Ibutilide (Corvert)
Lidocaine (Anestacon Topical, Xylocaine)
Mexiletine (Mexitil)

Procainamide (Pronestyl, Pronestyl SR, Procanbid)
Propafenone (Rythmol)
Quinidine (Quinidex, Quinaglute)
Sotalol (Betapace, Betapace AF)

Beta-Adrenergic Blockers

Acebutolol (Sectral)
Atenolol (Tenormin)
Atenolol & Chlorthalidone (Tenoretic)
Betaxolol (Kerlone)
Bisoprolol (Zebeta)

Carteolol (Cartrol, Ocupress Ophthalmic)
Carvedilol (Coreg, Coreg CR)
Labetalol (Trandate, Normodyne)

Metoprolol (Lopressor, Toprol XL)
Nadolol (Corgard)
Penbutolol (Levatol)
Pindolol (Visken)
Propranolol (Inderal)
Timolol (Blocadren)

Calcium Channel Antagonists

Amlodipine (Norvasc)
Diltiazem (Cardizem, Cartia XT, Dilacor, Diltia XT, Taztia XT, Tiamate, Tiazac)
Felodipine (Plendil)

Isradipine (DynaCirc)
Nicardipine (Cardene)
Nifedipine (Procardia, Procardia XL, Adalat, Adalat CC)

Nimodipine (Nimotop)
Nisoldipine (Sular)
Verapamil (Calan, Isoptin, Verelan)

Centrally Acting Antihypertensive Agents

Clonidine (Catapres)

Methyldopa (Aldomet)

Diuretics

Acetazolamide (Diamox)
Amiloride (Midamor)
Bumetanide (Bumex)
Chlorothiazide (Diuril)
Chlorthalidone (Hygroton)
Furosemide (Lasix)
Hydrochlorothiazide (HydroDIURIL, Esidrix)
Hydrochlorothiazide & Amiloride (Moduretic)
Hydrochlorothiazide & Spironolactone (Aldactazide)
Hydrochlorothiazide & Triamterene (Dyazide, Maxzide)
Indapamide (Lozol)
Mannitol
Metolazone (Mykrox, Zaroxolyn)
Spironolactone (Aldactone)
Torsemide (Demadex)
Triamterene (Dyrenium)

Inotropic/Pressor Agents

Digoxin (Digitek, Lanoxin, Lanoxicaps)
Dobutamine (Dobutrex)
Dopamine (Intropin)
Epinephrine (Adrenalin, Sus-Phrine, EpiPen)
Inamrinone (Inocor)
Isoproterenol (Isuprel)
Milrinone (Primacor)
Nesiritide (Natrecor)
Norepinephrine (Levophed)
Phenylephrine (Neo-Synephrine)

Antihypertensive Combination Agents

Amlodipine Besylate Benazepril Hydrochloride (Lotrel)
Isosorbide Dinitrate Hydralazine HCL (BiDil)

Lipid-Lowering Agents

Atorvastatin (Lipitor)
Cholestyramine (Questran)
Colesevelam (WelChol)
Colestipol (Colestid)
Ezetimibe (Zetia)
Fenofibrate (TriCor, Antara, Lipofen, Triglide)
Fluvastatin (Lescol)
Gemfibrozil (Lopid)
Lovastatin (Mevacor, Altocor)
Niacin (Niaspan)
Pravastatin (Pravachol)
Rosuvastatin (Crestor)
Simvastatin (Zocor)

Lipid-Lowering/Antihypertensive Combos

Amlodipine/Atorvastatin (Caduet)

Vasodilators

Alprostadil [Prostaglandin E$_1$] (Prostin VR)
Epoprostenol (Flolan)
Fenoldopam (Corlopam)
Hydralazine (Apresoline)
Iloprost (Ventavis)
Isosorbide Dinitrate (Isordil, Sorbitrate, Dilatrate-SR)
Isosorbide Mononitrate (Ismo, Imdur)
Minoxidil (Loniten, Rogaine)
Nitroglycerin (Nitrostat, Nitrolingual, Nitro-Bid Ointment, Nitro-Bid IV, Nitrodisc, Transderm-Nitro)
Nitroprusside (Nipride, Nitropress)
Tolazoline (Priscoline)
Treprostinil Sodium (Remodulin)

Miscellaneous Cardiovascular Agents

Aliskiren (Tekturna)   Conivaptan (Vaprisol)   Ranolazine (Ranexa)

CENTRAL NERVOUS SYSTEM AGENTS

Antianxiety Agents

Alprazolam (Xanax)
Buspirone (BuSpar)
Chlordiazepoxide
  (Librium, Mitran,
  Libritabs)
Clorazepate (Tranxene)

Diazepam (Valium,
  Diastat)
Doxepin (Sinequan,
  Adapin)
Hydroxyzine (Atarax,
  Vistaril)

Lorazepam (Ativan)
Meprobamate (Equanil,
  Miltown)
Oxazepam

Anticonvulsants

Carbamazepine
  (Tegretol)
Clonazepam (Klonopin)
Diazepam (Valium)
Ethosuximide
  (Zarontin)
Fosphenytoin (Cerebyx)
Gabapentin (Neurontin)

Lamotrigine (Lamictal)
Levetiracetam (Keppra)
Lorazepam (Ativan)
Oxcarbazepine
  (Trileptal)
Pentobarbital (Nembutal)
Phenobarbital

Phenytoin (Dilantin)
Tiagabine (Gabitril)
Topiramate (Topamax)
Valproic Acid (Depakene,
  Depakote)
Zonisamide (Zonegran)

Antidepressants

Amitriptyline (Elavil)
Bupropion (Wellbutrin,
  Zyban)
Citalopram (Celexa)
Desipramine (Norpramin)
Doxepin (Adapin)
Duloxetine (Cymbalta)
Escitalopram (Lexapro)

Fluoxetine (Prozac,
  Sarafem)
Fluvoxamine (Luvox)
Imipramine (Tofranil)
Mirtazapine (Remeron)
Nefazodone (Serzone)
Nortriptyline (Aventyl,
  Pamelor)

Paroxetine (Paxil)
Phenelzine (Nardil)
Selegiline, transdermal
  (Emsam)
Sertraline (Zoloft)
Trazodone (Desyrel)
Venlafaxine (Effexor,
  Effexor XR)

Antiparkinson Agents

Amantadine (Symmetrel)
Apomorphine (Apokyn)
Benztropine (Cogentin)
Bromocriptine (Parlodel)
Carbidopa/Levodopa
  (Sinemet)

Entacapone (Comtan)
Pramipexole (Mirapex)
Rasagiline mesylate
  (Azilect)
Ropinirole (Requip)

Selegiline (Eldepryl,
  Zelapar)
Tolcapone (Tasmar)
Trihexyphenidyl
  (Artane)

Antipsychotics

Aripiprazole (Abilify)
Chlorpromazine
  (Thorazine)
Clozapine (Clozaril,
  FazaClo)
Fluphenazine (Prolixin,
  Permitil)
Haloperidol (Haldol)
Lithium Carbonate
  (Eskalith, Lithobid)

Mesoridazine (Serentil)
Molindone (Moban)
Olanzapine (Zyprexa)
Paliperidone (Invega)
Perphenazine (Trilafon)
Prochlorperazine
  (Compazine)
Quetiapine (Seroquel,
  Seroquel XR)

Risperidone (Risperdal,
  Risperdal Consta,
  Risperdal M-Tab)
Thioridazine (Mellaril)
Thiothixene (Navane)
Trifluoperazine
  (Stelazine)
Ziprasidone (Geodon)

Sedative Hypnotics

Chloral Hydrate
  (Aquachloral,
  Supprettes)
Diphenhydramine
  (Benadryl)
Estazolam (ProSom)
Eszopiclone (Lunesta)

Flurazepam (Dalmane)
Hydroxyzine (Atarax,
  Vistaril)
Midazolam
Phenobarbital
Pentobarbital (Nembutal)
Propofol (Diprivan)

Ramelteon (Rozerem)
Quazepam (Doral)
Secobarbital (Seconal)
Temazepam (Restoril)
Triazolam (Halcion)
Zaleplon (Sonata)
Zolpidem (Ambien)

Miscellaneous CNS Agents

Atomoxetine HCL
  (Strattera)
Galantamine (Razadyne)
Interferon beta-1a (Rebif)
Lisdexamfetamine
  (Vyvanse)
Memantine (Namenda)

Methylphenidate, Oral
  (Concerta, Ritalin,
  Ritalin-SR, others)
Methylphenidate,
  Transdermal
  (Daytrana)
Natalizumab (Tysabri)

Nimodipine (Nimotop)
Rivastigmine (Exelon)
Sodium Oxybate
  (Xyrem)
Tacrine (Cognex)

DERMATOLOGIC AGENTS

Acitretin (Soriatane)
Acyclovir (Zovirax)
Alefacept (Amevive)
Amphotericin B
  (Fungizone)
Anthralin
  (Anthra-Derm)
Bacitracin, Topical
  (Baciguent)

Bacitracin & Polymyxin
  B, Topical (Polysporin)
Bacitracin, Neomycin, &
  Polymyxin B, Topical
  (Neosporin Ointment)
Bacitracin, Neomycin,
  Polymyxin B, &
  Hydrocortisone,
  Topical (Cortisporin)

Bacitracin, Neomycin,
  Polymyxin B, &
  Lidocaine, Topical
  (Clomycin)
Botulinum toxin type A
  (Botox Cosmetic)
Calcipotriene (Dovonex)
Capsaicin (Capsin,
  Zostrix)

Ciclopirox (Loprox)
Ciprofloxacin (Cipro)
Clindamycin (Cleocin)
Clotrimazole &
  Betamethasone
  (Lotrisone)
Dapsone, Topical (Aczone)
Dibucaine (Nupercainal)
Doxepin, Topical
  (Zonalon, Prudoxin)
Econazole (Spectazole)
Efalizumab (Raptiva)
Erythromycin, Topical
  (A/T/S, Eryderm,
  Erycette, T-Stat)
Finasteride (Propecia)
Gentamicin, Topical
  (Garamycin,
  G-Mycitin)
Imiquimod Cream, 5%
  (Aldara)
Isotretinoin [13-*cis*
  Retinoic Acid]
  (Accutane, Amnes-
  teem, Claravis, Sotret)
Ketoconazole (Nizoral)
Kunecatechins (Veregen)

Lactic Acid & Ammo-
  nium Hydroxide [Am-
  monium Lactate]
  (Lac-Hydrin)
Lindane (Kwell)
Lisdexamfetamine
  (Vyvanse)
Metronidazole (Flagyl,
  MetroGel)
Miconazole (Monistat)
Miconazole/Zinc
  Oxide/Petrolatum
  (Vusion)
Minocycline
  (Solodyn)
Minoxidil (Loniten,
  Rogaine)
Mupirocin (Bactroban)
Naftifine (Naftin)
Neomycin Sulfate
  (Myciguent)
Nystatin (Mycostatin)
Oxiconazole (Oxistat)
Penciclovir (Denavir)
Permethrin (Nix,
  Elimite)
Pimecrolimus (Elidel)

Podophyllin (Podocon-25,
  Condylox Gel 0.5%,
  Condylox)
Pramoxine (Anusol
  Ointment,
  ProctoFoam-NS)
Pramoxine & Hydrocor-
  tisone (Enzone,
  Proctofoam-HC)
Selenium Sulfide (Exsel
  Shampoo, Selsun Blue
  Shampoo, Selsun
  Shampoo)
Silver Sulfadiazine
  (Silvadene)
Steroids, Topical (Table 4)
Tacrolimus (Prograf,
  Protopic)
Tazarotene (Tazorac,
  Avage)
Terbinafine (Lamisil)
Tolnaftate (Tinactin)
Tretinoin, Topical
  [Retinoic Acid]
  (Retin-A, Avita,
  Renova)
Vorinostat (Zolinza)

DIETARY SUPPLEMENTS

Calcium Acetate
  (Calphron, Phos-Ex,
  PhosLo)
Calcium Glubionate
  (Neo-Calglucon)
Calcium Salts [Chloride,
  Gluconate,
  Gluceptate]
Cholecalciferol [Vitamin
  D_3] (Delta D)
Cyanocobalamin
  [Vitamin B_{12}]
  (Nascobal)

Ferric Gluconate
  Complex (Ferrlecit)
Ferrous Gluconate
  (Fergon)
Ferrous Sulfate
Fish Oil (Omacor, OTC)
Folic Acid
Iron Dextran (DexFerrum,
  INFeD)
Iron Sucrose (Venofer)
Magnesium Oxide
  (Mag-Ox 400)
Magnesium Sulfate

Multivitamins (Table 13)
Phytonadione [Vitamin
  K] (Aqua-MEPHY-
  TON)
Potassium Supplements
  (Kaon, Kaochlor,
  K-Lor, Slow-K,
  Micro-K, Klorvess)
Pyridoxine [Vitamin B_6]
Sodium Bicarbonate
  [$NaHCO_3$]
Thiamine [Vitamin B_1]

EAR (OTIC) AGENTS

Acetic Acid &
Aluminum Acetate
(Otic Domeboro)
Benzocaine &
Antipyrine
(Auralgan)
Ciprofloxacin, Otic
(Cipro HC Otic)
Neomycin, Colistin, &
Hydrocortisone
(Cortisporin-TC Otic
Drops)

Neomycin, Colistin,
Hydrocortisone, &
Thonzonium
(Cortisporin-TC
Otic Suspension)
Polymyxin B &
Hydrocortisone
(Otobiotic Otic)

Sulfacetamide &
Prednisolone
(Blephamide)
Triethanolamine
(Cerumenex)

ENDOCRINE SYSTEM AGENTS

Antidiabetic Agents

Acarbose (Precose)
Chlorpropamide
(Diabinese)
Glimepiride (Amaryl)
Glimepiride/pioglitazone
(Duetact)
Glipizide (Glucotrol)
Glyburide (DiaBeta,
Micronase,
Glynase)
Glyburide/Metformin
(Glucovance)

Insulins, Systemic
(Table 5)
Metformin (Glucophage)
Miglitol (Glyset)
Nateglinide (Starlix)
Pioglitazone (Actos)
Pioglitazone HCL/
Glimepiride (Duetact)
Pioglitazone/Metformin
(Actoplus Met)
Repaglinide (Prandin)
Rosiglitazone (Avandia)

Rosiglitazone/Metformin
(Avandamet)
Sitagliptin (Januvia)
Sitagliptin/Metformin
(Janumet)
Tolazamide (Tolinase)
Tolbutamide (Orinase)

Hormone & Synthetic Substitutes

Calcitonin (Cibacalcin,
Miacalcin)
Calcitriol (Rocaltrol,
Calcijex)
Cortisone Systemic,
Topical
Desmopressin (DDAVP,
Stimate)
Dexamethasone
(Decadron)

Fludrocortisone Acetate
(Florinef)
Fluoxymesterone
(Halotestin, Androxy)
Glucagon
Hydrocortisone Topical
& Systemic (Cortef,
Solu-Cortef)
Methylprednisolone
(Solu-Medrol)

Prednisolone
Prednisone
Testosterone (AndroGel,
Androderm, Striant,
Testim)
Vasopressin [Antidi-
uretic Hormone,
ADH] (Pitressin)

Hypercalcemia/Osteoporosis Agents

Etidronate Disodium
(Didronel)
Gallium Nitrate (Ganite)

Ibandronate Sodium
(Boniva)
Pamidronate (Aredia)

Zoledronic Acid
(Zometa)

Obesity

Sibutramine (Meridia)

Osteoporosis Agents

Alendronate (Fosamax)
Raloxifene (Evista)

Risedronate (Actonel)
Teriparatide (Forteo)

Zoledronic Acid
(Zometa)

Thyroid/Antithyroid

Levothyroxine
(Synthroid, Levoxyl)
Liothyronine (Cytomel)
Methimazole (Tapazole)

Potassium iodide [Lugol
Solution] (SSKI,
Thyro-Block)

Propylthiouracil [PTU]

Miscellaneous Endocrine Agents

Cinacalcet (Sensipar)
Demeclocycline
(Declomycin)

Diazoxide (Proglycem)

EYE (OPHTHALMIC) AGENTS

Glaucoma Agents

Acetazolamide (Diamox)
Apraclonidine (Iopidine)
Betaxolol, Ophthalmic
(Betopic)
Brimonidine (Alphagan P)
Brinzolamide (Azopt)
Carteolol (Cartrol,
Ocupress Ophthalmic)
Ciprofloxacin, Ophthalmic
(Ciloxan)
Cyclosporine, Ophthalmic
(Restasis)
Dipivefrin (Propine)
Dorzolamide (Trusopt)

Dorzolamide & Timolol
(Cosopt)
Echothiophate Iodine
(Phospholine
Ophthalmic)
Epinastine (Elestat)
Latanoprost (Xalatan)
Levobunolol (A-K Beta,
Betagan)
Levocabastine (Livostin)
Levofloxacin (Levaquin,
Quixin & Iquix
Ophthalmic)
Lodoxamide (Alomide)

Moxifloxacin (Vigamox)
Neomycin, Polymyxin,
& Hydrocortisone
(Cortisporin
Ophthalmic & Otic)
Norfloxacin (Chibroxin)
Ofloxacin (Ocuflox
Ophthalmic)
Rimexolone (Vexol
Ophthalmic)
Timolol, Ophthalmic
(Timoptic)
Trifluridine, Ophthalmic
(Viroptic)

Ophthalmic Antibiotics

Bacitracin, Ophthalmic (AK-Tracin Ophthalmic)
Bacitracin & Polymyxin B, Ophthalmic (AK-Poly-Bac Ophthalmic, Polysporin Ophthalmic)
Bacitracin, Neomycin, & Polymyxin B (AK Spore Ophthalmic, Neosporin Ophthalmic)
Bacitracin, Neomycin, Polymyxin B, & Hydrocortisone, Ophthalmic (AK Spore HC Ophthalmic, Cortisporin Ophthalmic)

Ciprofloxacin, Ophthalmic (Ciloxan)
Erythromycin, Ophthalmic (Ilotycin Ophthalmic)
Gentamicin, Ophthalmic (Garamycin, Genoptic, Gentacidin, Gentak)
Neomycin & Dexamethasone (AK-Neo-Dex Ophthalmic, NeoDecadron Ophthalmic)
Neomycin, Polymyxin B, & Dexamethasone (Maxitrol)
Neomycin, Polymyxin B, & Prednisolone (Poly-Pred Ophthalmic)

Ofloxacin (Floxin, Ocuflox Ophthalmic)
Silver Nitrate (Dey-Drop)
Sulfacetamide (Bleph-10, Cetamide, Sodium Sulamyd)
Sulfacetamide & Prednisolone (Blephamide)
Tobramycin, Ophthalmic (AKTob, Tobrex)
Tobramycin & Dexamethasone (TobraDex)
Trifluridine (Viroptic)

Miscellaneous Ophthalmic Agents

Artificial Tears (Tears Naturale)
Atropine
Cromolyn Sodium (Opticrom)
Cyclopentolate (Cyclogyl, Cyclate)
Cyclopentolate with Phenylephrine (Cyclomydril)
Cyclosporine Ophthalmic (Restasis)

Dexamethasone, Ophthalmic (AK-Dex Ophthalmic, Decadron Ophthalmic)
Emedastine (Emadine)
Ketorolac, Ophthalmic (Acular, Acular LS, Acular PF)
Ketotifen (Zaditor)
Lodoxamide (Alomide)
Naphazoline (Albalon, AK-Con, Naphcon, others)

Naphazoline & Pheniramine Acetate (Naphcon A)
Nepafenac (Nevanac)
Olopatadine (Patanol)
Pemirolast (Alamast)
Rimexolone (Vexol Ophthalmic)
Scopolamine Ophthalmic

GASTROINTESTINAL AGENTS

Antacids

Alginic Acid
(Gaviscon)
Aluminum Hydroxide
(Amphojel,
ALternaGEL)
Aluminum Hydroxide
with Magnesium
Carbonate
(Gaviscon)

Aluminum Hydroxide
with Magnesium
Hydroxide (Maalox)
Aluminum Hydroxide
with Magnesium
Hydroxide &
Simethicone
(Mylanta, Mylanta II,
Maalox Plus)

Aluminum Hydroxide
with Magnesium
Trisilicate (Gaviscon,
Gaviscon-2)
Calcium Carbonate
(Tums, Alka-Mints)
Magaldrate (Riopan,
Lowsium)
Simethicone (Mylicon)

Antidiarrheals

Bismuth Subsalicylate
(Pepto-Bismol)
Diphenoxylate with
Atropine (Lomotil,
Lonox)

Kaolin-Pectin (Kaodene,
Kao-Spen, Kapectolin,
Parepectolin)
Lactobacillus (Lactinex
Granules)

Loperamide (Imodium)
Octreotide (Sandostatin,
Sandostatin LAR)
Paregoric [Camphorated
Tincture of Opium]

Antiemetics

Aprepitant (Emend)
Chlorpromazine
(Thorazine)
Dimenhydrinate
(Dramamine)
Dolasetron (Anzemet)
Dronabinol (Marinol)
Droperidol (Inapsine)

Granisetron (Kytril)
Meclizine (Antivert)
Metoclopramide
(Reglan, Clopra,
Octamide)
Nabilone (Cesamet)
Ondansetron (Zofran)
Palonosetron (Aloxi)

Prochlorperazine
(Compazine)
Promethazine (Phenergan)
Scopolamine (Scopace)
Thiethylperazine
(Torecan)
Trimethobenzamide
(Tigan)

Antiulcer Agents

Cimetidine
(Tagamet)
Esomeprazole
(Nexium)
Famotidine (Pepcid,
Pepcid AC)

Lansoprazole
(Prevacid)
Nizatidine (Axid)
Omeprazole (Prilosec,
Zegerid)
Pantoprazole (Protonix)

Rabeprazole
(AcipHex)
Ranitidine Hydrochloride
(Zantac)
Sucralfate (Carafate)

Cathartics/Laxatives

Bisacodyl (Dulcolax)
Docusate Calcium (Surfak)
Docusate Potassium (Dialose)
Docusate Sodium (Doss, Colace)
Glycerin Suppository

Lactulose (Constulose, Generlac, Chronulac, Cephulac, Enulose)
Magnesium Citrate
Magnesium Hydroxide (Milk of Magnesia)
Mineral Oil

Polyethylene Glycol-Electrolyte Solution (GoLYTELY, CoLyte)
Psyllium (Metamucil, Serutan, EfferSyllium)
Sodium Phosphate (Visicol)
Sorbitol

Enzymes

Pancreatin (Pancrease, Cotazym, Creon, Ultrase)

Miscellaneous GI Agents

Alosetron (Lotronex)
Balsalazide (Colazal)
Budesonide (Entocort EC)
Dexpanthenol (Ilopan-Choline Oral, Ilopan)
Dibucaine (Nupercainal)
Dicyclomine (Bentyl)
Hydrocortisone, Rectal (Anusol-HC Suppository, Cortifoam Rectal, Proctocort)

Hyoscyamine (Anaspaz, Cystospaz, Levsin)
Hyoscyamine, Atropine, Scopolamine, & Phenobarbital (Donnatal)
Infliximab (Remicade)
Lubiprostone (Amitiza)
Mesalamine (Asacol, Lialda, Pentasa, Rowasa)
Metoclopramide (Reglan, Clopra, Octamide)
Misoprostol (Cytotec)

Neomycin Sulfate (Neo-Fradin, generic)
Olsalazine (Dipentum)
Pramoxine (Anusol Ointment, ProctoFoam-NS)
Pramoxine with Hydrocortisone (Enzone, ProctoFoam-HC)
Propantheline (Pro-Banthine)
Sulfasalazine (Azulfidine)
Vasopressin (Pitressin)

HEMATOLOGIC AGENTS

Anticoagulants

Ardeparin (Normiflo)
Argatroban (Acova)
Bivalirudin (Angiomax)
Dalteparin (Fragmin)

Enoxaparin (Lovenox)
Fondaparinux (Arixtra)
Heparin
Lepirudin (Refludan)

Protamine
Tinzaparin (Innohep)
Warfarin (Coumadin)

Antiplatelet Agents

Abciximab (ReoPro)
Aspirin (Bayer, Ecotrin,
St. Joseph's)
Clopidogrel (Plavix)

Dipyridamole (Persantine)
Dipyridamole & Aspirin
(Aggrenox)
Eptifibatide (Integrilin)

Reteplase (Retavase)
Ticlopidine (Ticlid)
Tirofiban (Aggrastat)

Antithrombotic Agents

Alteplase, Recombinant
[tPA] (Activase)
Aminocaproic Acid
(Amicar)
Anistreplase (Eminase)

Aprotinin (Trasylol)
Danaparoid (Orgaran)
Dextran 40 (Gentran 40,
Rheomacrodex)
Reteplase (Retavase)

Streptokinase (Streptase,
Kabikinase)
Tenecteplase (TNKase)
Urokinase (Abbokinase)

Hematopoietic Stimulants

Darbepoetin Alfa
(Aranesp)
Epoetin Alfa [Erythro-
poietin, EPO]
(Epogen, Procrit)

Filgrastim [G-CSF]
(Neupogen)
Oprelvekin (Neumega)
Pegfilgrastim (Neulasta)

Sargramostim
[GM-CSF] (Leukine)

Volume Expanders

Albumin (Albuminar,
Buminate,
Albutein)

Dextran 40
(Rheomacrodex)
Hetastarch (Hespan)

Plasma Protein Fraction
(Plasmanate)

Miscellaneous Hematologic Agents

Antihemophilic Factor
VIII (Monoclate)
Decitabine (Dacogen)

Desmopressin (DDAVP,
Stimate)
Lenalidomide (Revlimid)

Pentoxifylline (Trental)

IMMUNE SYSTEM AGENTS

Immunomodulators

Abatacept (Orencia)
Adalimumab (Humira)
Anakinra (Kineret)
Etanercept (Enbrel)
Interferon Alfa
(Roferon-A, Intron A)

Interferon Alfacon-1
(Infergen)
Interferon Beta-1b
(Betaseron)
Interferon Gamma-1b
(Actimmune)

Natalizumab (Tysabri)
Peg Interferon Alfa-2b
(PEG-Intron)

Immunosuppressive Agents

Azathioprine (Imuran)
Basiliximab (Simulect)
Cyclosporine (Sandimmune, NePO)
Daclizumab (Zenapax)
Lymphocyte Immune Globulin [Antithymocyte Globulin, ATG] (Atgam)

Muromonab-CD3 (Orthoclone OKT3)
Mycophenolic Acid (Myfortic)
Mycophenolate Mofetil (CellCept)

Sirolimus (Rapamune)
Steroids, Systemic (Table 3)
Tacrolimus (Prograf, Protopic)

Vaccines/Serums/Toxoids

Cytomegalovirus Immune Globulin [CMV-IG IV] (CytoGam)
Diphtheria, Tetanus Toxoids, & Acellular Pertussis Adsorbed, Hepatitis B (recombinant), & Inactivated Poliovirus Vaccine (IPV) Combined (Pediarix)
Haemophilus B Conjugate Vaccine (ActHIB, HibTITER, PedvaxHIB, ProHIBIt)
Hepatitis A Vaccine (Havrix, Vaqta)
Hepatitis A (Inactivated) & Hepatitis B Recombinant Vaccine (Twinrix)
Hepatitis B Immune Globulin (HyperHep, H-BIG)

Hepatitis B Vaccine (Engerix-B, Recombivax HB)
Human Papillomavirus (Types 6, 11, 16, 18) Recombinant Vaccine (Gardasil)
Immune Globulin, IV (Gamimune N, Sandoglobulin, Gammar IV)
Immune Globulin, Subcutaneous (Vivaglobin)
Influenza Vaccine (Fluarix, Flulaval, Fluzone, Fluvirin)
Influenza Virus Vaccine Live, Intranasal (FluMist)
Measles, Mumps, Rubella, and Varicella Virus Vaccine Live [MMRV] (ProQuad)

Meningococcal Conjugate Vaccine (Menactra)
Meningococcal Polysaccharide Vaccine (Menomune A/C/Y/W-135)
Pneumococcal 7-Valent Conjugate Vaccine (Prevnar)
Pneumococcal Vaccine, Polyvalent (Pneumovax-23)
Rotavirus Vaccine, live, oral, pentavalent (RotaTeq)
Tetanus Immune Globulin
Tetanus Toxoid
Varicella Virus Vaccine (Varivax)
Zoster Vaccine, live (Zostavax)

MUSCULOSKELETAL AGENTS

Antigout Agents

Allopurinol (Zyloprim, Lopurin, Aloprim)

Colchicine

Probenecid (Benemid)
Sulfinpyrazone

Muscle Relaxants

Baclofen (Lioresal Intrathecal)
Carisoprodol (Soma)
Chlorzoxazone (Paraflex, Parafon Forte DSC)

Cyclobenzaprine (Flexeril)
Cyclobenzaprine, extended release (Amrix)
Dantrolene (Dantrium)

Diazepam (Valium)
Metaxalone (Skelaxin)
Methocarbamol (Robaxin)
Orphenadrine (Norflex)

Neuromuscular Blockers

Atracurium (Tracrium)
Pancuronium (Pavulon)
Rocuronium (Zemuron)

Succinylcholine (Anectine, Quelicin, Sucostrin)

Vecuronium (Norcuron)

Miscellaneous Musculoskeletal Agents

Edrophonium (Tensilon, Enlon, Reversol)

Leflunomide (Arava)

Methotrexate (Rheumatrex)

OB/GYN AGENTS

Contraceptives

Copper IUD Contraceptive (ParaGard T 380A)
Drospirenone/Ethinyl Estradiol (YAZ)
Estradiol Cypionate & Medroxyprogesterone Acetate (Lunelle)
Etonogestrel Implant (Implanon)
Levonorgestrel intrauterine device (IUD) (Mirena)

Etonogestrel/Ethinyl Estradiol (NuvaRing)
Levonorgestrel Implant (Norplant)
Levonorgestrel/Ethinyl Estradiol (Seasonale)
Medroxyprogesterone (Provera, Depo-Provera)
Norgestrel (Ovrette)
Oral Contraceptives, Monophasic (Table 6)

Oral Contraceptives, Multiphasic (Table 6)
Oral Contraceptives, Progestin Only (Table 6)
Oral Contraceptives, Extended-Cycle Combination (Table 6)

Emergency Contraceptives

Ethinyl Estradiol & Levonorgestrel (Preven)

Levonorgestrel (Plan B)

Estrogen Supplementation

ESTROGEN ONLY

Drospirenone/Estradiol (Angelia)
Esterified Estrogens (Estratab, Menest)
Esterified Estrogens with Methyltestosterone (Estratest)

Estradiol (Estrace, others)
Estradiol gel (Elestrin)
Estradiol, Transdermal (Estraderm, Climara, Vivelle)
Estrogen, Conjugated (Premarin)

Estrogen, Conjugated-Synthetic (Cenestin, Enjuvia)
Esterified Estrogens (Estratab, Menest)

COMBINATION ESTROGEN/PROGESTIN

Esterified Estrogens with Methyltestosterone (Estratest, Estratest HS, Syntest DS, HS)
Estrogen, Conjugated with Medroxyprogesterone (Prempro, Premphase)
Estrogen, Conjugated with Methylprogesterone (Premarin with Methylprogesterone)

Estrogen, Conjugated with Methyltestosterone (Premarin with Methyltestosterone)
Estradiol/Levonorgestrel, Transdermal (Climara Pro)
Estradiol/Norethindrone acetate (FemHRT, Activella)

Norethindrone Acetate/Ethinyl Estradiol (Ethinyl Estradiol/Norethindrone Acetate)

Vaginal Preparations

Amino-Cerv pH 5.5 Cream
Lutrepulse

Miconazole (Monistat)
Nystatin (Mycostatin)

Terconazole (Terazol 7)
Tioconazole (Vagistat)

Miscellaneous Ob/Gyn Agents

Dinoprostone (Cervidil Vaginal Insert, Prepidil Vaginal Gel, Prostin E2)
Gonadorelin (Factrel)
Leuprolide (Lupron)
Lutropin Alfa (Luveris)

Magnesium Sulfate
Medroxyprogesterone (Provera, Depo-Provera)
Methylergonovine (Methergine)
Mifepristone [RU 486] (Mifeprex)

Oxytocin (Pitocin)
Terbutaline (Brethine, Bricanyl)

PAIN MEDICATIONS

Local Anesthetics (Table 2)

Benzocaine & Antipyrine
(Auralgan)
Bupivacaine (Marcaine)
Capsaicin (Capsin,
Zostrix)

Cocaine
Dibucaine
(Nupercainal)
Lidocaine (Anestacon
Topical, Xylocaine)

Lidocaine & Prilocaine
(EMLA, LMX)
Pramoxine (Anusol
Ointment, Procto-
Foam-NS)

Migraine Headache Medications

Acetaminophen with
Butalbital w/and w/o
Caffeine (Fioricet,
Medigesic, Repan,
Sedapap-10, Two-
Dyne, Triapin, Axocet,
Phrenilin Forte)

Almotriptan (Axert)
Aspirin & Butalbital
Compound (Fiorinal)
Aspirin with Butalbital,
Caffeine, & Codeine
(Fiorinal with
Codeine)

Eletriptan (Relpax)
Frovatriptan (Frova)
Naratriptan (Amerge)
Sumatriptan (Imitrex)
Zolmitriptan (Zomig)

Narcotic Analgesics

Acetaminophen with
Codeine
(Tylenol No. 3, 4)
Alfentanil (Alfenta)
Aspirin with Codeine
(Empirin No. 2, 3, 4)
Buprenorphine
(Buprenex)
Butorphanol (Stadol)
Codeine
Fentanyl (Sublimaze)
Fentanyl Iontophoretic
Transdermal System
(Ionsys)
Fentanyl, Transdermal
(Duragesic)
Fentanyl, Transmucosal
(Actiq, Fentora)

Hydrocodone &
Acetaminophen (Lorcet,
Vicodin, Hycet)
Hydrocodone & Aspirin
(Lortab ASA)
Hydrocodone & Ibupro-
fen (Vicoprofen)
Hydromorphone
(Dilaudid)
Levorphanol
(Levo-Dromoran)
Meperidine (Demerol)
Methadone (Dolophine)
Morphine (Avinza XR,
Duramorph, Infu-
morph, MS Contin,
Kadian SR, Oramorph
SR, Palladone, Rox-
anol)

Morphine, Liposomal
(DepoDur)
Nalbuphine (Nubain)
Oxycodone (OxyContin,
OxyIR, Roxicodone)
Oxycodone & Aceta-
minophen (Percocet,
Tylox)
Oxycodone & Aspirin
(Percodan, Percodan-
Demi)
Oxymorphone HCl
(Opana, Opana ER)
Pentazocine (Talwin)
Propoxyphene (Darvon)
Propoxyphene & Aceta-
minophen (Darvocet)
Propoxyphene & Aspirin
(Darvon Compound-65,
Darvon-N with Aspirin)

Nonnarcotic Analgesics

Acetaminophen [APAP]
(Tylenol)
Aspirin (Bayer, Ecotrin,
St. Joseph's)

Tramadol
(Ultram,
Ultram ER)

Tramadol/
Acetaminophen
(Ultracet)

Nonsteroidal Anti-inflammatory Agents

Celecoxib (Celebrex)
Diclofenac (Cataflam, Flector, Voltaren)
Diflunisal (Dolobid)
Etodolac
Fenoprofen (Nalfon)
Flurbiprofen (Ansaid, Ocufen)

Ibuprofen (Motrin, Rufen, Advil)
Indomethacin (Indocin)
Ketoprofen (Orudis, Oruvail)
Ketorolac (Toradol)
Meloxicam (Mobic)
Nabumetone (Relafen)

Naproxen (Aleve, Naprosyn, Anaprox)
Oxaprozin (Daypro)
Piroxicam (Feldene)
Sulindac (Clinoril)
Tolmetin (Tolectin)

Miscellaneous Pain Medications

Amitriptyline (Elavil)
Imipramine (Tofranil)

Pregabalin (Lyrica)
Tramadol (Ultram)

Ziconotide (Prialt)

RESPIRATORY AGENTS

Antitussives, Decongestants, & Expectorants

Acetylcysteine (Acetadote, Mucomyst)
Benzonatate (Tessalon Perles)
Codeine
Dextromethorphan (Mediquell, Benylin DM, PediaCare 1)
Guaifenesin (Robitussin)
Guaifenesin & Codeine (Robitussin AC, Brontex)

Guaifenesin & Dextromethorphan
Hydrocodone & Guaifenesin (Hycotuss Expectorant)
Hydrocodone & Homatropine (Hycodan, Hydromet)
Hydrocodone & Pseudoephedrine (Detussin, Histussin-D)

Hydrocodone, Chlorpheniramine, Phenylephrine, Acetaminophen, & Caffeine (Hycomine)
Potassium Iodide (SSKI, Thyro-Block)
Pseudoephedrine (Sudafed, Novafed, Afrinol)

Bronchodilators

Albuterol (Proventil, Ventolin, Volmax)
Albuterol & Ipratropium (Combivent)
Aminophylline
Arformoterol (Brovana)
Ephedrine
Epinephrine (Adrenalin, Sus-Phrine, EpiPen)

Formoterol (Foradil Aerolizer)
Isoproterenol (Isuprel)
Levalbuterol (Xopenex, Xopenex HFA)
Metaproterenol (Alupent, Metaprel)
Pirbuterol (Maxair)

Salmeterol (Serevent, Serevent Diskus)
Terbutaline (Brethine, Bricanyl)
Theophylline (Theo24, TheoChron)

Respiratory Inhalants

Acetylcysteine (Acetadote, Mucomyst)
Beclomethasone (Beconase, Vancenase Nasal Inhaler)
Beclomethasone (QVAR)
Beractant (Survanta)
Budesonide (Rhinocort, Pulmicort)
Budesonide/formoterol (Symbicort)

Calfactant (Infasurf)
Cromolyn Sodium (Intal, Nasalcrom, Opticrom)
Dexamethasone, Nasal (Dexacort Phosphate Turbinaire)
Flunisolide (AeroBid, Aerospan, Nasarel)
Fluticasone, Oral, Nasal (Flonase, Flovent)

Fluticasone Propionate & Salmeterol Xinafoate (Advair Diskus, Advair HFA)
Ipratropium (Atrovent HFA, Atrovent Nasal)
Nedocromil (Tilade)
Tiotropium (Spiriva)
Triamcinolone (Azmacort)

Miscellaneous Respiratory Agents

Alpha$_1$-Protease Inhibitor (Prolastin)

Dornase Alfa (Pulmozyme, Dnase)
Montelukast (Singulair)
Omalizumab (Xolair)

Zafirlukast (Accolate)
Zileuton (Zyflo)

URINARY/GENITOURINARY AGENTS

Alprostadil, Intracavernosal (Caverject, Edex)
Alprostadil, Urethral Suppository (Muse)
Ammonium Aluminum Sulfate [Alum]
Belladonna & Opium Suppositories (B & O Supprettes)
Bethanechol (Urecholine, Duvoid)
Darifenacin (Enablex)
Dimethyl Sulfoxide [DMSO] (Rimso 50)
Flavoxate (Urispas)
Hyoscyamine (Anaspaz, Cystospaz, Levsin)

Methenamine (Hiprex, Urex)
Neomycin-Polymyxin Bladder Irrigant [Neosporin GU Irrigant]
Nitrofurantoin (Macrodantin, Furadantin, Macrobid)
Oxybutynin (Ditropan, Ditropan XL)
Oxybutynin Transdermal System (Oxytrol)
Pentosan Polysulfate (Elmiron)
Phenazopyridine (Pyridium)

Potassium Citrate (Urocit-K)
Potassium Citrate & Citric Acid (Polycitra-K)
Sildenafil (Viagra)
Solifenacin (VESIcare)
Sodium Citrate/Citric Acid (Bicitra)
Tadalafil (Cialis)
Tolterodine (Detrol, Detrol LA)
Trimethoprim (Trimpex, Proloprim)
Trospium Chloride (Sanctura)
Vardenafil (Levitra)

Benign Prostatic Hyperplasia Medications

Alfuzosin (Uroxatral)
Doxazosin (Cardura, Cardura XL)

Dutasteride (Avodart)
Finasteride (Proscar)

Tamsulosin (Flomax)
Terazosin (Hytrin)

WOUND CARE

Becaplermin (Regranex Gel)

Silver Nitrate (Dey-Drop)

MISCELLANEOUS THERAPEUTIC AGENTS

Acamprosate (Campral)

Alglucosidase alfa (Myozyme)

Cilostazol (Pletal)

Drotrecogin Alfa (Xigris)

Eculizumab (Soliris)

Lanthanum Carbonate (Fosrenol)

Mecasermin (Increlex)

Megestrol Acetate (Megace)

Naltrexone (Depade, ReVia, Vivitrol)

Nicotine Gum (Nicorette, others)

Nicotine Nasal Spray (Nicotrol NS)

Nicotine, Transdermal (Habitrol, Nicoderm, Nicotrol, others)

Orlistat (Xenical, Alli [OTC])

Palifermin (Kepivance)

Potassium Iodide [Lugol Solution] (SSKI, Thyro-Block)

Sevelamer (Renagel)

Sodium Polystyrene Sulfonate (Kayexalate)

Talc (Sterile Talc Powder)

Varenicline (Chantix)

NATURAL & HERBAL AGENTS

Aloe Vera *Aloe barbadensis*

Arnica (*Arnica montana*)

Butcher's Broom (*Ruscus aculeatus*)

Bilberry *Vaccinium myrtillus*

Black Cohosh (*Cimicifuga racemosa*)

Bogbean *Menyanthes trifoliate*

Borage *Borago officinalis*

Bugleweed *Lycopus virginicus*

Capsicum *Capsicum frutescens*

Cascara Sagrada *Rhamnus purshiana*

Chamomile (*Matricaria recutita*)

Chondroitin Sulfate

Comfrey *Symphytum officinale*

Coriander *Coriandrum sativum*

Cranberry *Vaccinium macrocarpon*

Dong Quai (*Angelica polymorpha, sinensis*)

Echinacea (*Echinacea purpurea*)

Ephedra/Ma Huang

Evening Primrose Oil *Oenothera biennis*

Feverfew (*Tanacetum parthenium*)

Garlic (*Allium sativum*)

Gentian *Gentiana lutea*

Ginger (*Zingiber officinale*)

Ginkgo biloba

Ginseng (*Panax quinquefolius*)

Glucosamine Sulfate (chitosamine)

Green Tea *Camellia sinensis*

Guarana *Paullinia cupana*

Hawthorn (*Crataegus laevigata*)

Horsetail *Equisetum arvense*

Kava Kava (*Piper methysticum*)

Licorice (*Glycyrrhiza glabra*)

Melatonin (MEL)

Milk thistle (*Silybum marianum*)

Nettle *Urtica dioica*

Rue *Ruta graveolens*

Saw Palmetto (*Serenoa repens*)

Spirulina (*Spirulina* spp)

Stevia *Stevia rebaudiana*

St. John's Wort (*Hypericum perforatum*)

Tea Tree (*Melaleuca alternifolia*)

Valerian (*Valeriana officinalis*)

Yohimbine (*Pausinystalia yohimbe*)

GENERIC AND SELECTED BRAND DRUG DATA

Abacavir (Ziagen) [Antiretroviral/NRTI] WARNING: Allergy (fever, rash, fatigue, GI, resp) reported; stop drug immediately & do not rechallenge; lactic acidosis & hepatomegaly/steatosis reported **Uses:** *HIV Infxn* **Action:** Nucleoside RT Inhibitor **Dose:** *Adults.* 300 mg PO bid or 600 mg PO daily *Peds.* 8 mg/kg bid **Caution:** [C, –] CDC recommends HIV-infected mothers should not breast-feed (transmission risk) **Disp:** Tabs 300 mg; soln 20 mg/mL **SE:** See Warning, ↑ LFTs, fat redistribution **Interactions:** EtOH ↓ drug elimination and ↑ drug exposure **Labs:** Monitor LFTs, FBS, CBC & differential, BUN & Cr, triglycerides **NIPE:** ⊘ EtOH; monitor & teach pt about hypersensitivity Rxns; D/C drug immediately if hypersensitivity Rxn occurs and ⊘ rechallenge; take w/ or w/o food

Abatacept (Orencia) [Immunomodulator] **Uses:** *Mod/severe RA w/ inadequate response to one or more DMARDs* **Action:** Selective costimulation modulator, ↓ T-cell activation **Dose:** Initial 500 mg (<60 kg), 750 mg (60–100 kg); 1 g (>100 kg) IV over 30 min; repeat at 2 and 4 wk, then every 4 wk **Caution:** w/ TNF blockers [C, ?/–] COPD; h/o recurrent/localized/chronic, predisposition to Infxn **Contra:** w/ TNF antagonists (↑ Infxn) **Disp:** IV powder: 250 mg/10 mL **SE:** HA, URI, N, nasopharyngitis, Infxn, malignancy, inf Rxns/hypersensitivity (dizziness, HA, HTN), COPD exacerbations, cough, dyspnea **Interactions:** Do not give w/ live vaccines w/ or w/in 3 mo D/C Abatacept **NIPE:** Screen for TB prior to use; D/C if serious Infxn occurs

Abciximab (ReoPro) [Platelet-Aggregation Inhibitor/ Antiplatelet] **Uses:** *Prevent acute ischemic complications in PTCA*, MI **Action:** ↓ plt aggregation (glycoprotein IIb/IIIa inhibitor) **Dose:** *Unstable angina w/ planned PCI (ECC 2005):* 0.25 μg/kg bolus, then 10 μg/min cont inf × 18–24 h, stop 1 h after PCI; *PCI:* 0.25 mg/kg bolus 10–60 min pre-PTCA, then 0.125 μg/kg/min (max=10 μg/min) cont inf for 12 h **Caution:** [C, ?/–] **Contra:** Active or recent (w/in 6 wk) internal hemorrhage, CVA w/in 2 y or CVA w/ significant neurologic deficit, bleeding diathesis or PO anticoagulants w/in 7 d (unless PT<1.2 × control), ↓ plt (<100,000 cells/μL), recent trauma or major surgery (w/in 6 wk), CNS tumor, AVM, aneurysm, severe uncontrolled HTN, vasculitis, use of dextran prior to or during PTCA, allergy to murine proteins **Disp:** Inj 2 mg/mL **SE:** Allergic Rxns, bleeding, ↓ plt **Notes:** Use w/ heparin/ASA **Interactions:** May ↑ bleeding **W/** anticoagulants, antiplts, NSAIDs, thrombolytics **Labs:** Monitor CBC, PT, PTT, INR, guaiac stools, urine for blood **NIPE:** Monitor for ↑ bleeding & bruising; ⊘ shake vial or mix w/ another drug, ⊘ contact sports

25

Acamprosate (Campral) [Hypoglycemic/Alpha-glucosidase Inhibitor] Uses: *Maint abstinence from EtOH* Action: ↓ Glutamatergic transmission; modulates neuronal hyperexcitability; related to GABA Dose: 666 mg PO tid; CrCl 30–50 mL/min: 333 mg PO tid Caution: [C, ?/–] Contra: CrCl<30 mL/min Disp: Tabs 333 mg EC SE: N/D, depression, anxiety, insomnia Notes: Does not eliminate EtOH withdrawal Sx; continue even if relapse occurs Interactions: None Labs: ↑ BS, LFTs, uric acid; ↑ Hgb, Hct, plts NIPE: Caution w/ elderly & pts w/ h/o suicide ideations or depression; take w/o regard to food & swallow whole; ⊘ make-up missed dose or take >3 doses in 24 h

Acarbose (Precose) [Hypoglycemic/Alpha-Glucosidase Inhibitor] Uses: *Type 2 DM* Action: α-Glucosidase inhibitor; delays digestion of carbohydrates to ↓ glucose Dose: 25–100 mg PO tid w/ 1st bite of each meal; 50 mg tid (<60 kg); 100 mg tid (>60 kg) Caution: [B, ?] Avoid w/ CrCl <25 mL/min; can affect digoxin levels Contra: IBD, colonic ulceration, partial intestinal obst; cirrhosis Disp: Tabs 25, 50, 100 mg SE: Abd pain, D, flatulence, ↑ LFTs, hypersensitivity Rxn Notes: OK w/ sulfonylureas; Interactions: ↑ Hypoglycemic effect W/ juniper berries, ginseng, garlic, coriander, celery; ↓ effects W/ intestinal absorbents, digestive enzyme Preps, diuretics, corticosteroids, phenothiazides, estrogens, phenytoin, INH, sympathomimetics, CCBs, thyroid hormones; ↓ conc OF digoxin Labs: ✓ LFTs q3mo for 1st y, FBS, HbA1c, LFTs, Hgb & Hct, monitor digoxin levels NIPE: Take drug tid w/ 1st bite of food, ↓ GI side effects by ↓ dietary starch, treat hypoglycemia w/ dextrose instead of sucrose, continue diet & exercise program

Acebutolol (Sectral) [Antihypertensive, Antiarrhythmic/Beta-Blocker] Uses: *HTN, arrhythmias* angina Action: Blocks β-adrenergic receptors, β1, & ISA Dose: HTN: 200–800 mg/d; arrhythmia: 400–1200 mg/d ÷ doses; ↓ if CrCl <50 mL/min or elderly; initial 200–400 mg/d; max 800 mg/d Caution: [B, D in 2nd & 3rd tri, +] Can exacerbate ischemic heart Dz, do not D/C abruptly Contra: 2nd-, 3rd-degree heart block Disp: Caps 200, 400 mg SE: Fatigue, HA, dizziness, bradycardia Interactions: ↓ Antihypertensive effect W/ NSAIDs, salicylates, thyroid preps, anesthetics, antacids, α-adrenergic stimulants, ma-huang, ephedra, licorice; ↓ hypoglycemic effect OF glyburide; ↑ hypotensive response W/ other antihypertensives, nitrates, EtOH, diuretics, black cohash, hawthorn, goldenseal, parsley; ↑ bradycardia W/ digoxin, amiodarone; ↑ hypoglycemic effect OF insulin Labs: Monitor lipids, uric acid, K+, FBS, LFTs, thyroxin, ECG NIPE: Teach pt to monitor BP, pulse, S/Sxs CHF

Acetaminophen (APAP, N-acetyl-p-aminophenol) (Tylenol, other generic) [OTC] [Analgesic, Antipyretic] Uses: *Mild-moderate pain, HA, fever* Action: Nonnarcotic analgesic; ↓ CNS synth of prostaglandins & hypothalamic heat-regulating center Dose: Adults. 650 mg PO or PR q4–6h or 1000 mg PO q6h; max 4 g/24 h. Peds. <12 y 10–15 mg/kg/dose PO or PR q4–6h; max 2.6 g/24 h. See Table 1. Administer q6h if CrCl 10–50 mL/min & q8h if CrCl <10 mL/min

Caution: [B, +] Hepatotoxic in elderly & w/ EtOH use w/ >4 g/d; alcoholic liver Dz **Contra:** G6PD deficiency **Disp:** Tabs meltaway/dissolving 160 mg; tabs: 325, 500, 650 mg; chew tabs 80, 160 mg; Liq 100 mg/mL, 120 mg/2.5 mL, 120 mg/5 mL, 160 mg/5 mL, 167 mg/5 mL, 325 mg/5 mL, 500 mg/15 mL, 80 mg/0.8 mL; supp 80, 120, 125, 325, 650 mg **SE:** OD hepatotox at 10 g; 15 g can be lethal Rx w/ N-acetylcysteine **Notes:** No anti-inflammatory or plt-inhibiting action **Interactions:** ↑ Hepatotox **W/** EtOH, barbiturates, carbamazepine, INH, rifampin, phenytoin; ↑ risk of bleeding **W/** NSAIDs, salicylates, warfarin, feverfew, ginkgo biloba, red clover; ↓ absorption **W/** antacids, cholestyramine, colestipol **Labs:** Monitor LFTs, CBC, BUN, Cr, PT, INR; false ↑ urine 5-HIAA, urine glucose, serum uric acid; false ↓ serum glucose, amylase **NIPE:** Delayed absorption if given w/ food, ⊘ EtOH, teach S/Sxs hepatotox, consult health care provider if temp ↑ 103°F/>3 d

Acetaminophen + Butalbital ± Caffeine (Fioricet, Medigesic, Repan, Sedapap-10, Two-Dyne, Triapin, Axocet, Phrenilin Forte) [C-III] [Analgesic, Antipyretic/Barbiturate]

Uses: *Tension HA,* mild pain **Action:** Nonnarcotic analgesic w/ barbiturate **Dose:** 1–2 tabs or caps PO q4/6h PRN; ↓ in renal/hepatic impair; 4 g/24 h APAP max **Caution:** [C, D, +] Alcoholic liver Dz **Contra:** G6PD deficiency **Disp:** Caps *Dolgic Plus:* Butalbital 50 mg, caffeine 40 mg, APAP 750 mg; caps *Medigesic, Repan, Two-Dyne:* Butalbital 50 mg, caffeine 40 mg, APAP 325 mg; caps Axocet, Phrenilin Forte: Butalbital 50 mg + APAP 650 mg; caps: *Esgic-Plus, Zebutral:* Butalbital 50 mg, caffeine 40 mg, APAP 500 mg; Liq. *Dolgic LQ:* Butalbital 50 mg, caffeine 40 mg, APAP 325 mg/15mL; tabs *Medigesic, Fioricet, Repan:* Butalbital 50 mg, caffeine 40 mg, APAP 325 mg; *Phrenilin:* Butalbital 50 mg + APAP 325 mg; *Sedapap-10:* Butalbital 50 mg + APAP 650 mg **SE:** Drowsiness, dizziness, "hangover" effect **Interactions:** ↑ Effects *OF* benzodiazepines, opiate analgesics, sedatives/hypnotics, EtOH, methylphenidate hydrochloride; ↓ effects *OF* MAOIs, TCAs, corticosteroids, theophylline, OCPs, BBs, doxycycline **NIPE:** ⊘ EtOH & CNS depressants, may impair coordination, monitor for depression, use barrier protection contraception; butalbital is habit forming

Acetaminophen + Codeine (Tylenol No. 3, No. 4) [C-III, C-V] [Analgesic, Antipyretic/Opiate]

Uses: *Mild–moderate pain (No. 3); moderate–severe pain (No. 4)* **Action:** Combined APAP & narcotic analgesic **Dose:** **Adults.** 1–2 tabs q3–4h PRN (max dose APAP = 4 g/d). **Peds.** APAP 10–15 mg/kg/dose; codeine 0.5–1 mg/kg dose q4–6h (guide: 3–6 y, 5 mL/dose; 7–12 y, 10 mL/dose); ↓ in renal/hepatic impair **Caution:** [C, +] Alcoholic liver Dz **Contra:** G6PD deficiency **Disp:** Tabs 300 mg APAP + codeine; caps 325 mg APAP + codeine; susp (C-V) APAP 120 mg + codeine 12 mg/5 mL **SE:** Drowsiness, dizziness, N/V **Notes:** Codeine in No. 3=30 mg; No. 4=60 mg **Interactions:** ↑ Effects *OF* benzodiazepines, opiate analgesics, sedatives/hypnotics, EtOH, methylphenidate hydrochloride; ↓ effects *OF* MAOIs, TCAs, corticosteroids, theophylline, OCPs, BBs, doxycycline **NIPE:** ⊘ EtOH & CNS depressants, may impair coordination, monitor for depression, use barrier protection contraception; codeine may be habit forming

Acetazolamide (Diamox) [Anticonvulsant, Diuretic/Carbonic Anhydrase Inhibitor] Uses: *Diuresis, glaucoma, prevent high-altitude sickness, refractory epilepsy* **Action:** Carbonic anhydrase inhibitor; ↓ renal excretion of hydrogen & ↑ renal excretion of Na$^+$, K$^+$, HCO$_3^-$, H2O **Dose: Adults.** *Diuretic:* 250–375 mg IV or PO q24h. *Glaucoma:* 250–1000 mg PO q24h in ÷ doses. *Epilepsy:* 8–30 mg/kg/d PO in ÷ doses. *Altitude sickness:* 250 mg PO q8–12h or SR 500 mg PO q12–24h start 24–48 h before & 48 h after highest ascent. **Peds.** *Epilepsy:* 8–30 mg/kg/24 h PO in ÷ doses; max 1 g/d. *Diuretic:* 5 mg/kg/ 24 h PO or IV. *Alkalinization of urine:* 5 mg/kg/dose PO bid-tid. *Glaucoma:* 5–15 mg/kg/24 h PO in ÷ doses; max 1 g/d; ↓ dose w/CrCl 10–50 mL/min; avoid if CrCl <10 mL/min **Caution:** [C, +] **Contra:** Renal/hepatic failure, sulfa allergy **Disp:** Tabs 125, 250 mg; ER caps 500 mg; inj 500 mg/vial, powder for recons **SE:** Malaise, metallic taste, drowsiness, photosens, hyperglycemia **Interactions:** Causes ↑ effects *OF* amphetamines, quinidine, procainamide, TCAs, ephedrine; ↓ effects *OF* Li, phenobarbital, salicylates, barbiturates; ↑ K$^+$ loss *W*/ corticosteroids and amphotericin B **Labs:** Monitor serum electrolytes esp Na$^+$ & K$^+$, CBC, Cr, plt & intraocular pressure; false + for urinary protein, urinary urobilinogen; ↓ uptake; ↑ serum & urine glucose, uric acid, Ca^{2+}, serum ammonia **NIPE:** ↓ GI distress w/ food, monitor for S/Sxs metabolic acidosis, ↑ fluid to ↓ risk of kidney stones; ER forms not for epilepsy

Acetic Acid & Aluminum Acetate (Otic Domeboro) [Astringent/ Anti-infective] Uses: *Otitis externa* **Action:** Anti-infective **Dose:** 4–6 gtt in ear(s) q2–3h **Caution:** [C, ?] **Contra:** Perforated tympanic membranes **Disp:** 2% Otic soln **SE:** Local irritation **NIPE:** Burning w/ instillation or irrigation

Acetylcysteine (Acetadote, Mucomyst) [Mucolytic/Amino acid derivative] Uses: *Mucolytic, antidote to APAP hepatotox/OD* adjuvant Rx chronic bronchopulm Dzs & CF* prevent contrast-induced renal dysfunction. **Action:** Splits mucoprotein disulfide linkages; restores glutathione in APAP OD to protect liver **Dose: Adults & Peds.** *Nebulizer:* 3–5 mL of 20% soln diluted w/ equal vol of H$_2$O or NS tid-qid. *Antidote:* PO or NG: 140 mg/kg load, then 70 mg/kg q4h × 17 doses. (Dilute 1:3 in carbonated beverage or OJ) *Acetadote:* 150 mg/kg IV over 15 min, then 50 mg/kg over 4 h, then 100 mg/kg over 16 h; *Prevention:* 600 mg PO bid × 2 d **Caution:** [C, ?] **Disp:** Soln, inhaled, & oral 10%, 20%; Acetadote IV soln 20% **SE:** Bronchospasm (inhal), N/V, drowsiness, anaphylactoid Rxns w/ IV **Notes:** Activated charcoal adsorbs PO acetylcysteine for APAP ingestion; start Rx for APAP OD w/in 6–8 h **Interactions:** Discolors rubber, Fe, Cu, Ag; incompatible *W/* multiple antibiotics—administer drugs separately **Labs:** Monitor ABGs & pulse oximetry w/ bronchospasm **NIPE:** Inform pt of ↑ productive cough, clear airway before aerosol administration, ↑ fluids to liquefy secretions, unpleasant odor will disappear & may cause N/V

Acitretin (Soriatane) [Retinoid] WARNING: Must not be used by females who are pregnant or intend to become pregnant during therapy or for up to 3 y after D/C of therapy; EtOH must not be ingested during therapy or for 2 mo following cessation of therapy; do not donate blood for 3 y following cessation **Uses:** *Severe psoriasis*; other keratinization disorders (lichen planus, etc) **Action:** Retinoid-like activity **Dose:** 25–50 mg/d PO, w/ main meal; ↑ if no response by 4 wk to 75 mg/d **Caution:** [X, -] Renal/hepatic impair; in women of reproductive potential **Contra:** See Warning **Disp:** Caps 10, 25 mg **SE:** Cheilitis, skin peeling, alopecia, pruritus, rash, arthralgia, GI upset, photosens, thrombocytosis, hypertriglyceridemia **Interactions:** ↑ 1/2 life W/ EtOH use, ↑ hepatotox W/ MTX, ↓ effects OF progestin-only contraceptives **Labs:** Monitor LFTs, lipids, FBS, HbA1c **NIPE:** Use effective contraception; ⊘ donate blood for 3 y after Rx, teach pt S/Sxs pancreatitis; patient agreement/informed consent prior to use

Acyclovir (Zovirax) [Antiviral/Synthetic Purine Nucleoside]
Uses: *Herpes simplex & zoster Infxns* **Action:** Interferes w/ viral DNA synth **Dose:** *Adults.* Dose on IBW if obese >125% IBW PO: Initial genital herpes: 200 mg PO q4h while awake, 5 caps/d × 10 d or 400 mg PO tid × 7–10 d. *Chronic suppression:* 400 mg PO bid. *Intermittent Rx:* As initial Rx, except Rx for 5 d, or 800 mg PO bid, at prodrome. *Herpes zoster:* 800 mg PO 5×/d for 7–10 d. *IV:* 5–10 mg/kg/dose IV q8h. *Topical: Initial herpes genitalis:* Apply q3h (6×/d) for 7 d. *Peds.* 5–10 mg/kg/dose IV or PO q8h or 750 mg/m²/24 h ÷ q8h. *Chickenpox:* 20 mg/kg/dose PO qid; ↓ W/ CrCl <50 mL/min **Caution:** [B, +] **Contra:** Hypersensitivity to compound **Disp:** Caps 200 mg; tabs 400, 800 mg; susp 200 mg/5 mL; inj 500 mg/vial; 1000, inj soln 25 mg/mL, 50 mg/mL; oint 5% & cream 5% **SE:** Dizziness, lethargy, confusion, rash, inflammation at IV site; **Interactions:** ↑ CNS SE W/ MTX & zidovudine, ↑ blood levels W/ probenecid **Labs:** Monitor BUN, SCr, LFTs, CBC; transient ↑ Cr/BUN **NIPE:** Start immediately w/ Sxs, ↑ hydration w/ IV dose, ↑ risk cervical cancer w/ genital herpes, ↑ length of Rx in immunocompromised pts, PO better than topical for herpes genitalis

Adalimumab (Humira) [Antirheumatic/TNF Alpha Blocker]
WARNING: Cases of TB have been observed; ✓ TB skin test prior to use; Hep B reactivation possible, invasive fungal and other opportunistic Infxns have been reported **Uses:** *Moderate-severe RA w/ an inadequate response to one or more DMARDs* Active arthritis w/ psoriatic arthritis **Action:** TNF-a inhibitor **Dose:** 40 mg SQ qowk; may ↑ 40 mg qwk if not on MTX **Caution:** [B, ?/-] Serious Infxns & sepsis reported **SE:** Prefilled 0.8 mL (40 mg) syringe **SE:** Inj site Rxns, serious Infxns, neurologic events, malignancies **Notes:** Refrigerate prefilled syringe, rotate inj sites, OK w/ other DMARDs **Interactions:** ↑ Effects W/ MTX **Labs:** May ↑ lipids, alk phosp, **NIPE:** ⊘ Exposure to Infxn; ⊘ admin live-virus vaccines

Adefovir (Hepsera) [Antiviral/Acyclic Nucleotide Analogue]
WARNING: Acute exacerbations of hepatitis may occur following D/C therapy (monitor LFTs); chronic use may lead to nephrotox w/ underlying renal impair (monitor renal Fxn); HIV resistance may emerge; lactic acidosis & severe hepatomegaly

w/ steatosis reported alone or in combo w/ other antiretrovirals **Uses:** *Chronic active Hep B* **Action:** Nucleotide analog **Dose:** CrCl >50 mL/min: 10 mg PO daily; CrCl 20–49 mL/min: 10 mg PO q48h; CrCl 10–19 mL/min: 10 mg PO q72h; HD: 10 mg PO q7d postdialysis; adjust w/ CrCl <50 mL/min **Caution:** [C, -] **Disp:** Tabs 10 mg **SE:** Asthenia, HA, abd pain; see Warning **Interactions:** See Warning **Labs:** LFTs, BUN, Cr, creatine kinase, amylase **NIPE:** Effects on fetus & baby not known ⊘ breast-feed; use barrier contraception

Adenosine (Adenocard) [Antiarrhythmic/Nucleoside] Uses: *PSVT*; including w/ WPW **Action:** Class IV antiarrhythmic; slows AV node conduction **Dose:** *Adults.* 6 mg over 1–3 s, then 20 mL NS bolus, elevate extremity; repeat 12 mg in 1–2 min PRN *(ECC 2005) Peds.* 0.05 mg/kg IV bolus; may repeat q1–2min to 0.3 mg/kg max **Caution:** [C, ?] **Contra:** 2nd- or 3rd-degree AV block or SSS (w/o pacemaker); recent MI or cerebral hemorrhage **Disp:** Inj 3 mg/mL **SE:** Facial flushing, HA, dyspnea, chest pressure, ↓ BP **Interactions:** ↓ Effects **W/** theophylline, caffeine, guarana; ↑ effects **W/** dipyridamole; ↑ risk **OF** hypotension & chest pain **W/** nicotine; ↑ risk **OF** bradycardia **W/** BBs; ↑ risk **OF** heart block **W/** carbamazepine; ↑ risk **OF** ventricular fibrillation **W/** digitalis glycosides **Labs:** Monitor ECG during administration **NIPE:** Monitor BP & pulse during therapy, monitor resp status ↑ risk of bronchospasm in asthmatics, discard unused or unclear soln; doses >12 mg not OK; can cause monentary asystole when administered

Albumin (Albuminar, Buminate, Albutein) [Plasma Volume Expander] Uses: *Plasma volume expansion for shock* (eg, burns, hemorrhage) **Action:** Maint plasma colloid oncotic pressure **Dose:** *Adults.* Initial 25 g IV; then based on response; 250 g/48h max *Peds.* 0.5–1 g/kg/dose; inf at 0.05–0.1 g/min **Caution:** [C, ?] Severe anemia; cardiac, renal, or hepatic insuff due to protein load & hypervolemia **Contra:** CHF **Disp:** Soln 5%, 25% **SE:** Chills, fever, CHF, tachycardia, ↓ BP, hypervolemia **Interactions:** Atypical Rxns **W/** ACEI withhold 24 h prior to albumin administration **Labs:** ↑ Alk phosp; monitor HMG, Hct, electrolytes, serum protein **NIPE:** Monitor BP & D/C if hypotensive, monitor intake & output, admin to all blood types; Contains 130–160 mEq Na$^+$/L; may cause pulm edema

Albuterol (Proventil, Ventolin, Volmax) [Bronchodilator/ Adrenergic] Uses: *Asthma; prevent exercise-induced bronchospasm* **Action:** β-adrenergic sympathomimetic bronchodilator; relaxes bronchial smooth muscle **Dose:** *Adults. Inhaler:* 2 inhal q4–6h PRN; 1 Rotacap inhaled q4–6h. *PO:* 2–4 mg PO tid-qid. *Neb:* 1.25–5 mg (0.25–1 mL of 0.5% soln in 2–3 mL of NS) tid-qid. *Peds. Inhaler:* 2 inhal q4–6h. *PO:* 0.1–0.2 mg/kg/dose PO; max 2–4 mg PO tid; *Neb:* 0.05 mg/kg (max 2.5 mg) in 2–3 mL of NS tid-qid **Caution:** [C, +] **Disp:** Tabs 2, 4 mg; XR tabs 4, 8 mg; syrup 2 mg/5 mL; 90 μg/dose met-dose inhaler; soln for neb 0.083, 0.5% **SE:** Palpitations, tachycardia, nervousness, GI upset **Interactions:** ↑ Effects **W/** other sympathomimetics; ↑ CV effects

W/ MAOI, TCA, inhaled anesthetics; ↓ effects W/ BBs; ↓ effectiveness OF insulin, oral hypoglycemics, digoxin **Labs:** Transient ↑ in serum glucose after inhalation; transient ↓ K+ after inhalation **NIPE:** Monitor HR, BP, ABGs, s&s bronchospasm & CNS stimulation; instruct on use of inhaler, must use as 1st inhaler, & rinse mouth after use

Albuterol & Ipratropium (Combivent, DuoNeb) [Bronchodilator/Adrenergic, Anticholinergic] Uses: *COPD* Action:
Combo of β-adrenergic bronchodilator & quaternary anticholinergic **Dose:** 2 inhal qid; neb 3 mL q6h **Caution:** [C, +] **Contra:** Peanut/soybean allergy **Disp:** Metdose inhaler, 18 μg ipratropium & 103 μg albuterol/puff; nebulization (DuoNeb) ipratropium 0.5 mg & albuterol 2.5 mg/3 mL 0.042%, 0.21% **SE:** Palpitations, tachycardia, nervousness, GI upset, dizziness, blurred vision **Interactions:** ↑ Effects W/ anticholinergics, including ophthalmic meds; ↓ effects W/ herb jaborandi tree, pill-bearing spurge **NIPE:** See Albuterol; may cause transient blurred vision/irritation or urinary changes

Aldesleukin [IL-2] (Proleukin) [Immunomodulator/Antineoplastic] WARNING: (Use restricted to pts w/ nl pulm & cardiac Fxn Uses:
Met RCC & melanoma **Action:** Acts via IL-2 receptor; many immunomodulatory effects **Dose:** 600,000 IU/kg q8h × 14 doses days 1–5 and days 15–19 of 28-d cycle (FDA-approved dose/schedule for RCC); other schedules (eg, "high dose" 24 × 10⁶ IU/m² IV q8h on days 1–5 & 12–16) **Caution:** [C, ?/-] **Contra:** Organ allografts **Disp:** Powder for recons 22 × 10⁶ IU, when reconstituted 18 million IU/mL = 1.1 mg/mL **SE:** Flu-like synd (malaise, fever, chills); N/V/D, ↑ bilirubin; capillary leak synd w/ ↓ BP, pulm edema, fluid retention, & wt gain; renal & mild hematologic tox (↓ HgB, plt,WBC), eosinophilia; cardiac tox (ischemia, atrial arrhythmias); neuro tox (CNS depression, somnolence, delirium, rare coma); pruritic rashes, urticaria, & erythroderma common. **Notes:** Cont inf ↑ risk severe ↓ BP & fluid retention **Interactions:** May ↑ tox OF cardiotoxic, hepatotoxic, myelotoxic, & nephrotoxic drugs; ↑ hypotension W/ antihypertensive drugs; ↓ effects W/ corticosteroids; acute Rxn W/ iodinated contrast media up to several months after inf; CNS effects W/ psychotropics **Labs:** May cause ↑ alkaline phosphatase, bilirubin, BUN, SCr, LFTs **NIPE:** Thoroughly explain serious side effects of drug & that some side effects are expected; ⊘ EtOH, NSAIDs, ASA

Alefacept (Amevive) [Antipsoriatic/Immunosuppressive]
WARNING: Must monitor CD4 before each dose; w/hold if <250; D/C if <250 × 1 month **Uses:** *Moderate/severe chronic plaque psoriasis* **Action:** Fusion protein inhibitor **Dose:** 7.5 mg IV or 15 mg IM once wk × 12 wk **Caution:** [B, ?/-] PRG registry; associated w/ serious Infxn **Contra:** Lymphopenia, HIV **Disp:** 7.5, 15-mg powder for recons vials **SE:** Pharyngitis, myalgia, inj site Rxn, malignancy, Infxn **Interactions:** No studies performed **Labs:** Monitor WBCs, CD4+ T lymphocyte counts **NIPE:** ↑ Risk of Infxn; ⊘ exposure to Infxns; inj site inflammation; rotate sites; IV and IM different formulations; may repeat course 12 wk later if CD4 OK

Alendronate (Fosamax, Fosamax Plus D) [Antiosteoporotic]

Uses: *Rx & prevent osteoporosis male & female, Rx steroid-induced osteoporosis, Paget Dz* **Action:** ↓ Nl & abnormal bone resorption **Dose:** *Osteoporosis:* Rx: 10 mg/d PO or 70 mg qwk; Fosamax plus D 1 tab qwk. *Steroid-induced osteoporosis:* Rx: 5 mg/d PO. *Prevention:* 5 mg/d PO or 35 mg qwk. Paget Dz: 40 mg/d PO **Caution:** [C, ?] Not OK if CrCl <35 mL/min, w/ NSAID use **Contra:** Esophageal anomalies, inability to sit/stand upright for 30 min, ↓ Ca²⁺ **Disp:** Tabs 5, 10, 35, 40, 70 mg, soln 70 mg/75 mL, Foxamax plus D: Alendronate 70 mg and cholecalciferol 2800 IU **SE:** GI disturbances, esophageal irritation, HA, pain, jaw osteonecrosis (w/ dental procedures, chemo) **Notes:** Take 1st thing in AM w/ H₂O (8 oz) >30 min before 1st food/beverage of the day. Do not lie down for 30 min after. Ca²⁺ & vitamin D supl necessary for regular tab **Interactions:** ↓ Absorption W/ antacids, Ca supls, Fe, food; ↑ risk of upper GI bleed W/ ASA & NSAIDs **Labs:** May cause transient ↑ serum Ca & phosphate **NIPE:** Adequate Ca & vitamin D supl needed, ↑ wt-bearing activity, ↓ smoking, EtOH use

Alfentanil (Alfenta) [Narcotic Analgesic] [C-II]

Uses: *Adjunct in the maint of anesthesia; analgesia* **Action:** Short-acting narcotic analgesic **Dose:** *Adults & Peds >12 y.* 3–75 μg/kg (IBW) IV inf; total depends on duration of procedure **Caution:** [C, +/–] ↑ ICP, resp depression **Disp:** Inj 500 μg/mL **SE:** Bradycardia, ↓ BP arrhythmias, peripheral vasodilation, ↑ ICP, drowsiness, resp depression **Interactions:** ↓ Effect W/ phenothiazines; ↑ effects W/ BBs, CNS depressants, erythromycin **NIPE:** Monitor HR, BP, resp rate

Alfuzosin (Uroxatral) [Selective Alpha Adrenergic Antagonist]

WARNING: May prolong QTc interval **Uses:** *BPH* **Action:** α-Blocker **Dose:** 10 mg PO daily immediately after the same meal **Caution:** [B, –] **Contra:** w/ CYP3A4 inhibitors; moderate-severe hepatic impair **Disp:** Tabs 10 mg **SE:** Postural ↓ BP, dizziness, HA, fatigue **Interactions:** ↑ Effects W/ atenolol, azole antifungals, cimetidine, ritonavir; ↑ effects *OF* antihypertensives **NIPE:** Not indicated for use in women or children; take w/ food; ↑ risk of postural hypotension; ⊘ take other meds that prolong QT interval. ⊘ cut or crush XR tablet; Fewest reports of ejaculatory disorders compared w/ similar drugs

Alginic Acid + Aluminum Hydroxide & Magnesium Trisilicate (Gaviscon) [Antacid] [OTC]

Uses: *Heartburn*; hiatal hernia pain **Action:** Protective layer blocks gastric acid **Dose:** 2–4 tabs or 15–30 mL PO qid followed by H₂O; **Caution:** [B, –] Avoid in renal impair or Na⁺-restricted diet **Disp:** Tabs, susp **SE:** D, constipation **Interactions:** ↓ Absorption OF tetracyclines

Alglucosidase alfa (Myozyme) [Recombinant Acid Alpha-Glucosidase]

WARNING: Life-threatening anaphylactic Rxns have occurred w/ inf; appropriate medical support measures should be immediately available **Uses:** *Rx Pompe Dz* **Action:** Degrades glycogen in lysosomes **Dose:** 20 mg/kg IV q2wk over 4 h (see insert) **Caution:** [B,?/–] Illness at time of inf may

↑ inf Rxns **Disp:** Powder 50 mg/vial **SE:** Hypersensitivity, fever, rash, D,V, gastroenteritis, pneumonia, URI, cough, respiratory distress, Infxns, cardiorespiratory failure, cardiac arrhythmia w/ general anesthesia

Aliskiren (Tekturna) [Direct Renin Inhibitor] WARNING: May cause injury and death to a developing fetus; D/C immediately when pregnancy is detected **Uses:** HTN **Action:** Direct renin inhibitor **Dose:** 150–300 mg PO day **Caution:** [C (1st tri), D (2nd & 3rd tri), ?]; w/ severe renal impair **Disp:** Tabs 150, 300 mg **SE:** D, abd pain, dyspepsia, GERD, cough, ↑ K⁺, angioedema, ↓ BP

Allopurinol (Zyloprim, Lopurin, Aloprim) [Xanthine Oxidase Inhibitor] **Uses:** *Gout, hyperuricemia of malignancy, uric acid urolithiasis* **Action:** ↓ Uric acid production **Dose:** *Adults. PO:* Initial 100 mg/d; usual 300 mg/d; max 800 mg/d. *IV:* 200–400 mg/m²/d (max 600 mg/24 h); (after meal w/ plenty of fluid) *Peds.* Only for hyperuricemia of malignancy if <10 y: 10 mg/kg/24 h PO or 200 mg/m²/d IV ÷ q6–8h; max 600 mg/24 h; ↓ in renal impair **Caution:** [C, M] **Disp:** Tabs 100, 300 mg; inj 500 mg/30 mL (Aloprim) **SE:** Rash, N/V, renal impair, angioedema **Notes:** Aggravates acute gout; begin after acute attack resolves; IV dose of 6 mg/mL final conc as single daily inf or ÷ 6-, 8-, or 12-h intervals **Interactions:** ↑ Effect *OF* theophylline, oral anticoagulants; ↑ hypersensitivity Rxns *W/* ACEIs, thiazide diuretics; ↑ risk of rash *W/* ampicillin/amoxicillin; ↑ bone marrow depression *W/* cyclophosphamide, azathioprine, mercaptopurine; ↓ effects *W/* EtOH **Labs:** ↑ Alkaline phosphatase, bilirubin, LFTs **NIPE:** ↑ fluids to 2–3 L/d, take pc, may ↑ drowsiness

Almotriptan (Axert) [Serotonin 5-HT1 Receptor Agonist] **Uses:** *Rx acute migraine* **Action:** Vascular serotonin receptor agonist **Dose:** *Adults. PO:* 6.25–12 mg PO, repeat in 2 h PRN; 2 dose/24h max PO dose; max 12 or 24 mg/d **Caution:** [C, ?/–] **Contra:** Angina, ischemic heart Dz, coronary artery vasospasm, hemiplegic or basilar migraine, uncontrolled HTN, ergot use, MAOI use w/in 14 d **Disp:** Tabs 6.25, 12.5 mg **SE:** N, somnolence, paresthesias, HA, dry mouth, weakness, numbness, coronary vasospasm, HTN **Interactions:** ↑ Serotonin effects *OF* SSRIs, ↑ vasoactive action *OF* ergot derivatives & 5-HT agonists, ↑ effects *W/* erythromycin, ketoconazole, itraconazole, MAOIs, ritonavir, verapamil **NIPE:** ⊘ Ergot compounds or 5-HT agonist within 24 h of almotriptan; ⊘ use if pregnant or breast-feeding; concurrent with SSRIs may cause serotonin synd; use only during migraine headache attack; avoid driving if drug causes drowsiness

Alosetron (Lotronex) [Selective 5-HT3 Receptor Antagonist] WARNING: Serious GI side effects, some fatal, including ischemic colitis reported. May be prescribed only through participation in the prescribing program for Lotronex **Uses:** *Severe diarrhea-predominant IBS in women who fail conventional therapy* **Action:** Selective 5-HT₃ receptor antagonist **Dose:** *Adults.* 0.5 mg PO bid; titrate to 1 mg bid max; D/C after 4 wk at max dose if Sxs not controlled **Caution:** [B, ?/–] **Contra:** h/o chronic/severe constipation, GI obst, strictures, toxic megacolon, GI perforation, adhesions, ischemic/ulcerative colitis, Crohn Dz, diverticulitis, thrombophlebitis, hypercoagulability **Disp:** Tabs 0.5, 1 mg **SE:** Constipation, abd pain, N **Notes:** D/C immediately if constipation or Sxs of ischemic colitis develop; pt must sign informed consent prior to use "patient–health care provider agreement" **Interactions:** ↑ Risk constipation W/ other drugs that ↓ GI motility, inhibits *N*-acetyltransferase, & may influence metabolism of INH, procainamide, hydralazine **Labs:** Monitor for ↑ ALT, AST, alk phosp, bilirubin **NIPE:** Administer w/o regard to food, eval effectiveness >4 wk

Alpha$_1$-Protease Inhibitor (Prolastin) [Respiratory Agent/ Alpha Protease Inhibitor Replacement] Uses: *α$_1$-Antitrypsin deficiency*; pancinar emphysema **Action:** Replace human α$_1$-protease inhibitor **Dose:** 60 mg/kg IV once/wk **Caution:** [C, ?] **Contra:** Selective IgA deficiencies w/ known IgA antibodies **Disp:** Inj 500 mg/20 mL, 1000 mg/40 mL powder for inj **SE:** Fever, dizziness, flulike Sxs, allergic Rxns **Labs:** Monitor for ↑ ALT, AST **NIPE:** Inf over 30 min, ⊘ mix w/ other drugs, use w/in 3 h of reconstitution

Alprazolam (Xanax, Niravam) [Anxiolytic/Benzodiazepine] [C-IV] Uses: *Anxiety & panic disorders*, anxiety w/ depression **Action:** Benzodiazepine; antianxiety agent **Dose:** *Anxiety:* Initial, 0.25–0.5 mg tid; ↑ to response; ↓ in elderly, debilitated, hepatic impair **Caution:** [D, –] **Contra:** NAG, concomitant itra/ ketoconazole **Disp:** Tabs 0.25, 0.5, 1, 2 mg; *Xanax XR* 0.5, 1, 2, 3 mg; *Niravam* (orally disintegrating tabs) 0.25, 0.5, 1, 2 mg; soln 1 mg/mL **SE:** Drowsiness, fatigue, memory impair, sexual dysfunction, paradoxical Rxns **Interactions:** ↑ CNS depression W/ EtOH, other CNS depressants, narcotics, MAOIs, anesthetics, antihistamines, theophylline, herbs: kava kava, valerian; ↑ effect W/ OCPs, cimetidine, INH, disulfiram, omeprazole, valproic acid, ciprofloxacin, erythromycin, clarithromycin, phenytoin, verapamil, grapefruit juice; ↑ risk OF ketoconazole, itraconazole, digitalis tox, ↓ effectiveness OF levodopa; ↓ effect W/ carbamazepine, rifampin, rifabutin, barbiturates, cigarette smoking **Labs:** ↑ Alkaline phosphatase, may cause ↓ Hct & neutropenia **NIPE:** Monitor for resp depression; avoid abrupt D/C after prolonged use

Alprostadil [Prostaglandin E$_1$] (Prostin VR) [Vasodilator/ Prostaglandin] **WARNING:** Apnea in up to 12% of neonates especially <2 kg at birth Uses: *Conditions ductus arteriosus blood flow must be maintained* sustain pulm/systemic circulation until OR (eg, pulm atresia/stenosis, transposition, etc) **Action:** Vasodilator (ductus arteriosus very sensitive), plt inhibitor **Dose:** 0.05 μg/kg/min IV; ↓ to lowest that maintains response **Caution:** [X, –] **Contra:** Neonatal resp distress synd **Disp:** Inj 500 μg/mL **SE:** Cutaneous vasodilation, Sz-like activity, jitteriness, ↑ temp, thrombocytopenia, ↓ BP; may cause apnea **Interactions:** ↑ Effects OF anticoagulants & antihypertensives, ↓ effects OF cyclosporine **Labs:** ↓ Ca^{2+}, fibrinogen **NIPE:** Dilute drug before administration, refrigerate & discard >24 h, central line preferred, flushing indicates catheter malposition, apnea & bradycardia indicates drug overdose, keep intubation kit at bedside

Alprostadil, Intracavernosal (Caverject, Edex) [GU Agent/Prostaglandin] Uses: *Erectile dysfunction* Action: Relaxes smooth muscles, dilates cavernosal arteries, ↑ lacunar spaces and blood entrapment Dose: 2.5–60 µg intracavernosal; titrate in office Caution: [X, –] Contra: ↑ Risk of priapism (eg, sickle cell); penile deformities/implants; men in whom sexual activity inadvisable Disp: Caverject: 5, 10, 20, 40 µg powder for inj vials ± diluent syringes 10, 20, 40 µg amp. Caverject impulse: Self-contained syringe (29 gauge) 10 & 20 µg. Edex: 10, 20, 40 µg cartridges SE: Local pain w/ inj Interactions: ↑ Effects OF anticoagulants & antihypertensives, ↓ effects OF cyclosporine Labs: ↓ Fibrinogen NIPE: Vaginal itching and burning in female partners, ⊘ inj >3 ×/wk or closer than 24 h/dose; Counsel about priapism, penile fibrosis, hematoma risks, titrate dose in office

Alprostadil, Urethral Suppository (Muse) [GU Agent/Prostaglandin] Uses: *Erectile dysfunction* Action: Urethral absorption; vasodilator, relaxes smooth muscle of corpus cavernosa Dose: 125–1000 µg system 5–10 min prior to sexual activity; may repeat ×1/24 hr; titrate in office Caution: [X, –] Contra: ↑ priapism risk (eg, sickle cell) penile deformities/implants; men in whom sexual activity inadvisable Disp: 125, 250, 500, 1000 µg w/ transurethral delivery system SE: ↓ BP, dizziness, syncope, penile/testicular pain, urethral burning/bleeding, priapism Interactions: ↑ Effects OF anticoagulants & antihypertensives, ↓ effects OF cyclosporine Labs: ↓ Fibrinogen NIPE: No more than 2 supp/24 h, urinate prior to use; titrate dose in office

Alteplase, Recombinant [tPA] (Activase) [Plasminogen Activator/Thrombolytic Enzyme] Uses: *AMI, PE, acute ischemic stroke, & CV cath occlusion* Action: Thrombolytic; binds fibrin in thrombus, initiates fibrinolysis Dose: AMI: 15 mg IV over 1–2 min, then 0.75 mg/kg (max 50 mg) over 30 min, then 0.5 mg/kg over next 60 min (max 35 mg)(ECC 2005) Stroke: 0.09 mg/kg IV over 1 min, then 0.81 mg/kg; max 90 mg) inf over 60 min (ECC 2005) Cath occlusion: 10–29 mg 1 mg/mL; ≥30 mg 2 mg/mL Caution: [C, ?] Contra: Active internal bleeding; uncontrolled HTN (SBP=>185 mm Hg/DBP=>110 mm Hg); recent (w/in 3 mo) CVA, GI bleed, trauma; intracranial or intraspinal surgery or Dz (AVM/aneurysm/subarachnoid hemorrhage); prolonged cardiac massage); intracranial neoplasm; suspected aortic dissection; bleeding/hemostatic defects, Sz at the time of stroke Disp: Powder for inj 2, 50, 100 mg SE: Bleeding, bruising (eg, venipuncture sites), ↓ BP Interactions: ↑ Risk of bleeding W/ heparin, ASA, NSAIDs, abciximab, dipyridamole, eptifibatide, tirofiban; ↓ effects W/ nitroglycerine Labs: ↓ Fibrinogen, monitor PT/PTT NIPE: Compress venipuncture site at least 30 min, bed rest during inf; give heparin to prevent reocclusion; in AMI, doses of >150 mg associated w/ intracranial bleeding

Altretamine (Hexalen) [Antineoplastic/Alkylating Agent] WARNING: BM suppression, neurotox common Uses: *Epithelial ovarian CA* Action: Unknown; cytotoxic agent, unknown alkylating agent; ↓ nucleotide incorporation into DNA/RNA Dose: 260 mg/m²/d in 4 ÷ doses for 14–21 d of a 28-d Rx cycle;

dose ↑ to 150 mg/m²/d for 14 d in multiagent regimens (per protocols); after meals and at bedtime **Caution:** [D, ?/–]. **Contra:** Preexisting BM depression or neurologic tox **Disp:** Caps 50 mg **SE:** V/D, cramps; neurologic (peripheral neuropathy, CNS depression); minimally myelosuppressive **Interactions:** ↓ Effect W/ phenobarbital, ↓ antibody response W/ live vaccines, ↑ risk of tox W/ cimetidine & hypotension W/ MAOIs, ↑ BM depression W/ radiation **Labs:** Monitor CBC, ↑ alkaline phosphatase, BUN, SCr **NIPE:** Use barrier contraception, take w/ food, routine neuro exams

Aluminum Hydroxide (Amphojel, AlternaGEL) [OTC] [Antacid/Aluminum Salt] Uses: *Relief of heartburn, upset or sour stomach, or acid indigestion*; supl to Rx of hyperphosphatemia **Action:** Neutralizes gastric acid; binds PO_4^{-2} **Dose:** *Adults.* 10–30 mL or 300–1200 mg PO q4–6h. *Peds.* 5–15 mL PO q4–6h or 50–150 mg/kg/24 h PO ÷ q4–6h (hyperphosphatemia) **Caution:** [C, ?] **Disp:** Tabs 300, 600 mg; susp 320, 600 mg/5 mL **SE:** Constipation **Interactions:** ↓ Absorption & effects OF allopurinol, benzodiazepines, corticosteroids, chloroquine, cimetidine, digoxin, INH, phenytoin, quinolones, ranitidine, tetracycline **Labs:** ↑ Serum gastrin, ↓ serum phosphate **NIPE:** Separate other drug administration by 2 h, ↑ effectiveness if liquid form; OK in renal failure

Aluminum Hydroxide + Magnesium Carbonate (Gaviscon Extra Strength, Liquid) [OTC] [Antacid/Aluminum & Magnesium Salts] Uses: *Relief of heartburn, acid indigestion* **Action:** Neutralizes gastric acid **Dose:** *Adults.* 15–30 mL PO pc & hs. *Peds.* 5–15 mL PO qid or PRN; avoid in renal impair **Caution:** ↑ Mg²⁺ (w/ renal insuff) [C, ?] **Disp:** Liq w/ AlOH 95 mg/ MgCO₃ 358 mg/15 mL; Extra strength Liq AlOH 254 mg/Mg carbonate 237 mg/15mL; chew tabs AlOH 160 mg/MgCO₃ 105 mg **SE:** Constipation, D **Interactions:** In addition to AlOH ↓ effects OF histamine blockers, hydantoins, nitrofurantoin, phenothiazines, ticlopidine, ↑ effects OF quinidine, sulfonylureas **NIPE:** ↑ fiber; qid doses best given pc & hs; may affect absorption of some drugs, take 2–3 h apart to ↓ effect

Aluminum Hydroxide + Magnesium Hydroxide (Maalox) [OTC] [Antacid/Aluminum & Magnesium Salts] Uses: *Hyperacidity* (peptic ulcer, hiatal hernia, etc) **Action:** Neutralizes gastric acid **Dose:** *Adults.* 10–20 mL or 2–4 tabs PO qid or PRN. *Peds.* 5–15 mL PO qid or PRN **Caution:** [C, ?] **Disp:** Tabs, susp **SE:** May cause ↑ Mg²⁺ in renal insuff, constipation, D **Interactions:** In addition to AlOH, ↓ effects OF digoxin, quinolones, phenytoin, Fe supl, & ketoconazole **NIPE:** ⊘ Concurrent drug use; separate by 2 h; doses qid best given pc & hs

Aluminum Hydroxide + Magnesium Hydroxide & Simethicone (Mylanta, Mylanta II, Maalox Plus) [OTC] [Antacid/Aluminum & Magnesium Salts] Uses: *Hyperacidity w/ bloating* **Action:** Neutralizes gastric acid & defoaming **Dose:** *Adults.* 10–20 mL or 2–4 tabs PO qid or PRN *Peds.* 5–15 mL PO qid or PRN; avoid in renal impair

Caution: [C, ?] **Disp:** Tabs, susp, Liq **SE:** ↑ Mg^{2+} in renal insuff, D, constipation **Interactions:** In addition to AlOH, ↓ effects *OF* digoxin, quinolones, phenytoin, Fe supl, and ketoconazole **NIPE:** ⊘ Concurrent drug use; separate by 2 h; Mylanta II contains 2 × AlOH & MgOH of Mylanta

Aluminum Hydroxide + Magnesium Trisilicate (Gaviscon, Regular Strength) [OTC] [Antacid/Aluminum & Magnesium Salts] **Uses:** *Relief of heartburn, upset or sour stomach, or acid indigestion* **Action:** Neutralizes gastric acid **Dose:** Chew 2–4 tabs qid; avoid in renal impair **Caution:** [C, ?] **Contra:** Mg^{2+}, sensitivity **Disp:** AlOH 80 mg/Mg trisilicate 20 mg/tab **SE:** ↑ Mg^{2+} in renal insuff, constipation, D **Interactions:** In addition to AlOH, ↓ effects *OF* digoxin, quinolones, phenytoin, Fe supl, & ketoconazole **NIPE:** ⊘ Concurrent drug use; separate by 2 h

Amantadine (Symmetrel) [Antiviral, Antiparkinsonian/ AntiCholinergic-Like Medium] **Uses:** *Rx or prophylaxis influenza A, parkinsonism, & drug-induced EPS* (Note: Do not use for Influenza A in the US—increased resistance.) **Action:** Prevents release of infectious viral nucleic acid into host cell; releases dopamine from intact dopaminergic terminals **Dose:** *Adults. Influenza A:* 200 mg/d PO or 100 mg PO bid. *Parkinsonism:* 100 mg PO daily-bid. *Peds. 1–9 y:* 4.4–8.8 mg/kg/24 h to 150 mg/24 h max ÷ doses daily-bid. *10–12 y:* 100–200 mg/d in 1–2 ÷ doses; ↓ in renal impair **Caution:** [C, M] **Disp:** Caps 100 mg; tabs 100 mg; soln 50 mg/5 mL **SE:** Orthostatic ↓ BP, edema, insomnia, depression, irritability, hallucinations, dream abnormalities; **Interactions:** ↑ Effects *W/* HCTZ, triamterene, amiloride, pheasant's eye herb, scopolia root, benztropine **Labs:** ↑ BUN, SCr, CPK, alkaline phosphatase, bilirubin, LDH, AST, ALT **NIPE:** ⊘ Discontinue abruptly, take at least 4 h before sleep if insomnia occurs, eval for mental status changes, take w/ meals, ⊘ EtOH

Amifostine (Ethyol) [Antineoplastic/Thiophosphate Cytoprotective] **Uses:** *Xerostomia prophylaxis during RT (head, neck, ovarian, non–small-cell lung CA); ↓ renal tox w/ repeated cisplatin* **Action:** Prodrug, dephosphorylated by alkaline phosphatase to active thiol metabolite **Dose:** 910 mg/m²/d 15-min IV inf 30 min prior to chemo **Caution:** [C, +/–] CV disease **Disp:** 500-mg vials powder, reconstitute in NS **SE:** Transient ↓ BP (>60%), N/V, flushing w/ hot or cold chills, dizziness, ↓ Ca^{2+}, somnolence, sneezing **Notes:** Does not ↓ effectiveness of cyclophosphamide + cisplatin chemo **Interactions:** ↑ Effects *W/* antihypertensives **Labs:** ↓ Ca levels **NIPE:** Monitor BP, ensure adequate hydration, infuse over 15 min w/ pt supine

Amikacin (Amikin) [Antibiotic/Aminoglycoside] **Uses:** *Serious gram(-) bacterial Infxns* & mycobacteria **Action:** Aminoglycoside; ↓ protein synth *Spectrum:* Good gram(–) bacterial coverage: *Pseudomonas* & *Mycobacterium* sp **Dose:** *Adults & Peds. Conventional:* 5–7.5 mg/kg/dose q8h; once daily; 15–20 mg/kg q24h; ↑ interval w/ renal impair. *Neonates <1200 g, 0–4 wk:* 7.5 mg/kg/dose q12–18h. *Postnatal age <7 d, 1200–2000 g:* 7.5 mg/kg/dose q12h;

>*2000 g:* 10 mg/kg/dose q12h. *Postnatal age >7 d, 1200–2000 g:* 7 mg/kg/dose q8h; *>2000 g:* 7.5–10 mg/kg/dose q8h **Caution:** [C, +/–] Avoid w/ diuretics **Disp:** 50 mg/mL, 250 mg/mL **SE:** Nephro/oto/neurotox, neuromuscular blockage, resp paralysis **Notes:** May be effective in gram(-) bacteria resistant to gent & tobra; follow Cr; *Levels: Peak* 30 min after inf; *Trough* <0.5h before next dose; *Therapeutic: Peak* 20–30 µg/mL, *Trough* <8 µg/mL; *Toxic Peak* >35 µg/mL; *1/2 life:* 2 h **Interactions:** ↑ Risk *OF* ototox and nephrotox *W/* acyclovir, amphotericin B, cephalosporins, cisplatin, loop diuretics, methoxyflurane, polymyxin B, vancomycin; ↑ neuromuscular blocking effect *W/* muscle relaxants & anesthetics **Labs:** ↑ BUN, SCr, AST, ALT, serum alkaline phosphatase, bilirubin, LDH **NIPE:** ↑ Fluid consumption.

Amiloride (Midamor) [Potassium Sparing Diuretic] Uses: *HTN, CHF, & thiazide-induced ↓ K^+* **Action:** K^+-sparing diuretic; interferes w/ K^+/Na^+ exchange in distal tubule **Dose:** *Adults.* 5–10 mg PO daily **Peds.** 0.625 mg/kg/d; ↓ in renal impair **Caution:** [B, ?] **Contra:** ↑ K^+, SCr >1.5, BUN >30, diabetic neuropathy **Disp:** Tabs 5 mg **SE:** ↑ K^+; HA, dizziness, dehydration, impotence **Interactions:** ↑ Risk of hyperkalemia *W/* ACE-I, K-sparing diuretics, NSAIDs, & K salt substitutes; ↑ effects *OF* Li, digoxin, antihypertensives, amantadine; ↑ risk of hypokalemia *W/* licorice **Labs:** monitor K^+ **NIPE:** Take w/ food, I&O, daily wt, ⊘ salt substitutes, bananas, oranges

Aminocaproic Acid (Amicar) [Antithrombotic Agent/ Carboxylic acid derivative] Uses: *Excessive bleeding from systemic hyperfibrinolysis & urinary fibrinolysis* **Action:** ↓ Fibrinolysis; via inhibition of TPA substances **Dose:** *Adults.* 5 g IV or PO (1st h) followed by 1–1.25 g/h IV or PO (max dose/d: 30 g) **Peds.** 100 mg/kg IV (1st h) then 1 g/m²/h; max 18 g/m²/d; ↓ in renal failure **Caution:** [C, ?] Upper urinary tract bleeding **Contra:** DIC **Disp:** Tabs 500, syrup 250 mg/mL, inj 250 mg/mL **SE:** ↓ BP, bradycardia, dizziness, HA, fatigue, rash, GI disturbance, ↓ plt Fxn **Notes:** Administer × 8 h or until bleeding controlled; not for upper urinary tract bleeding **Interactions:** ↑ Coagulation *W/* estrogens & OCP **Labs:** ↑ K^+ levels, false ↑ urine amino acids **NIPE:** Creatine kinase monitoring w/ long-term use, eval for thrombophlebitis & difficulty urinating

Amino-Cerv pH 5.5 Cream [Cervical Hydrating Agent] Uses: *Mild cervicitis*, postpartum cervicitis/cervical tears, postcauterization, postcryosurgery, postconization **Action:** Hydrating agent; removes excess keratin in hyperkeratotic conditions **Dose:** 1 Applicatorle intravag hs × 2–4 wk **Caution:** [C, ?] w/ viral skin Infxn **Disp:** Vaginal cream **SE:** Stinging, local irritation **NIPE:** AKA carbamide or urea; contains 8.34% urea, 0.5% sodium propionate, 0.83% methionine, 0.35% cystine, 0.83% inositol, benzalkonium chloride

Aminoglutethimide (Cytadren) [Adrenal Steroid Inhibitor] Uses: *Cushing synd* adrenocortical carcinoma, breast CA & CAP **Action:** ↓ Adrenal steroidogenesis & conversion of androgens to estrogens; aromatase inhibitor **Dose:** Initial 250 mg PO 4 × d, titrate q1–2wks max 2 g/d; w/ hydrocortisone

20–40 mg/d; ↓ in renal insuff **Caution:** [D, ?] **Disp:** Tabs 250 mg **SE:** Adrenal insuff ("medical adrenalectomy"), hypothyroidism, masculinization, ↓ BP, V, rare hepatotox, rash, myalgia, fever **Interactions:** ↓ Effects *W/* dexamethasone & hydrocortisone, ↓ effects *OF* warfarin, theophylline, medroxyprogesterone **NIPE:** Masculinization reversible after D/C drug, ⊘ PRG

Aminophylline [Bronchodilator/Xanthine Derivative] Uses:
Asthma, COPD & bronchospasm **Action:** Relaxes smooth muscle (bronchi, pulm vessels); stimulates diaphragm **Dose: Adults.** *Acute asthma:* Load 6 mg/kg IV, then 0.4–0.9 mg/kg/h IV cont inf. *Chronic asthma:* 24 mg/kg/24 h PO ÷ q6h. **Peds.** Load 6 mg/kg IV, then 1 mg/kg/h IV cont inf; ↓ in hepatic insuff & w/ certain drugs (macrolide & quinolone antibiotics, cimetidine, & propranolol) **Caution:** [C, +] Uncontrolled arrhythmias, HTN, Sz disorder, hyperthyroidism, peptic ulcers **Disp:** Tabs 100, 200 mg; PR tabs 100, 200 mg, soln 105 mg/5 mL, inj 25 mg/mL **SE:** N/V, irritability, tachycardia, ventricular arrhythmias, Szs **Notes:** Individualize dosage; Level 10–20 µg/mL, tox >20 µg/mL; aminophylline 85% theophylline; erratic rectal absorption **Interactions:** ↓ Effects *OF* Li, phenytoin, adenosine; ↓ effects *W/* phenobarbital, aminoglutethamide, barbiturates, rifampin, ritonavir, thyroid meds; ↑ effects *W/* cimetidine, ciprofloxacin, erythromycin, INH, OCP, verapamil, tobacco, charcoal-broiled foods, St. John's Wort **Labs:** ↑ Uric acid levels, falsely ↑ levels *W/* furosemide, probenecid, acetaminophen, coffee, tea, cola, chocolate **NIPE:** ⊘ Chew or crush time-released caps & take on empty stomach, immediate release can be taken w/ food, ↑ fluids 2 L/d, tobacco ↑ drug elimination

Amiodarone (Cordarone, Pacerone) [Ventricular Antiarrhythmic/Adrenergic Blocker] Uses:
Recurrent VF or hemodynamically unstable VT, supraventricular arrhythmias, AF **Action:** Class III antiarrhythmic (Table 10) **Dose: Adults.** *Ventricular arrhythmias: IV:* 15 mg/min for 10 min, then 1 mg/min ×6 h, maint 0.5 mg/min cont inf or *PO: Load:* 800–1600 mg/d PO ×1–3 wk. *Maint:* 600–800 mg/d PO for 1 mo, then 200–400 mg/d. *Supraventricular arrhythmias: IV:* 300 mg IV over 1 h, then 20 mg/kg for 24 h, then 600 mg PO daily for 1 wk, maint 100–400 mg daily or *PO: Load:* 600–800 mg/d PO for 1–4 wk. *Maint:* Slow ↓ to 100–400 mg daily *(ECC 2005). Cardiac arrest:* 300 mg IV push; 150 mg IV push 3–5 min PRN. *Refractory pulseless VT, VF:* 5 mg/kg rapid IV bolus. *Perfusing arrhythmias: Load:* 5 mg/kg IV/IO over 20–60 min (repeat, max 15 mg/kg). **Peds.** 10–15 mg/kg/24 h ÷ q12h PO for 7–10 d, then 5 mg/kg/24 h ÷ q12h or daily (infants/neonates require ↑ loading); ↓ w/ liver insuff **Caution:** [D, –] **Contra:** Sinus node dysfunction, 2nd-/3rd-degree AV block, sinus bradycardia (w/o pacemaker), iodine sensitivity **Disp:** Tabs 100, 200, 300, 400 mg; inj 50 mg/mL **SE:** Pulm fibrosis, exacerbation of arrhythmias, prolongs QT interval; CHF, hypo/hyperthyroidism, liver failure, corneal microdeposits, optic neuropathy/ neuritis, peripheral neuropathy, photosens **Notes:** IV conc of >0.2 mg/mL via a central catheter; *Levels: Trough:* Just before next dose *Therapeutic:* 1–2.5 µg/mL; *Toxic:* >2.5 µg/mL; *1/2 life:* 30–100 h **Interactions:** ↑ Serum levels *OF* digoxin,

quinidine, procainamide, flecainide, phenytoin, warfarin, theophylline, cyclosporine; ↑ levels W/ cimetidine, indinavir, ritonavir; ↓ levels W/ cholestyramine, rifampin, St. John's Wort; ↑ cardiac effects W/ BBs, CCB **Labs:** ↑ LFTs, ↑ T_4 & RT_3, ANA titer, ↓ T_3 **NIPE:** Monitor cardiac rhythm, BP, LFTs, thyroid Fxn, ophthalmologic exam; ↑ photosensitivity—use sunscreen; take w/ food

Amitriptyline (Elavil) [Antidepressant/TCA] **WARNING:** Antidepressants may ↑ suicide risk; consider risks/benefits of use. Monitor patients closely **Uses:** *Depression*; peripheral neuropathy, chronic pain, tension HAs **Action:** TCA; ↓ reuptake of serotonin & norepinephrine by presynaptic neurons **Dose: Adults.** Initial, 30–50 mg PO hs; may ↑ to 300 mg hs. **Peds.** Not OK <12 y unless for chronic pain; initial 0.1 mg/kg PO hs, ↑ over 2–3 wk to 0.5–2 mg/kg PO hs; taper to D/C **Caution:** [D,+/–] CV Dz, seizures, NAG, hepatic impair **Contra:** w/ MAOIs, during acute MI recovery **Disp:** Tabs 10, 25, 50, 75, 100, 150 mg; inj 10 mg/mL **SE:** Strong anticholinergic SEs; OD may be fatal; urine retention, sedation, ECG changes, photosens **Notes:** *Levels: Therapeutic:* 120–150 ng/mL; *Toxic:* >500 mg/mL **Interactions:** ↓ Effects W/ carbamazepine, phenobarbital, rifampin, cholestyramine, colestipol, tobacco; ↑ effects W/ cimetidine, quinidine, indinavir, ritonavir, CNS depressants, SSRIs, haloperidol, OCPs, BBs, phenothiazines, EtOH, evening primrose oil; ↑ effects OF amphetamines, anticholinergics, epinephrine, hypoglycemics, phenylephrine **Labs:** ↑ Glucose, false ↑ carbamazepine levels **NIPE:** ↑ Photosensitivity—use sunscreen, appetite, & craving for sweets; ⊘ D/C abruptly, may turn urine blue-green

Amlodipine (Norvasc) [Antihypertensive, Antianginal/CCB] **Uses:** *HTN, stable or unstable angina* **Action:** CCB; relaxes coronary vascular smooth muscle **Dose:** 2.5–10 mg/d PO; ↓ w/ hepatic impair **Caution:** [C, ?] **Disp:** Tabs 2.5, 5, 10 mg **SE:** Peripheral edema, HA, palpitations, flushing **Interactions:** ↑ Effect OF hypotension W/ antihypertensives, fentanyl, nirates quinidine, EtOH, grapefruit juice; ↑ risk OF neurotox W/ lithium; ↓ effects W/ NSAIDs **Labs:** Monitor BUN, Cr, LFTs **NIPE:** Take w/o regard to meals

Amlodipine/Atorvastatin (Caduet) [Antianginal, Antihypertensive, Antilipemic/CCB, HMG-CoA Reductase Inhibitor] **Uses:** *HTN, chronic stable/vasospastic angina, control cholesterol & triglycerides* **Action:** CCB & HMG-CoA reductase inhibitor **Dose:** Amlodipine 2.5–10 mg w/ Atorvastatin 10–80 mg PO daily **Caution:** [X, –] **Contra:** Active liver Dz, ↑ LFT **Disp:** Tabs Amlodipine/Atorvastatin: 2.5/10, 2.5/20, 2.5/40, 5/10, 5/20, 5/40, 5/80, 10/10, 10/20, 10/40, 10/80 mg **SE:** Peripheral edema, HA, palpitations, flushing, myopathy, arthralgia, myalgia, GI upset **Interactions:** ↑ Hypotension W/ fentanyl, nitrates, EtOH, quinidine, other antihypertensives, grapefruit juice; ↑ effects W/ diltiazem, erythromycin, H_2 blockers, proton pump inhibitors, quinidine; ↓ effects W/ NSAIDs, barbiturates, rifampin **Labs:** Monitor LFTs and CPK **NIPE:** ⊘ D/C abruptly, ↑ photosensitivity—use sunscreen; rare risk of rhabdomyolysis; instruct patient to report muscle pain/weakness

Ammonium Aluminum Sulfate [Alum] [OTC] [GU Astringent]
Uses: *Hemorrhagic cystitis when saline bladder irrigation fails* Action: Astringent Dose: 1–2% soln w/ constant NS bladder irrigation Caution: [+/–] Disp: Powder for recons SE: Encephalopathy possible; can precipitate & occlude catheters Labs: Monitor aluminum levels, especially in renal insuff NIPE: Safe to use w/o anesthesia & w/ vesicoureteral reflux

Amoxicillin (Amoxil, Polymox) [Antibiotic/Aminopenicillin]
Uses: *Ear, nose, & throat, lower resp, skin, UTI from susceptible gram(+) bacteria* endocarditis prophylaxis Action: β-Lactam antibiotic; ↓ cell wall synth Spectrum: Gram(+) (Streptococcus sp, Enterococcus sp); some gram(–) (H. influenzae, E. coli, N. gonorrhoeae, H. pylori, & P. mirabilis) Dose: Adults. 250–500 mg PO tid or 500–875 mg bid. Peds. 25–100 mg/kg/24 h PO ÷ q8h. 200–400 mg PO bid (equivalent to 125–250 mg tid); ↓ in renal impair Caution: [B, +] Disp: Caps 250, 500 mg; chew tabs 125, 200, 250, 400 mg; susp 50 mg/mL, 125, 200, 250, 400 mg/5 mL; tabs 500, 875 mg SE: D; skin rash Interactions: ↑ Effects OF warfarin, ↑ effects W/ probenecid, disulfiram, ↑ risk of rash W/ allopurinol, ↓ effects OF OCP, ↓ effects W/ tetracyclines, chloramphenicol Labs: ↑ Serum alkaline phosphatase, LDH, LFTs, false + direct Coombs test NIPE: Space med over 24 h, avoid for super Infxn, use barrier contraception; cross hypersensitivity w/ PCN; many E. coli strains resistant; chew tabs contain pheylalanine

Amoxicillin & Clavulanic Acid (Augmentin, Augmentin 600 ES, Augmentin XR) [Antibiotic/Aminopenicillin, Beta-lactamase Inhibitor] Uses: *Ear, lower resp, sinus, UTI, skin Infxns caused by β-lactamase-producing H. influenzae, S. aureus, & E. coli* Action: Combo β-lactam antibiotic & β-lactamase inhibitor. Spectrum: Gram(+) same as amox alone, MSSA; gram(–) as w/ amox alone, β-lactamase-producing H. influenzae, Klebsiella sp, M. catarrhalis Dose: Adults. 250–500 mg PO q8h or 875 mg q12h; XR 2000 mg PO q12h. Peds. 20–40 mg/kg/d as amoxicillin PO ÷ q8h or 45 mg/kg/d ÷ q12h; ↓ in renal impair; take w/ food Caution: [B, enters breast milk] Disp: Supplied (as amox/clav): Tabs 250/125, 500/125, 875/125 mg; chew tabs 125/31.25, 200/28.5, 250/62.5, 400/57 mg; susp 125/31.25, 250/62.5, 200/28.5, 400/57 mg/5 mL; susp: ES 600/42.9 mg/5 mL; XR tab 1000/62.5 mg SE: Abd discomfort, N/V/D, allergic Rxn, vaginitis Notes: Do not substitute two 250-mg tabs for one 500-mg tab (OD of clavulanic acid); max clavulanic acid 125 mg/dose Interactions: ↑ Effects OF warfarin, ↑ effects W/ probenecid, disulfiram, ↑ risk of rash W/ allopurinol, ↓ effects OF OCP, ↓ effects W/ tetracyclines, chloramphenicol Labs: ↑ Serum alkaline phosphatase, LDH, LFTs, false + direct Coombs test NIPE: Space med over 24/h, eval for super Infxn, use barrier contraception

Amphotericin B (Amphocin) [Antifungal/Polyene Macrolide]
Uses: *Severe, systemic fungal Infxns; oral & cutaneous candidiasis* Action: Binds ergosterol in the fungal membrane to alter permeability Dose: Adults & Peds. Test dose: 1 mg IV adults or 0.1 mg/kg to 1 mg IV in children; then 0.25–1.5 mg/kg/24 h IV

over 2–6 h (range 25–50 mg/d or qod). Total dose varies w/ indication. *PO:* 1 mL qid **Caution:** [B, ?] **Disp:** Powder for inj 50 mg/vial **SE:** ↓ K⁺/Mg²⁺ from renal wasting; anaphylaxis reported, HA, fever, chills, nephrotox, ↓ BP, anemia, rigors **Notes:** ? ↓ In renal impair; pretreatment w/ APAP & antihistamines (Benadryl) ↓ SE **Interactions:** ↑ Nephrotoxic effects **W/** antineoplastics, cyclosporine, furosemide, vancomycin, aminoglycosides, ↑ hypokalemia **W/** corticosteroids, skeletal muscle relaxants **Labs:** Monitor Cr/LFTs/K/Mg; ↑ serum bilirubin, serum cholesterol **NIPE:** Monitor CNS effects & ⊘ take hs

Amphotericin B Cholesteryl (Amphotec) [Antifungal/Polyene Macrolide]

Uses: *Aspergillosis if intolerant/refractory to conventional amphotericin B*, systemic candidiasis **Action:** Binds cell membrane sterols, alters permeability **Dose:** *Adults & Peds.* Test dose 1.6–8.3 mg, over 15–20 min, then 3–4 mg/kg/d; 1 mg/kg/h inf; ↓ w/ renal insuff **Caution:** [B, ?] **Disp:** Powder for inj 50 mg, 100 mg/vial **SE:** Anaphylaxis; fever, chills, HA, nephrotox, ↓ BP, anemia **Notes:** Do not use in-line filter **Interactions:** See Amphotericin B **Labs:** Monitor LFTs, electrolytes; ↓ K⁺, ↓ Mg²⁺

Amphotericin B Lipid Complex (Abelcet) [Antifungal/Polyene Macrolide]

Uses: *Refractory invasive fungal Infxn in pts intolerant to conventional ampho B* **Action:** Binds cell membrane sterols, alters permeability **Dose:** *Adults & Peds.* 5 mg/kg/d IV single daily dose; 2.5 mg/kg/h inf **Caution:** [B, ?] **Disp:** Inj 5 mg/mL **SE:** Anaphylaxis; fever, chills, HA, nephrotox, ↓ BP, anemia **Notes:** Filter w/ 5-µm needle; do not mix in electrolyte-containing solns; if inf >2 h, manually mix bag **Interactions:** See Amphotericin B **Labs:** ↓ K⁺, ↓ Mg²⁺

Amphotericin B Liposomal (AmBisome) [Antifungal/Polyene Macrolide]

Uses: *Refractory invasive fungal Infxn w/ intolerance to conventional ampho B; cryptococcal meningitis in HIV; empiric for febrile neutropenia; visceral leishmaniasis* **Action:** Binds cell membrane sterols, changes membrane permeability **Dose:** *Adults & Peds.* 3–6 mg/kg/d, inf 60–120 min; **Caution:** [B, ?] **Disp:** Powder inj 50 mg **SE:** Anaphylaxis, fever, chills, HA, nephrotox, ↓ BP, anemia **Notes:** Filter w/ 1- µm filter; ? ↓ in renal insuff **Interactions:** See Amphotericin B **Labs:** ↓ K⁺, ↓ Mg²⁺

Ampicillin (Amcill, Omnipen) [Antibiotic/Aminopenicillin]

Uses: *Resp, GU, or GI tract Infxns, meningitis due to gram(-) & (+) bacteria; SBE prophylaxis* **Action:** β-Lactam antibiotic; ↓ cell wall synth. **Spectrum:** Gram(+) (*Streptococcus* sp, *Staphylococcus* sp, *Listeria* sp); gram(–) (*Klebsiella* sp, *E. coli, H. influenzae, P. mirabilis, Shigella* sp, *Salmonella* sp) **Dose:** *Adults.* 500 mg–2 g IM or IV q6h or 250–500 mg PO q6h. *Peds. Neonates <7 d:* 50–100 mg/kg/24 h IV ÷ q8h. *Term infants:* 75–150 mg/kg/24 h ÷ q6–8h IV or PO. *Children >1 mo:* 100–200 mg/kg/24 h ÷ q4–6h IM or IV; 50–100 mg/kg/24 h ÷ q6h PO up to 250 mg/dose. *Meningitis:* 200–400 mg/kg/24 h ÷ q4–6h IV; ↓ in renal impair; take on empty stomach **Caution:** [B, M] Cross hypersensitivity w/ PCN **Disp:** Caps 250, 500 mg; susp 100 mg/5 mL (reconstituted drops); 125 mg/5 mL,

250 mg/5 mL; powder for inj 125 mg, 250 mg, 500 mg, 1 g, 2 g, 10 g/vial **SE:** D, skin rash, allergic Rxn **Notes:** Many *E. coli* strains resistant **Interactions:** ↓ Effects *OF* OCP & atenolol, ↓ effects *W/* chloramphenicol, erythromycin, tetracycline, & food; ↑ effects *OF* anticoagulants & MTX; ↑ risk of rash *W/* allopurinal; ↑ effects *W/* probenecid & disulfiram **Labs:** ↑ LFTs, serum protein, serum theophylline, serum uric acid; ↓ serum estrogen, serum cholesterol, serum folate; false + direct Coombs test, urine glucose, & urine amino acids **NIPE:** Take on empty stomach & around the clock; may cause candidal vaginitis; use barrier contraception

Ampicillin-Sulbactam (Unasyn) [Antibiotic/Aminopenicillin & Beta-Lactamase Inhibitor]

Uses: *Gynecologic, intra-abd, skin Infxns due to β-lactamase-producing *S. aureus*, *Enterococcus* sp, *H. influenzae*, *P. mirabilis*, & *Bacteroides* sp* **Action:** β-lactam antibiotic & β-lactamase inhibitor. **Spectrum:** Gram(+) & (−) as for amp alone; also *Enterobacter*, *Acinetobacter*, *Bacteroides* **Dose:** *Adults.* 1.5–3 g IM or IV q6h. *Peds.* 100–200 mg ampicillin/kg/d (150–300 mg Unasyn) q6h; ↓ w/ renal insuff **Caution:** [B, M] **Disp:** Powder for inj 1.5, 3 g/vial, 15 g bulk package **SE:** Allergic Rxns, rash, D, inj site pain **Notes:** A 2:1 ratio Ampicillin:Sulbactam **Interactions:** See Ampicillin

Amprenavir (Agenerase) [Antiviral/HIV Protease Inhibitor]

WARNING: PO soln contra in children <4 y, Asians, Eskimos, Native Americans (polypropylene glycol tox) **Uses:** *HIV Infxn* **Action:** Protease inhibitor; prevents virion maturation **Dose:** *Adults.* 1200 mg bid. *Peds.* 20 mg/kg bid or 15 mg/kg tid to 2400 mg/d; ↓ w/ hepatic insuff **Caution:** [C, ?] CDC recommends HIV-infected mothers not to breast-feed; h/o sulfonamide allergy **Contra:** *E. coli*–derived proteins allergy, acute Infxn, <18 y **Disp:** Caps 50, 150 mg; soln 15 mg/mL **SE:** Life-threatening rash, hyperglycemia, hypertriglyceridemia, fat redistribution, N/V/D, depression **Notes:** Caps & soln unequal contain vitamin E > RDA; **Interactions:** ↑ Effects *W/* abacavir, cimetidine, delavirdine, indinavir, itraconazole, ketoconazole, macrolides, ritonavir, zidovudine, grapefruit juice; ↑ effects *OF* cisapride, clozapine, ergotamine, loratadine, nelfinavir, dapsone, pimozide, rifabutin, saquinavir, sildenafil, terfenadine, triazolam, warfarin, zidovudine, HMG-CoA reductase inhibitors; ↓ effects *W/* antacids, barbiturates, carbamazepine, nevirapine, phenytoin, rifampin, St. John's Wort, high-fat food; ↓ effects *OF* OCP **Labs:** ↑ Serum glucose, cholesterol, & triglyceride levels **NIPE:** Use barrier contraception, may take w/ food other than high-fat food, ⊘ take vitamin E

Anakinra (Kineret) [Antirheumatic/Immunomodulator]

WARNING: Associated w/ ↑ incidence of serious Infxn; D/C w/ serious Infxn **Uses:** *Reduce S/Sxs of moderate/severe active RA, failed 1 or more DMARD* **Action:** Human IL-1 receptor antagonist **Dose:** 100 mg SQ daily; w/ CrCl <30 mL/min, QOD **Caution:** [B, ?] **Contra:** *E. coli*–derived proteins allergy, active Infxn, <18 y **Disp:** 100-mg prefilled syringes; 100 mg (0.67 mL/vial) **SE:** Neutropenia especially w/ TNF-blocking agents, inj site Rxn, Infxn **Interactions:** ↓ Effects

OF immunizations; ↑ risk of Infxns if combined W/ TNF-blocking drugs **Labs:** ↓ WBCs, plts, absolute neutrophil count **NIPE:** Store drug in refrigerator, ⊘ light exposure, & discard unused portion; ⊘ use soln if discolored or has particulate matter

Anastrozole (Arimidex) [Antineoplastic/Nonsteroidal Aromatase Inhibitor] Uses: *Breast CA: postmenopausal w/ met breast CA, adjuvant Rx postmenopausal early hormone-receptor(+) breast CA* **Action:** Selective nonsteroidal aromatase inhibitor, ↓ circ estradiol **Dose:** 1 mg/d **Caution:** [D, ?] **Contra:** PRG **Disp:** Tabs 1 mg **SE:** D, HTN, flushing, ↑ bone/tumor pain, HA, somnolence **Interactions:** None noted **Labs:** ↑ GTT, LFTs, alkaline phosphatase, total & LDL cholesterol; No effect on adrenal corticosteroids or aldosterone **NIPE:** May ↓ fertility & cause fetal damage, eval for pain & administer adequate analgesia, may cause vaginal bleeding first few weeks

Anidulafungin (Eraxis) [Antifungal/Echinocandin] Uses: *Candidemia, esophageal candidiasis, other Candida sp Infxn (peritonitis, intraabd abscess)* **Action:** Echinocandin; ↓ cell wall synth. *Spectrum: C. albicans, C. glabrata, C. parapsilosis, C. tropicalis* **Dose:** *Candidemia, others:* 200 mg IV × 1, then 100 mg IV daily (Tx 14 d after last + culture); *Esophageal candidiasis:* 100 mg IV × 1, then 50 mg IV daily (Tx >14 d and 7 d after resoln of Sx); 1.1 mg/min max inf rate **Caution:** [C, ?/–] **Contra:** Echinocandin hypersensitivity **Disp:** Powder 50 mg/vial, 100 mg/vial **SE:** Generally safe, histamine-mediated inf Rxns (urticaria, flushing, ↓ BP, dyspnea, etc), fever, N/V/D, HA, hepatitis, worsening hepatic failure **Labs:** ↑ LFTs, ↓ K+ **NIPE:** ↓ Inf rate to <1.1 mg/min w/ inf Rxns

Anistreplase (Eminase) [Antithrombotic Agent/Plasminogen Activator] Uses: *AMI* **Action:** Thrombolytic; activates conversion of plasminogen to plasmin, ↑ thrombolysis **Dose:** 30 units IV over 2–5 min *(ECC 2005)* **Caution:** [C, ?] **Contra:** Active internal bleeding, h/o CVA, recent (<2 mo) intracranial or intraspinal surgery/trauma/neoplasm, AVM, aneurysm, bleeding diathesis, severe HTN **Disp:** 30 units/vial **SE:** Bleeding, ↓ BP, hematoma **Notes:** Ineffective if readministered >5 d after the previous dose of anistreplase or streptokinase, or streptococcal Infxn (production of antistreptokinase Ab) **Interactions:** ↑ Risk of hemorrhage W/ warfarin, oral anticoagulants, ASA, NSAIDs, dipyridamole; ↓ effectiveness W/ aminocaproic acid **Labs:** ↓ Plasminogen & fibrinogen, ↑ transaminase level, thrombin time, aPTT & PT **NIPE:** Store powder in refrigerator & use w/in 30 min of reconstitution, initiate therapy ASAP after MI, monitor S/Sxs internal bleeding

Anthralin (Anthra-Derm) [Keratolytic Dermatologic Agent] Uses: *Psoriasis* **Action:** Keratolytic **Dose:** Apply daily **Caution:** [C, ?] **Contra:** Acutely inflamed psoriatic eruptions, erythroderma **Disp:** Cream, oint 0.1, 0.25, 0.4, 0.5, 1% **SE:** Irritation; hair/fingernails/skin discoloration **Interactions:** ↑ Tox if used immediately after long-term topical corticosteroid therapy **NIPE:** May stain fabric; external use only; ⊘ sunlight-medicated areas

Antihemophilic Factor [AHF, Factor VIII] (Monoclate) [Anti-hemophilic] Uses: *Classic hemophilia A, von Willebrand Dz* Action: Provides factor VIII needed to convert prothrombin to thrombin Dose: *Adults & Peds.* 1 AHF unit/kg ↑ factor VIII level @2%, units required = (kg) (desired factor VIII ↑ as % nl) × (0.5); Prevent spontaneous hemorrhage = 5% nl; Hemostasis after trauma/surgery = 30% nl; Head injuries, major surgery, or bleeding = 80–100% nl Caution: [C, ?] Disp: ✓ Each vial for units contained, powder for recons SE: Rash, fever, HA, chills, N/V Notes: Determine % nl factor VIII before dosing Interactions: None Labs: Monitor CBC & direct Coombs test NIPE: ⊘ ASA, immunize against Hep B, DC if tachycardic

Antithymocyte Globulin (See Lymphocyte Immune Globulin,) [Immunosuppressive Agent]

Apomorphine (Apokyn) [Antiparkinsonian/Dopamine Agonist] WARNING: Do not administer IV Uses: *Acute, intermittent hypomobility ("off") episodes of Parkinson Dz* Action: Dopamine agonist Dose: *Adults.* 0.2-mL SQ test dose under medical supervision; if BP OK, initial 0.2 mL (2 mg) SQ during "off" periods; only 1 dose per "off" period; titrate dose; 0.6 mL (6 mg) max single doses; use w/ antiemetic; ↓ in renal impair Caution: [C, +/–] Avoid EtOH; antihypertensives, vasodilators, cardio or cerebrovascular Dz, hepatic impair Contra: 5HT3 antagonists, sulfite allergy Disp: Inj 10 mg/mL, 3-mL pen cartridges; 2-mL amp SE: Emesis, syncope, QT prolongation, orthostatic ↓ BP, somnolence, ischemia, injection site Rxn, abuse potential, dyskinesia, fibrotic conditions, priapism Interactions:↑ Risk of hypotension W/ alosetron, dolasetron, granisetron, ondansetron, palonosetron Labs: ECG—monitor for prolongation of QT interval NIPE: Daytime somnolence may limit activities; trimethobenzamide 300 mg tid PO or other non–5HT3 antagonist antiemetic given 3 d prior to & up to 2 mo following initiation

Apraclonidine (Iopidine) [Glaucoma Agent/Alpha-Adrenergic Agonist] Uses: *Glaucoma, postop intraocular HTN* Action: α_2-Adrenergic agonist Dose: 1–2 gtt of 0.5% tid; 1 gtt before and after surgical procedure Caution: [C, ?] Contra: w/ MAOI Disp: 0.5, 1% soln SE: Ocular irritation, lethargy, xerostomia Interactions: ↓ Intraocular pressure W/ pilocarpine or topical BBs NIPE: Monitor CV status of pts w/ CAD, potential for dizziness

Aprepitant (Emend) [Centrally Acting Antiemetic] Uses *Prevents N/V assoc w/ emetogenic CA chemo (eg, cisplatin) (use in combo w/ other antiemetics)* Action: Substance P/neurokinin 1(NK_1) receptor antagonist Dose: 125 mg PO day 1, 1 h before chemo, then 80 mg PO q AM days 2 & 3 Caution: [B, ?/–]; substrate & mod CYP3A4 inhibitor; CYP2C9 inducer (Table 11) Contra: Use w/ pimozide, Disp: Caps 40, 80, 125 mg SE: Fatigue, asthenia, hiccups Interactions: ↑ Effects W/ clarithromycin, diltiazem, itraconazole, ketoconazole, nefazodone, nelfinavir, ritonavir, troleandomycin; ↑ effects OF alprazolam, astemizole, cisapride, dexamethasone, methylprednisolone, midazolam, pimozide, terfenadine, triazolam & chemotherapeutic agents, eg, docetaxel, etoposide, ifosfamide, imatinib, irinotecan, paclitaxel, vinblastine, vincristine, vinorelbine; ↓ effects W/ paroxetine, rifampin; ↓ effects OF OCPs, paroxetine, phenytoin, tolbutamide, warfarin **Labs:** ↑ ALT, AST, BUN, alkaline phosphatase, leukocytes **NIPE:** Use barrier contraception, take w/o regard to food

Aprotinin (Trasylol) [Antithrombotic Agent/Protease Inhibitor]
WARNING: May cause fatal anaphylactic Rxns **Uses:** *↓ Loss during CABG* **Action:** Protease inhib, antifibrinolytic **Dose:** 1-mL IV test dose; *High dose:* 2 million KIU load, 2 million KIU to prime pump, then 500,000 KIU/h until surgery ends; *Low dose:* 1 million KIU load, 1 million KIU to prime pump, then 250,000 KIU/h until surgery ends; 7 million KIU max total **Caution:** [B, ?] Thromboembolic Dz requiring anticoagulants/blood factor administration **Contra:** Previous use <12 mo (↑ anaphylactic risk) **Disp:** Inj 1.4 mg/mL (10,000 KIU/mL) **SE:** AF, MI, CHF, dyspnea, **Notes:** 1000/KIU = 0.14 mg aprotinin **Interactions:** ↑ Clotting time W/ heparin, ↓ effects OF fibrinolytics, captopril **Labs:** Monitor aPTT, ACT, CBC, BUN, Cr; postop ↑ Cr **NIPE:** Monitor cardiac and pulmonary status during inf

Arformoterol (Brovana) [Long acting Beta 2 agonist]
WARNING: Long-acting β-2 agonists may ↑ risk of asthma related death **Uses:** *COPD maint* **Action:** LA β-2 agonist, relaxes airway smooth muscles **Dose:** 15 µg neb bid, 30 µg/d max **Caution:** [C, ?] w/ CV disease, ↓ **Contra:** Not for acute asthma; component hypersensitivity; peds; w/ phenothiazines **Disp:** 15 µg/2 mL nebulizer **SE:** chest/back pain, D, sinusitis, leg cramps, dyspnea, rash, flu-synd, ↑ BP, arrhythmias, heart block ↓K⁺

Argatroban (Acova) [Anticoagulant/Thrombin inhibitor]
Uses: *Prevent/Tx thrombosis in HIT, PCI in pts w/ risk of HIT* **Action:** Anticoagulant, direct thrombin inhibitor **Dose:** 2 µg/kg/min IV; adjust until aPTT 1.5–3 × baseline not to exceed 100 s; 10 µg/kg/min max; ↓ w/ hepatic impair **Caution:** [B, ?] Avoid PO anticoagulants, ↑ bleeding risk; avoid use w/ thrombolytics **Contra:** Overt major bleed **Disp:** Inj 100 mg/mL **SE:** AF, cardiac arrest, cerebrovascular disorder, ↓ BP, VT, N/V/D, sepsis, cough, renal tox, **Note:** Steady state in 1–3 h **Interactions:** ↑ Risk of bleeding W/ anticoagulants, feverfew, garlic, ginger, ginkgo, ↑ risk of intracranial bleed W/ thrombolytics **Labs:** ↑ aPTT, PT, INR, ACT, thrombin time; ↓ Hgb **NIPE:** Report ↑ bruising & bleeding, ⊘ breast-feed

Aripiprazole (Abilify) [Antipsychotic/Psychotropic] **WARNING:** Increased mortality in elderly with dementia-related psychosis **Uses:** *Schizophrenia* **Action:** Dopamine & serotonin antagonist **Dose:** Adults. 10–15 mg PO daily; 5.25–15 mg for acute agitation ↓ dose W/ CYP3A4/CYP2D6 inhibitors (Table 11); ↑ dose W/ CYP3A4 inducer **Caution:** [C, –] **Disp:** Tabs 2, 5, 10, 15, 20, 30 mg; Discmelt (disint. tabs 10, 15, 20, 30 mg, soln 1 mg/mL, inj 7.5 mg/mL **SE:** Neuroleptic malignant synd, tardive dyskinesia, orthostatic ↓ BP, cognitive & motor impair **Interactions:** ↑ Effects W/ ketoconazole, quinidine, fluoxetine, paroxetine, ↓ effects W/ carbamazepine **Labs:** ↑ Glucose **NIPE:** ⊘ Breast-feed, consume EtOH, or use during PRG; use barrier contraception; ↑ fluid intake

Artificial Tears (Tears Naturale) [OTC] [Ocular Lubricant]
Uses: *Dry eyes* **Action:** Ocular lubricant **Dose:** 1–2 gtt tid-qid **Disp:** OTC soln

l-Asparaginase (Elspar, Oncaspar) [Antineoplastic/Protein Synthesis Inhibitor] **Uses:** *ALL* (in combo w/ other agents) **Action:** Protein synth inhibitor **Dose:** 500–20,000 IU/m²/d for 1–14 d (Per protocols) **Caution:** [C, ?] **Contra:** Active/h/o pancreatitis **Disp:** Inj powder for recons 10,000 units **SE:** Allergy 20–35% (urticaria to anaphylaxis); rare GI tox (mild N, anorexia, pancreatitis) ↑ glucose, coagulopathy; **Interactions:** ↑ Effects W/ prednisone, vincristine; ↓ effects OF MTX, sulfonylureas, insulin **Labs:** Monitor glucose & pt/plt; ↓ T₄ & T₄-binding globulin, serum albumin, total cholesterol, plasma fibrinogen; ↑ BUN, glucose, uric acid, LFTs, alkaline phosphatase **NIPE:** ↑ Fluid intake, monitor for bleeding, monitor I&O and wt, ○ EtOH or ASA; test dose recommended

Aspirin (Bayer, Ecotrin, St. Joseph's) [OTC] [Antipyretic, Analgesic/Salicylate] **Uses:** *Angina, CABG, PTCA, carotid endarterectomy, ischemic stroke, TIA, MI, arthritis, pain,* HA, *fever*, inflammation, Kawasaki Dz **Action:** Prostaglandin inhibitor **Dose:** *Adults. Pain, fever:* 325–650 mg q4–6h PO or PR. *RA:* 3–6 g/d PO in ÷ doses. *Plt inhibitor:* 81–325 mg PO daily. *Prevent MI:* 81(preferred)–325 mg PO daily. *Acute Coronary Syndrome (ECC 2005):* 160–325 mg PO ASAP (chewing preferred at onset) *Peds. Antipyretic:* 10–15 mg/kg/dose PO or PR q4h up to 80 mg/kg/24 h. *RA:* 60–100 mg/kg/24 h PO ÷ q4–6h (keep levels 15–30 mg/dL); avoid w/ CrCl <10 mL/min, severe liver Dz **Caution:** [C, M] Linked to Reye synd; avoid w/ viral illness in children **Contra:** Allergy to ASA, chickenpox/flu Sxs, synd of nasal polyps, angioedema, & bronchospasm to NSAIDs **Disp:** Tabs 325, 500 mg; chew tabs 81 mg; EC tabs 81, 162, 325, 500, 650, 975 mg; SR tabs 650, 800 mg; effervescent tabs 325, 500 mg; supp 125, 200, 300, 600 mg **SE:** GI upset & erosion **Notes:** Salicylate levels *Therapeutic:* 100–250 μg/mL. *Toxic:* >300 μg/mL **Interactions:** ↑ Effects W/ anticoagulants, ammonium chloride, antibiotics, ascorbic acid, furosemide, methionine, nizatidine, NSAIDs, verapamil, EtOH, feverfew, garlic, ginkgo biloba, horse chestnut, kelpware (black-tang), prickly ash, red clover; ↓ effects W/ antacids, activated charcoal, corticosteroids, griseofulvin, NaHCO₃, ginseng, food; ↑ effects OF ACEI, hypoglycemics, insulin, Li, MTX, phenytoin, sulfonamides, valproic acid; ↓ effects OF BBs, probenecid, spironolactone, sulfinpyrazone **Labs:** False-results of urinary glucose & urinary ketone tests, serum albumin, total serum phenytoin, T₃ & T₄ **NIPE:** D/C 1 wk prior to surgery; avoid/limit EtOH; Chronic ASA use may result in ↓ folic acid, Fe-deficiency anemia, & hypernatremia; ○ foods ↑ salicylate, eg curry powder, paprika, licorice, prunes, raisins, tea; take ASA w/ food or milk; report S/xss bleeding/GI pain/ringing in ears

Aspirin & Butalbital Compound (Fiorinal) [C-III] [Analgesic & Barbiturate] **Uses:** *Tension HA*, pain **Action:** Combo barbiturate & analgesic **Dose:** 1–2 PO q4h PRN, max 6 tabs/d; avoid w/ CrCl <10 mL/min & severe liver Dz **Caution:** [C (D w/ prolonged use or high doses at term), ?] **Contra:**

ASA allergy, GI ulceration, bleeding disorder, porphyria, synd of nasal polyps, angioedema, & bronchospasm to NSAIDs **Disp:** Caps (Fiorgen PF, Lanorinal), Tabs (Lanorinal) ASA 325 mg/butalbital 50 mg/caffeine 40 mg **SE:** Drowsiness, dizziness, GI upset, ulceration, bleeding; see Aspirin **Additional Interactions:** ↑ Effect *OF* benzodiazepines, CNS depressants, chloramphenicol, methylphenidate, propoxyphene, valproic acid; ↓ effects *OF* BBs, corticosteroids, chloramphenicol, cyclosporines, doxycycline, griseofulvin, haloperidol, OCPs, phenothiazines, quinidine, TCAs, theophylline, warfarin **NIPE:** Butalbital habit-forming; D/C 1 wk prior to surgery, use barrier contraception, ⊘ EtOH

Aspirin + Butalbital, Caffeine, & Codeine (Fiorinal + Codeine) [C-III] [Analgesic & Barbiturate & Narcotic]   **Uses:** Mild *pain,* HA, especially when associated w/ stress **Action:** Sedative analgesic, narcotic analgesic **Dose:** 1–2 tabs (caps) PO q4–6h PRN max 6/d **Caution:** [D, ?] **Contra:** Allergy to ASA and codeine; synd of nasal polyps, angioedema & bronchospasm to NSAIDs **Disp:** Cap/tab contains 325 mg ASA, 40 mg caffeine, 50 mg of butalbital, 30 mg of codeine **SE:** Drowsiness, dizziness, GI upset, ulceration, bleeding; see Aspirin + Butalbital **Additional Interactions:** ↑ Effects *W/* narcotic analgesics, MAOIs, neuromuscular blockers; ↓ effects *W/* tobacco smoking; ↑ effects *OF* digitoxin, phenytoin, rifampin; ↑ resp & CNS depression *W/* cimetidine **Labs:** ↑ Plasma amylase & lipase **NIPE:** D/C 1 wk prior to surgery; avoid/limit EtOH; May cause constipation, ↑ fluids & fiber, take w/ milk to ↓ GI distress

Aspirin + Codeine (Empirin No. 3, 4) [C-III] [Narcotic Analgesic]   **Uses:** Mild to *moderate pain* **Action:** Combined effects of ASA & codeine **Dose:** *Adults.* 1–2 tabs PO q4–6h PRN. *Peds.* ASA 10 mg/kg/dose; codeine 0.5–1 mg/kg/dose q4h **Caution:** [D, M] **Contra:** Allergy to ASA/codeine, PUD, bleeding, anticoagulant Rx, children w/ chickenpox or flu Sxs, synd of nasal polyps, angioedema, & bronchospasm to NSAIDs **Disp:** Tabs 325 mg of ASA & codeine (Codeine in No. 3=30 mg, No. 4=60 mg) **SE:** Drowsiness, dizziness, GI upset, ulceration, bleeding; see Aspirin **Additional Interactions** ↑ Effects *W/* narcotic analgesics, MAOIs, neuromuscular blockers, ↓ effects *W/* tobacco smoking; ↑ effects *OF* digitoxin, phenytoin, rifampin; ↑ resp & CNS depression *W/* cimetidine **Labs:** ↑ Plasma amylase & lipase **NIPE:** D/C 1 wk prior to surgery; avoid/limit EtOH; May cause constipation, ↑ fluids & fiber, take w/ milk to ↓ GI distress

Atazanavir (Reyataz) [Antiretroviral/HIV-1 Protease Inhibitor]   **WARNING:** Hyperbilirubinemia may require drug D/C **Uses:** *HIV-1 Infxn* **Action:** Protease inhibitor **Dose:** 400 mg PO daily w/ food; when given w/ efavirenz 600 mg, administer atazanavir 300 mg + ritonavir 100 mg once/d; separate doses from buffered didanosine administration; ↓ in hepatic impair **Caution:** [B, –]; **Contra:** w/ midazolam, triazolam, ergots, pimozide **Disp:** Caps 100, 150, 200, 300 mg **SE:** HA, N/V/D, rash, abd pain, DM, photosens, ↑ PR interval **Notes:** May have less adverse effect on cholesterol **Interactions:** ↑ Effects *W/* amprenavir, clarithromycin, indinavir, lamivudine, lopinavir, ritonavir, saquinavir, stavudine,

tenofovir, zalcitabine, zidovudine; ↑ effects *OF* amiodarone, atorvastatin, CCBs, clarithromycin, cyclosporine, diltiazem, irinotecan, lidocaine, lovastatin, OCPs, rifabutin, quinidine, saquinavir, sildenafil, simvastatin, sirolimus, tacrolimus, TCAs, warfarin; ↓ effects *W/* antacids, antimycobacterials, efavirenz, esomeprazole, H₂ receptor antagonists, lansoprazole, omeprazole, rifampin, St. John's Wort **Labs:** ↑ ALT, AST, total bilirubin, amylase, lipase, serum glucose, ↓ Hgb, neutrophils **NIPE:** CDC recommends HIV-infected mothers not to breast-feed; take w/ food; will not cure HIV or ↓ risk of transmission; use barrier contraception; ↑ risk of skin and/or scleral yellowing

Atenolol (Tenormin) [Antihypertensive, Antianginal/Beta-Blocker]
Uses: *HTN, angina, MI* **Action:** β-Adrenergic receptor blocker **Dose:** *HTN & angina:* 50–100 mg/d PO. *AMI:* 5 mg IV × 2 over 10 min, then 50 mg PO bid if tolerated; ↓ in renal impair; 5 mg IV over 5 min; in 10 min, 5 mg slow IV; if tolerated in 10 min, start 50 mg PO, then 50 mg PO BID *(ECC 2005)* **Caution:** [D, M] DM, bronchospasm; abrupt D/C can exacerbate angina & ↑ MI risk **Contra:** Bradycardia, cardiogenic shock, cardiac failure, 2nd-/3rd-degree AV block **Disp:** Tabs 25, 50, 100 mg; inj 5 mg/10 mL **SE:** Bradycardia, ↓ BP, 2nd-/3rd-degree AV block, dizziness, fatigue **Interactions:** ↑ Effects *W/* other antihypertensives especially diltiazem & verapamil, nitrates, EtOH; ↑ bradycardia *W/* adenosine, digitalis glycosides, dipyridamole, physostigmine, tacrine; ↓ effects *W/* ampicillin, antacids, NSAIDs, salicylates; ↑ effects *OF* lidocaine; ↓ effects *OF* dopamine, glucagons, insulin, sulfonylureas **Labs:** ↑ ANA titers, BUN, glucose, serum lipoprotein, K⁺, triglyceride, uric acid levels; ↓ HDL **NIPE:** May mask S/Sxs hypoglycemia, may ↑ sensitivity to cold, may ↑ depression, wheezing, orthostatic hypotension

Atenolol & Chlorthalidone (Tenoretic) [Antihypertensive, Antianginal/Beta-Blocker & Diuretic]
Uses: *HTN* **Action:** β-Adrenergic blockade w/ diuretic **Dose:** 50–100 mg/d PO; ↓ in renal impair **Caution:** [D, M] DM, bronchospasm **Contra:** See Atenolol; anuria, sulfonamide cross-sensitivity **Disp:** *Tenoretic 50:* Atenolol 50 mg/chlorthalidone 25 mg; *Tenoretic 100:* Atenolol 100 mg/chlorthalidone 25 mg **SE:** Bradycardia, ↓ BP, 2nd- or 3rd-degree AV block, dizziness, fatigue; see Atenolol Additional **Interactions:** ↑ Effects *W/* other antihypertensives; ↓ effects *W/* cholestyramine, NSAIDs; ↑ effects *OF* Li, digoxin, ↓ effects *OF* sulfonylureas **Labs:** False ↓ urine esriol; ↑ CPK, serum ammonia, amylase, Ca²⁺, Cl⁻, K⁺, cholesterol, glucose; ↓ serum Cl⁻, Mg²⁺, K⁺, Na⁻ **NIPE:** Take in AM to prevent nocturia, use sunblock >SPF 15, photosensitivity, monitor S/Sxs gout

Atomoxetine (Strattera) [ADHD/Selective Norepinephrine Reuptake Inhibitor]
WARNING: Severe liver injury may rarely occur; D/C w/ jaundice or ↑LFT, ↑ frequency of suicidal thoughts **Uses:** *ADHD* **Action:** Selective norepinephrine reuptake inhibitor **Dose:** *Adults & children >70 kg.* 40 mg × 3 d, ↑ to 80–100 mg ÷ daily-bid. *Peds <70 kg.* 0.5 mg/kg × 3 d, then

↑ 1.2 mg/kg daily or bid (max 1.4 mg/kg or 100 mg) **Caution:** [C, ?/–] **Contra:** NAG, w/ or w/in 2 wk of D/C an MAOI **Disp:** Caps 5, 10, 18, 25, 40, 60, 80, 100 mg **SE:** ↑ BP, tachycardia, wt loss, sexual dysfunction **NIPE:** ↓ Dose w/ hepatic insuff or in combo w/ CYP2D6 inhibitors (Table 11)

Atorvastatin (Lipitor) [Antilipemic/HMG-CoA Reductase Inhibitor] Uses: *↑ Cholesterol & triglycerides* Action: HMG-CoA reductase inhibitor **Dose:** Initial 10 mg/d, may ↑ to 80 mg/d **Caution:** [X, –] **Contra:** Active liver Dz, unexplained ↑ LFT **Disp:** Tabs 10, 20, 40, 80 mg **SE:** Myopathy, HA, arthralgia, myalgia, GI upset; **Interactions:** ↑ Effects *W/* azole antifungals, erythromycin, nefazodone, protease inhibitors, grapefruit juice; ↓ effects *W/* antacids, bile acid sequestrants; ↑ effects *OF* digoxin, levothyroxine, OCPs **Labs:** Monitor LFTs due to ↑ LFTs, CPK, ↓ lipid levels **NIPE:** Instruct patient to report unusual muscle pain or weakness; ⊘ EtOH, breast-feeding, or while PRG

Atovaquone (Mepron) [Antiprotozoal] Uses: *Rx & prevention PCP* Action: ↓ nucleic acid & ATP synth **Dose:** *Rx:* 750 mg PO bid for 21 d. *Prevention:* 1500 mg PO once/d (w/ meals) **Caution:** [C, ?] **Disp:** Susp 750 mg/5 mL **SE:** Fever, HA, anxiety, insomnia, rash, N/V **Interactions:** ↓ Effects *W/* metoclopramide, rifabutin, rifampin, tetracycline **Labs:** Monitor LFTs w/ long-term use **NIPE:** ↑ Absorption w/ meal esp ↑ fat

Atovaquone/Proguanil (Malarone) [Antimalarial] Uses: *Prevention or Rx P. falciparum malaria* Action: Antimalarial **Dose:** *Adults: Prevention:* 1 tab PO 2 d before, during, & 7 d after leaving endemic region; *Rx:* 4 tabs PO single dose daily × 3 d. *Peds.* See insert **Caution:** [C, ?] **Contra:** CrCl <30 mL/min **Disp:** Tab atovaquone 250 mg/proguanil 100 mg; peds 62.5/25 mg **SE:** HA, fever, myalgia **Interactions:** ↓ Effects *W/* metoclopramide, rifabutin, rifampin, tetracycline **Labs:** Monitor LFTs w/ long-term use **NIPE:** ↑ Absorption w/ meal esp ↑ fat

Atracurium (Tracrium) [Skeletal Muscle Relaxant/Neuromuscular Blocker] Uses: *Anesthesia adjunct to facilitate ET intubation* Action: Nondepolarizing neuromuscular blocker **Dose:** *Adults & Peds.* 0.4–0.5 mg/kg IV bolus, then 0.08–0.1 mg/kg q20–45 min PRN **Caution:** [C, ?] **Disp:** Inj 10 mg/mL **SE:** Flushing **Notes:** Pt must be intubated & on controlled ventilation; use adequate amounts of sedation & analgesia; **Interactions:** ↑ Effects *W/* general anesthetics, aminoglycosides, bacitracin, BBs, β-agonists, clindamycin, CCBs, diuretics, lidocaine, Li, MgSO₄, narcotic analgesics, procainamide, quinidine, succinylcholine, trimethaphan, verapamil; ↓ effects *W/* Ca, carbamazepine, phenytoin, theophylline, caffeine **Labs:** Monitor BUN, Cr, LFTs **NIPE:** Drug does not effect consciousness or pain, inability to speak until drug wears off

Atropine (AtroPen) [Antiarrhythmic/Anticholinergic] **WARNING:** Primary protection against exposure to chemical nerve agent and insecticide poisoning is the wearing of specially designed protective garments Uses: *Preanesthetic; symptomatic bradycardia & asystole, organophosphate (insecticide) and acetylcholinesterase (nerve agent) inhibitor antidote; cycloplegic* Action: Antimuscarinic;

blocks acetylcholine at parasympathetic sites, cycloplegic **Dose:** *Adults. (2005 ECC):* Asystole or PEA: 1 mg IV/IO push. Repeat every 3–5 min (if asystole persists) to 0.03–0.04 mg/kg max. *Bradycardia:* 0.5–1.0 mg IV every 3–5 min as needed; max 0.03–0.04 mg/kg; ET 2–3 mg in 10 mL NS. *Preanesthetic:* 0.3–0.6 mg IM. *Poisoning:* 1–2 mg IV bolus, repeat Q 3–5 min PRN to reverse effects *Peds. (ECC 2005):* 0.01–0.03 mg/kg IV q2–5min, max 1 mg, min dose 0.1 mg. *Preanesthetic:* 0.01 mg/kg/dose SC/IV (max 0.4 mg). *Poisoning:* 0.05 mg/kg IV, repeat Q 3–5 min PRN to reverse effects **Caution:** [C, +] **Contra:** NAG **Disp:** inj 0.05, 0.1, 0.3, 0.4, 0.5, 0.8, 1 mg/mL; *AtroPen AutoInjector:* 0.5, 1, 2 mg/dose; MDI 0.36 mg/inhal **SE:** Flushing, mydriasis, tachycardia, dry mouth & nose, blurred vision, urinary retention, constipation, psychosis **Notes:** SLUDGE (salivation, lacrimation, urination, diaphoresis, gastrointestinal motility, emesis) are Sx of organophosphate poisoning; AutoInjector limited distribution **Interactions:** ↑ Effects *W/* amantadine, antihistamines, disopyramide, procainamide, quinidine, TCA, thiazides, betel palm, squaw vine; ↓ effects *W/* antacids, levodopa; ↓ effects *OF* phenothiazines **Labs:** ↓ Gastric motility & emptying may affect results of upper GI series **NIPE:** Monitor I&O, ↑ fluids & oral hygiene, wear dark glasses to ↓ photophobia

Atropine, ophthalmic (Isopto Atropine, generic) [Antiarrhythmic/Anticholinergic] Uses: *Cycloplegic refraction, uveitis, amblyopia * **Action:** Antimuscarinic; cycloplegic, dilates pupils **Dose:** *Adults. Refraction:* 1–2 gtt 1 h before; *Uveitis:* 1–2 gtt daily-qid *Peds.* 1 gtt in nonamblyotic eye daily **Caution:** [C, +] **Contra:** Glaucoma **Disp:** 15-mL bottle 1% ophthal soln **SE:** Local irritation, burning, blurred vision, light sensitivity; **Interactions:** ↑ Effects *W/* amantadine, antihistamines, disopyramide, procainamide, quinidine, TCA, thiazides, betel palm, squaw vine; ↓ effects *W/* antacids, levodopa; ↓ effects *OF* phenothiazines **NIPE:** Compress lacrimal sac 2–3 min after instillation; effects can last 1–2 weeks; increased risk of photophobia

Atropine/pralidoxime (DuoDote) [Antiarrhythmic/Anticholinergic/Antidote] **WARNING:** For use by personnel with appropriate training; wear protective garments; do not rely solely on medication; evacuation and decontamination as soon as possible Uses: *Nerve agent and insecticide poisoning* **Action:** Atropine blocks effects of excess acetylcholine; pralidoxime reactivates acetylcholinesterase inactivated by organophosphorus poisoning **Dose:** 1 injection in midlateral thigh; if symptoms progress or are severe, give 2 additional injections **Caution:** [C, ?] **Contra:** **Disp:** AutoInjector 2.1 mg atropine/60 mg pralidoxime **SE:** Dry mouth, blurred vision, dry eyes, photophobia, confusion, HA, tachycardia, flushing, urinary retention, constipation, abd pain N/V, emesis **Interactions:** ↑ Effects *W/* amantadine, antihistamines, disopyramide, procainamide, quinidine, TCA, thiazides, betel palm, squaw vine; ↑ effects *OF* barbiturates; ↓ effects *W/* antacids, levodopa; ↓ effects *OF* phenothiazines **Labs:** ↑ ALT, AST, Cr **NIPE:** Severe Sx of poisoning include confusion, dyspnea with copious secretions, weakness & twitching, involuntary urination and defecation, convulsions, unconsciousness

Azathioprine (Imuran) [Immunosuppressant/Purine Antagonist] **WARNING:** May ↑ neoplasia w/ chronic use; mutagenic and hematologic tox possible **Uses:** *Adjunct to prevent renal transplant rejection, RA*, SLE, Crohn Dz, ulcerative colitis* **Action:** Immunosuppressive; antagonizes purine metabolism **Dose:** *Adults & Peds.* 1–3 mg/kg/d IV or PO; Crohn & ulcerative colitis, start 50 mg/d, ↑ 100–250 mg/d; ↓ w/ renal insuff **Caution:** [D, ?] **Contra:** PRG **Disp:** Tabs 25, 50, 75, 100 mg; inj 100 mg powder for recons **SE:** GI intolerance, fever, chills, leukopenia, thrombocytopenia **Interactions:** ↑ Effects *W/* allopurinol; ↑ effects *OF* antineoplastic drugs, cyclosporine, myelosuppressive drugs, MTX; ↑ risk *OF* severe leucopenia *W/* ACEI; ↓ effects *OF* nondepolarizing neuromuscular blocking drugs, warfarin **Labs:** Monitor BUN, Cr, CBC, LFTs during therapy **NIPE:** Handle inj w/ cytotoxic precautions; do not administer live vaccines on drug; dose per local transplant protocol, usually start 1–3 d pretransplant ⊘ PRG, breast-feeding

Azelastine (Astelin, Optivar) [Antihistamine/H1-Receptor Antagonist] **Uses:** *Allergic rhinitis (rhinorrhea, sneezing, nasal pruritus); allergic conjunctivitis* **Action:** Histamine H1-receptor antagonist **Dose:** *Nasal:* 2 sprays/nostril bid. *Ophth:* 1 gtt in each affected eye bid **Caution:** [C, ?/–] **Contra:** Component sensitivity **Disp:** Nasal 137 µg/spray; ophth soln 0.05% **SE:** Somnolence, bitter taste **Interactions:** ↑ Effects *W/* cimetidine; ↑ effects *OF* EtOH, CNS depressants **Labs:** ↑ AST, ↓ skin reactions to antigen skin tests **NIPE:** Systemically absorbed; clear nares before admin; prime pump before use

Azithromycin (Zithromax) [Antibiotic/Macrolide] **Uses:** *Community-acquired pneumonia, pharyngitis, otitis media, skin Infxns, non-gonococcal (chlamydial) urethritis, chancroid & PID; Rx & prevention of MAC in HIV* **Action:** Macrolide antibiotic; bacteriostatic; ↓ protein synth. *Spectrum:* Chlamydia sp, H. ducreyi, H. influenzae, Legionella sp, M. catarrhalis, M. pneumoniae, M. hominis, N. gonorrhoeae, S. aureus, S. agalactiae, S. pneumoniae, S. pyogenes **Dose:** *Adults.* Resp tract Infxns: PO: Cap 500 mg day 1, then 250 mg/d PO × 4 d. Sinusitis 500 mg/d PO × 3 d. IV: 500 mg × 2 d, then 500 mg PO × 7–10 d or 500 mg IV daily × 2 d, then 500 mg/d PO × 7–10 d Nongonococcal urethritis: 1 g PO × 1. Gonorrhea, uncomplicated 2 mg PO × 1; Prevent MAC: 1200 mg PO once/wk. *Peds.* Otitis media: 10 mg/kg PO day 1, then 5 mg/kg/d days 2–5. Pharyngitis: 12 mg/kg/d PO × 5 d (susp on empty stomach; tabs OK w/ or w/o food; ↓ w/ CrCl <10 mL/min **Caution:** [B, +] **Disp:** Tabs 250, 500, 600 mg; Z-Pack (5-d, 250 mg); Tri-Pak (500-mg tabs × 3); susp 1-g; single-dose packet (ZMAX) ER susp. (2 g); susp 100, 200 mg/5 mL; powder for recons 500, 2.5-mg ophtn soln 1% **SE:** GI upset, metallic taste **Interactions:** ↓ Effects *W/* Al- & Mg-containing antacids, atovaquone, food (suspension); ↑ effects *OF* alfentanil, barbiturates, bromocriptine, carbamazepine, cyclosporine, digoxin, disopyramide, ergot alkaloids, phenytoin, pimozide, terfenadine, theophylline, triazolam, warfarin; ↓ effects *OF* penicillins **Labs:** May ↑ serum bilirubin, alkaline phosphatase, BUN, Cr,

CPK, glucose, K+, LFTs, LDH, PT; may ↓ WBC, plt count, serum folate **NIPE:** Monitor S/Sxs super Infxns, use sunscreen & protective clothing

Aztreonam (Azactam) [Antibiotic/Monobactam] Uses: *Aerobic gram(-) UTIs, lower resp, intra-abd, skin, gynecologic Infxns & septicemia* **Action:** Monobactam. ↓ Cell wall synth. *Spectrum:* Gram(-) (*Pseudomonas* sp, *E. coli, Klebsiella* sp, *H. influenzae, Serratia* sp, *Proteus* sp, *Enterobacter* sp, *Citrobacter* sp) **Dose:** *Adults.* 1–2 g IV/IM q6–12h. *Peds.* Premature: 30 mg/kg/dose IV q12h. *Term & children:* 30 mg/kg/dose q6–8h; ↓ in renal impair **Caution:** [B, +] **Disp:** Inj (soln), 1 g, 2 g/ 50 mL Inj powder for recons 500 mg 1 g, 2 g **SE:** N/V/D, rash, pain at injection site **Interactions:** ↑ Effects *W/* probenecid, aminoglycosides, β-lactam antibiotics; ↓ effects *W/* cefoxitin, chloramphenicol, imipenem **Labs:** ↑ LFTs, alkaline phosphatase, SCr, PT, PTT, & + direct Coombs test **NIPE:** No gram(+) or anaerobic activity; OK in PCN-allergic pts; Monitor S/Sxs super Infxn, taste changes w/ IV administration

Bacitracin, Ophthalmic (AK-Tracin Ophthalmic); Bacitracin & Polymyxin B, Ophthalmic (AK Poly Bac Ophthalmic, Polysporin Ophthalmic); Bacitracin, Neomycin, & Polymyxin B, Ophthalmic (AK Spore Ophthalmic, Neosporin Ophthalmic); Bacitracin, Neomycin, Polymyxin B, & Hydrocortisone, Ophthalmic (AK Spore HC Ophthalmic, Cortisporin Ophthalmic) [Antibiotic/Anti-Inflammatory] Uses: *Steroid-responsive inflammatory ocular conditions* **Action:** Topical antibiotic w/ anti-inflammatory **Dose:** Apply q3–4h into conjunctival sac **Caution:** [C, ?] **Contra:** Viral, mycobacterial, fungal eye Infxn **Disp:** See Bacitracin, Topical equivalents, below **Interactions:** ↑ Effects *W/* neuromuscular blocking agents, anesthetics, nephrotoxic drugs **NIPE:** May cause blurred vision

Bacitracin, Topical (Baciguent); Bacitracin & Polymyxin B, Topical (Polysporin); Bacitracin, Neomycin, & Polymyxin B, Topical (Neosporin Ointment); Bacitracin, Neomycin, Polymyxin B, & Hydrocortisone, Topical (Cortisporin); Bacitracin, Neomycin, Polymyxin B, & Lidocaine, Topical (Clomycin) [Antibiotic/Anti-Inflammatory/Analgesic] Uses: Prevent/Rx of *minor skin Infxns* **Action:** Topical antibiotic w/ added components (anti-inflammatory & analgesic) **Dose:** Apply sparingly bid-qid **Caution:** [C, ?] **Disp:** Bacitracin 500 units/g oint; Bacitracin 500 units/polymyxin B sulfate 10,000 units/g oint & powder; Bacitracin 400 units/neomycin 3.5 mg/polymyxin B 5000 units/g oint; Bacitracin 400 units/neomycin 3.5 mg/polymyxin B 5000 units/hydrocortisone 10 mg/g oint; Bacitracin 500 units/neomycin 3.5 mg/polymyxin B 5000 units/lidocaine 40 mg/g oint **NIPE:** Systemic & irrigation forms available, but not generally used due to potential tox

Baclofen (Lioresal Intrathecal, generic) [Antispasmodic/ Skeletal Muscle Relaxant] WARNING: IT abrupt D/C can lead to organ failure, rhabdomyolysis, & death Uses: *Spasticity due to severe chronic disorders (eg, MS, ALS, or spinal cord lesions)*, trigeminal neuralgia, hiccups **Action:** Centrally acting skeletal muscle relaxant; ↓ transmission of monosynaptic & polysynaptic cord reflexes **Dose:** *Adults.* Initial, 5 mg PO tid; ↑ q3d to effect; max 80 mg/d. *Intrathecal:* Via implantable pump (see insert) *Peds.* 2–7 y: 10–15 mg/d ÷ q8h; titrate, max 40 mg/d. >8 y: Max 60 mg/d. *IT:* Via implantable pump; ↓ in renal impair; w/ food or milk **Caution:** [C, +] Epilepsy, neuropsychiatric disturbances; **Disp:** Tabs 10, 20 mg; IT inj 50 µg/mL 10 mg/20 mL, 10 mg/5 mL **SE:** Dizziness, drowsiness, insomnia, ataxia, weakness, ↓ BP **Interactions:** ↑ CNS depression *W/* CNS depressants, MAOIs, EtOH, antihistamines, opioid analgesics, sedatives, hypnotics; ↑ effects *OF* antihypertensives, clindamycin, guanabenz; ↑ risk of resp paralysis & renal failure *W/* aminoglycosides **Labs:** ↑ Serum glucose, AST, ammonia, alkaline phosphatase; ↓ bilirubin **NIPE:** Take oral meds w/ food; ⊘ EtOH

Balsalazide (Colazal) [Anti-inflammatory/GI Drug] Uses: *Ulcerative colitis* **Action:** 5-ASA derivative, anti-inflammatory, ↓ leukotriene synth **Dose:** 2.25 g (3 caps) tid × 8–12 wk **Caution:** [B, ?] Severe renal/hepatic failure **Contra:** Mesalamine or salicylates hypersensitivity **Disp:** Caps 750 mg **SE:** Dizziness, HA, N, angioacytosis, pancytopenia, renal impair, allergic Rxns **Notes:** Daily dose of 6.75 g = to 2.4 g mesalamine **Interactions:** Oral antibiotics may interfere *W/* mesalamine release in the colon **Labs:** ↑ Bilirubin, CPK, LFTs, LDH, **NIPE:** ⊘ If ASA allergy; take w/ food & swallow capsule whole

Basiliximab (Simulect) [Immunosuppressant/Monoclonal Antibody] **WARNING:** Administer only under the supervision of a provider experienced in immunosuppression therapy in an appropriate facility **Uses:** *Prevent acute transplant rejection* **Action:** IL-2 receptor antagonists **Dose:** *Adults.* 20 mg IV 2 h before transplant, then 20 mg IV 4 d post. *Peds.* 12 mg/m² ↑ to max of 20 mg 2 h prior to transplant; same dose IV 4 d post **Caution:** [B, ?/–] Avoid w/ other immunosuppressants **Contra:** Hypersensitivity to murine proteins **Disp:** *Inj:* powder for recons 10, 20 mg **SE:** Edema, HTN, HA, dizziness, fever, pain, Infxn, GI effects, electrolyte disturbances **Notes:** A murine/human MoAb **Interactions:** May ↑ immunosuppression *W/* other immunosuppressive drugs **Labs:** ↑ Cholesterol, BUN, Cr, lipids, uric acid; ↓ serum Mg phosphate, plts, Hgb, Hct, Ca²⁺, or ↓ glucose, K⁺; **NIPE:** Monitor for Infxns, hypersensitivity Rxns, IV dose over 20–30 min

BCG [Bacillus Calmette-Guérin] (TheraCys, Tice BCG) [Antineoplastic, Antituberculotic] Uses: *Bladder carcinoma (superficial)*, TB prophylaxis **Action:** Immunomodulator **Dose:** Bladder CA, 1 vial prepared & instilled in bladder for 2 h. Repeat once/wk for 6 wk; then 1 treatment at 3, 6, 12, 18, & 24 mo after initial therapy **Caution:** [C, ?] Asthma **Contra:** Immunosuppression, UTI, steroid use, acute illness, fever of unknown origin, w/ traumatic catheterization or UTI **Disp:** Inj powder for recons 81 mg (10.5 ± 8.7 × 10⁸ CFU vial) (TheraCys), 50 mg (1–8 × 10⁸ CFU/vial) (Tice BCG) **SE:** *Intravesical:* Hematuria, urinary frequency, dysuria, bacterial UTI, rare BCG sepsis **Notes:** Routine

US adult BCG immunization not rec; occasionally used in high-risk children who are PPD(-) & cannot take INH, dispose/void in toilet with chlorine bleach; **Interactions:** ↓ Effects W/ antimicrobials, immunosuppressives, radiation **Labs:** Prior BCG may cause false + PPD **NIPE:** Monitor for S/Sxs systemic Infxn, report persistent pain on urination or blood in urine

Becaplermin (Regranex Gel) [Growth Factor] Uses: Adjunct to local wound care w/ *diabetic foot ulcers* **Action:** Recombinant PDGF, enhances granulation tissue **Dose:** Based on lesion; 11/3-in ribbon from 2-g tube, 2/3-in ribbon from 15-g tube/in × in^2 of ulcer; apply & cover w/ moist gauze; rinse after 12 h; do not reapply; repeat in 12 h **Caution:** [C, ?] **Contra:** Neoplasm/or active site Infxn **Disp:** 0.01% gel in 2-, 15-g tubes **SE:** Erythema, local pain; **Interactions:** None known **NIPE:** Dosage recalculated q1–2 wk; Use w/ good wound care; wound must be vascularized

Beclomethasone (Beconase) [Anti-inflammatory/Corticosteroid] Uses: *Allergic rhinitis* refractory to antihistamines & decongestants; *nasal polyps* **Action:** Inhaled steroid **Dose:** *Adults & Peds 6–12. Aqueous inhal:* 1–2 sprays/nostril twice daily **Caution:** [C, ?] **Disp:** Nasal met-dose inhaler **SE:** Local irritation, burning, epistaxis **Notes:** Nasal spray delivers 42 μg/dose **Interactions:** None noted **NIPE:** Prior use of decongestant nasal gtt if edema or secretions, may cause headache

Beclomethasone (QVAR) [Antiasthmatic/Synthetic Corticosteroid] Uses: Chronic *asthma* **Action:** Inhaled corticosteroid **Dose:** *Adults & Peds. 5–11 y:* 40–160 μg 1–4 inhal bid; initial 40–80 μg inhal bid if on bronchodilators alone; 40–160 μg w/ other inhaled steroids; 320 μg bid max; taper to lowest effective dose bid rinse mouth/throat after **Caution:** [C, ?] **Contra:** Acute asthma **Disp:** PO met-dose inhaler; 40, 80 μg/inhal **SE:** HA, cough, hoarseness, oral candidiasis **Notes:** Not effective for acute asthma **Interactions:** None noted **NIPE:** Use inhaled bronchodilator prior to inhaled steroid, rinse mouth after inhaled steroid

Belladonna & Opium Suppositories (B&O Supprettes) [C-II] [Antispasmodic, Analgesic] Uses: *Bladder spasms; moderate/severe pain* **Action:** Antispasmodic, analgesic **Dose:** 1 supp PR q6h PRN; 15A=30 mg powdered opium/16.2 mg belladonna extract; 16A=60 mg powdered opium/16.2 mg belladonna extract **Caution:** [C, ?] **Contra:** Glaucoma, resp dep **Disp:** Supp 15A, 16A **SE:** Anticholinergic (eg, sedation, urinary retention, constipation) **Interactions:** ↑ Effects W/ CNS depressants, TCAs; ↓ effects W/ phenothiazines **Labs:** ↑ LFTs **NIPE:** ⊘ Refrigerate; moisten finger & supp before insertion; may cause blurred vision

Benazepril (Lotensin) [Antihypertensive/ACEI] Uses: *HTN*, DN, CHF **Action:** ACE inhibitor **Dose:** 10–40 mg/d PO **Caution:** [C (1st tri), D (2nd & 3rd tri), +] **Contra:** Angioedema, h/o edema, bilateral RAS **Disp:** Tabs 5, 10, 20, 40 mg **SE:** Symptomatic ↓ BP w/ diuretics; dizziness, HA, nonproductive cough **Interactions:** ↑ Effects W/ α-blockers, diuretics, capsaicin; ↓ effects W/ NSAIDs, ASA; ↑ effects OF insulin, Li; ↑ risk of hyperkalemia W/ trimethoprim & K-sparing diuretics **Labs:** ↑ BUN, SCr, K⁺; ↓ hemoglobin; ECG changes **NIPE:** Persistent cough and/or taste changes may develop; ⊘ PRG, D/C if angioedema

Benzocaine & Antipyrine (Auralgan) [Otic Anesthetic] Uses: *Analgesia in severe otitis media* **Action:** Anesthetic w/ local decongestant **Dose:** Fill ear & insert a moist cotton plug; repeat 1–2 h PRN **Caution:** [C, ?] **Contra:** w/ perforated eardrum **Disp:** Soln 5.4% antipyrine, 1.4% benzocaine **SE:** Local irritation; **Interactions:** May ↓ effects OF sulfonamides

Benzonatate (Tessalon Perles) [Antitussive] Uses: Symptomatic relief of *cough* **Action:** Anesthetizes the stretch receptors in the resp passages **Dose:** *Adults & Peds.* >10 y: 100 mg PO tid (max 600 mg/d) **Caution:** [C, ?] **Disp:** Caps 100, 200 mg **SE:** Sedation, dizziness, GI upset **Interactions:** ↑ CNS depression W/ antihistamines, EtOH, hypnotics, opioids, sedatives **NIPE:** ↑ Fluid intake to liquefy secretions; Do not chew or puncture the caps

Benztropine (Cogentin) [Antiparkinsonian/Anticholinergic] Uses: *Parkinsonism & drug-induced extrapyramidal disorders* **Action:** Partially blocks striatal cholinergic receptors **Dose:** *Adults.* 0.5–6 mg PO, IM, or IV in ÷ doses/d to 4 mg/day max *Peds.* >3 y: 0.02–0.05 mg/kg/dose 1–2/d **Caution:** [C, ?] **Contra:** <3 y, myasthenia gravis **Disp:** Tabs 0.5, 1, 2 mg; inj 1 mg/mL **SE:** Anticholinergic side effects **Notes:** Physostigmine 1–2 mg SC/IV to reverse severe Sxs **Interactions:** ↑ Sedation and depressant effects W/ EtOH & CNS depressants; ↑ anticholinergic effects W/ antihistamines, phenothiazines, quinidine, disopyramide, TCAs, MAOIs; ↑ effect OF digoxin; ↓ effect OF levodopa; ↓ effects W/ antacids and antidiarrheal drugs **NIPE:** May ↑ susceptibility to heat stroke, take w/ meals to avoid GI upset

Beractant (Survanta) [Lung Surfactant] Uses: *Prevention & Rx of RDS in premature infants* **Action:** Replaces pulm surfactant **Dose:** 100 mg/kg via ET tube; repeat 3 × q6h PRN; max 4 doses/48 h **Disp:** Susp 25 mg of phospholipid/mL **SE:** Transient bradycardia, desaturation, apnea **Notes:** Administer via 4-quadrant method **Interactions:** None noted **NIPE:** ↑ Risk of nosocomial sepsis after Rx w/ this drug

Betaxolol (Kerlone) [Antihypertensive/Beta-Blocker] Uses: *HTN* **Action:** Competitively blocks β-adrenergic receptors, β₁ **Caution:** [C (1st tri), D (2nd or 3rd tri), +/–] **Contra:** Sinus bradycardia, AV conduction abnormalities, uncompensated cardiac failure **Dose:** 5–20 mg/d **Disp:** Tabs 10, 20 mg **SE:** Dizziness, HA, bradycardia, edema, CHF **Interactions:** ↑ Effects W/ anticholinergics, verapamil, general anesthetics; ↓ effects W/ thyroid drugs, amphetamine, cocaine, ephedrine, epinephrine, norepinephrine, phenylephrine, pseudoephedrine, NSAIDs; ↑ effects OF insulin, digitalis glycosides; ↓ effects OF theophylline, dopamine, glucagon **Labs:** ↑ BUN, serum lipoprotein, glucose, K⁺, triglyceride, uric acid, ANA titers **NIPE:** May ↑ sensitivity to cold, ⊘ D/C abruptly

Betaxolol, Ophthalmic (Betoptic) [Beta-Blocker] Uses: Open-angle glaucoma **Action:** Competitively blocks β-adrenergic receptors, β_1 **Dose:** 1–2 gtt bid **Caution:** [C (1st tri), D (2nd or 3rd tri), ?/–] **Disp:** Soln 0.5%; susp 0.25% **SE:** Local irritation, photophobia; see Betaxolol **+ NIPE:** Use sunglasses to ↓ exposure, may cause photophobia, review installation procedures

Bethanechol (Urecholine, Duvoid, others) [Urinary Tract Stimulant/Cholinergic Agonist] Uses: *Neurogenic bladder atony w/ retention*, acute *postop* & postpartum functional *(nonobst) urinary retention* **Action:** Stimulates cholinergic smooth muscle receptors in bladder & GI tract **Dose:** *Adults.* 10–50 mg PO tid-qid or 2.5–5 mg SQ tid-qid & PRN. *Peds.* 0.6 mg/kg/24 h PO ÷ tid-qid or 0.15–2 mg/kg/d SQ ÷ 3–4 × (take on empty stomach) **Caution:** [C, ?/–] **Contra:** BOO, PUD, epilepsy, hyperthyroidism, bradycardia, COPD, AV conduction defects, parkinsonism, ↓ BP, vasomotor instability **Disp:** Tabs 5, 10, 25, 50 mg; inj 5 mg/mL **SE:** Abd cramps, D, salivation, ↓BP **Notes:** Do not use IM/IV **Interactions:** ↑ Effects W/ BBs, tacrine, cholinesterase inhibitors; ↓ effects W/ atropine, anticholinergic drugs, procainamide, quinidine, epinephrine **Labs:** ↑ In serum AST, ALT, amylase, lipase, bilirubin **NIPE:** May cause blurred vision, monitor I&O, take on an empty stomach

Bevacizumab (Avastin) [Antineoplastic/Monoclonal Antibody] **WARNING:** Associated w/ GI perforation, wound dehiscence, & fatal hemoptysis Uses: *Met colorectal ca, w/ 5-FU NSCLC w/ paclitaxel and carboplatin* **Action:** Vascular endothelial GF inhibitor **Dose:** *Adults.* Colon: 5 mg/kg or 10 mg/kg IV q14d; *NSCLC:* 15 mg/kg q21d; 1st dose over 90 min; 2nd over 60 min, 3rd over 30 min if tolerated **Caution:** [C, –] Do not use w/in 28 d of surgery if time for separation of drug & anticipated surgical procedures is unknown; D/C w/ serious adverse events **Disp:** 100 mg/4 mL, 400 mg/16 mL vials **SE:** Wound dehiscence, GI perforation, tracheoesophageal fistula, hemoptysis, hemorrhage, HTN, proteinuria, CHF, inf Rxns, D, leukopenia, thromboembolism **Labs:** Monitor for ↑ proteinuria; NIPE: Monitor for ↑ BP

Bicalutamide (Casodex) [Antineoplastic/Nonsteroidal Antiandrogen] Uses: *Advanced CAP (met)* (w/ GnRH agonists [eg, leuprolide, goserelin]) **Action:** Nonsteroidal antiandrogen **Dose:** 50 mg/d **Caution:** [X, ?] **Contra:** Women **Disp:** Caps 50 mg **SE:** Hot flashes, loss of libido, impotence, D/N/V, gynecomastia **Interactions:** ↑ Effects *OF* anticoagulants, TCAs, phenothiazides; ↓ effects *OF* antipsychotic drugs **Labs:** ↑ LFTs, alkaline phosphatase, bilirubin, BUN, Cr; ↓ Hgb, WBCs **NIPE:** Monitor PSA, may experience hair loss

Bicarbonate (See Sodium Bicarbonate)

Bisacodyl (Dulcolax) [OTC] [Stimulant Laxative] Uses: *Constipation; preop bowel prep* **Action:** Stimulates peristalsis **Dose:** *Adults.* 5–15 mg PO or 10 mg PR PRN. *Peds.* <2y: 5 mg PR PRN. >2 y: 5 mg PO or 10 mg PR PRN (do not chew tabs or give w/in 1 h of antacids or milk) **Caution:** [B, ?] **Contra:** Acute abdomen or bowel obst, appendicitis, gastroenteritis **Disp:** EC tabs 5 mg;

DR tab 5 mg; supp 10 mg, enema soln 10 mg/30 mL **SE:** Abd cramps, proctitis, & inflammation w/ suppositories **Interactions:** Antacids & milk ↑ dissolution *OF* EC causing abd irritation **Labs:** ↑ Phosphate, Na; ↓ Ca, Mg, K⁺ **NIPE:** ↑ Fluid intake & high-fiber foods, ⊘ take w/ milk or antacids

Bismuth Subcitrate/Metronidazole/Tetracycline (Pylera) [Antibacterial/Antiprotozoal] WARNING: Metronidazole carcinogenic in mice and rats; avoid use unless absolutely necessary. **Uses:** **H. pylori Infxn w/ omeprazole** **Action:** eradication of *H. pylori*, **Dose:** 3 caps 4 × d w/ omeprazole 20 mg 2× d for 10 d **Caution:** [D, –] **Contra:** Pregnancy, childhood to 8 yr (tetracycline during tooth development causes teeth discoloration), w/ renal/hepatic impair, component hypersensitivity **Disp:** Caps w/ 140 mg bismuth subcitrate potassium, 125 mg metronidazole, and 125 mg tetracycline hydrochloride **SE:** Stool abnormality, D, dyspepsia, abd pain, HA, flu-like synd, taste perversion, vaginitis, dizziness; see SE for each component **Interactions:** See multiple drug interactions for each component **Labs:** ↓ neutrophils, WBC; **NIPE:** EtOH use may cause disulfiram-like reaction; possible occurrence of metallic taste & reddish-brown urine; take with food.

Bismuth Subsalicylate (Pepto-Bismol) [Antidiarrheal/ Adsorbent] [OTC] Uses: Indigestion, N, & **D**; combo for Rx of **H. pylori* Infxn* **Action:** Antisecretory & anti-inflammatory **Dose:** *Adults.* 2 tabs or 30 mL PO PRN (max 8 doses/24 h). *Peds. 3–6 y:* 1/3 tab or 5 mL PO PRN (max 8 doses/24 h). *6–9 y:* 2/3 tab or 10 mL PO PRN (max 8 doses/24 h). *9–12 y:* 1 tab or 15 mL PO PRN (max 8 doses/24 h) **Caution:** [C, D (3rd tri), –] Avoid w/ renal failure; h/o severe GI bleed **Contra:** Influenza or chickenpox (↑ risk of Reye synd), ASA allergy (see Aspirin) **Disp:** Chew tabs 262 mg; Caplets 262 mg, Liq 262, 525 mg/15 mL, susp 262 mg/15 mL **SE:** May turn tongue & stools black **Interactions:** ↑ Effects *OF* ASA, MTX, valproic acid; ↓ effects *OF* tetracyclines; ↓ effects *W/* corticosteroids, probenecid **Labs:** ↑ Lipid levels; may interfere w/ GI tract x-rays **NIPE:** May darken tongue & stool, chew tab, ⊘ swallow whole

Bisoprolol (Zebeta) [Antihypertensive/Beta-Blocker] Uses: **HTN** **Action:** Competitively blocks β₁-adrenergic receptors **Dose:** 2.5–10 mg/d (max dose 20 mg/d); ↓ w/ renal impair **Caution:** [C (D 2nd & 3rd tri). +/–] **Contra:** Sinus bradycardia, AV conduction abnormalities, uncompensated cardiac failure **Disp:** Tabs 5, 10 mg **SE:** Fatigue, lethargy, HA, bradycardia, edema, CHF **Notes:** Not dialyzed; **Interactions:** ↑ Bradycardia *W/* adenosine, amiodarone, digoxin, dipyridamole, neostigmine, physostigmine, tacrine; ↑ effects *W/* cimetidine, fluoxetine, prazosin; ↓ effects *W/* NSAIDs, rifampin; ↓ effects *OF* theophylline, glucagon **Labs:** ↑Alkaline phosphatase, BUN, cholesterol, glucose, K⁺, triglycerides, uric acid **NIPE:** ⊘ D/C abruptly, may mask S/Sxs hypoglycemia, take w/o regard to food

Bivalirudin (Angiomax) [Anticoagulant/Direct Thrombin Inhibitor] Uses: **Anticoagulant w/ ASA in unstable angina undergoing PTCA,

PCI or in patients undergoing PCI w/ or at risk of HIT/HITTS* **Action:** Anticoagulant, thrombin inhibitor **Dose:** 0.75 mg/kg IV bolus, then 1.75 mg/kg/h for duration of procedure and up to 4 h post; ✓ ACT 5 min after bolus, may repeat 0.3 mg/kg bolus if necessary (give w/ ASA 300–325 mg/d; start pre-PTCA) **Caution:** [B, ?] **Contra:** Major bleeding **Disp:** Powder 250 mg for inj **SE:** Bleeding, back pain, N, HA **Interactions:** ↑ Risk of bleeding **W/** heparin, warfarin, oral anticoagulants **Labs:** ↑ PT, PTT **NIPE:** Monitor venipuncture site for bleeding; instruct pt to watch for bleeding, bruising, or tarry stool

Bleomycin Sulfate (Blenoxane) [Antineoplastic/Antibiotic]

Uses: *Testis CA; Hodgkin Dz & NHLs; cutaneous lymphomas; & squamous cell CA (head & neck, larynx, cervix, skin, penis); malignant pleural effusion sclerosing agent* **Action:** Induces DNA breakage (scission) **Dose:** (Per protocols); ↓ w/ renal impair **Caution:** [D, ?] Severe pulm Dz (pulm fibrosis) **Disp:** Inj: Powder for recons 15, 30 units **SE:** Hyperpigmentation (skin staining) & allergy (rash to anaphylaxis); fever in 50%; lung tox (idiosyncratic & dose related); pneumonitis w/ fibrosis; Raynaud phenomenon, N/V **Notes:** Test dose 1 unit, especially in lymphoma pts; lung tox w/ total dose >400 units or single dose >30 units **Interactions:** ↑ Effects **W/** cisplatin & other antineoplastic drugs; ↓ effects **OF** digoxin & phenytoin **Labs:** ↑ Uric acid, WBC; monitor BUN, Cr, pulmonary Fxn tests **NIPE:** Eval lungs for adventious sounds; transient hair loss; ⊘ immunizations, breastfeeding; use contraception method

Bortezomib (Velcade) [Antineoplastic/Proteosome Inhibitor]

WARNING: May worsen preexisting neuropathy **Uses:** *Rx multiple myeloma or mantel cell lymphoma with one previous Rx* **Action:** Proteasome inhibitor **Dose:** 1.3 mg/m² bolus IV 2 ×/wk × 2 wk, w/ 10-day rest period (=1 cycle); ↓ dose w/ hematologic tox, neuropathy **Caution:** [D, ?/–] w/drugs CYP450 metabolized (Table 11) **Disp:** 3.5-mg vial **SE:** Asthenia, GI upset, anorexia, dyspnea, HA, orthostatic ↓ BP, edema, insomnia, dizziness, rash, pyrexia, arthralgia, neuropathy **Interactions:** ↑ Risk of peripheral neuropathy **W/** amiodarone, antivirals, INH, nitrofurantoin, statins; ↑ risk hypotension **W/** antihypertensives; ↑ effects **W/** cimetidine, clarithromycin, diltiazem, disulfiram, erythromycin, fluoxetine, propoxyphene, verapamil, zafirlukast; ↓ effects **W/** amiodarone, carbamazepine, phenobarbital, phenytoin, rifampin **Labs:** ↓ HMG, Hct, neutrophils, plts **NIPE:** ⊘ PRG or breastfeeding; use contraception; caution w/ driving due to fatigue/dizziness; ↑ fluids if C/O N/V

Botulinum Toxin Type A (Botox, Botox Cosmetic) [Neuromuscular Blocker/Neurotoxin]

Uses: *Glabellar lines (cosmetic), blepharospasm, cervical dystonia, axillary hyperhidrosis, strabismus* **Action:** ↓ Acetylcholine release from nerve endings, ↓ neuromuscular transmission and local muscle activity; neurotoxin **Dose:** *Adults:* Glabellar lines (cosmetic): 0.1 mL IM × 5 sites q3–4mo; Blepharospasm: 1.25–2.5 units IM/site q3mo; max 200 units/30 d cum dose; Cervical dystonia: 198–300 units IM divided <100 units into sternocleidomastoid; *Hyperhidrosis, axillary:* 50 units intradermal/axilla divided; *Strabismus:* 1.25–2.5 units IM/site q3mo; inject extraocular muscles w/ EMG guidance *Peds: Blepharospasm >12 y:* see Adults; *Cervical dystonia >16 y:* 198–300 units IM ÷ among affected muscles; use <100 units in sternocleidomastoid; *Strabismus >12 y:* 1.25–2.5 units IM/site q3mo; 25 units/site max; inject extraocular muscles w/ EMG guidance **Caution:** [C, ?] w/ neurologic Dz **Contra:** hypersensitivity to components, infect at inj site **Disp:** powder for reconst **SE:** Anaphylaxis, erythema multiforme, dysphagia, dyspnea, syncope, HA, NAG; **Interactions:** ↑ Effects **W/** aminoglycosides, clindamycin, lincomycin, Mg sulfate, neuromuscular blockers, quinidine; **NIPE:** may cause inj site pain

Brimonidine (Alphagan P) [Alpha Agonist/Glaucoma Agent]

Uses: *Open-angle glaucoma, ocular HTN* **Action:** α_2-Adrenergic agonist **Dose:** 1 gtt in eye(s) tid (wait 15 min to insert contacts) **Caution:** [B, ?] **Contra:** MAOI therapy **Disp:** 0.15, 0.1% soln **SE:** Local irritation, HA, fatigue; **Interactions:** ↑ Effects **OF** antihypertensives, BBs, cardiac glycosides, CNS depressants; ↓ effects **W/** TCAs **NIPE:** ⊘ EtOH, insert soft contact lenses 15 + min after drug use

Brinzolamide (Azopt) [Carbonic Anhydrase Inhibitor/Glaucoma Agent]

Uses: *Open-angle glaucoma, ocular HTN* **Action:** Carbonic anhydrase inhibitor **Dose:** 1 gtt in eye(s) tid **Caution:** [C, ?] **Contra:** Sulfonamide allergy **Disp:** 1% susp **SE:** Blurred vision, dry eye, blepharitis, taste disturbance **Interactions:** ↑ Effects **W/** oral carbonic anhydrase inhibitors **Labs:** Check LFTs, BUN, Cr **NIPE:** ⊘ Use drug if ↓ renal & hepatic studies or allergies to sulfonamides; shake well before use; insert soft contact lenses 15 + min after drug use; wait 10 min before use of other topical ophthalmic drugs

Bromocriptine (Parlodel) [Antiparkinson/Dopamine Receptor Agonist]

Uses: *Parkinson Dz, hyperprolactinemia, acromegaly, pituitary tumors* **Action:** Direct-acting on the striatal dopamine receptors; ↓ prolactin secretion **Dose:** Initial, 1.25 mg PO bid; titrate to effect, w/ food **Caution:** [B, ?] **Contra:** Severe ischemic heart Dz or PVD **Disp:** Tabs 2.5 mg; caps 5 mg **SE:** ↓ BP, Raynaud phenomenon, dizziness, N, hallucinations; **Interactions:** ↑ Effects **W/** erythromycin, fluvoxamine, nefazodone, sympathomimetics; ↓ effects **W/** phenothiazines, antipsychotics; **Labs:** ↑ BUN, AST, ALT, CPK, alkaline phosphatase, uric acid **NIPE:** ⊘ Breast-feeding, PRG, OCPs; drug may cause intolerance to EtOH, return of menses & suppression of galactorrhea may take 6–8 wk; take drug with meals

Budesonide (Rhinocort Aqua, Pulmicort) [Anti-inflammatory/Glucocorticoid]

Uses: *Allergic & nonallergic rhinitis, asthma* **Action:** Steroid **Dose:** *Adults:* Rhinocort Aqua 1–4 sprays/nostril/d; Turbuhaler 1–4 inhal bid; Pulmicort Flexhaler 1–2 inhal bid *Peds:* Rhinocort Aqua intranasal 1–2 sprays/nostril/d; Pulmicort Turbuhaler 1–2 inhal bid, Respules: 0.25–0.5 mg daily or bid (Rinse mouth after PO use) **Caution:** [C, ?/–] **Disp:** Met-dose Turbuhaler, 200 μg/inhalation; Flexhaler 90, 180 μg/inh,; Respules 0.25, 0.5 mg/2 mL;

Rhinocort Aqua 32 µg/spray **SE:** HA, cough, hoarseness, *Candida* Infxn, epistaxis **Interactions:** ↑ Effects W/ ketoconazole, itraconazole, ritonavir, indinavir, saquinavir, erythromycin, and & grapefruit juice; **NIPE:** Shake inhaler well before use, rinse mouth & wash inhaler after use, swallow capsules whole, ⊘ exposure chickenpox or measles.

Budesonide, oral (Entocort EC) [Anti-inflammatory, Corticosteroid]
Uses: *Mild-moderate Crohn Dz* **Action:** Steroid, anti-inflammatory **Dose:** *Adults:* Initial, 9 mg PO qAM to 8 wk max: maint 6 mg PO qAM taper by 3 mo; avoid grapefruit juice **Contra:** Active TB and fungal Infxn **Caution:** [C, ?/–] DM, glaucoma, cataracts, HTN, CHF **Disp:** Caps 3 mg ER **SE:** HA, cough, hoarseness, *Candida* Infxn, epistaxis; **Interactions:** ↑ effects W/ erythromycin, indinavir, itraconazole, ketoconazole, ritonavir, grapefruit; **Labs:** ↑ Alkaline phosphatase, C-reactive protein, ESR, WBC; ↓ HMG, Hct **NIPE:** Do not cut/crush/chew caps

Budesonide/formoterol (Symbicort) [Anti-inflammatory, Bronchodilator/Beta-2-Agonist]
WARNING: Long-acting β₂ agonists may ↑ risk of asthma-related death **Uses:** *Asthma maintenance* **Action:** Steroid w/ LA β₂-agonist **Dose:** *Adult and Peds. >12 y:* 2 inhal BID **Caution:** [C, ?] w/ transfer from systemic to inhal steroids **Contra:** acute attack **Disp:** Inhal 80/4.5, 160/4.5 **SE:** Allergic Rxns, HA, tremor, ↑ BP & HR, ↑ Infxn risk, throat irritation, growth ↓ in children **Interactions:** ↑ Effects W/ adrenergics; ↑ hypokalemic effects W/ cardiac glycosides, diuretics, steroids; ↑ risk of ventricular arrhythmias W/ MAOIs, TCA, quinidine, phenothiazines; ↓ effects W/ β-blockers **Labs:** ↑ Serum glucose; ↓ K⁺ **NIPE:** ⊘ EtOH

Bumetanide (Bumex) [Diuretic/Loop]
Uses: *Edema from CHF, hepatic cirrhosis, & renal Dz* **Action:** Loop diuretic; ↓ reabsorption of Na⁺ & Cl⁻, in ascending loop of Henle & the distal tubule **Dose:** *Adults.* 0.5–2 mg/d PO; 0.5–1 mg IV/IM q8–24h (max 10 mg/d) for PO and IV. *Peds.* 0.015–0.1 mg/kg/d PO, q6–24h **Caution:** [D, ?] **Contra:** Anuria, hepatic coma, severe electrolyte depletion **Disp:** Tabs 0.5, 1, 2 mg; inj 0.25 mg/mL **SE:** ↓ K⁺, ↓ Na⁺, ↑ Cr, ↑ uric acid, dizziness, ototox **Notes:** Monitor fluid & lytes **Interactions:** ↑ Effects W/ antihypertensives, thiazides, nitrates, EtOH, clofibrate; ↑ effects *OF* Li, warfarin, thrombolytic drugs, anticoagulants; ↑ K⁺ loss W/ carbenoxolone, corticosteroids, terbutaline; ↑ ototox W/ aminoglycosides, cisplatin; ↓ effects W/ cholestyramine, colestipol, NSAIDs, probenecid, barbiturates, phenytoin **Labs:** ↑ T₄, T₃, BUN, serum glucose, Cr, uric acid; ↓ serum K⁺, Ca²⁺, Mg⁺ **NIPE:** Take drug w/ food, take early to prevent nocturia, daily wt

Bupivacaine (Marcaine) [Anesthetic]
Uses: *Local, regional, & spinal anesthesia, local & regional analgesia* **Action:** Local anesthetic **Dose:** *Adults & Peds.* Dose dependent on procedure (tissue vascularity, depth of anesthesia, etc) (Table 2) **Caution:** [C, ?] **Contra:** Severe bleeding, ↓ BP, shock & arrhythmias, local Infxns at anesthesia site, septicemia **Disp:** Inj 0.25, 0.5, 0.75%

SE: ↓ BP, bradycardia, dizziness, anxiety **Interactions:** ↑ Effects *W/* BBs, hyaluronidase, ergot-type oxytocics, MAOI, TCAs, phenothiazines, vasopressors, CNS depressants; ↓ effects *W/* chloroprocaine **NIPE:** Anesthetized area has temporary loss of sensation & Fxn

Buprenorphine (Buprenex) [C-V] [Analgesic/Opioid Agonist-Antagonist] Uses: *Moderate/severe pain* **Action:** Opiate agonist-antagonist **Dose:** 0.3–0.6 mg IM or slow IV push q6h PRN **Caution:** [C, ?/–] **Disp:** 0.3 mg/mL **SE:** Sedation, ↓ BP, resp depression **Notes:** Withdrawal if opioid-dependent **Interactions:** ↑ Effects of resp & CNS depression *W/* EtOH, opiates, benzodiazepines, TCAs, MAOIs, other CNS depressants **Labs:** ↓ Alkaline phosphatase, HMG, Hct, erythrocyte count **NIPE:** ⊘ EtOH & other CNS depressants

BuPropion (Wellbutrin, Wellbutrin SR, Wellbutrin XL, Zyban) [Antidepressant/Smoking Cessation/Aminoketone]
WARNING: Closely monitor for worsening depression or emergence of suicidality, increased suicidal behavior in young adults **Uses:** *Depression, adjunct to smoking cessation* ADHD **Action:** Weak inhibitor of neuronal uptake of serotonin & norepinephrine; ↑ neuronal dopamine reuptake **Dose:** *Depression:* 100–450 mg/d ÷ bid-tid; SR 150–200 mg bid; XR 150–450 mg daily. *Smoking cessation (Zyban, Wellbutrin XR):* 150 mg/d × 3 d, then 150 mg bid × 8–12 wk, last dose not after 6 PM; ↓ renal/hepatic impair **Caution:** [C, ?/–] **Contra:** Sz disorder, h/o anorexia nervosa or bulimia, MAOI, w/in 14 d, abrupt D/C of EtOH or sedatives **Disp:** Tabs 75, 100 mg; SR tabs 50, 100, 150, 200 mg; XR tabs 150, 300 mg; Zyban 150 mg tabs **SE:** Szs, agitation, insomnia, HA, tachycardia **Notes:** Avoid EtOH and other CNS depressants, SR and XR do not cut/chew/crush **Interactions:** ↑ Effects *W/* cimetidine, levodopa, MAOIs; ↑ risk of Szs *W/* EtOH, phenothiazines, antidepressants, theophylline, TCAs, or abrupt withdrawal of corticosteroids, benzodiazepines **Labs:** ↓ Prolactin level **NIPE:** Drug may cause Szs, take 3–4 wk for full effect, ⊘ EtOH or abrupt D/C

Buspirone (BuSpar) [Anxiolytic] **WARNING:** Closely monitor for worsening depression or emergence of suicidality **Uses:** *Short-term relief of *anxiety* **Action:** Antianxiety; antagonizes CNS serotonin receptors **Dose:** Initial: 7.5 mg PO bid; ↑ by 5 mg q2–3d to effect; usual 20–30 mg/d; max 60 mg/d **Contra:** w/ MAOI **Caution:** [B, ?/–] Avoid w/ severe hepatic/renal insuff **Disp:** Tabs ÷ dose 5, 10, 15, 30 mg **SE:** Drowsiness, dizziness, HA, N, EPS, serotonin synd, hostility, depression **Notes:** No abuse potential or physical/psychologic dependence **Interactions:** ↑ Effects *W/* erythromycin, clarithromycin, itraconazole, ketoconazole, diltiazem, verapamil, grapefruit juice; ↓ effects *W/* carbamazepine, rifampin, phenytoin, dexamethasone, phenobarbital, fluoxetine **Labs:** ↑ Glucose; ↓ WBC, plts **NIPE:** ↑ Sedation w/ EtOH, therapeutic effects may take up to 4 wk

Busulfan (Myleran, Busulfex) [Antineoplastic/Alkylating Drug] Uses: *CML*, preparative regimens for allogeneic & ABMT in high doses **Action:** Alkylating agent **Dose:** (Per protocol) **Caution:** [D, ?] **Disp:** Tabs 2 mg, inj 60 mg/10 mL **SE:** ↓ BM, pulm fibrosis, N (w/ high-dose), gynecomastia, adrenal insuff, & skin hyperpigmentation **Interactions:** ↑ Effects W/ acetaminophen; ↑ BM suppression W/ antineoplastic drugs & radiation therapy; ↑ uric acid levels W/ probenecid & sulfinpyrazone; ↓ effects W/ itraconazole, phenytoin **Labs:** ↑ Glucose, ALT, bilirubin, BUN, Cr, uric acid; monitor CBC, LFTs **NIPE:** ⊘ Immunizations, PRG, breast-feeding; ↑ fluids; use barrier contraception; ↑ risk of hair loss, rash, darkened skin pigment; ↑ susceptibility to Infx

Butorphanol (Stadol) [C-IV] [Analgesic/Opiate Agonist-Antagonist] Uses: *Anesthesia adjunct, pain* & migraine HA **Action:** Opiate agonist-antagonist w/ central analgesic actions **Dose:** 1–4 mg IM or IV q3–4h PRN. *Migraine:* 1 spray in 1 nostril, repeat × 1 60–90 min, then q3–4h ↓ in renal impair **Caution:** [C (D if high dose or prolonged use at term), +] **Disp:** Inj 2 mg/mL; nasal 1 mg/spray **SE:** Drowsiness, dizziness, nasal congestion **Interactions:** ↑ Effects W/ EtOH, antihistamines, cimetidine, CNS depressants, phenothiazines, barbiturates, skeletal-muscle relaxants, MAOIs; ↓ effects OF opiates **Labs:** ↑ Serum amylase & lipase **NIPE:** ⊘ EtOH or other CNS depressants; May induce withdrawal in opioid dependency

Calcipotriene (Dovonex) [Keratolytic] Uses: *Plaque psoriasis* **Action:** Keratolytic **Dose:** Apply bid **Caution:** [C, ?] **Contra:** ↑ Ca²⁺; vitamin D tox; do not apply to face **Disp:** Cream; oint; soln 0.005% **SE:** Skin irritation, dermatitis **Interactions:** None noted **Labs:** Monitor serum Ca **NIPE:** Wash hands after application or wear gloves to apply, D/C drug if ↑ Ca

Calcitonin (Fortical, Miacalcin) [Hypocalcemic, Bone Resorption Inhibitor/Thyroid Hormone] Uses: *Paget Dz of bone, ↑ Ca²⁺, osteogenesis imperfecta, *postmenopausal osteoporosis* **Action:** Polypeptide hormone **Dose:** *Paget Dz:* 100 units/d IM/SC initial, 50 units/d or 50–100 units q1–3d maint. ↑ Ca²⁺ 4 units/kg IM/SC q12h; ↑ to 8 units/kg q12h, max q6h. *Osteoporosis:* 100 units/qod IM/SQ; intranasal 200 units = 1 nasal spray/d **Caution:** [C, ?] **Disp:** Spray, nasal 200 units/activation; inj, salmon 200 units/mL (2 mL) **SE:** Facial flushing, N, inj site edema, nasal irritation, polyuria **Notes:** For nasal spray alternate nostrils daily; **Interactions:** Prior treatment w/ alendronate, risedronate, etidronate or pamidronate may ↓ effects of calcitonin **Labs:** ↓ Serum Li; monitor serum Ca and alkaline phosphatase **NIPE:** Allergy skin test prior to use; take at bedtime to <N/V; flushing > inj is transient; nausea > inj will < w/ continued treatment

Calcitriol (Rocaltrol, Calcijex) [Antihypocalcemic/Vitamin D Analog] Uses: *Reduction of ↑ PTH levels, ↓ Ca²⁺ on dialysis* **Action:** 1,25-Dihydroxycholecalciferol (vitamin D analog) **Dose:** *Adults. Renal failure:* 0.25 μg/d PO, ↑ 0.25 μg/d q4–6wk PRN; 0.5 μg 3 ×/wk IV, ↑ PRN. *Hypoparathyroidism:* 0.5–2 μg/d. **Peds.** *Renal failure:* 15 ng/kg/d, ↑ PRN; maint 30–60 ng/kg/d. *Hypoparathyroidism:* <5 y, 0.25–0.75 μg/d. >6 y: 0.5–2 μg/d **Caution:** [C, ?] **Contra:** ↑ Ca²⁺; vitamin D tox **Disp:** Inj 1, 2 μg/mL (in 1-mL); caps 0.25, 0.5 μg;

sol 1 μg/mL **SE:** ↑ Ca^{2+} **Interactions:** ↑ Effect *W/* thiazide diuretics; ↓ effect *W/* cholestyramine, colestipol, ketoconazole **Labs:** Monitor for ↑ Ca^{2+}, cholesterol, BUN, AST, ALT; ↓ alkaline phosphatase **NIPE:** ⊘ Mg-containing antacids or supls

Calcium Acetate (PhosLo) [Calcium Supplement, Anti-Arrhythmic/Mineral, Electrolyte] Uses: *ESRD-associated hyperphosphatemia* **Action:** Ca^{2+} supl w/o aluminum to ↓ PO_4^{2-} absorption **Dose:** 2–4 tabs PO w/ meals **Caution:** [C, ?] **Contra:** ↑ Ca^{2+} **Disp:** Gelcap 667 mg **SE:** Can ↑ Ca^{2+}, hypophosphatemia, constipation **Interactions:** ↑ Effects *OF* quinidine; ↓ effects *W/* large intake of dietary fiber, spinach, rhubarb; ↓ effects *OF* atenolol, CCB, etidronate, tetracyclines, fluoroquinolones, phenytoin, Fe salts, thyroid hormones **Labs:** Monitor for ↑ Ca^{2+}; ↓ Mg2+ **NIPE:** ⊘ EtOH, caffeine, tobacco; separate Ca supls and other meds by 1–2 h

Calcium Carbonate (Tums, Alka-Mints) [Antacid, Calcium Supplement/Mineral, Electrolyte] [OTC] Uses: *Hyperacidity associated w/ peptic ulcer Dz, hiatal hernia, etc* **Action:** Neutralizes gastric acid **Dose:** 500 mg–2 g PO PRN; ↓ in renal impair **Caution:** [C, ?] **Disp:** Chew tabs 350, 420, 500, 550, 750, 850 mg; susp **SE:** ↑ Ca^{2+}, ↓PO^{-4} constipation **Interactions:** ↑ Effect *OF* tetracyclines, fluoroquinolones, Fe salts, & ASA; ↓ Ca absorption *W/* high intake of dietary fiber **Labs:** Monitor for ↑ Ca^{2+}, ↓ Mg^{2+} **NIPE:** ↑ Fluids, may cause constipation, ⊘ EtOH, caffeine, tobacco; separate Ca supls and other meds by 1–2 h, chew tabs well

Calcium Glubionate (Neo-Calglucon) [OTC] [Calcium Supplement, Anti-Arrhythmic/Mineral, Electrolyte] Uses: *Rx & prevent Ca deficiency* **Action:** Ca^{2+} supl **Dose:** *Adults.* 6–18 g/d ÷ doses. *Peds.* 600–2000 mg/kg/d ÷ qid (9 g/d max); ↓ in renal impair **Caution:** [C, ?] **Contra:** ↑ Ca^{2+} **Disp:** OTC syrup 1.8 g/5 mL = elemental Ca 115 mg/5 mL **SE:** ↑ Ca^{2+}, ↓ PO^{-4} constipation; **Interactions:** ↑ Effects *OF* quinidine; ↓ effect *OF* tetracyclines; ↓ Ca absorption *W/* high intake of dietary fiber **Labs:** ↑ Ca^{2+}, ↓ Mg^{2+} **NIPE:** ⊘ EtOH, caffeine, tobacco, separate Ca supls and other meds by 1–2 h

Calcium Salts (Chloride, Gluconate, Gluceptate) [Calcium Supplement, Anti-Arrhythmic/Mineral, Electrolyte] Uses: *Ca^{2+} replacement*, VF, Ca^{2+} blocker tox, Mg^{2+} intox, tetany, *hyperphosphatemia in ESRD* **Action:** Ca^{2+} supl/replacement **Dose:** *Adults. Replacement:* 1–2 g/d PO. *Tetany:* 1 g CaCl over 10–30 min; repeat in 6 h PRN; *Hyperkalemia/calcium channel blocker overdose:* 8–16 mg/kg (usually 5–10 mL) IV; 2–4 mg/kg (usually 2 mL) IV before IV Ca blockers *(ECC 2005).* *Peds. Replacement:* 200–500 mg/kg/24 h PO or IV ÷ qid. *Cardiac emergency:* 100 mg/kg/dose IV gluconate salt q10min. *Tetany:* 10 mg/kg CaCl over 5–10 min; repeat in 6 h or use inf (200 mg/kg/d max). *Adult & Peds.* ↓ Ca^{2+} due to citrated blood inf: 0.45 mEq Ca/100 mL citrated blood inf (↓ in renal impair) **Caution:** [C, ?] **Contra:** ↑ Ca^{2+} **Disp:** CaCl inj 10% = 100 mg/mL = Ca 27.2 mg/mL = 10-mL amp; Ca gluconate inj 10% = 100 mg/mL = Ca 9 mg/mL; tabs 500 mg = 45 mg Ca, 650 mg = 58.5 mg Ca,

975 mg = 87.75 mg Ca, 1 g = 90 mg Ca; Ca gluceptate inj 220 mg/mL = 18 mg/mL Ca SE: Bradycardia, cardiac arrhythmias, $\uparrow Ca^{2+}$ **Notes:** CaCl 270 mg (13.6 mEq) elemental Ca/g, & calcium gluconate 90 mg (4.5 mEq) Ca/g. **RDA for Ca:** Adults = 800 mg/d; Peds = <6 mo, 360 mg/d, 6 mo–1 y, 540 mg/d, 1–10 y, 800 mg/d, 10–18 y, 1200 mg/d **Interactions:** $\uparrow$ Effects *OF* quinidine and digitalis; $\downarrow$ effects *OF* tetracyclines, quinolones, verapamil, CCBs, Fe salts, ASA, atenolol; $\downarrow$ Ca absorption *W/* high intake of dietary fiber **Labs:** Monitor for $\uparrow Ca^{2+}$, $\downarrow Mg^{2+}$ **NIPE:** $\bigcirc$ EtOH, caffeine, tobacco; separate Ca supls and other meds by 1–2 h

Calfactant (Infasurf) [RDS Agent/Surfactant] Uses: *Prevention & Rx of RSD in infants* **Action:** Exogenous pulm surfactant **Dose:** 3 mL/kg instilled into lungs. Can retreat for a total of 3 doses given 12 h apart **Caution:** [?, ?] **Disp:** Intratracheal susp 35 mg/mL **SE:** Monitor for cyanosis, airway obst, bradycardia during administration **Interactions:** None noted **NIPE:** Only for intratracheal use; $\bigcirc$ Reconstitute, dilute, or shake vial; refrigerate & keep away from light; no need to warm soln prior to use

Candesartan (Atacand) [Antihypertensive/ARB] Uses: *HTN*, DN, CHF **Action:** Angiotensin II receptor antagonist **Dose:** Z-32 mg/d (usual 16 mg/d) **Caution:** [C (1st tri), D (2nd & 3rd tri), –] **Contra:** Primary hyperaldosteronism; bilateral RAS **Disp:** Tabs 4, 8, 16, 32 mg **SE:** Dizziness, HA, flushing, angioedema **Interactions:** $\uparrow$ Effects *W/* cimetidine; $\uparrow$ risk of hyperkalemia *W/* amiloride, spironolactone, triamterene, K supls, trimethoprim; $\uparrow$ effects *OF* Li; $\downarrow$ effects *W/* phenobarbital, rifampin **Labs:** $\uparrow$ BUN, Cr, K^+, LFTs, uric acid; monitor for albuminuria, hyperglycemia, triglyceridemia, uricemia **NIPE:** $\bigcirc$ Breast-feeding or PRG, use barrier contraception, may take 4–6 wk for full effect, adequate fluid intake, take w/o regard to food

Capsaicin (Capsin, Zostrix, others) [OTC] [Topical Anesthetic/ Analgesic] Uses: Pain due to *postherpetic neuralgia*, chronic neuralgia, *arthritis, diabetic neuropathy*, postop pain, psoriasis, intractable pruritus **Action:** Topical analgesic **Dose:** Apply tid-qid **Caution:** [C, ?] **Disp:** OTC creams; gel; lotions; roll-ons **SE:** Local irritation, neurotox, cough **Note:** Weeks to onset of action **Interactions:** May $\uparrow$ cough *W/* ACEIs **NIPE:** External use only, $\bigcirc$ contact w/ eyes or broken/irritated skin, apply w/ gloves, transient stinging/burning

Captopril (Capoten, others) [Antihypertensive/ACEI] Uses: *HTN, CHF, MI*, LVD, DN **Action:** ACE inhibitor **Dose:** *Adults. HTN:* Initial, 25 mg PO bid-tid; $\uparrow$ to maint q1–2wk by 25-mg increments/dose (max 450 mg/d) to effect. *CHF:* Initial, 6.25–12.5 mg PO tid; titrate PRN. *LVD:* 50 mg PO tid. *DN:* 25 mg PO tid. *Peds. Infants <2 mo:* 0.05–0.5 mg/kg/dose PO q8–24h. *Children:* Initial, 0.3–0.5 mg/kg/dose PO; $\uparrow$ to 6 mg/kg/d max in 2–4 divided doses; 1 h before meals **Caution:** [C (1st tri); D (2nd & 3rd tri) +]; unknown effects in renal impair **Contra:** h/o angioedema, bilateral RAS **Disp:** Tabs 12.5, 25, 50, 100 mg **SE:** Rash, proteinuria, cough, $\uparrow K^+$ **Interactions:** $\uparrow$ Effects *W/* antihypertensives, diuretics, nitrates, probenecid, black catechu; $\downarrow$ effects *W/* antacids, ASA, NSAIDs, food; ↑ effects *OF* digoxin, insulin, oral hypoglycemics, Li **Labs:** False + urine acetone; may ↑ urine protein, serum BUN, Cr, K⁺, prolactin, LFTs; may ↓ HMG, Hct, RBC, WBC, plt **NIPE:** ⊘ PRG, breast-feeding, K-sparing diuretics; take w/o food, give 1 h < meals; may take 2 wk for full therapeutic effect

Carbamazepine (Tegretol XR, Carbatrol, Epitol) [Anticonvulsant/Analgesic]   WARNING: Aplastic anemia & agranulocytosis have been reported w/ carbamazepine **Uses:** *Epilepsy, trigeminal neuralgia*, EtOH withdrawal **Action:** Anticonvulsant **Dose:** *Adults.* Initial, 200 mg PO bid; or 100 mg 4 ×/d as susp; ↑ by 200 mg/d; usual 800–1200 mg/d ÷ doses. *Peds. <6 y:* 5 mg/kg/d, ↑ to 10–20 mg/kg/d ÷ in 2–4 doses. *6–12 y:* Initial, 100 mg PO bid or 10 mg/kg/24 h PO ÷ daily-bid; ↑ to maint 20–30 mg/kg/24 h ÷ tid-qid; ↓ in renal impair; take w/ food **Caution:** [D, +] **Contra:** MAOI use, h/o BM suppression **Disp:** Tabs 100, 200, 300, 400 mg; chew tabs 100 mg, 200 mg; XR tabs 100, 200, 400 mg; caps ER 100, 200, 300 mg; susp 100 mg/5 mL SE: Drowsiness, dizziness, blurred vision, N/V, rash, ↓ Na⁺, leukopenia, agranulocytosis **Notes:** *Trough:* Just before next dose. *Therapeutic: Peak* 8–12 μg/mL (monotherapy), 4–8 (polytherapy). *Toxic trough* > 12 μg/mL. *1/2 life:* 15–20 h; generic products not interchangeable, administer susp in 3–4 ÷ doses daily **Interactions:** ↑ Effects *W/* cimetidine, clarithromycin, danazol, diltiazem, felbamate, fluconazole, fluoxetine, fluvoxamine, INH, itraconazole, ketoconazole, macrolides, metronidazole, propoxyphene, protease inhibitors, valproic acid, verapamil, grapefruit juice; ↑ effects *OF* Li, MAOIs; ↓ effects *W/* phenobarbital, phenytoin, primidone, plantain; ↓ effects *OF* benzodiazepines, corticosteroids, cyclosporine, doxycycline, felbamate, haloperidol, OCPs, phenytoin, theophylline, thyroid hormones, TCAs, warfarin **Labs:** ↑ BUN, eosinophil count; ↓ HMG, Hct, WBC, plts, LFTs, thyroid hormones **NIPE:** Take w/ food; may cause photosensitivity—use sunscreen; use barrier contraception; abrupt withdrawal may cause Sz; ⊘ breast-feeding or PRG

Carbidopa/Levodopa (Sinemet, Parcopa) [Antiparkinsonian/Dopamine Agonist]   **Uses:** *Parkinson Dz* **Action:** ↑ CNS dopamine levels **Dose:** 25/100 mg bid-qid; ↑ as needed (max 200/2000 mg/d) **Caution:** [C, ?] **Contra:** NAG, suspicious skin lesion (may activate melanoma), melanoma, MAOI use **Disp:** Tabs (mg carbidopa/mg levodopa) 10/100, 25/100, 25/250; tabs SR (mg carbidopa/mg levodopa) 25/100, 50/200; ODT (oral disintegrating tab) 10/100, 25/100, 25/250. **SE:** Psychiatric disturbances, orthostatic ↓ BP, dyskinesias, cardiac arrhythmias **Interactions:** ↑ Risk of hypotension *W/* antihypertensives; ↑ risk of HTN *W/* MAOIs; ↑ effects *W/* antacids; ↓ effects *W/* anticholinergics, anticonvulsants, benzodiazepines, haloperidol, Fe, methionine, papaverine, phenothiazines, phenytoin, pyridoxine, reserpine, spiramycin, tacrine, thioxanthenes, high-protein food **Labs:** ↑ Alkaline phosphatase, aspartate aminotransferase, bilirubin, BUN, uric acid ↓ HMG, plts, WBCs **NIPE:** Darkened urine & sweat may result, ⊘ crush or chew SR tabs, take w/o food; muscle or eyelid twitching may suggest tox

Carboplatin (Paraplatin) [Antineoplastic/Alkylating Agent]

WARNING: Administration only by provider experienced in cancer chemotherapy; BM suppression possible, Anaphylaxis may occur **Uses:** *Ovarian*, lung, head & neck, testicular, urothelial, & brain *CA, NHL* & allogeneic ABMT in high doses **Action:** DNA cross-linker; forms DNA-platinum adducts **Dose:** 360 mg/m^2 (ovarian carcinoma); AUC dosing 4–7 mg/mL (Culvert formula: mg = AUC × [25 + calculated GFR]); adjust based on plt count, CrCl, & BSA (Egorin formula); up to 1500 mg/m^2 used in ABMT setting (per protocols) **Caution:** [D, ?] **Contra:** Severe BM suppression, excessive bleeding **Disp:** Inj 50, 150, 450 mg vial (10 mg/mL) **SE:** Anaphylaxis, ↓ BM, N/V/D, nephrotox, hematuria, neurotox, **Notes:** Physiologic dosing based on Culvert or Egorin formula allows ↑ doses w/ ↓ tox **Interactions:** ↑ Myelosuppression W/ myelosuppressive drugs; ↑ hematologic effects W/ BM suppressants; ↑ bleeding W/ ASA; ↑ nephrotox W/ nephrotoxic drugs; ↓ effects *OF* phenytoin **Labs:** Monitor for ↑ LFTs, BUN, Cr; ↓ Mg^{2+}, K$^+$, Na$^+$, Ca^{2+}, HMG, Hct, neutrophils, plts, RBC, WBC **NIPE:** ⊘ Use w/ Al needles or IV administration sets, PRG, breast-feeding; antiemetics prior to admin may prevent N/V, maintain adequate food & fluid intake

Carisoprodol (Soma) [Skeletal Muscle Relaxant/Carbamate Derivative]

Uses: *Adjunct to sleep & physical therapy to relieve painful musculoskeletal conditions* **Action:** Centrally acting skeletal muscle relaxant **Dose:** 350 mg PO tid-qid **Caution:** [C, M] Tolerance may result; w/ renal/hepatic impair **Contra:** Allergy to meprobamate; acute intermittent porphyria **Disp:** Tabs 350 mg **SE:** CNS depression, drowsiness, dizziness, tachycardia **Interactions:** ↑ Effects W/ CNS depressants, phenothiazines, EtOH **NIPE:** Avoid EtOH & other CNS depressants; available in combo w/ ASA or codeine; ⊘ breast-feeding; take w/ food if GI upset

Carmustine [BCNU] (BiCNU, Gliadel) [Antineoplastic, Alkylating Agent]

Uses: *Primary brain tumors, melanoma, Hodgkin lymphoma & NHLs, multiple myeloma, & induction for allogeneic & ABMT in high doses; adjunct to surgery in pts w/ recurrent glioblastoma* **Action:** Alkylating agent; nitrosourea forms DNA cross-links to inhibit DNA **Dose:** 150–200 mg/m^2 q6–8wk single or ÷ dose daily inj over 2 d; 20–65 mg/m^2 q4–6wk; 300–900 mg/m^2 in BMT (per protocols) **Caution:** [D, ?] Renal/hepatic impair **Contra:** ↓ BM, PRG **Disp:** Inj 100 mg/vial; wafer: 7.7 mg **SE:** ↓BP, N/V, ↓ WBC & plt, phlebitis, facial flushing, hepatic/renal dysfunction, pulm fibrosis, optic neuroretinitis; hematologic tox may persist 4–6 wk after dose **Notes:** Do not give course more frequently than q6wk (cumulative tox) **Interactions:** ↑ Bleeding W/ ASA, anticoagulants, NSAIDs; ↑ hepatic dysfunction W/ etoposide; ↑ suppression of BM W/ cimetidine, radiation or additional antineoplastics; ↓ effects *OF* phenytoin, digoxin; ↓ pulmonary Fxn **Labs:** ↑ AST, alkaline phosphatase, bilirubin; ↓ HMG, Hct, WBC, RBC, plt counts; monitor PFTs **NIPE:** ⊘ PRG, breast-feeding, exposure to Infxns, ASA products; ✓ baseline PFTs

Carteolol (Cartrol, Ophthalmic) [Beta-Blocker/Glaucoma Agent] Uses: *HTN, ↑ intraocular pressure, chronic open-angle glaucoma* **Action:** Blocks β-adrenergic receptors (β₁, β₂), mild ISA **Dose:** Ophth 1 gt in eye(s) bid **Caution:** [C (1st tri); D (2nd & 3rd tri), ?/–] Cardiac failure, asthma **Contra:** Sinus bradycardia; heart block >1st degree; bronchospasm **Disp:** Ophth soln 1% **SE:** Drowsiness, sexual dysfunction, bradycardia, edema, CHF; ocular: conjunctival hyperemia, anisocoria, keratitis, eye pain; **Interactions:** ↑ Effects W/ amiodarone, adenosine, barbiturates, CCBs, clonidine, digoxin, dipyridamole, fluoxetine, rifampin, tacrine, nitrates, EtOH; ↑ α-adrenergic effects W/ amphetamines, cocaine, ephedrine, epinephrine, phenylephrine; ↑ effects OF theophylline; ↓ effects W/ antacids, NSAIDs, thyroid drugs; ↓ effects OF hypoglycemics, theophylline, dopamine **Labs:** ↑ BUN, uric acid, K⁺, serum lipoprotein, triglycerides, glucose **NIPE:** Ophthalmic drug may cause photophobia & risk of burning; may ↑ cold sensitivity, mental confusion; no value in CHF

Carvedilol (Coreg, Coreg CR) [Antihypertensive/Alpha-1- & Beta-Blocker] Uses: *HTN, mild to severe CHF, LV dysfunction post MI* **Action:** Blocks adrenergic receptors, β₁, β₂, a₁ **Dose:** HTN: 6.25–12.5 mg bid. CHF: 3.125–25 mg bid; w/ food to minimize ↓ BP **Caution:** [C (1st tri); D (2nd & 3rd tri), ?/–] asthma, DM **Contra:** Decompensated CHF, 2nd-/3rd-degree heart block, SSS, severe bradycardia w/o pacemaker, asthma, severe hepatic impair **Disp:** Tabs 3.125, 6.25, 12.5, 25 mg **SE:** Dizziness, fatigue, hyperglycemia, may mask/potentiate hypoglycemia, bradycardia, edema, hypercholesterolemia **Interactions:** ↑ Effects W/ cimetidine, clonidine, MAOIs, reserpine, verapamil, fluoxetine, paroxetine, EtOH; ↑ effects OF digoxin, hypoglycemics, cyclosporine, CCBs; ↓ effects W/ rifampin, NSAIDs **Labs:** ↑ LFTs, K⁺, triglycerides, uric acid, BUN, Cr, alkaline phosphatase, glucose; ↓ pt, INR, plts **NIPE:** Do not D/C abruptly; food slows absorption but reduces risk of dizziness; may cause dry eyes w/ contact lenses

Caspofungin (Cancidas) [Antifungal/Echinocandin] Uses: *Invasive aspergillosis refractory/intolerant to standard therapy, esophageal candidiasis* **Action:** Echinocandin; ↓ fungal cell wall synth; highest activity in regions of active cell growth **Dose:** 70 mg IV load day 1, 50 mg/d IV; slow inf; ↓ in hepatic impair **Caution:** [C, ?/–] Do not use w/ cyclosporine; not studied as initial therapy **Contra:** Allergy to any component **Disp:** Inj 50, 70 mg powder for reconsti **SE:** Fever, HA, N/V, thrombophlebitis at site **Interactions:** ↑ Effects W/ cyclosporine; ↓ effects W/ carbamazepine, dexamethasone, efavirenz, nelfinavir nevirapine, phenytoin, rifampin; ↓ effect OF tacrolimus **Labs:** ↑ LFTs, serum alkaline phosphatase, eosinophils, PT, urine protein & RBCs; ↓ K⁺, Hgb, Hct **NIPE:** Monitor during inf; infuse slowly over 1 h & ⊘ mix w/ other drugs; limited experience beyond 2 wk of therapy

Cefaclor (Ceclor, Raniclor) [Antibiotic/Cephalosporin-2nd Generation] Uses: *Bacterial Infxns of the upper & lower resp tract, skin, bone, urinary tract, abdomen, gynecologic system* **Action:** 2nd-gen cephalosporin; ↓ cell wall synth

Spectrum: More gram(–) activity than 1st-gen cephalosporins; effective against gram(+) (*S. aureus*); good gram(–) coverage against *H. influenzae* **Dose:** *Adults.* 250–500 mg PO tid; XR 375–500 mg bid. **Peds.** 20–40 mg/kg/d PO ÷ 8–12 h; ↓ renal impair **Caution:** [B, +] **Contra:** Cephalosporin allergy **Disp:** Caps 250, 500 mg; Tabs ER 375, 500 mg chew tabs 125, 187, 250, 375 mg; susp 125, 187, 250, 375 mg/5 mL **SE:** D, rash, eosinophilia, ↑ transaminases **Interactions:** ↑ Bleeding **W/** anticoagulants; ↑ nephrotox **W/** aminoglycosides, loop diuretics; ↑ effects **W/** probenecid; ↓ effects **W/** antacids, chloramphenicol **Labs:** ↑ LFTs, alkaline phosphatase, bilirubin, BUN, Cr; ↓ Hgb, Hct, plts, WBC; false + direct Coombs test **NIPE:** Take w/ food to <GI upset; monitor for super Infxn, ⊘ antacids within 2 hr of XR tabs

Cefadroxil (Duricef) [Antibiotic/Cephalosporin-1st Generation]
Uses: *Infxns of skin, bone, upper & lower resp tract, urinary tract* **Action:** 1st-gen cephalosporin; ↓ cell wall synth. *Spectrum:* Good gram(+) coverage (group A β-hemolytic *Streptococcus, Staphylococcus*); gram(–) (*E. coli, Proteus, Klebsiella*) **Dose:** *Adults.* 1–2 g/d PO, 2 ÷ doses **Peds.** 30 mg/kg/d ÷ bid; ↓ in renal impair **Caution:** [B, +] **Contra:** Cephalosporin allergy **Disp:** Caps 500 mg; tabs 1 g; susp 125, 250, 500 mg/5 mL **SE:** N/V/D, rash, eosinophilia **Interactions:** ↑ Nephrotox **W/** aminoglycosides, loop diuretics; ↑ effects **W/** probenecid **Labs:** ↑ LFTs, alkaline phosphatase, bilirubin, LDH, GGT, eosinophils, BUN, Cr; ↓ Hgb, Hct, plts, WBC false + direct Coombs test **NIPE:** Take w/ food to <GI upset; monitor for super Infxn

Cefazolin (Ancef, Kefzol) [Antibiotic/Cephalosporin-1st Generation]
Uses: * Infxns of skin, bone, upper & lower resp tract, urinary tract* **Action:** 1st-gen cephalosporin; ↓ cell wall synth. *Spectrum:* Good coverage gram(+) bacilli & cocci, (*Streptococcus, Staphylococcus* [except *Enterococcus*]); some gram(–) (*E. coli, Proteus, Klebsiella*) **Dose:** *Adults.* 1–2 g IV q8h **Peds.** 25–100 mg/kg/d IV ÷ q6–8h; ↓ in renal impair **Caution:** [B, +] **Contra:** Cephalosporin allergy **Disp:** Inj: 500 mg, 1, 10, 20 g **SE:** D, rash, eosinophilia, ↑ LFT, inj site pain **Notes:** Widely used for surgical prophylaxis **Interactions:** ↑ Bleeding **W/** anticoagulants; ↑ nephrotox **W/** aminoglycosides, loop diuretics; ↑ effects **W/** probenecid; ↓ effects **W/** antacids, chloramphenicol **Labs:** ↑ LFTs, alkaline phosphatase, bilirubin, LDH, GGT, eosinophils, BUN, Cr; false + direct Coombs test **NIPE:** take w/ food to <GI upset; monitor for super Infxn; monitor renal Fxn

Cefdinir (Omnicef) [Antibiotic/Cephalosporin-3rd Generation]
Uses: *Infxns of the resp tract, skin, bone, & urinary tract* **Action:** 3rd-gen cephalosporin; ↓ cell wall synth. *Spectrum:* Many gram(+) & (–) organisms; more active than cefaclor & cephalexin against *Streptococcus, Staphylococcus*; some anaerobes **Dose:** *Adults.* 300 mg PO bid or 600 mg/d PO. **Peds.** 7 mg/kg PO bid or 14 mg/kg/d PO; ↓ in renal impair **Caution:** [B, +] w/ PCN-sensitive pts, serum sicknesslike Rxns reported **Contra:** Hypersensitivity to cephalosporins **Disp:** Caps 300 mg; susp 125, 250 mg/5 mL **SE:** Anaphylaxis, D, rare pseudomembranous

colitis **Interactions:** ↑ Bleeding **W/** anticoagulants; ↑ nephrotox **W/** aminoglycosides, loop diuretics; ↑ effects **W/** probenecid; ↓ effects **W/** antacids, chloramphenicol; ↓ effects **W/** Fe supls **Labs:** ↑ LFTs, alkaline phosphatase, bilirubin, LDH, GGT, eosinophils, BUN, Cr; ↓ HMG, Hct, plts, WBC; false + direct Coombs test **NIPE:** Take w/ food to <GI upset; monitor for super Infxn; stools may initially turn red in color; instruct pt to report persistant diarrhea; ⊘ antacids within 2 h of this drug; suspension contains sugar

Cefditoren (Spectracef) [Antibiotic/Cephalosporin-3rd Generation] Uses: *Acute exacerbations of chronic bronchitis, pharyngitis, tonsillitis; skin Infxns* **Action:** 3rd-gen cephalosporin; ↓ cell wall synth. *Spectrum:* Good gram(+) (*Streptococcus* & *Staphylococcus*); gram(−) (*H. influenzae, M. catarrhalis*) **Dose:** *Adults & Peds >12 y: Skin:* 200 mg PO bid × 10 d. *Chronic bronchitis, pharyngitis, tonsillitis:* 400 mg PO bid × 10 d; avoid antacids w/in 2 h; take w/ meals; ↓ in renal impair **Caution:** [B, ?] Renal/hepatic impair **Contra:** Cephalosporin/PCN allergy, milk protein, or carnitine deficiency **Disp:** 200-mg tabs **SE:** HA, N/V/D, colitis, nephrotox, hepatic dysfunction, Stevens-Johnson synd, toxic epidermal necrolysis, allergic Rxns **Notes:** Causes renal excretion of carnitine; tablets contain milk protein **Interactions:** ↑ Bleeding **W/** anticoagulants; ↑ nephrotox **W/** aminoglycosides, loop diuretics; ↑ effects **W/** probenecid; ↓ effects **W/** antacids, chloramphenicol **Labs:** ↑ LFTs, Hct, PT; false + direct Coombs test **NIPE:** High-fat meal will increase bioavailability; monitor for super Infxn; report persistent D; ⊘ antacids within 2 h of this drug;

Cefepime (Maxipime) [Antibiotic/Cephalosporin-4th Generation] Uses: *UTI, pneumonia, febrile neutropenia, skin/soft tissue Infxns* **Action:** 4th-gen cephalosporin; ↓ cell wall synth. *Spectrum:* gram(+) *S. pneumoniae, S. aureus,* gram(−) *K. pneumoniae, E. coli, P. aeruginosa, Enterobacter* sp **Dose:** *Adults.* 1–2 g IV q6-12h. *Peds.* 50 mg/kg q8h for febrile neutropenia; 50 mg/kg bid for skin/soft tissue Infxns; ↓ in renal impair **Caution:** [B, +] **Contra:** Cephalosporin allergy **Disp:** Inj 500 mg, 1, 2 g **SE:** Rash, pruritus, N/V/D, fever, HA, (+) direct Coombs test w/o hemolysis **Notes:** Give IM or IV **Interactions:** ↑ Nephrotox **W/** aminoglycosides, loop diuretics; ↑ effects **W/** probenecid **Labs:** ↑ LFTs; ↓ HMG, Hct, PT; false + direct Coombs test **NIPE:** Monitor for super Infxn; report persistent D; monitor inf site for inflammation

Cefixime (Suprax) [Antibiotic/Cephalosporin-3rd Generation] Uses: *Infxns of the resp tract, skin, bone, & urinary tract* **Action:** 3rd-gen cephalosporin; ↓ cell wall synth. *Spectrum: S. pneumoniae, S. pyogenes, H. influenzae,* & Enterobacteriaceae **Dose:** *Adults.* 400 mg PO daily-bid. *Peds.* 8–20 mg/kg/d PO ÷ daily-bid; ↓ in renal impair **Caution:** [B, +] **Contra:** Cephalosporin allergy **Disp:** Susp 100 mg/5 mL, 200 mg/5 mL **SE:** N/V/D, flatulence, & abd pain **Notes:** Monitor renal & hepatic Fxn; use susp for otitis media **Interactions:** ↑ Nephrotox **W/** aminoglycosides, loop diuretics; ↑ effects **W/** nifedipine, probenecid **Labs:** ↑ LFTs, alkaline phosphatase, bilirubin, LDH, GGt, eosinophils, BUN, Cr;

↓ HMG, Hct, plts, WBC; false + direct Coombs test **NIPE:** monitor for super Infxn; after mixing suspension it is stable for 14 d without refrigeration

Cefoperazone (Cefobid) [Antibiotic/Cephalosporin-3rd Generation]

Uses: *Rx Infxns of the resp, skin, urinary tract, sepsis* **Action:** 3rd-gen cephalosporin; ↓ bacterial cell wall synth. *Spectrum:* Gram(−) (eg, *E. coli*, *Klebsiella* sp), *P. aeruginosa* but < ceftazidime; gram(+) variable against *Streptococcus* & *Staphylococcus* sp **Dose:** *Adults.* 2–4 g/d IM/IV ÷ q8–12h (12 g/d max). *Peds.* (Not approved) 100–150 mg/kg/d IM/IV ÷ bid-tid (12 g/d max); ↓ in renal/hepatic impair **Caution:** [B, +] May ↑ bleeding risk **Contra:** Cephalosporin allergy **Disp:** Powder for inj 1, 2, 10 g **SE:** D, rash, eosinophilia, ↑ LFTs, hypoprothrombinemia, & bleeding (due to MTT side chain) **Notes:** May interfere w/ warfarin **Interactions:** ↑ Bleeding *W/* anticoagulants; ↑ nephrotox *W/* aminoglycosides, loop diuretics **Labs:** ↑ LFTs, eosinophils, BUN, Cr; ↓ HMG, Hct, plts; **NIPE:** Monitor for super Infxn

Cefotaxime (Claforan) [Antibiotic/Cephalosporin-3rd Generation]

Uses: *Rx Infxns of resp tract, skin, bone, urinary tract, meningitis, sepsis* **Action:** 3rd-gen cephalosporin; ↓ cell wall synth. *Spectrum:* Most gram(−) (not *Pseudomonas* sp), some gram(+) cocci (not *Enterococcus* sp); many PCN-resistant pneumococci **Dose:** *Adults.* 1–2 g IV q4–12h. *Peds.* 50–200 mg/kg/d IV ÷ q 4–12h; ↓ dose renal/hepatic impair **Caution:** [B, +] Arrhythmia w/ rapid inj; w/ colitis **Contra:** Cephalosporin allergy **Disp:** Powder for inj 500 mg, 1, 2, 10, 20 g, premixed inf 20 mg/mL, 40 mg/mL **SE:** D, rash, pruritus, colitis, eosinophilia, ↑ transaminases **Interactions:** ↑ Nephrotox *W/* aminoglycosides, loop diuretics; ↓ effects *W/* probenecid **Labs:** ↑ LFTs, alkaline phosphatase, bilirubin, LDH, GGt, eosinophils, BUN, Cr; ↓ HMG, Hct, plts, WBC **NIPE:** Monitor for super Infxn; IM inj deep into large muscle mass; rotate infusion sites

Cefotetan (Cefotan) [Antibiotic/Cephalosporin-2nd Generation]

Uses: *Rx Infxns of the upper & lower resp tract, skin, bone, urinary tract, abdomen, & gynecologic system* **Action:** 2nd-gen cephalosporin; ↓ cell wall synth. *Spectrum:* Less active against gram(+); anaerobes including *B. fragilis*; gram(−), including *E. coli*, *Klebsiella* sp, *Proteus* sp **Dose:** *Adults.* 1–3 g IV q12h. *Peds.* 20–40 mg/kg/divided IV ÷ q12h; ↓ w/ renal impair **Caution:** [B, +] May ↑ bleeding risk; w/ h/o of PCN allergies, w/ other nephrotoxic drugs **Contra:** Cephalosporin allergy **Disp:** Powder for inj 1, 2, 10 g **SE:** D, rash, eosinophilia, ↑ transaminases, hypoprothrombinemia, & bleeding (due to MTT side chain) **Notes:** May interfere w/ warfarin **Interactions:** ↑ Bleeding *W/* anticoagulants; ↑ nephrotox *W/* aminoglycosides, loop diuretics **Labs:** ↑ LFTs, eosinophils; ↓ HMG, Hct, plts **NIPE:** Monitor for super Infxn; rotate inf sites

Cefoxitin (Mefoxin) [Antibiotic/Cephalosporin-2nd Generation]

Uses: *Rx Infxns of the upper & lower resp tract, skin, bone, urinary tract, abdomen, & gynecologic system* **Action:** 2nd-gen cephalosporin; ↓ cell wall synth. *Spectrum:* Good gram(−) against enteric bacilli (ie, *E. coli*, *Klebsiella* sp, &

Proteus sp); anaerobic *B. fragilis* Dose: **Adults.** 1–2 g IV q6–8h. **Peds.** 80–160 mg/kg/d ÷ q4–6h; ↓ in renal impair **Caution:** [B, +] **Contra:** Cephalosporin allergy **Disp:** Powder for inj 1, 2, 10 g **SE:** D, rash, eosinophilia, ↑ transaminases **Interactions:** ↑ Nephrotox **W/** aminoglycosides, loop diuretics; ↑ effects **W/** probenecid **Labs:** ↑ LFTs, alkaline phosphatase, bilirubin, LDH, GGT, eosinophils, BUN, Cr; ↓ HMG, Hct, plts **NIPE:** Monitor for super Infxn, report persistent D

Cefpodoxime (Vantin) [Antibiotic/Cephalosporin-3rd Generation]
Uses: *Rx resp, skin, & urinary tract Infxns* **Action:** 3rd-gen cephalosporin; ↓ cell wall synth. *Spectrum: S. pneumoniae* or non-β-lactamase-producing *H. influenzae*; acute uncomplicated *N. gonorrhoeae*; some uncomplicated gram(–) (*E. coli, Klebsiella* sp, *Proteus* sp) **Dose: Adults.** 100–400 mg PO q12h. **Peds.** 10 mg/kg/d PO ÷ bid; ↓ in renal impair, w/ food **Caution:** [B, +] **Contra:** Cephalosporin allergy **Disp:** Tabs 100, 200 mg; susp 50, 100 mg/5 mL **SE:** D, rash, HA, eosinophilia, ↑ transaminases **Notes:** Drug interactions w/ agents that ↑ gastric pH **Interactions:** ↑ Nephrotox **W/** aminoglycosides, loop diuretics; ↑ effects **W/** probenecid; ↓ effects **W/** antacids, chloramphenicol **Labs:** ↑ LFTs, alkaline phosphatase, bilirubin, LDH, GGT, eosinophils, BUN, Cr; ↓ HMG, Hct, plts; false + direct Coombs test; **NIPE:** Food will ↑ absorption & < GI upset, monitor for super Infxn; ⊘ take within 2 hr of antacids

Cefprozil (Cefzil) [Antibiotic/Cephalosporin-2nd Generation]
Uses: *Rx resp tract, skin, & urinary tract Infxns* **Action:** 2nd-gen cephalosporin; ↓ cell wall synth. *Spectrum:* Active against MSSA, strep, & gram(–) bacilli (*E. coli, Klebsiella* sp, *P. mirabilis, H. influenzae, Moraxella* sp) **Dose: Adults.** 250–500 mg PO daily-bid. **Peds.** 7.5–15 mg/kg/d PO ÷ bid; ↓ in renal impair **Caution:** [B, +] **Contra:** Cephalosporin allergy **Disp:** Tabs 250, 500 mg; susp 125, 250 mg/5 mL **SE:** D, dizziness, rash, eosinophilia, ↑ transaminases **Notes:** Use higher doses for otitis & pneumonia **Interactions:** ↑ Nephrotox **W/** aminoglycosides, loop diuretics; ↑ effects **W/** probenecid; ↓ effects **W/** antacids, chloramphenicol **Labs:** ↑ LFTs, alkaline phosphatase, bilirubin, LDH, GGT, eosinophils, BUN, Cr; ↓ HMG, Hct, plts **NIPE:** Food will ↑ absorption & < GI upset, monitor for super Infxn; ⊘ take within 2 h of antacids; stable after reconsitution for 14 d—keep refrigerated

Ceftazidime (Fortaz, Tazicef) [Antibiotic/Cephalosporin-3rd Generation]
Uses: *Rx resp tract, skin, bone, urinary tract Infxns, meningitis, & septicemia* **Action:** 3rd-gen cephalosporin; ↓ cell wall synth. *Spectrum: P. aeruginosa*, good gram(–) activity **Dose: Adults.** 500–2 g IV/IM q8–12h. **Peds.** 30–50 mg/kg/dose IV q8h; ↓ in renal impair **Caution:** [B, +] PCN sensitivity **Contra:** Cephalosporin allergy **Disp:** Powder for inj 500 mg, 1, 2, 6 g **SE:** D, rash, eosinophilia, ↑ transaminases **Notes:** Use only for proven or strongly suspected Infxn to ↓ development of drug resistance **Interactions:** ↑ Nephrotox **W/** aminoglycosides, loop diuretics; ↑ effects **W/** probenecid; ↓ effects **W/** antacids, chloramphenicol

Labs: ↑ LFTs, alkaline phosphatase, bilirubin, LDH, GGT, eosinophils, BUN, Cr; ↓ HMG, Hct, plts **NIPE:** Food will ↑ absorption & < GI upset, monitor for super Infxn; ⊘ take within 2 h of antacids; stable after reconsitution for 14 d—keep refrigerated

Ceftibuten (Cedax) [Antibiotic/Cephalosporin-3rd Generation] Uses: *Rx resp tract, skin, urinary tract Infxns & otitis media* **Action:** 3rd-gen cephalosporin; ↓ cell wall synth. *Spectrum: H. influenzae & M. catarrhalis*; weak against *S. pneumoniae* **Dose:** *Adults.* 400 mg/d PO. *Peds.* 9 mg/kg/d PO; ↓ in renal impair; take on empty stomach (susp) **Caution:** [B, +] **Contra:** Cephalosporin allergy **Disp:** Caps 400 mg; susp 90 mg/5 mL **SE:** D, rash, eosinophilia, ↑ transaminases **Interactions:** ↑ Nephrotox *W/* aminoglycosides, loop diuretics; ↑ effects *W/* probenecid; ↓ effects *W/* antacids, chloramphenicol **Labs:** ↑ LFTs, alkaline phosphatase, bilirubin, LDH, GGT, eosinophils, BUN, Cr; ↓ HMG, Hct, plts **NIPE:** Take oral suspension 1 h < or 2 h > a meal; monitor for super Infxn; stable after reconsitution for 14 d—keep refrigerated

Ceftizoxime (Cefizox) [Antibiotic/Cephalosporin-3rd Generation] Uses: *Rx resp tract, skin, bone, & urinary tract Infxns, meningitis, septicemia* **Action:** 3rd-gen cephalosporin; ↓ cell wall synth. *Spectrum:* Good gram(−) bacilli (not *Pseudomonas* sp), some gram(+) cocci (not *Enterococcus* sp), & some anaerobes **Dose:** *Adults.* 1–4g IV q8–12h. *Peds.* 150–200 mg/kg/d IV ÷ q6–8h; ↓ in renal impair **Caution:** [B, +] **Contra:** Cephalosporin allergy **Disp:** Inj 1, 2, 10 g **SE:** D, fever, rash, eosinophilia, thrombocytosis, ↑ transaminases **Interactions:** ↑ Nephrotox *W/* aminoglycosides, loop diuretics; ↑ effects *W/* probenecid; **Labs:** ↑ LFTs, alkaline phosphatase, bilirubin, LDH, GGT, eosinophils, BUN, Cr; ↓ HMG, Hct, plts **NIPE:** Monitor for super Infxn; stable after reconsitution for 1 d at room temperature and 4 d if refrigerated; IM injection deep into large muscle mass

Ceftriaxone (Rocephin) [Antibiotic/Cephalosporin-3rd Generation] Uses: *Resp tract (pneumonia), skin, bone, urinary tract Infxns, meningitis, & septicemia* **Action:** 3rd-gen cephalosporin; ↓ cell wall synth. *Spectrum:* Moderate gram(+); excellent against β-lactamase producers **Dose:** *Adults.* 1–2 g IV/IM q12–24h. *Peds.* 50–100 mg/kg/d IV/IM ÷ q12–24h; ↓ in renal impair **Caution:** [B, +] **Contra:** Cephalosporin allergy; hyperbilirubinemic neonates **Disp:** Powder for inj 250 mg, 500 mg, 1, 2, 10 g; premixed 10, 20, 40 mg/mL **SE:** D, rash, leukopenia, thrombocytosis, eosinophilia, ↑ transaminases **Interactions:** ↑ Nephrotox *W/* aminoglycosides, loop diuretics; ↑ effects *W/* probenecid **Labs:** ↑ LFTs, alkaline phosphatase, bilirubin, LDH, GGT, eosinophils, BUN, Cr; ↓ HMG, Hct, plts **NIPE:** Monitor for super Infxn, solutions are stable for 24 h at room temperature after dilution; IM injections deep into large muscle mass

Cefuroxime (Ceftin [PO], Zinacef [parenteral]) [Antibiotic/Cephalosporin-2nd Generation] Uses: *Upper & lower resp tract, skin, bone, urinary tract, abdomen, gynecologic Infxns* **Action:** 2nd-gen cephalosporin; ↓ cell wall synth. *Spectrum:* Staphylococci, group B streptococci, *H. influenzae*, *E. coli*, *Enterobacter* sp, *Salmonella* sp, & *Klebsiella* sp **Dose:** **Adults.** 750 mg–1.5 g IV q6h or 250–500 mg PO bid. **Peds.** 100–150 mg/kg/d IV ÷ q8h or 20–30 mg/kg/d PO ÷ bid; ↓ in renal impair; take w/ food **Caution:** [B, +] **Contra:** Cephalosporin allergy **Disp:** Tabs 125, 250, 500 mg; susp 125, 250 mg/ 5 mL; powder for inj 750 mg, 1.5, 7.5 g **SE:** D, rash, eosinophilia, ↑ LFTs **Notes:** Cefuroxime film-coated tabs & susp not bioequivalent; do not substitute on a mg/mg basis; IV crosses blood–brain barrier **Interactions:** ↑ Nephrotox W/ aminoglycosides, loop diuretics; ↑ effects W/ probenecid; ↑ effects W/ Al & Mg antacids **Labs:** ↑ LFTs, alkaline phosphatase, bilirubin, LDH, GGT, eosinophils, BUN, Cr; ↓ HMG, Hct, plts **NIPE:** Monitor for super Infxn; high-fat meals increased drug bioavailability; give suspension with food; IM injections deep into large muscle mass

Celecoxib (Celebrex) [Anti-Inflammatory/COX-2 Inhibitor]

WARNING: ↑ Risk of serious CV thrombotic events, MI & stroke, can be fatal; ↑ risk of serious GI adverse events including bleeding, ulceration, & perforation of the stomach or intestines; can be fatal **Uses:** *Osteoarthritis & RA, ankylosing spondylitis; acute pain, primary dysmenorrhea; preventive in familial adenomatous polyposis* **Action:** NSAID; ↓ COX-2 pathway **Dose:** 100–200 mg/d or bid; FAP: 400 mg PO bid; ↓ w/ hepatic impair; take w/ food/milk **Caution:** [C/D (3rd tri), ?] w/ renal impair **Contra:** Sulfonamide allergy, periop CABG **Disp:** Caps 100, 200 400 mg **SE:** See Warning; GI upset, HTN, edema, renal failure, HA **Interactions:** ↑ Effects W/ fluconazole; ↑ effects OF Li; ↑ risks of GI upset &/or bleeding W/ ASA, NSAIDs, warfarin, EtOH; ↓ effects W/ Al- & Mg-containing antacids, ↓ effects OF thiazide diuretics, loop diuretics, ACEIs **Labs:** ↑ LFTs, BUN, Cr, CPK, alkaline phosphatase; monitor for hypercholesterolemia, hyperglycemia, hypokalemia, hypophosphatemia, albuminuria, hematuria **NIPE:** Take w/ food if GI distress; watch for Sxs of GI bleed; no effect on plt/bleeding time; can affect drugs metabolized by P-450 pathway

Cephalexin (Keflex, Pranixine Disperdose) [Antibiotic/ Cephalosporin-1st Generation]

Uses: *Skin, bone, upper/lower resp tract, urinary tract Infxns* **Action:** 1st-gen cephalosporin; ↓ cell wall synth. *Spectrum:* Streptococcus sp, Staphylococcus sp, E. coli, Proteus sp, & Klebsiella sp **Dose:** **Adults.** 250–1000 mg PO qid. **Peds.** 25–100 mg/kg/d PO ÷ qid; ↓ in renal impair; (on empty stomach) **Caution:** [B, +] **Contra:** Cephalosporin allergy **Disp:** Caps 250, 500 mg; tabs for oral susp 100, 125, 250 mg; susp 125, 250 mg/5 mL **SE:** D, rash, eosinophilia, ↑ LFTs **Interactions:** ↑ Nephrotox W/ aminoglycosides, loop diuretics; ↑ effects W/ probenecid **Labs:** ↑ LFTs, alkaline phosphatase, bilirubin, LDH, GGT, eosinophils, BUN, Cr; ↓ HMG, Hct, plts **NIPE:** Food will ↑ absorption and < GI upset; monitor for super Infxn; oral suspension stable for 14 d after reconstitution if refrigerated

Cephradine (Velosef) [Antibiotic/Cephalosporin-1st Generation] Uses: *Respiratory, GU, GI, skin, soft tissue, bone, & joint Infxns* Action: 1st-gen cephalosporin; ↓ cell wall synth. *Spectrum:* Gram(+) bacilli & cocci (not *Enterococcus* sp); some gram(−) (*E. coli, Proteus* sp, *Klebsiella* sp) Dose: *Adults.* 250–500 mg q6–12h (8 g/d max). *Peds >9 mo.* 25–100 mg/kg/d ÷ bid-qid (4 g/d max); ↓ in renal impair Caution: [B, +] Contra: Cephalosporin allergy Disp: Caps: 250, 500 mg; powder for susp 125, 250 mg/5 mL SE: Rash, eosinophilia, ↑ LFTs, N/V/D Interactions: ↑ Nephrotox W/ aminoglycosides, loop diuretics; ↑ effects W/ probenecid Labs: ↑ LFTs, alkaline phosphatase, bilirubin, LDH, GGT, eosinophils, BUN, Cr; ↓ HMG, Hct, plts NIPE: Food will ↑ absorption and < GI upset; monitor for super Infxn; oral suspension stable for 14 d after reconstitution if refrigerated

Cetirizine (Zyrtec, Zyrtec D) [Allergy/Antihistamine] Uses: *Allergic rhinitis & other allergic Sxs including urticaria* Action: Nonsedating antihistamine Dose: *Adults & Children >6 y.* 5–10 mg/d. Zyrtec D 5/120 mg PO bid whole *Peds.* 6–11 mo: 2.5 mg daily. 12–23 mo: 2.5 mg daily-bid; ↓ in renal/hepatic impair Caution: [B, ?/−] Elderly & nursing mothers; >10 mg/d may cause drowsiness Contra: Allergy to cetirizine, hydroxyzine Disp: Tabs 5, 10 mg; chew tabs 5, 10 mg; syrup 5 mg/5 mL; *Zyrtec D:* Tabs 5/120 mg (cetirizine/pseudoephedrine) SE: HA, drowsiness, xerostomia Interactions: ↑ Effects W/ anticholinergics, CNS depressants, theophylline, EtOH Labs: May cause false−/allergy skin tests NIPE: ⊘ take w/ EtOH or CNS depressants; can cause sedation; sun exposure can cause photosensitivity

Cetuximab (Erbitux) [Antineoplastic/Recombinant Monoclonal Antibody] WARNING: Severe inf Rxns including rapid onset of airway obst (bronchospasm, stridor, hoarseness), urticaria, & ↓ BP; permanent D/C required; ↑ risk sudden death and cardiopulm arrest Uses: *EGFR + met colorectal CA w/wo irinotecan, unresectable head/neck SCC w/ RT; monotherapy in met head/neck cancer* Action: Human/mouse recombinant MoAb; binds EGFR, ↓ tumor cell growth Dose: Per protocol; load 400 mg/m^2 IV over 2 h; 250 mg/m^2 given over 1 h 1 × wk Caution: [C, −] Disp: Inj 100 mg/50 mL SE: Acneform rash, asthenia/malaise, N/V/D, abd pain, alopecia, inf Rxn, derm tox, interstitial lung disease, fever, sepsis, dehydration, kidney failure, PE Notes: Assess tumor for EGFR before Rx; pretreat w/ diphenhydramine; w/ mild SE ↓ inf rate by 50% NIPE: Monitor for inf reactions for 1 h after inf; during 1st 2 wk observe for skin tox; limit sun exposure

Charcoal, Activated (Superchar, Actidose, Liqui-Char) [Adsorbent] Uses: *Emergency poisoning by most drugs & chemicals (see Contra)* Action: Adsorbent detoxicant Dose: Give w/ 70% sorbitol (2 mL/kg); repeated use of sorbitol not OK *Adults. Acute intox:* 30–100 g/dose. *GI dialysis:* 20–50 g q6h for 1–2 d. *Peds 1–12 y. Acute intox:* 1–2 g/kg/dose. *GI dialysis:* 5–10 g/dose q4–8h

Caution: [C, ?] May cause V (hazardous w/ petroleum & caustic ingestions); do not mix w/ dairy **Contra:** Not effective for cyanide, mineral acids, caustic alkalis, organic solvents, iron, EtOH, methanol poisoning, Li; do not use sorbitol in pts w/ fructose intolerance, intestinal obst, nonintact GI tracts **Disp:** Powder, Liq, caps **SE:** Some Liq dosage forms in sorbitol base (a cathartic); V/D, black stools, constipation **Notes:** Charcoal w/ sorbitol not OK in children <1 y; monitor for ↓ K+ & Mg²⁺; protect airway in lethargic/comatose pts **Interactions:** ↓ Effects if taken w/ ice cream, milk, sherbet; ↓ effects *OF* digoxin & absorption of other oral meds, ↓ effects *OF* syrup of ipecac **NIPE:** Most effective if given w/in 30 min of acute poisoning, only give to conscious patients

Chloral Hydrate (Aquachloral, Supprettes) [C-IV] [Sedative/Hypnotic/CNS Depressant]
Uses: *Short-term nocturnal & preop sedation* **Action:** Sedative hypnotic; active metabolite trichloroethanol **Dose: Adults.** *Hypnotic:* 500 mg–1 g PO or PR 30 min hs or before procedure. *Sedative:* 250 mg PO or PR tid. **Peds.** *Hypnotic:* 20–50 mg/kg/24 h PO or PR 30 min hs or before procedure. *Sedative:* 5–15 mg/kg/dose q8h; avoid w/ CrCl <50 mL/min or severe hepatic impair **Contra:** [C, +] Porphyria & neonates, long-term care facility residents **Contra:** Allergy to components; severe renal, hepatic or cardiac Dz **Disp:** Caps 500 mg; syrup 250, 500 mg/5 mL; supp 324, 648 mg **SE:** GI irritation, drowsiness, ataxia, dizziness, nightmares, rash **Interactions:** ↑ Effects *W/* antihistamines, barbiturates, paraldehyde, CNS depressants, opiate analgesics, EtOH; ↑ effects *OF* anticoagulants **Labs:** ↑ Eosinophils, BUN; ↓ WBCs **NIPE:** ⊘ Take w/ EtOH, CNS depressants; ⊘ chew or crush caps; May accumulate; tolerance may develop >2 wk; taper dose; mix syrup in H₂O or fruit juice

Chlorambucil (Leukeran) [Antineoplastic/Alkylating Agent]
WARNING: Myelosuppressive, carcinogenic, teratogenic, associated with infertility **Uses:** *CLL, Hodgkin Dz, Waldenström macroglobulinemia* **Action:** Alkylating agent (nitrogen mustard) **Dose:** (Per protocol) 0.1–0.2 mg/kg/d for 3–6 wk or 0.4 mg/kg/dose q2wk **Caution:** [D, ?] Sz disorder & BM suppression; affects human fertility **Contra:** Previous resistance; alkylating agent allergy; w/ live vaccines **Disp:** Tabs 2 mg **SE:** ↓ BM, CNS stimulation, N/V, drug fever, rash, secondary leukemias, alveolar dysplasia, pulm fibrosis, hepatotox **Interactions:** ↑ BM suppression *W/* antineoplastic drugs and immunosuppressants; ↑ risk of bleeding *W/* ASA, anticoagulants **Labs:** ↑ Urine and serum uric acid, ALT, alkaline phosphatase; ↓ HMG, Hct, neutrophil, plts, RBCs, WBCs **NIPE:** ⊘ PRG, breast-feeding, Infxn; ↑ fluids to 2–3 L/d; monitor lab work periodically & CBC w/ differential weekly during drug use; may cause hair loss; ↓ dose if pt has received radiation

Chlordiazepoxide (Librium, Mitran, Libritabs) [C-IV] [Anxiolytic, Sedative/Hypnotic/Benzodiazepine]
Uses: *Anxiety, tension, EtOH withdrawal*, & preop apprehension **Action:** Benzodiazepine; antianxiety agent **Dose: Adults.** *Mild anxiety:* 5–10 mg PO tid-qid or PRN. *Severe anxiety:* 25–50 mg IM, IV, or PO q6–8h or PRN. **Peds** >6 y. 0.5 mg/kg/24 h PO or

IM ÷ q6–8h; ↓ in renal impair, elderly **Caution:** [D, ?] Resp depression, CNS impair, h/o of drug dependence; avoid in hepatic impair **Contra:** Preexisting CNS depression, NAG **Disp:** Caps 5, 10, 25 mg; inj 100 mg **SE:** Drowsiness, CP, rash, fatigue, memory impair, xerostomia, wt gain **Interactions:** ↑ Effects *W/* antidepressants, antihistamines, anticonvulsants, barbiturates, general anesthetics, MAOIs, narcotics, phenothiazines cimetidine, disulfiram, fluconazole, itraconazole, ketoconazole, OCPs, INH, metoprolol, propoxyphene, propranolol, valproic acid, EtOH, grapefruit juice, kava kava, valerian; ↑ effects *OF* digoxin, phenytoin; ↓ effects *W/* aminophylline, antacids, carbamazepine, theophylline, rifampin, rifabutin, tobacco; ↓ effects *OF* levodopa **Labs:** ↑ LFTs, alkaline phosphatase, bilirubin, triglycerides; ↓ granulocytes **NIPE:** ⊘ EtOH, PRG, breast-feeding; risk of photosensitivity—use sunscreen, orthostatic hypotension, tachycardia; erratic IM absorption

Chlorothiazide (Diuril) [Antihypertensive/Thiazide Diuretic]

Uses: *HTN, edema* **Action:** Thiazide diuretic **Dose:** *Adults.* 500 mg–1 g PO daily-bid; 100–1000 mg/d IV (for edema only). *Peds >6 mo.* 20–30 mg/kg/24 h PO ÷ bid; 4 mg/kg/d IV; OK w/ food **Caution:** [D, +] **Contra:** Cross-sensitivity to thiazides/sulfonamides, anuria **Disp:** Tabs 250, 500 mg; susp 250 mg/5 mL; inj 500 mg/vial **SE:** ↓ K⁺, Na⁺, dizziness, hyperglycemia, hyperuricemia, hyperlipidemia, photosens **Interactions:** ↑ Effects *W/* ACEI, amphotericin B, corticosteroids; ↑ effects *OF* diazoxide, Li, MTX; ↓ effects *W/* colestipol, cholestyramine, NSAIDs; ↓ effects *OF* hypoglycemics **Labs:** ↑ CPK, ammonia, amylase, Ca²⁺, Cl⁻, cholesterol, glucose, Mg²⁺, K⁺, Na⁺, uric acid **NIPE:** Do not use IM/SQ; take early in the day to avoid nocturia; monitor for gout, hyperglycemia, photosensitivity—use sunscreen, I&O, weight

Chlorpheniramine (Chlor-Trimeton, others) [OTC] [Antihistamine/Propylamine]

Uses: *Allergic rhinitis* common cold **Action:** Antihistamine **Dose:** *Adults.* 4 mg PO q4–6h or 8–12 mg PO bid of SR *Peds.* 0.35 mg/kg/24 h PO ÷ q4–6h or 0.2 mg/kg/24 h SR **Caution:** [B, ?/–] BOO; NAG; hepatic insuff **Contra:** Allergy **Disp:** Tabs 4 mg; chew tabs 2 mg; SR tabs 8, 12 mg **SE:** Anticholinergic SE & sedation common, postural ↓ BP, QT changes, extrapyramidal Rxns, photosens **Interactions:** ↑ Effects *W/* other CNS depressants, EtOH, opioids, sedatives, MAOIs, atropine, haloperidol, phenothiazines, quinidine, disopyramide; ↑ effects *OF* epinephrine; ↓ effects *OF* heparin, sulfonylureas **Labs:** False–w/ allergy testing **NIPE:** Stop drug 4 d prior to allergy testing, take w/ food if GI distress; do not cut/crush/chew ER forms; recent deaths in <2 y assoc w/ cough and cold meds [*MMWR* 2007 56(01):1–4]

Chlorpromazine (Thorazine) [Antipsychotic, Antiemetic/Phenothiazine]

Uses: *Psychotic disorders, N/V*, apprehension, intractable hiccups **Action:** Phenothiazine antipsychotic; antiemetic **Dose:** *Adults. Psychosis:* 10–25 mg PO bid-tid (usual 30–800 mg/d in ÷ doses). *Severe Sxs:* 25 mg IM/IV initial; may repeat in 1–4 h; then 25–50 mg PO or PR tid. *Hiccups:* 25–50 mg PO bid-tid. *Children >6 mo. Psychosis & N/V:* 0.5–1 mg/kg/dose PO q4–6h or IM/IV q6–8h **Caution:** [C, ?/-] Safety in children <6 mo not established; Szs, avoid w/ hepatic impair, BM suppression **Contra:** Cross-sensitivity w/ phenothiazines; NAG **Disp:** Tabs 10, 25, 50, 100, 200 mg; conc 30, 100 mg/mL; syrup 10 mg/5 mL; inj 25 mg/mL **SE:** Extrapyramidal SE & sedation; α-adrenergic blocking properties; ↓ BP; ↑ QT interval **Interactions:** ↑ Effects *W/* amodiaquine, chloroquine, sulfadoxine–pyrimethamine, antidepressants, narcotic analgesics, propranolol, quinidine, BBs, MAOIs, TCAs, EtOH, kava kava; ↑ effects *OF* anticholinergics, centrally acting antihypertensives, propranolol, valproic acid; ↓ effects *W/* antacids, antidiarrheals, barbiturates, Li, tobacco; ↓ effects *OF* anticonvulsants, guanethidine, levodopa, Li, warfarin **Labs:** False + urine bilirubin; false + or – PRG test; ↑alk phos, bilirubin, CK, GGT, eosinophil count; ↓ HMG, Hct, granulocytes, plts, WBC **NIPE:** Do not D/C abruptly; dilute PO conc in 2–4 oz of Liq; Risk of photosensitivity—use sunscreen; risk of tardive dyskinesia; take w/ food if GI upset; may darken urine

Chlorpropamide (Diabinese) [Hypoglycemic/Sulfonylurea]

Uses: *Type 2 DM* **Action:** Sulfonylurea; ↑ pancreatic insulin release; ↑ peripheral insulin sensitivity; ↓ hepatic glucose output **Dose:** 100–500 mg/d w/ food, ↓ hepatic impairment **Caution:** [C, ?/-] CrCl <50 mL/min; ↓ in hepatic impair **Contra:** Cross-sensitivity w/ sulfonamides **Disp:** Tabs 100, 250 mg **SE:** HA, dizziness, rash, photosens, hypoglycemia, SIADH **Interactions:** ↑ Effects *W/* ASA, NSAIDs, anticoagulants, BBs, chloramphenicol, guanethidine, insulin, MAOIs, rifampin, sulfonamides, EtOH, juniper berries, ginseng, garlic, fenugreek, coriander, dandelion root, celery, bitter melon, ginkgo biloba; ↓ effects *W/* diazoxide, thiazide diuretics **Labs:** ↑ Alk phos, bilirubin, BUN, Cr, cholesterol; ↓ glucose HMG, Hct, plts, WBC **NIPE:** EtOH (disulfiram-like Rxn)

Chlorthalidone (Hygroton, others) [Antihypertensive/Thiazide Diuretic]

Uses: *HTN* **Action:** Thiazide diuretic **Dose:** *Adults.* 25–100 mg PO daily. *Peds.* (Not approved) 2 mg/kg/dose PO 3×/wk or 1–2 mg/kg/d PO; ↓ in renal impair; OK w/ food, milk **Caution:** [D, +] **Contra:** Cross-sensitivity w/ thiazides or sulfonamides; anuria **Disp:** Tabs 15, 25, 50 mg **SE:** ↓ K⁺, dizziness, photosens, hyperglycemia, hyperuricemia, sexual dysfunction **Interactions:** ↑ Effects *W/* ACEIs, diazoxide; ↑ effects *OF* digoxin, Li, MTX; ↓ effects *W/* cholestyramine, colestipol, NSAIDs; ↓ effects *OF* hypoglycemics; ↓ K⁺ *W/* amphotericin B, carbenoxolone, corticosteroids **Labs:** ↑ Bilirubin, Ca²⁺, Cr, uric acid; ↑ glucose in diabetics; ↓ Mg²⁺, K⁺, Na⁺ **NIPE:** May take w/ food, and milk, take early in day, use sunscreen; ↑ K⁺ rich foods in diet

Chlorzoxazone (Paraflex, Parafon Forte DSC, others) [Skeletal Muscle Relaxant/ANS Drug]

Uses: *Adjunct to rest & physical therapy to relieve discomfort associated w/ acute, painful musculoskeletal conditions* **Action:** Centrally acting skeletal muscle relaxant **Dose:** *Adults.* 250–500 mg PO tid-qid. *Peds.* 20 mg/kg/d in 3–4 ÷ doses **Caution:** [C, ?] Avoid EtOH & CNS depressants **Contra:** Severe liver Dz **Disp:** Tabs 250, 500 mg

SE: Drowsiness, tachycardia, dizziness, hepatotox, angioedema **Interactions:** ↑ Effects *W/* antihistamines, CNS depressants, MAOIs, TCAs, opiates, EtOH, watercress **Labs:** ↑ Alk phos, bilirubin; monitor LFTs **NIPE:** Urine may turn reddish purple or orange

Cholecalciferol [Vitamin D₃] (Delta D) [Vitamin/Dietary Supplement] **Uses:** Dietary supl to Rx vitamin D deficiency **Action:** ↑ Intestinal Ca²⁺ absorption **Dose:** 400–1000 IU/d PO **Caution:** [A (D doses above the RDA), +] **Contra:** ↑ Ca²⁺, hypervitaminosis, allergy **Disp:** Tabs 400, 1000 IU **SE:** Vitamin D tox (renal failure, HTN, psychosis) **Notes:** 1 mg cholecalciferol = 40,000 IU vitamin D activity **Interactions:** ↑ Risk of arrhythmias *W/* cardiac glycosides; ↓ effects *W/* cholestyramine, colestipol, mineral oil, orlistat, phenobarbital, phenytoin **Labs:** ↑ BUN, Ca, cholesterol, Cr, LFTs, urine urea **NIPE:** Vitamin D is fat soluble; mineral oil interferes with vitamin D absorption; vitamin D is needed for Ca absorption

Cholestyramine (Questran, Prevalite) [Antilipemic, Bile Acid Sequestrant] **Uses:** *Hypercholesterolemia; Rx pruritus associated w/ partial biliary obst; D associated w/ excess fecal bile acids* pseudomembranous colitis **Action:** Binds intestinal bile acids, forms insoluble complexes **Dose:** *Adults.* Titrate: 4 g/d-bid ↑ to max 24 g/d & 6 doses/d. *Peds.* 240 mg/kg/d in 3 ÷ doses **Caution:** [C, ?] Constipation, phenylketonuria **Contra:** Complete biliary or bowel obst; hypolipoproteinemia types III, IV, V **Disp:** 4 g of cholestyramine resin/9 g powder; w/ aspartame: 4 g resin/5 g powder (Light) 4 g resin/6.4 g powder **SE:** Constipation, abd pain, bloating, HA, rash **Interactions:** ↓ Effects *OF* acetaminophen, amiodarone, anticoagulants, ASA, cardiac glycosides, clindamycin, corticosteroids, diclofenac, fat-soluble vitamins, gemfibrozil, glipizide, Fe salts, MTX, methyldopa, nicotinic acid, penicillins, phenobarbital, phenytoin, propranolol, thiazide diuretics, tetracyclines, thyroid drugs, troglitazone, warfarin if given with this drug; **Labs:** ↑ Alkaline phosphatase, prothromin time; ↓ cholesterol, folic acid, HMG, Hct **NIPE:** ↑ Fluids, take other drugs 1–2 h before or 6 h after; OD may cause GI obst; mix 4 g in 2–6 oz of noncarbonated beverage

Ciclesonide (Omnaris) [Corticosteroid] **Uses:** Allergic rhinitis **Action:** Nasal corticosteroid **Dose:** *Adults and Peds >12 y:* 2 sprays each nostril 1 × d **Caution:** [C,?/–] w/ ketoconazole **Contra:** Component allergy **Disp:** Intranasal spray susp, 50 µg/spray, 120 doses **SE:** adrenal suppression, delayed nasal wound healing, URI, HA, ear pain, epistaxis **NIPE:** ↑ Risk viral Dz (eg, chickenpox), delayed growth in children

Ciclopirox (Loprox, Penlac) [Antifungal/Antibiotic] **Uses:** *Tinea pedis, tinea cruris, tinea corporis, cutaneous candidiasis, tinea versicolor, tinea rubrum* **Action:** Antifungal antibiotic; cellular depletion of essential substrates &/or ions **Dose:** *Adults & Peds >10 y.* Massage into affected area bid. *Onychomycosis:* Apply to nails daily, with removal every 7 d **Caution:** [B, ?] **Contra:** Component sensitivity **Disp:** Cream 0.77%, gel 0.77%, topical sus 0.77%, shampoo 1%, nail lacquer 8% **SE:** Pruritus, local irritation, burning **Interactions:** None noted **NIPE:** Nail lacquer may take 6 mo to see improvement; cream/gel/lotion see improvement by 4 wk; D/C w/ irritation; avoid dressings; gel best for athlete's foot

Cidofovir (Vistide) [Antiviral/Inhibits DNA synthesis]
WARNING: Renal impair is the major tox. Follow administration instructions **Uses:** *CMV retinitis w/ HIV* **Action:** Selective inhibition of viral DNA synth **Dose:** *Rx:* 5 mg/kg IV over 1 h once/wk for 2 wk w/ probenecid. *Maint:* 5 mg/kg IV once/2 wk w/ probenecid (2 g PO 3 h prior to cidofovir, then 1 g PO at 2 h & 8 h after cidofovir); ↓ in renal impair **Caution:** [C, –] SCr >1.5 mg/dL or CrCl = 55 mL/min or urine protein >100 mg/dL; w/ other nephrotoxic drugs **Contra:** Probenecid or sulfa allergy **Disp:** Inj 75 mg/mL **SE:** Renal tox, chills, fever, HA, N/V/D, thrombocytopenia, neutropenia **Interactions:** ↑ Nephrotox *W/* aminoglycosides, amphotericin B, foscarnet, IV pentamidine, NSAIDs, vancomycin; ↑ effects *W/* zidovudine **Labs:** ↑ SCr, BUN, alkaline phosphatase, LFTs, urine protein; ↓ Ca, HMG, Hct, neutrophils, plts; monitor for hematuria, glycosuria, hypocalcemia, hyperglycemia, hypokalemia, hyperlipidemia **NIPE:** Coadminister oral probenecid w/ each dose to < GI target; possible hair loss; hydrate w/ NS prior to each inf

Cilostazol (Pletal) [Antiplatelet, Arterial Vasodilator/Phosphodiesterase Inhibitor] **Uses:** *Reduce Sxs of intermittent claudication* **Action:** Phosphodiesterase III inhibitor; ↑'s cAMP in plts & blood vessels, vasodilation & inhibit plt aggregation **Dose:** 100 mg PO bid, 1/2 h before or 2 h after breakfast & dinner **Caution:** [C, +/–] ↓ dose w/ drugs that inhibit CYP3A4 & CYP2C19 (Table 11) **Contra:** CHF, hemostatic disorders, active pathologic bleeding **Disp:** Tabs 50, 100 mg **SE:** HA, palpitation, D **Interactions:** ↑ Effects *W/* diltiazem, macrolides, omeprazole, fluconazole, itraconazole, ketoconazole, sertraline, grapefruit juice; ↑ effects *OF* ASA; ↓ effects *W/* cigarette smoking; **Labs:** ↑ HDL; ↓ triglycerides **NIPE:** Take on empty stomach; may take up to 12 wk to ↓ cramping pain; may cause dizziness

Cimetidine (Tagamet) (Tagamet HB, Tagamet DS OTC) [Antiulcerative/H₂-Receptor Antagonist] **Uses:** *Duodenal ulcer; ulcer prophylaxis in hypersecretory states, (eg, trauma, burns); & GERD* **Action:** H₂-receptor antagonist **Dose:** *Adults. Active ulcer:* 2400 mg/d IV cont inf or 300 mg IV q6h; 400 mg PO bid or 800 mg hs. *Maint:* 400 mg PO hs. *GERD:* 300–600 mg PO q6h; maint 800 mg PO hs. *Peds. Infants:* 10–20 mg/kg/24 h PO or IV ÷ q6–12h. *Children:* 20–40 mg/kg/24 h PO or IV ÷ q6h; ↓ w/ renal insuff & in elderly **Caution:** [B, +] Many drug interactions (P-450 system) **Contra:** Component sensitivity **Disp:** Tabs 200, 300, 400, 800 mg; Liq 300 mg/5 mL; inj 300 mg/2 mL **SE:** Dizziness, HA, agitation, thrombocytopenia, gynecomastia **Interactions:** ↑ Effects *OF* benzodiazepines, disulfram, flecainide, INH, lidocaine, OCPs, sulfonylureas, warfarin, theophylline, phenytoin, metronidazole, triamterene, procainamide, quinidine, propranolol, diazepam, nifedipine, TCAs, procainamide, tacrine, carbamazepine, valproic acid, xanthines; ↓ effects *W/* antacids, tobacco; ↓ effects *OF* digoxin, ketoconazole, cefpodoxime, indomethacin, tetracyclines **Labs:** ↑ Cr, LFTs; ↓ HMG, Hct, neutrophils, plt counts **NIPE:** Take w/ meals; monitor for gynecomastia, breast pain, impotence; take 1 h before or 2 h after antacids; avoid EtOH

Cinacalcet (Sensipar) [Hyperparathyroidism Agent/Calcimimetic]

Uses: *Secondary hyperparathyroidism in CRF; ↑ Ca²⁺ in parathyroid carcinoma* **Action:** ↓ PTH by ↑ Ca-sensing receptor sensitivity **Dose:** *Secondary hyperparathyroidism:* 30 mg PO daily; titrate q2–4wk based on Ca & PTH levels; swallow whole; take w/ food *Parathyroid carcinoma:* 30 mg PO bid; titrate q2–4wk based on Ca & PTH levels; swallow whole; take w/ food **Caution:** [C, ?/–] w/ seizures, adjust w/ CYP3A4 inhibitors (Table 11) **Disp:** Tabs 30, 60, 90 mg **SE:** N/V/D, myalgia, dizziness, ↓ Ca²⁺ **Interactions:** ↑ Effects W/ CYP3A4 inhibitors such as ketoconazole, itraconazole, erythromycine; ↑ effects *OF* drugs metabolized at CYP2D6 such as TCA, thioridazine, flecainide, vinblastine **Labs:** Monitor Ca²⁺, PO₄⁻², PTH **NIPE:** Must take drug with vitamin D and/or phosphate binders; ↑ concentrations of drug if taken w/ food

Ciprofloxacin (Cipro, Cipro XR, Proquin XR) [Antibiotic/Fluoroquinolone]

Uses: *Rx lower resp tract, sinuses, skin & skin structure, bone/joints, & urinary tract Infxns including prostatitis* **Action:** Quinolone antibiotic; ↓ DNA gyrase. *Spectrum:* Broad gram(+) & (–) aerobics; little *Streptococcus* sp; good *Pseudomonas* sp, *E. coli, B. fragilis, P. mirabilis, K. pneumoniae, C. jejuni,* or *Shigella* sp **Dose:** *Adults.* 250–750 mg PO q12h; XR 500–1000 mg PO q24h; or 200–400 mg IV q12h; in renal impair **Caution:** [C, ?/–] Children <18 y **Contra:** Component sensitivity **Disp:** Tabs 100, 250, 500, 750 mg; tabs XR 500, 1000 mg; susp 5 g/100 mL, 10 g/100 mL; inj 200, 400 mg; premixed piggyback 200 mg/100 mL **SE:** Restlessness, N/V/D, rash, ruptured tendons, ↑ LFTs **Interactions:** ↑ Effects W/ probenecid; ↑ effects *OF* diazepam, theophylline, caffeine, metoprolol, propranolol, phenytoin, warfarin; ↓ effects W/ antacids, didanosine, Fe salts, Mg, sucralfate, Na bicarbonate, Zn **Labs:** ↑ LFTs, alkaline phosphatase, serum bilirubin, LDH, BUN, SCr, K⁺, PT, triglycerides; ↓ plts, WBC **NIPE:** ⊘ Give to children <18 y; ↑ fluids to 2–3 L/d, may cause photosensitivity—use sunscreen; avoid antacids; reduce/restrict caffeine intake

Ciprofloxacin, Ophthalmic (Ciloxan) [Antibiotic/Fluoroquinolone Opthalmic Agent]

Uses: *Rx & prevention of ocular Infxns (conjunctivitis, blepharitis, corneal abrasions)* **Action:** Quinolone antibiotic; ↓ DNA gyrase **Dose:** 1–2 gtt in eye(s) q2h while awake for 2 d then 1–2 gtt q4h while awake for 5 d, oint 1/2″ ribbon in eye 3 × d × 2 d, then 2 × d × 5 d **Caution:** [C, ?/–] **Contra:** Component sensitivity **Disp:** Soln 3.5 mg/mL; oint 0.3%, 35g **SE:** Local irritation **Interactions:** None reported **NIPE:** Limited systemic absorption

Ciprofloxacin, Otic (Cipro HC Otic) [Antibiotic/Fluoroquinolone Otic Agent]

Uses: *Otitis externa* **Action:** Quinolone antibiotic; ↓ DNA gyrase **Dose:** *Adult & Peds >1 mo.* 1–2 gtt in ear(s) bid for 7 d **Caution:** [C, ?/–] **Contra:** Perforated tympanic membrane, viral Infxns of the external canal **Disp:** Susp ciprofloxacin 0.2% & hydrocortisone 1% **SE:** HA, pruritus **NIPE:** 1st-choice therapy for otitis externa

Cisplatin (Platinol, Platinol AQ) [Antineoplastic/Alkylating Agent] Uses: *Testicular, SCLC, NSCLC, bladder, ovarian, breast, head & neck, & penile CAs; osteosarcoma; ped brain tumors* Action: DNA-binding; denatures double helix; intrastrand cross-linking Dose: 10–20 mg/m²/d for 5 d q3wk; 50–120 mg/m² q3–4wk; (per protocols); ↓ w/ renal impair Caution: [D, –] Cumulative renal tox may be severe; ✓ Mg²⁺, lytes before & w/in 48 h after cisplatin Contra: Platinum-containing compound allergy; ↓ BM, hearing impair, preexisting renal insuff Disp: Inj 1 mg/mL SE: Allergic Rxns, N/V, nephrotox (↑ w/ admin of other nephrotoxic drugs; minimize by NS inf & mannitol diuresis), high-frequency hearing loss in 30%, peripheral "stocking glove"-type neuropathy, cardiotox (ST, T-wave changes), ↓ Mg²⁺, mild↓ BM, hepatotox; renal impair dose-related & cumulative Notes: Give taxanes before platinum derivatives Interactions: ↑ Effects *OF* antineoplastic drugs and radiation therapy; ↑ ototox *W/* loop diuretics; ↑ nephrotox *W/* aminoglycosides, amphotericin B, vancomycin; ↓ effects *W/* Na thiosulfate; ↓ effects *OF* phenytoin Labs: ↑ BUN, Cr, serum bilirubin, AST, uric acid; ↓ Ca²⁺, Mg²⁺, phosphate, Na⁺, K⁺, RBC, WBC, plts NIPE: May cause infertility, ⊘ immunizations or products with ASA; instruct pt to report signs of Infxn and tinnitus

Citalopram (Celexa) [Antidepressant/SSRI] WARNING: Closely monitor for worsening depression or emergence of suicidality, particularly in patients <24 y Uses: *Depression* Action: SSRI Dose: Initial 20 mg/d, may ↑ to 40 mg/d; ↓ in elderly & hepatic/renal insuff Caution: [C, +/–] h/o of mania, Szs & pts at risk for suicide Contra: MAOI or w/in 14 d of MAOI use Disp: Tabs 10, 20, 40 mg; dist tabs 10, 20, 40 mg; cap 10, 20, 40 mg; Soln 10 mg/5 mL SE: Somnolence, insomnia, anxiety, xerostomia, diaphoresis, sexual dysfunction Notes: May cause ↓ Na⁺/SIADH Interactions: ↑ Effects *W/* azole antifungals, cimetidine, Li, macrolides, EtOH; ↑ effects *OF* BBs, carbamazepine, CNS drugs, warfarin; ↓ effects *W/* carbamazepine; ↓ effects *OF* phenytoin; may cause fatal Rxn *W/* MAOIs Labs: ↑ LFTs NIPE: ⊘ PRG, breast-feeding, use barrier contraception

Cladribine (Leustatin) [Antineoplastic Agent/Purine Nucleoside Analog] Uses: *HCL, CLL, NHLs, progressive MS* Action: Induces DNA strand breakage; interferes w/ DNA repair/synth; purine nucleoside analog Dose: 0.09–0.1 mg/kg/d cont IV inf for 1–7 d (Per protocols) Caution: [D, ?/–] Causes neutropenia & Infxn Contra: Component sensitivity Disp: Inj 1 mg/mL SE: ↓ BM, T-lymphocyte ↓ may be prolonged (26–34 wk), fever in 46%, tumor lysis synd, Infxns (especially lung & IV sites), rash (50%), HA, fatigue Interactions: ↑ Risk of bleeding *W/* anticoagulants, NSAIDs, salicylates, ↑ risk of nephrotox *W/* amphotericin B Labs: Monitor CBC, LFTs, SCr NIPE: ⊘ PRG, breast-feeding; consider prophylactic allopurinol

Clarithromycin (Biaxin, Biaxin XL) [Antibiotic/Macrolide] Uses: *Upper/lower resp tract; skin/skin structure Infxns, H. pylori Infxns, & Infxns caused by nontuberculosis (atypical) Mycobacterium sp; prevention of MAC*

Infxns in HIV-Infxn* **Action:** Macrolide antibiotic, ↓ protein synth. *Spectrum:* H. influenzae, M. catarrhalis, S. pneumoniae, M. pneumoniae, & H. pylori **Dose:** *Adults.* 250–500 mg PO bid or 1000 mg (2 × 500 mg XR tab)/d. *Mycobacterium:* 500 mg PO bid. *Peds >9 mo.* 7.5 mg/kg/dose PO bid; ↓ in renal/hepatic impair **Caution:** [C, ?] Antibiotic-associated colitis; rare QT prolongation & ventricular arrhythmias, including torsades de pointes **Contra:** Macrolide allergy; w/ raniti-dine in pts w/ h/o of porphyria or CrCl <25 mL/min **Disp:** Tabs 250, 500 mg; susp 125, 250 mg/5 mL; 500, 1000 mg XR tab **SE:** ↑QT interval, causes metallic taste, N/D, abd pain, HA, rash **Interactions:** ↑ Effects *W/* amprenavir, indinavir, nelfi-navir, ritonavir; ↑ effects *OF* atorvastatin, buspirone, clozapine, colchicine, di-azepam, felodipine, itraconazole, lovastatin, simvastatin, methylprednisolone, theophylline, phenytoin, quinidine, digoxin, carbamazepine, triazolam, warfarin, ergotamine, alprazolam, valproic acid; ↓ effects *W/* EtOH; ↓ effects *OF* penicillins, zafirlukast **Labs:** ↑ Serum AST, ALT, GTT, alkaline phosphatase, LDH, total bilirubin, BUN, Cr, PT, INR; ↓ WBC **NIPE:** May take w/ food; do not refrigerate susp & discard >14 d

Clemastine Fumarate (Tavist, Dayhist, Antihist-1) [OTC] [Antihistamine]

Uses: *Allergic rhinitis & Sxs of urticaria* **Action:** Antihista-mine **Dose:** *Adults & Peds. >12 y:* 1.34 mg bid–2.68 mg tid; max 8.04 mg/d. *<6 y:* 0.335–0.67 mg/d ÷ into (max 1.34 mg/d) 2–3 d. *6–12 y:* 0.67–1.34 mg bid (max 4.02 /d) **Caution:** [C, M] BOO: Do not take w/ MAOI **Contra:** NAG **Disp:** Tabs 1.34, 2.68 mg; syrup 0.67 mg/5 mL **SE:** Drowsiness, dyscoordination, epigastric distress, urinary retention **Interactions:** ↑ Effects *W/* CNS de-pressants, MAOIs, EtOH; ↓ effects *OF* heparin, sulfonylureas

Clindamycin (Cleocin, Cleocin-T, Others) [Antibiotic/Lincomycin Derivative]

WARNING: Pseudomembranous colitis may range from mild to life threatening **Uses:** *Rx aerobic & anaerobic Infxns; topical for severe acne & vaginal Infxns* **Action:** Bacteriostatic; interferes w/ protein synth. *Spectrum:* Streptococci sp, Pneumococci sp, Staphylococci sp, & gram(+) & (–) anaerobes; no activity against gram(–) aerobes **Dose:** *Adults. PO:* 150–450 mg PO q6–8h. *IV:* 300–600 mg IV q6h or 900 mg IV q8h. *Vaginal:* 1 applicator hs for 7 d. *Topical:* Apply 1% gel, lotion, or soln bid. *Peds. Neonates:* (Avoid use; contains benzyl al-cohol) 10–15 mg/kg/24 h ÷ q8–12h. *Children >1 mo:* 10–30 mg/kg/24 h ÷ q6–8h, to a max of 1.8 g/d PO or 4.8 g/d IV. *Topical:* Apply 1%, gel, lotion, or soln bid; ↓ in severe hepatic impair **Caution:** [B, +] Can cause fatal colitis **Contra:** h/o pseudomembranous colitis **Disp:** Caps 75, 150, 300 mg; susp 75 mg/5 mL; inj 300 mg/2 mL; vaginal cream 2%; topical sol 1%; gel 1%, lotion 1%, vaginal supp 100 mg **SE:** D may be C. difficile pseudomembranous colitis, rash, ↑ LFTs **Interactions:** Effects of neuromuscular blockage *W/* tubocurarine, pancuronium; ↓ effects *W/* erythromycin, kaolin, foods w/ sodium cyclamate **Labs:** Monitor CBC, LFTs, BUN, Cr; ↓ WBC,plts **NIPE:** D/C drug w/ D, eval for C. difficile; ⊘ intercourse, tampons, douches while using vaginal cream; take oral meds w/ 8 oz water

Clofarabine (Clolar) [Antineoplastic; Purine Nucleoside Antimetabolite] **Uses:** Rx relapsed/refractory ALL after at least 2 regimens in children 1–21 y **Action:** Antimetabolite; ↓ ribonucleotide reductase w/ false nucleotide base-inhibiting DNA synth **Dose:** 52 mg/m² IV over 2 h daily × 5 d (repeat q2–6wk); per protocol **Caution:** [D, –] **Disp:** Inj 20 mg/20 mL **SE:** N/V/D, anemia, leukopenia, thrombocytopenia, neutropenia, Infxn **Interactions:** ↑ Additive risk W/ hepatotoxic or nephrotoxic drugs **Labs:** ↑ AST, ALT, Cr, HMG, Hct **NIPE:** Pts at risk for tumor lysis synd—monitor serum uric acid, phosphate, Ca & Cr bid for 2–3 d after starting chemotherapy; monitor for systemic inflammatory response synd (SIRS)/capillary leak synd; hydrate well

Clonazepam (Klonopin) [C-IV] [Anticonvulsant/Benzodiazepine] **Uses:** *Lennox-Gastaut synd, akinetic & myoclonic Szs, absence Szs, panic attacks*, restless legs synd, neuralgia, parkinsonian dysarthria, bipolar disorder **Action:** Benzodiazepine; anticonvulsant **Dose:** *Adults.* 1.5 mg/d PO in 3 ÷ doses; ↑ by 0.5–1 mg/d q3d PRN up to 20 mg/d. *Peds.* 0.01–0.03 mg/kg/24 h PO ÷ tid; ↑ to 0.1–0.2 mg/kg/24 h ÷ tid; avoid abrupt D/C **Caution:** [D, M] Elderly pts, resp Dz, CNS depression, severe hepatic impair, NAG **Contra:** Severe liver Dz, acute NAG **Disp:** Tabs 0.5, 1, 2 mg, Oral disintegrating tabs 0.125, 0.25, 0.5, 1, 2 mg **SE:** CNS side effects, including drowsiness, dizziness, ataxia, memory impair **Interactions:** ↑ CNS depression W/ antidepressants, antihistamines, opiates, benzodiazepines; ↑ effects W/ cimetidine, disulfiram, fluoxetine, INH, itraconazole, ketoconazole, metoprolol, valproic acid, EtOH, kava kava, valerian; ↓ effects W/ phenytoin **Labs:** ↑ LFTs, ↓ WBC, plts **NIPE:** ⊘ D/C abruptly; can cause retrograde amnesia; a CYP3A4 substrate

Clonidine, Oral (Catapres) [Antihypertensive/Centrally Acting Sympatholytic] **Uses:** *HTN*; opioid, EtOH, & tobacco withdrawal **Action:** Centrally acting α-adrenergic stimulant **Dose:** *Adults.* 0.1 mg PO bid, adjust daily by 0.1–0.2-mg increments (max 2.4 mg/d). *Peds.* 5–10 μg μg/kg/d ÷ q8–12h (max 0.9 mg/d); ↓ in renal impair **Caution:** [C, +/–] Avoid w/ β-blocker **Contra:** Component sensitivity **Disp:** Tabs 0.1, 0.2, 0.3 mg **SE:** drowsiness, orthostatic ↓ BP, xerostomia, constipation, bradycardia, dizziness **Interactions:** ↑ Sedation W/ CNS depressants; ↓ antihypertensive effects W/ amphetamines, BB, MAOIs TCA **Labs:** ↑ Glucose **NIPE:** More effective for HTN if combined w/ diuretics; withdraw slowly, rebound HTN w/ abrupt D/C of doses >0.2 mg bid

Clonidine, Transdermal (Catapres TTS) [Antihypertensive/Centrally Acting Sympatholytic] **Uses:** *HTN* **Action:** Centrally acting α-adrenergic stimulant **Dose:** 1 patch q7d to hairless area (upper arm/torso); titrate to effect; ↓ w/ severe renal impair **Caution:** [C, +/–] Avoid w/ β-blocker, withdraw slowly **Contra:** Component sensitivity **Disp:** TTS-1, TTS-2, TTS-3 (delivers 0.1, 0.2, 0.3 mg, respectively, of clonidine/d for 1 wk) **SE:** Drowsiness, orthostatic ↓ BP, xerostomia, constipation, bradycardia **Interactions:** ↑ Sedation W/ CNS depressants; ↓ antihypertensive effects W/ amphetamines, BB, MAOIs TCA

Labs: ↑ Glucose, CK **NIPE:** Do not D/C abruptly (rebound HTN) Doses >2 TTS-3 usually not associated w/ ↑ efficacy; steady state in 2–3 d

Clopidogrel (Plavix) [Antiplatelet/Platelet Aggregation Inhibitor] **Uses:** *Reduce atherosclerotic events*, administer ASAP in ECC setting w/ high risk ST depression or T wave inversion **Action:** ↓ Plt aggregation **Dose:** 75 mg/d; 300–600 mg PO × 1 dose can be used to load pts; 300 mg PO, then 75 mg daily 1–9 mo *(ECC 2005)* **Caution:** [B, ?] Active bleeding; risk of bleeding from trauma & other; TTP; liver Dz **Contra:** Coagulation disorders, active/or intracranial bleeding; CABG planned w/in 5–7 d **Disp:** Tabs 75 mg **SE:** ↑ Bleeding time, GI intolerance, HA, dizziness, rash, thrombocytopenia **Interactions:** ↑ Risk of GI bleed W/ ASA, NSAIDs, heparin, warfarin, feverfew, garlic, ginger, ginkgo biloba; ↑ effects *OF* phenytoin, tamoxifen, tolbutamide **Labs:** ↑ LFTs; ↓ plts, WBC; D/C drug 1 wk prior to surgery; plt aggregation to baseline 5 d after D/C, plt transfusion to reverse acutely

Clorazepate (Tranxene) [C-IV] [Anxiolytic, Anticonvulsant, Sedative/Hypnotic/Benzodiazepine] **Uses:** *Acute anxiety disorders, acute EtOH withdrawal Sxs, adjunctive therapy in partial Szs* **Action:** Benzodiazepine; antianxiety agent **Dose:** *Adults.* 15–60 mg/d PO single or ÷ doses. *Elderly & debilitated pts:* Initial 7.5–15 mg/d in ÷ doses. *EtOH withdrawal: Day 1:* Initial 30 mg; then 30–60 mg ÷ doses; *Day 2:* 45–90 mg ÷ doses; *Day 3:* 22.5–45 mg ÷ doses; *Day 4:* 15–30 mg ÷ doses. *Peds.* 3.75–7.5 mg/dose bid to 60 mg/d max ÷ bid-tid **Caution:** [D, ?/–] Elderly; h/o depression **Contra:** NAG; not OK <9 y of age **Disp:** Tabs 3.75, 7.5, 15 mg; Tabs-SD (daily) 11.25, 22.5 mg **SE:** CNS depressant effects (drowsiness, dizziness, ataxia, memory impair), ↓ BP **Interactions:** ↑ Effects W/ antidepressants, antihistamines, barbiturates, MAOIs, opiates, phenothiazines, cimetidine, disulfiram, EtOH; ↓ effects *OF* levodopa; ↓ effects W/ rifampin, ginkgo, tobacco **Labs:** ↑ Alk phosp; monitor pts w/ renal/hepatic impair (drug may accumulate) **NIPE:** ⊘ D/C abruptly; may cause dependence

Clotrimazole (Lotrimin, Mycelex, Others) [OTC] [Antifungal] **Uses:** *Candidiasis & tinea Infxns* **Action:** Antifungal; alters cell wall permeability. *Spectrum:* Oropharyngeal candidiasis, dermatophytes, superficial mycoses, cutaneous candidiasis, & vulvovaginal candidiasis **Dose:** *PO: Prophylaxis:* One troche dissolved in mouth tid *Rx:* One troche dissolved in mouth 5 × d for 14 d. *Vaginal 1% cream:* 1 applicator full hs for 7 d. *2% cream:* 1 applicator full hs for 3 d *Tabs:* 100 mg vaginally hs for 7 d or 200 mg (2 tabs) vaginally hs for 3 d or 500-mg tabs vaginally hs once. *Topical:* Apply bid 10–14 d **Caution:** [B, (C if PO), ?] Not for systemic fungal Infxn; safety in children <3 y not established **Contra:** Component allergy **Disp:** 1% cream; soln; lotion; troche 10 mg; vaginal tabs 100, 500 mg; vaginal cream 1%, 2% **SE:** *Topical:* Local irritation; *PO:* N/V **Interactions:** ↑ Effects of cyclosporine, tacrolimus; ↓ effects of spermicides **Labs:** ↑ LFTs **NIPE:** PO prophylaxis immunosuppressed pts

Clotrimazole & Betamethasone (Lotrisone) [Antifungal, Anti-inflammatory] Uses: *Fungal skin Infxns* Action: Imidazole antifungal & anti-inflammatory. *Spectrum:* Tinea pedis, cruris, & corpora Dose: *Pts = 17 y:* Apply & massage into area bid for 2–4 wk Caution: [C, ?] Varicella Infxn Contra: Children <12 y Disp: Cream 15, 45 g; lotion 30 mL SE: Local irritation, rash NIPE: Not for diaper dermatitis or under occlusive dressings

Clozapine (Clozaril & FazaClo) [Antipsychotic/Dibenzodiazepine Derivative] WARNING: Myocarditis, agranulocytosis, Szs, & orthostatic ↓ BP associated w/ clozapine; ↑ mortality in elderly w/ dementia-related psychosis Uses: *Refractory severe schizophrenia*; childhood psychosis Action: "Atypical" TCA Dose: 25 mg daily-bid initial; ↑ to 300–450 mg/d over 2 wk; maint lowest dose possible; do not D/C abruptly Caution: [B, +/–] Monitor for psychosis & cholinergic rebound Contra: Uncontrolled epilepsy; comatose state; WBC <3500 cells/mm^3 and ANC <2000 cells/mm^3 before Rx or <3000 cells/mm^3 during Rx Disp: Orally disint tabs 25 mg, 100 mg; tabs 25, 100 mg SE: Sialorrhea, tachycardia, drowsiness, ↑ wt, constipation, incontinence, rash, Szs, CNS stimulation, hyperglycemia Notes: Avoid activities where sudden loss of consciousness could cause harm; benign temperature ↑ may occur during the 1st 3 wk of Rx, weekly CBC mandatory 1st 6 mo, then qowk Interactions: ↑ Effects W/ clarithromycin, cimetidine, erythromycin, fluoxetine, paroxetine, quinidine, sertraline; ↑ depressant effects W/ CNS depressants, EtOH; ↑ effects OF digoxin, warfarin; ↓ effects W/ carbamazepine, phenytoin, primidone, phenobarbital, valproic acid, St. John's Wort, nutmeg, caffeine; ↓ effects OF phenytoin Labs: Monitor WBCs NIPE: ↑ Risk of developing agranulocytosis

Cocaine [C-II] [Narcotic analgesic] Uses: *Topical anesthetic for mucous membranes* Action: Narcotic analgesic, local vasoconstrictor Dose: Lowest topical amount that provides relief; 1 mg/kg max Caution: [C, ?] Contra: PRG Disp: Topical soln & various preparations 4–10%; powder SE: CNS stimulation, nervousness, loss of taste/smell, chronic rhinitis, CV tox, abuse potential Interactions: ↑ Effects W/ MAOIs, ↑ risk of HTN & arrhythmias W/ epinephrine NIPE: Use only on PO, laryngeal, & nasal mucosa; do not use on extensive areas of broken skin

Codeine [C-II] [Analgesic, Antitussive/Opioid] Uses: *Mild-moderate pain; symptomatic relief of cough* Action: Narcotic analgesic; ↓ cough reflex Dose: *Adults. Analgesic:* 15–20 mg PO or IM qid PRN. *Antitussive:* 10–20 mg PO q4h PRN; max 120 mg/d. *Peds. Analgesic:* 0.5–1 mg/kg/dose PO q4–6h PRN. *Antitussive:* 1–1.5 mg/kg/24 h PO ÷ q4h; max 30 mg/24 h. *Max:* 60 mg/dose; ↓ in renal/hepatic impair Caution: [C, (D if prolonged use or high dose at term), +] Contra: Component sensitivity Disp: Tabs 15, 30, 60 mg; soln 15 mg/5 mL; inj 15, 30 mg/mL SE: Drowsiness, constipation, ↓ BP Notes: 120 mg IM = 10 mg IM morphine Interactions: ↑ CNS depression W/ CNS depressants, antidepressants, MAOIs, TCAs, barbiturates, benzodiazepines, muscle relaxants, phenothiazines, cimetidine, antihistamines, sedatives, EtOH; ↑ effects *OF* digitoxin, phenytoin, rifampin; ↓ effects *W/* nalbuphine, pentazocine, tobacco **Labs:** ↑ amylase, lipase, ↑ urine morphine **NIPE:** Usually combined w/ APAP for pain or w/ agents (eg, terpin hydrate) as an antitussive

Colchicine [Antigout Agent/Colchicum Alkaloid]

Uses: *Acute gouty arthritis & prevention of recurrences; familial Mediterranean fever*; primary biliary cirrhosis **Action:** ↓ migration of leukocytes; ↓ leukocyte lactic acid production **Dose:** *Initial:* 0.6–1.2 mg PO, then 0.6 mg q1–2h until relief or GI SE develop (max 8 mg/d); do not repeat for 3 d. *IV:* 1–3 mg, then 0.5 mg q6h until relief (max 4 mg/d); do not repeat for 7 d. *Prophylaxis:* PO: 0.6 mg/d or 3–4 d/wk; ↓ renal impair **Caution:** [D, +] Elderly **Contra:** Serious renal, GI, hepatic, or cardiac disorders; blood dyscrasias **Disp:** Tabs 0.6 mg; inj 1 mg/2 mL **SE:** N/V/D, abd pain, BM suppression, hepatotox; local Rxn w/ SQ/IM **Notes:** Colchicine 1–2 mg IV w/in 24–48 h of an acute attack diagnostic/therapeutic in monoarticular arthritis **Interactions:** ↑ Risk of leukopenia *W/* phenylbutazone; ↓ effects *W/* loop diuretics; ↓ effects *OF* vitamin B_{12} **Labs:** ↑ Alk phos, ALT, AST; ↓ cholesterol, HMG, Hct, plts; false + urine Hgb & RBCs **NIPE:** ⊘ EtOH

Colesevelam (WelChol) [Antilipemic/Bile Acid Sequestrant]

Uses: *Reduction of LDL & total cholesterol alone or in combo w/ an HMG-CoA reductase inhibitor* **Action:** Bile acid sequestrant **Dose:** 3 tabs PO bid w/ meals **Caution:** [B, ?] Severe GI motility disorders; in patients w/ triglycerides >300 mg/dL (may ↑ levels); use not established in peds **Contra:** Bowel obst **Disp:** Tabs 625 mg **SE:** Constipation, dyspepsia, myalgia, weakness **Interactions:** ↓ Vitamin absorption **Labs:** Monitor lipids **NIPE:** Take w/ food and Liq; may ↓ absorption of fat-soluble vitamins

Colestipol (Colestid) [Antilipemic/Bile Acid Sequestrant]

Uses: *Adjunct to ↓ serum cholesterol in primary hypercholesterolemia, relieve pruritus associate with ↑ bile acids* **Action:** Binds intestinal bile acids to form insoluble complex **Dose:** *Granules:* 5–30 g/d ÷ 2–4 doses; *Tabs:* 2–16 g/d daily-bid **Caution:** [C, ?] Avoid w/ high triglycerides, GI dysfunction **Contra:** Bowel obst **Disp:** Tabs 1 g; granules 5, 7.5, 300, 450, 500 g **SE:** Constipation, abd pain, bloating, HA **Interactions:** ↓ Absorption *OF* numerous drugs especially anticoagulants, cardiac glycosides, digitoxin, digoxin, phenobarbital, penicillin G, tetracycline, thiazide diuretics, thyroid drugs **Labs:** ↑ Alk phos; PT prolonged **NIPE:** Take other meds 1 h before or 4 h after colestipol; do not use dry powder; mix w/ beverages, cereals, etc; may ↓ absorption of other medications and fat-soluble vitamins

Conivaptan HCL (Vaprisol) [Hyponatremic Agent/Vasopressin Receptor Antagonist]

Uses: Euvolemic hyponatremia **Action:** Dual arginine vasopressin V_{1A}/V_2 receptor antagonist **Dose:** 20 mg IV × 1 over 30 min, then 20 mg cont IV inf over 24 h; 20 mg/d cont IV inf for 1–3 more d; may ↑ to 40 mg/d if Na^+ not responding; 4 d max use; use large vein, change site q24h

Caution: [C; ?/–] Rapid ↑ Na⁺ (>12 mEq/L/24 h) may cause osmotic demyelination synd; impaired renal/hepatic Fxn; may ↑ digoxin levels; CYP3A4 inhibitor (Table 11) **Contra:** Hypovolemic hyponatremia; w/ CYP3A4 inhibitors **Disp:** Ampule 20 mg/4 mL **SE:** Inf site Rxns, HA, N/V/D, constipation, ↓ K⁺, orthostatic ↓ BP, thirst, dry mouth, pyrexia, pollakiuria, polyuria, Infxn **Interactions:** ↑ Effects *OF* amlodipine, digoxin, midazolam, simvastatin, & CYP3A4 inhibitors such as clarithromycin, itraconazole, ketoconazole, ritonavir **Labs:** May ↑ digoxin; ↓ K⁺, Na⁺, Mg²⁺; monitor Na⁺; D/C w/ very rapid ↑ Na⁺ **NIPE:** Monitor volume and neurologic status; mix only w/ 5% dextrose; D/C w/ very rapid ↑ Na⁺; monitor Na⁺, volume and neurologic status

Copper IUD Contraceptive (ParaGard T 380A) [Contraceptive]

Uses: *Contraception, long-term (up to 10 y)* **Action:** ?, Interfere w/ sperm survival/transport **Dose:** Insert any time during menstrual cycle; replace @ 10 y max **Caution:** [C, ?] Remove w/ intrauterine PRG, increased risk of comps w/ PRG and device in place **Contra:** Acute PID or in high-risk behavior, postpartum endometritis, cervicitis **Disp:** 52 mg IUD **SE:** PRG, ectopic PRG, pelvic Infxn immunocompromise, embedment, perforation expulsion, Wilson Dz, fainting w/ insert, vaginal bleeding, expulsion **NIPE:** Counsel patient does not protect against STD/HIV; see insert for detailed instructions; 99% effective

Cortisone   See Steroids, and Tables 3 & 4

Cromolyn Sodium (Intal, NasalCrom, Opticrom, others) [Antiasthmatic/Mast Cell Stabilizer]

Uses: *Adjunct to the Rx of asthma; prevent exercise-induced asthma; allergic rhinitis; ophth allergic manifestations*; food allergy **Action:** Antiasthmatic; mast cell stabilizer **Dose: Adults & Children >12 y:** *Inhal:* 20 mg (as powder in caps) inhaled qid or met-dose inhaler 2 puffs qid. *PO:* 200 mg qid 15–20 min ac, up to 400 mg qid. *Nasal instillation:* Spray once in each nostril 2–6 × /d. *Ophth:* 1–2 gtt in each eye 4–6 × /d. **Peds.** *Inhal:* 2 puffs qid of met-dose inhaler. *PO: Infants <2 y:* (Not OK) 20 mg/kg/d in 4 ÷ doses. *2–12 y:* 100 mg qid ac **Caution:** [B, ?] **Contra:** Acute asthmatic attacks **Disp:** PO conc 100 mg/5 mL; soln for neb 20 mg/2 mL; met-dose inhaler; nasal soln 40 mg/mL; ophth soln 4% **SE:** Unpleasant taste, hoarseness, coughing **Interactions:** None noted **Labs:** Monitor pulmonary Fxn tests **NIPE:** No benefit in acute Rx; 2–4 wk for max effect in perennial allergic disorders

Cyanocobalamin [Vitamin B₁₂] (Nasocobal) [Vitamin B/Dietary Supplement]

Uses: *Pernicious anemia & other vitamin B₁₂ deficiency states; ↑ requirements due to PRG; thyrotoxicosis; liver or kidney Dz* **Action:** Dietary vitamin B₁₂ supl **Dose: Adults.** 100 μg/d IM or SQ daily; intranasal: 500 μgμg once/wk for pts in remission, for 5–10 d, then 100 μg IM 2 × /wk for 1 mo, then 100 μg IM monthly. **Peds.** Use 0.2 μg/kg × 2 d test dose; if OK 30–50 μg/d/M for 2 or more wk (total 10 μg) then maint 100 mg/mo **Caution:** [A (C if dose exceeds RDA), +] **Contra:** Allergy to cobalt; hereditary optic nerve atrophy; Leber Dz **Disp:** Tabs 50, 100, 250, 500, 1000, 2500, 5000 μg; inj 100, 1000 μg/mL;

intranasal (Nasocobal) gel 500 μg/0.1 mL **SE:** Itching, D, HA, anxiety **Interactions:** ↓ Effects due to malabsorption of B_{12} **W/** aminosalicylic acid, aminoglycosides, chloramphenicol, EtOH **Labs:** ↓ K^+ levels **NIPE:** PO absorption erratic and not recommended; OK for use **W/** hyperalimentation

Cyclobenzaprine (Flexeril) [Skeletal Muscle Relaxant/ANS Agent] **Uses:** *Relief of muscle spasm* **Action:** Centrally acting skeletal muscle relaxant; reduces tonic somatic motor activity **Dose:** 5–10 mg PO bid-qid (2–3 wk max) **Caution:** [B, ?] Shares the toxic potential of the TCAs; urinary hesitancy, NAG **Contra:** Do not use concomitantly or w/in 14 d of MAOIs; hyperthyroidism; heart failure; arrhythmias **Disp:** Tabs 5, 7.5, 10 mg **SE:** Sedation & anticholinergic effects **Interactions:** ↑ Effects of CNS depression **W/** CNS depressants, TCAs, barbiturates, EtOH; ↑ risk of HTN & convulsions **W/** MAOIs **NIPE:** ↑ Fluids & fiber for constipation; may inhibit mental alertness or physical coordination

Cyclobenzaprine, extended release (Amrix) [Skeletal Muscle Relaxant/ANS Agent] **Uses:** *Muscle spasm* **Action:** ? Centrally acting long-term muscle relaxant **Dose:** 15–30 mg PO daily 2–3 wk; 30 mg/d max **Caution:** [B, ?/–] w/ urinary retention, NAG, w/ EtOH/CNS depressant **Contra:** MAOI w/in 14 d, elderly, arrhythmias, heart block, CHF, MI recovery phase, ↑thyroid **Disp:** Caps 15, 30 ER **SE:** Dry mouth, drowsiness, dizziness, HA, N, blurred vision, dysgeusia **Interactions:** ↑ Effects of CNS depression **W/** CNS depressants, TCAs, barbiturates, EtOH; ↑ risk of HTN & convulsions **W/** MAOIs **NIPE:** ↑ Fluids & fiber constipation; may inhibit mental alertness or physical coordination; avoid abrupt D/C w/ long-term use

Cyclopentolate ophthalmic (Cyclogyl, Cylate) [Anticholinergic/Cycloplegic Mydriatic Agent] **Uses:** *Cycloplegia, mydriasis* **Action:** Cycloplegic mydriatic, anticholinergic inhibits iris sphincter and ciliary body **Dose:** *Adults.* 1 gtt in eye 40–50 min preprocedure, may repeat × 1 in 5–10 min **Peds.** As adults, children 0.5–1.0%; infants use 0.5% **Caution:** [C (may cause late-term fetal anoxia/bradycardia), +/–], Premature infants HTN, Down synd, elderly, **Contra:** NAG **Disp:** Ophth soln 0.5, 1, 2% **SE:** Tearing, HA, irritation, eye pain, photophobia, arrhythmia, tremor, ↑ IOP, confusion **Interactions:** ↓ Effects *OF* carbachol, cholinesterase inhibitors, pilocarpine **NIPE:** Burning sensation when instilled; compress lacrimal sac for several min after dose; heavily pigmented irises may require ↑ strength; peak 25–75 min, cycloplegia 6–24 h, mydriasis up to 24 h; 2% soln may result in psychotic Rxns and behavioral disturbances in peds

Cyclopentolate with Phenylephrine (Cyclomydril) [Anticholinergic/Cycloplegic Mydriatic, Alpha-Adrenergic Agonist] **Uses:** * **Action:** Cycloplegic mydriatic, α-adrenergic agonist w/ anticholinergic to inhibit iris sphincter **Dose:** 1 gtt in eye q5–10min (max 3 doses) 40–50 min preprocedure **Caution:** [C (may cause late-term fetal anoxia/bradycardia), +/–] HTN, w/ elderly w/ CAD, **Contra:** NAG **Disp:** Ophth soln cyclopentolate 0.2%/phenlephrine 1% (2, 5 mL) **SE:** Tearing, HA, irritation, eye pain, photophobia, arrhythmia, tremor **NIPE:** Compress lacrimal sac for several min after dose; heavily pigmented irises may require ↑ strength; peak 25–75 min, cycloplegia 6–24 h, mydriasis up to 24 h

Cyclophosphamide (Cytoxan, Neosar) [Antineoplastic/ Alkylating Agent]

Uses: *Hodgkin Dz & NHLs; multiple myeloma; small-cell lung, breast, & ovarian CAs; mycosis fungoides; neuroblastoma; retinoblastoma; acute leukemias; allogeneic & ABMT in high doses; severe rheumatologic disorders* **Action:** Converted to acrolein & phosphoramide mustard, the active alkylating moieties **Dose:** (Per protocol) 500–1500 mg/m²; single dose at 2- to 4-wk intervals; 1.8 g/m² to 160 mg/kg (or @ 12 g/m² in 75-kg individual) in the BMT setting (per protocols); ↓ renal impair **Caution:** [D, ?] w/ BM suppression, hepatic insuff **Contra:** Component sensitivity **Disp:** Tabs 25, 50 mg; inj 500 mg, 1g, 2g **SE:** ↓ BM; hemorrhagic cystitis, SIADH, alopecia, anorexia; N/V; hepatotox; rare interstitial pneumonitis; irreversible testicular atrophy possible; cardiotox rare; 2nd malignancies (bladder, ALL), risk 3.5% at 8 y, 10.7% at 12 y **Interactions:** ↑ Effects **W/** allopurinol, cimetidine, phenobarbital, rifampin; ↑ effects **OF** succinylcholine, warfarin; ↓ effects **OF** digoxin **Labs:** May ↑ uric acid level; ↑ HMG, Hct, plts, RBC, WBCs **NIPE:** May cause sterility, hair loss, ⊘ PRG, breast-feeding, immunizations; hemorrhagic cystitis prophylaxis: continuous bladder irrigation & mesna uroprotection; encourage hydration, long-term bladder Ca screening

Cyclosporine (Sandimmune, NeOral, Gengraf) [Immuno-suppressant/Polypeptide Antibiotic]

WARNING: ↑ Risk neoplasm, ↑ risk skin malignancies, ↑ risk HTN and nephrotox **Uses:** *Organ rejection in kidney, liver, heart, & BMT w/ steroids; RA; psoriasis* **Action:** Immunosuppressant; reversible inhibition of immunocompetent lymphocytes **Dose:** **Adults & Peds.** **PO:** 15 mg/kg/d 12 h pretransplant; after 2 wk, taper by 5 mg/wk to 5–10 mg/kg/d. **IV:** If NPO, give 1/3 PO dose IV; ↓ in renal/hepatic impair **Caution:** [C, ?] Dose-related risk of nephrotox/hepatotox; live, attenuated vaccines may be less effective **Contra:** Renal impair; uncontrolled HTN **Disp:** Caps 25, 50, 100 mg; PO soln 100 mg/mL; inj 50 mg/mL **SE:** May ↑ BUN & Cr & mimic transplant rejection; HTN; HA; hirsutism **Notes:** *Levels: Trough:* Just before next dose. *Therapeutic: Variable* 150–300 ng/mL (RIA) **Interactions:** ↑ Effects **W/** azole antifungals, allopurinol, amiodarone, anabolic steroids, CCBs, cimetidine, chloroquine, clarithromycin, clonidine, diltiazem, macrolides, metoclopramide, nicardipine, NSAIDs, OCPs, ticlopidine, grapefruit juice; ↑ nephrotox **W/** aminoglycosides, amphotericin B, acyclovir, colchicine, enalapril, ranitidine, sulfonamides; ↑ risk **OF** digoxin tox; ↑ risk of hyperkalemia **W/** diuretics, ACEIs; ↓ effects **W/** barbiturates, carbamazepine, INH, nafcillin, pyrazinamide, phenytoin, rifampin, sulfonamides, St. John's Wort, alfalfa sprouts, astragalus, echinacea, licorice; ↓ effects **OF** immunizations **Labs:** ↑ SCr, BUN, LFTs, LDL,glucose; ↓ HMG, plts, WBCs **NIPE:** Monitor for hyperglycemia, hyperkalemia, hyperuricemia, risk of photosensitivity—use sunscreen; administer in glass container; NeOral & Sandimmune not interchangeable

Cyclosporine ophthalmic (Restasis) [Immunosuppressant/ Anti-inflammatory]

Uses: *↑ Tear production suppressed due to ocular inflammation* **Action:** Immune modulator, anti-inflammatory **Dose:** 1 gtt bid each eye 12 h apart; OK w/ artificial tears, allow 15 min between **Caution:** [C, –] **Contra:** Ocular Infxn, component allergy **Disp:** Single-use vial 0.05% **SE:** Ocular burning/hyperemia **NIPE:** ⊘ Children <16 y; may insert contact lenses 15 min after installation; mix vial well

Cyproheptadine (Periactin) [Antihistamine, Antipruritic]

Uses: *Allergic Rxns; itching* **Action:** Phenothiazine antihistamine; serotonin antagonist **Dose:** *Adults.* 4–20 mg PO ÷ q8h; max 0.5 mg/kg/d. *Peds.* 2–6 y: 2 mg bid-tid (max 12 mg/24 h). 7–14 y: 4 mg bid-tid; ↓ in hepatic impair **Caution:** [B, ?] BPH **Contra:** Neonates or <2 y; NAG; BOO; acute asthma; GI obst **Disp:** Tabs 4 mg; syrup 2 mg/5 mL **SE:** Anticholinergic, drowsiness **Interactions:** ↑ Effects *W/* CNS depressants, MAOIs, EtOH; ↓ effects *OF* epinephrine, fluoxetine **Labs:** False—allergy skin testing **NIPE:** ↑ Risk photosensitivity—use sunscreen, take w/ food if GI distress; may stimulate appetite

Cytarabine [ARA-C] (Cytosar-U) [Antineoplastic/Antimetabolite]

WARNING: Administration by experienced physician in properly equipped facility; potent myelosuppressive agent **Uses:** *Acute leukemias, CML, NHL; IT for leukemic meningitis or prophylaxis* **Action:** Antimetabolite; interferes w/ DNA synth **Dose:** 100–150 mg/m²/d for 5–10 d (low dose); 3 g/m² q12h for 8–12 doses (high dose); 1 mg/kg 1–2/wk (SQ maint); 5–70 mg/m² up to 3/wk IT (per protocols); ↓ in renal/hepatic impair **Caution:** [D, ?] w/ marked BM suppression, ↓ dosage by ↓ the number of days of administration **Contra:** Component sensitivity **Disp:** Inj 100, 500 mL, 1, 2 g also 20, 100 mg/mL **SE:** ↓ BM, N/V/D, stomatitis, flulike Sx, rash on palms/soles, hepatic/cerebellar dysfunction, noncardiogenic pulm edema, neuropathy, fever **Interactions:** ↓ Effects *OF* digoxin, flucytosine **Labs:** ↑ Uric acid, ↓ HMG, Hct, plts, RBCs, WBCs **NIPE:** ⊘ EtOH, NSAIDs, ASA, PRG, breast-feeding, immunizations; little use in solid tumors; high-dose tox limited by corticosteroid ophth soln

Cytarabine Liposome (DepoCyt) [Antineoplastic/Antimetabolite]

WARNING: Can cause chemical arachnoiditis (N/V/HA, fever) ↓ severity w/ dexamethasone. Administer by experienced physician in properly equipped facility **Uses:** *Lymphomatous meningitis* **Action:** Antimetabolite; interferes w/ DNA synth **Dose:** 50 mg IT q14d for 5 doses, then 50 mg IT q28d × 4 doses; use dexamethasone prophylaxis **Caution:** [D, ?] May cause neurotox; blockage to CSF flow may ↑ the risk of neurotox; use in peds not established **Contra:** Active meningeal Infxn **Disp:** IT inj 50 mg/5 mL **SE:** Neck pain/rigidity, HA, confusion, somnolence, fever, back pain, N/V, edema, neutropenia, ↓ plt, anemia **Interactions:** ↓ Effects *OF* digoxin, flucytosine **Labs:** ↑ Uric acid, ↓ HMG, Hct, plts, RBCs, WBCs **NIPE:** ⊘ EtOH, NSAIDs, ASA, PRG, breast-feeding, immunizations; cytarabine liposomes are similar in microscopic appearance to WBCs; caution in interpreting CSF studies

Cytomegalovirus Immune Globulin [CMV-IG IV] (CytoGam) [Immune Globulin] Uses: *Attenuation CMV Dz associated w/ transplantation* **Action:** Exogenous IgG antibodies to CMV **Dose:** 150 mg/kg/dose w/in 72 h of transplant, for 16 wk posttransplant; see insert **Caution:** [C, ?] Anaphylactic Rxns; renal dysfunction **Contra:** Allergy to immunoglobulins; IgA deficiency **Disp:** Inj 50 mg/mL **SE:** Flushing, N/V, muscle cramps, wheezing, HA, fever **Interactions:** ↓ Effects *OF* live virus vaccines **NIPE:** IV only; administer by separate line; do not shake; administer immunizations at least 3 mo after CMV-IG

Dacarbazine (DTIC) [Antineoplastic/Alkylating Agent]
WARNING: Causes hematopoietic depression, hepatic necrosis, may be carcinogenic, teratogenic **Uses:** *Melanoma, Hodgkin Dz, sarcoma* **Action:** Alkylating agent; antimetabolite as a purine precursor; ↓ protein synth, RNA, & especially DNA **Dose:** 2–4.5 mg/kg/d for 10 consecutive d or 250 mg/m²/d for 5 d (Per protocols); ↓ in renal impair **Caution:** [C, ?] In BM suppression; renal/hepatic impair **Contra:** Component sensitivity **Disp:** Inj 100, 200, 500 mg **SE:** ↓ BM, N/V, hepatotox, flu-like Sx, ↓ BP, photosens, alopecia, facial flushing, facial paresthesias, urticaria, phlebitis at inj site **Interactions:** ↑ Risk of bleeding *W/* anticoagulants, ASA; ↓ effects *W/* phenobarbital, phenytoin **Labs:** ↑ AST, ALT; ↓ plts, RBCs, WBCs **NIPE:** Risk of photosensitivity—use sunscreen, hair loss, Infxn; avoid extravasation

Daclizumab (Zenapax) [Immunosuppressant/Immunomodulator] **WARNING:** Administer under skilled supervision in equipped facility **Uses:** *Prevent acute organ rejection* **Action:** IL-2 receptor antagonist **Dose:** 1 mg/kg/dose IV; 1st dose pretransplant, then 4 doses 14 d apart post-transplant **Caution:** [C, ?] **Contra:** Component sensitivity **Disp:** Inj 5 mg/mL **SE:** Hyperglycemia, edema, HTN, ↓ BP, constipation, HA, dizziness, anxiety, nephrotox, pulm edema, pain, anaphylaxis/hypersensivity; **Interactions:** ↑ Risk of mortality *W/* corticosteroids, cyclosporine, mycophenolate mofetil; **NIPE:** ⊘ Immunizations, Infxns, ↑ fluid intake; Administer w/in 4 h of preparation

Dactinomycin (Cosmegen) [Antineoplastic/Antibiotic]
WARNING: Administer under skilled supervision in equipped facility; powder and soln toxic, corrosive, mutagenic, carcinogenic, & teratogenic, avoid exposure and use precautions **Uses:** *Choriocarcinoma, Wilms tumor, Kaposi and Ewing sarcoma, rhabdomyosarcoma, uterine and testicular CA* **Action:** DNA intercalating agent **Dose:** *Adult:* 0.5 mg/kg/d for 5 d; 2 mg/wk for 3 consecutive wk; 15 μg/kg or 0.45 mg/m²/d (max 0.5 mg) for 5 d q3–8wk *Peds: Sarcoma* (per protocols); ↓ in renal impair **Caution:** [C, ?] **Contra:** Concurrent/recent chickenpox or herpes zoster; infants <6 mo **Disp:** Inj 0.5 mg **SE:** Myelo/immunosuppression, severe N/V, alopecia, acne, hyperpigmentation, radiation recall phenomenon, tissue damage w/ extrav, hepatotox **Interactions:** ↑ Effects of BM suppressants, radiation therapy; ↓ effects of vitamin K **Labs:** Monitor CBC; ↓ HMG, Hct, plts, RBCs, WBCs **NIPE:** ⊘ PRG, breast-feeding; risk of irreversible infertility, reversible hair loss, ↑ fluids to 2–3 L/d

Dalteparin (Fragmin) [Anticoagulant/Low Molecular Weight Heparin] WARNING: ↑ Risk of spinal/epidural hematoma with LP Uses: *Unstable angina, non-Q-wave MI, prevention of ischemic comps due to clot formation in pts on concurrent ASA, prevent & Rx DVT following surgery* **Action:** LMW heparin **Dose:** *Angina/MI:* 120 units/kg (max 10,000 units) SQ q12h w/ ASA. DVT prophylaxis: 2500–5000 units SC 1–2 h preop, then daily for 5–10 d. *Systemic anticoagulation:* 200 units/kg/d SQ or 100 units/kg bid SQ **Caution:** [B, ?] In renal/hepatic impair, active hemorrhage, cerebrovascular Dz, cerebral aneurysm, severe HTN **Contra:** HIT; pork product allergy; w/ mifepristone **Disp:** Inj 2500 units (16 mg/0.2 mL), 5000 units (32 mg/0.2 mL), 7500 units (48 mg/0.3 mL), 10,000 units (64 mg/mL), 25,000 units/mL (3.8 mL); prefilled vials: 10,000 units/mL (9.5 mL) **SE:** Bleeding, pain at site, ↓ plt **Interactions:** ↑ Bleeding *W/* oral anticoagulants, plt inhibitors, warfarin, garlic, ginger, ginkgo biloba, ginseng, chamomile **Labs:** ↑ AST, ALT; monitor CBC & plts **NIPE:** ⊘ Give IM or IV; administer Subq OK route only

Dantrolene (Dantrium) [Skeletal Muscle Relaxant/Hydantoin Derivative] WARNING: Hepatotox reported; D/C after 45 d if no benefit observed Uses: *Rx spasticity due to upper motor neuron disorders (eg, spinal cord injuries, stroke, CP, MS); malignant hyperthermia* **Action:** Skeletal muscle relaxant **Dose:** *Adults. Spasticity:* 25 mg PO daily; ↑ 25 mg to effect to 100 mg max PO qid PRN. *Peds.* 0.5 mg/kg/dose bid; ↑ by 0.5 mg/kg to effect, to 3 mg/kg/dose max qid PRN. *Adults & Peds. Malignant hyperthermia: Rx:* Continuous rapid IV, start 1 mg/kg until Sxs subside or 10 mg/kg is reached. *Postcrisis F/U:* 4–8 mg/kg/d in 3–4 ÷ doses for 1–3 d to prevent recurrence **Caution:** [C, ?] Impaired cardiac/pulm Fxn **Contra:** Active hepatic Dz; where spasticity needed to maintain posture or balance **Disp:** Caps 25, 50, 100 mg; powder for inj 20 mg/vial **SE:** Hepatotox, ↑ LFTs, drowsiness, dizziness, rash, muscle weakness, D/N/V pleural effusion w/ pericarditis, D, blurred vision, hepatitis **Interactions:** ↑ Effects *W/* CNS depressants, antihistamines, opiates, EtOH; ↑ risk of hepatotox *W/* estrogens; ↑ risk of CV collapse & ventricular fib *W/* CCBs; ↓ plasma protein binding *W/* clofibrate, warfarin **Labs:** ↑ LFTs **NIPE:** ↑ Risk of photosensitivity—use sunscreen; ⊘ EtOH

Dapsone, Oral [Antileprotic, Antimalarial] Uses: *Rx & prevent PCP; toxoplasmosis prophylaxis; leprosy* **Action:** Unknown; bactericidal **Dose:** *Adults.* PCP prophylaxis 50–100 mg/d PO; Rx PCP 100 mg/d PO w/ TMP 15–20 mg/kg/d for 21 d. *Peds.* PCP prophylaxis alternated dose: (>1 mo) 4 mg/kg/dose once/wk (max 200 mg); Prophylaxis of PCP 1–2 mg/kg/24 h PO daily; max 100 mg/d **Caution:** [C, +] G6PD deficiency; severe anemia **Contra:** Component sensitivity **Disp:** Tabs 25, 100 mg **SE:** Hemolysis, methemoglobinemia, agranulocytosis, rash, cholestatic jaundice **Notes:** Absorption ↑ by an acidic environment; for leprosy, combine w/ rifampin & other agents **Interactions:** ↑ Effects *W/* probenecid, trimethoprim; ↓ effects *W/* activated charcoal, rifampin **Labs:** Monitor CBC, LFTs **NIPE:** ↑ Risk of photosensitivity—use sunscreen

Dapsone, topical (Aczone) [Antileprotic, Antimalarial] Uses: *Topical for acne vulgaris* Action: Unknown; bactericidal Dose: Apply pea-sized amount and rub into areas BID; wash hands after Caution: [C, +] G6PD deficiency; severe anemia Contra: Component sensitivity Disp: 5% gel SE: Skin oiliness/peeling, dryness erythema Labs: Monitor CBC; check G6PD levels and monitor G6PD if deficient NIPE: Not for oral, ophthalmic, or intravag use

Daptomycin (Cubicin) [Antibiotic/Cyclic Lipopeptide Antibacterial] Uses: *Complicated skin/skin structure Infxns due to gram(+) organisms* S. aureus, bacteremia, right-sided MSA, MRSA endocarditis Action: Cyclic lipopeptide; rapid membrane depolarization & bacterial death. Spectrum: S. aureus (including MRSA), S. pyogenes, S. agalactiae, S. dysgalactiae subsp Equisimilis & E. faecalis (vancomycin-susceptible strains only) Dose: Bacteremia: 4 mg/kg IV daily × 7–14 d (over 30 min); 6mg/kg IV daily for 2–6 wk; Endocarditis: 6 mg/kg q 48; ↓ w/ CrCl < 30 mL/min/ or Dialysis: 4 mg/kg q48h Contra: [B, ?] w/ HMG-CoA inhibitors Disp: Inj 250, 500 mg/10 mL SE: Anemia, constipation, N/V/D, HA, rash, site Rxn, muscle pain/weakness, edema, cellulitis, hypo/hyperglycemia, ↑ alkaline phosphatase, cough, back pain, abd pain, ↓ K⁺, anxiety, chest pain, sore throat, cardiac failure, confusion, Candida Infxns Notes: Consider D/C HMG-CoA reductase inhibitors to ↓ myopathy risk Interactions: ↑ Effects OF anticoagulants; ↓ effects OF tobramycin; ↓ effects W/ tobramycin Labs: monitor CPK baseline and weekly, LFTs, PT, INR; ↑ alkaline phosphatase, CPK, LFTs; ↓ HMG, Hct, K⁺ NIPE: Monitor for pseudomembranous colitis; safety & efficacy not established in pts <18 y

Darbepoetin Alfa (Aranesp) [Antianemic/Hematopoietic] WARNING: Associated with ↑ CV, thromboembolic events and/or mortality; D/C if HB >12 g/dL; may increase tumor progression and death in cancer patients Uses: *Anemia associated w/ CRF*, anemia in nonmyeloid malignancy w/ concurrent chemo Action: ↑ Erythropoiesis, recombinant erythropoietin variant Dose: 0.45 µg/kg single IV or SQ qwk; titrate, do not exceed target Hgb of 12 g/dL; use lowest doses possible, see insert to convert from Epogen Caution: [C, ?] May ↑ risk of CV &/or neurologic SE in renal failure; HTN; w/ h/o Szs Contra: Uncontrolled HTN, component allergy Disp: 25, 40, 60, 100, 200, 300, µg/mL, 150 µg/0.075 mL in polysorbate or albumin excipient SE: May ↑ cardiac risk, CP, hypo/hypertension, N/V/D, myalgia, arthralgia, dizziness, edema, fatigue, fever, ↑ risk Infxn Interactions: None noted Labs: Monitor weekly CBC until stable NIPE: Longer 1/2-life than Epogen; monitor BP & for Sz activity, shaking vial inactivates drug

Darifenacin (Enablex) [Antispasmodic/Anticholinergic] Uses: *OAB* Urinary antispasmodic, Action: Muscarinic receptor antagonist Dose: 7.5 mg/d PO; 15 mg/d max (7.5 mg/d w/ moderate hepatic impair or w/ CYP3A4 inhibitors); w/ drugs metabolized by CYP2D) (Table 11); swallow whole Caution: [C, ?/–] w/ hepatic impair Contra: Urinary/gastric retention, uncontrolled NAG, paralytic ileus Disp: Tabs ER 7.5 mg, 15 mg SE: Xerostomia/eyes, constipation, dyspepsia, abd pain, retention, abnormal vision, dizziness, asthenia

Interactions: ↑ Effects W/ clarithromycin, itraconazole, ketoconazole, ritonavir, nelfinavir, ↑ effects OF digoxin, flecainide, TCAs, thioridazine **Labs:** Monitor LFTs **NIPE:** Take W/ or W/O food & swallow whole; drug will relieve symptoms but not treat cause; may cause heat prostration d/t < sweating

Darunavir (Prezista) [Antiretroviral/Protease Inhibitor]
Uses: *Rx HIV w/ resistance to multiple protease inhibitors* **Action:** HIV-1 protease inhibitor **Dose:** 600 mg PO BID, administer w/ ritonavir 100 mg BID **Caution:** [B, ?/–] h/o sulf allergy, CYP3A4 substrate, increase or decrease levels of many medications **Contra:** w/ astezole, terfadine, dihydroergotamine, ergonovine, ergotamine, methylergonovine, pimozide, midazolam, triazolam **Supplied:** Tabs 300 mg **SE:** Central redistribution of fat (metabolic synd), N **Interactions:** ↑ Effects OF amiodarone, atorvastatin, bepridil, clarithromycin, cyclosporine, dihydropyridine, felodipine, HMG-CoA reductase inhibitors (statins), itraconazole, ketoconazole, lidocaine, nifedipine, pravastatin, quinidine, sildenafil, tacrolimus, trazodone, vardenafil; ↓ effects W/ carbamazepine, phenobarbital, phenytoin, rifabutin, rifampin, efavirenz, St. John's Wort; ↓ effects OF methadone, rifampin, SSRI, trazodone, warfarin **Labs:** ↑ Amylase, glucose; cholesterol, triglycerides, LFTs, uric acid; ↓ WBCs, neutrophils **NIPE:** Administer w/ ritonavir and food

Dasatinib (Sprycel) [Antineoplastic/Protein-Tyrosin Kinase Inhibitor] **Uses:** CML, Ph + ALL **Action:** Multi tyrosine kinase inhibitor **Dose:** 70 mg PO bid; adjust w/ CYP3A inhibitors/inducers (Table 11) **Caution:** [D, ?/–] **Contra:** None **Disp:** Tabs 20, 50, 70 mg **SE:** ↓ BM, edema, fluid retention, pleural effusions, N/V/D, abd pain, bleeding, fever, ↑ QT **Interactions:** ↑ Effects W/ atazanavir, clarithromycin, erythromycin, indinavir, itraconazole, ketoconazole, nefazodone, nelfinavir, ritonavir, saquinavir, telithromycin; ↓ effects W/ antacids, carbamazepine, dexamethasone, phenobarbital, phenytoin, rifampicin, St. John's Wort **Labs:** ↑ LFTs, Cr, uric acid, troponin levels; ↓ plts, RBC, neutrophils; monitor CBC weekly for 2 mo, then monthly **NIPE:** ⊘ Chew or crush tabs

Daunorubicin (Daunomycin, Cerubidine) [Antineoplastic/Anthracycline] **WARNING:** Cardiac Fxn should be monitored due to potential risk for cardiac tox & CHF, renal/hepatic dsfxn **Uses:** *Acute leukemias* **Action:** DNA intercalating agent; ↓ topoisomerase II; generates oxygen free radicals **Dose:** 45–60 mg/m²/d for 3 consecutive d; 25 mg/m²/wk (per protocols); ↓ in renal/hepatic impair **Caution:** [D, ?] **Contra:** Component sensitivity **Disp:** Inj 20, 50 mg **SE:** ↓ BM, mucositis, N/V, alopecia, radiation recall phenomenon, hepatotox (hyperbilirubinemia), tissue necrosis w/ extrav, cardiotox (1–2% CHF w/ 550 mg/m² cumulative dose) **Notes:** Prevent cardiotox w/ dexrazoxane (when pt received >300 mg/m of daunorubicin cum dose); for IV use only; admin allopurinol prior to ↓ risk of hyperuricemia **Interactions:** ↑ Risk of cardiotox W/ cyclophosphamide; ↑ myelosuppression W/ antineoplastic agents; ↓ response to live virus vaccines **Labs:** ↓ Neutrophils, plts **NIPE:** ⊘ ASA, NSAIDs, EtOH, PRG, breast-feeding, immunizations; risk of hair loss

Decitabine (Dacogen) Uses: *MDS* Action: Inhibits DNA methyltransferase Dose: 15 mg/m^2 cont inf over 3 h; repeat q8h × 3 d; repeat cycle q6wk, min 4 cycles; delay Tx and ↓ dose if inadequate hematologic recovery at 6 wk (see label protocol) Caution: [D, ?/–]; avoid PRG; males should not father a child during or 2 mo after; renal/hepatic impair Disp: Powder 50 mg/vial SE: Neutropenia, febrile neutropenia, thrombocytopenia, anemia, leukopenia, peripheral edema, petechiae, N/V/D, constipation, stomatitis, dyspepsia, cough, fever, fatigue, ↑ LFTs & bili, hyperglycemia, Infxn, HA Labs: ↑ LFTs, bili, glucose; check CBC and plt before each cycle & PRN NIPE: May premedicate w/ antiemetic; ⊘ PRG; males should not father a child during or 2 mo after use

Delavirdine (Rescriptor) [Antiretroviral/NNRTI] Uses: *HIV Infxn* Action: Nonnucleoside RT inhibitor Dose: 400 mg PO tid Caution: [C, ?] CDC recommends HIV-infected mothers not to breast-feed (transmission risk); w/ renal/hepatic impair Contra: Use w/ drugs dependent on CYP3A for clearance (Table 11) Disp: Tabs 100, 200 mg SE: Fat redistribution, immune reconstitution synd, HA, fatigue, rash, ↑ transaminases, N/V/D Interactions: ↑ Effects W/ fluoxetine; ↑ effects OF benzodiazepines, cisapride, clarithromycin, dapsone, ergotamine, indinavir, lovastatin, midazolam, nifedipine, quinidine, ritonavir, simvastatin, terfenadine, triazolam, warfarin; ↓ effects W/ antacids, barbiturates, carbamazepine, cimetidine, famotidine, lansoprazole, nizatidine, phenobarbital, phenytoin, ranitidine, rifabutin, rifampin; ↓ effects OF dianosine Labs: ↑ AST, ALT, ↓ HMG, Hct, plts, neutrophil counts, WBC NIPE: Take w/o regard to food

Deferasirox (Exjade) [Iron Chelator] Uses: *Chronic iron overload due to transfusion in patients >2 y* Action: Oral iron chelator Dose: Initial: 20 mg/kg PO/d; adjust by 5–10 mg/kg q3–6mo based on monthly ferritin; 30 mg/kg/d max; on empty stomach 30 min before food; hold dose if ferritin <500 µg/L, dissolve in water, orange, apple juice (<1 g/3.5 oz; >1 g in 7 oz) drink immediately; resuspend residue and swallow; do not chew, swallow whole tabs or take w/ Al-containing antacids Caution: [B, ?/–] Disp: Tabs for oral susp 125, 250, 500 mg SE: N/V/D, abd pain, skin rash, HA, fever, cough, Infxn, hearing loss, dizziness, cataracts, retinal disorders, ↑ IOP, lens opacities, dizziness Notes: ARF, peripheral cytopenia possible Labs: ↑ Cr, LFTs; ✓ Cr weekly 1st mo then Q month, ✓monitor CBC; monthly Cr, urine protein, LFTs NIPE: Do not combine w/ other iron chelator therapies; dose to nearest whole tablet; auditory and ophthalmic testing initially and q12 mo

Demeclocycline (Declomycin) [Antibiotic] Uses: *SIADH* Action: Antibiotic, antagonizes ADH action on renal tubules Dose: 300–600 mg PO q12h on empty stomach; ↓ in renal failure; avoid antacids Caution: [D, +] Avoid in hepatic/renal impair & children Contra: Tetracycline allergy Disp: Tabs 150, 300 mg SE: D, abd cramps, photosens, DI Interactions: Effects OF digoxin, anticoagulants; ↓ effects W/ antacids, Bi salts, Fe, Na bicarbonate, barbiturates, carbamazepine, hydantoins, food; ↓ effects *OF* OCPs, penicillin **Labs:** False—urine glucose; monitor CBC, LFTs, BUN, Cr **NIPE:** Risk of photosensitivity—use sunscreen & avoid sunlight

Desipramine (Norpramin) [Antidepressant/TCA] WARNING: Closely monitor for worsening depression or emergence of suicidality **Uses:** *Endogenous depression*, chronic pain, peripheral neuropathy **Action:** TCA; ↑ synaptic serotonin or norepinephrine in CNS **Dose:** 75–200 mg/d single or ÷ dose; usually single hs dose (max 300 mg/d); ↓ dose in elderly **Caution:** [C, ?/–] CV Dz, Sz disorder, hypothyroidism **Contra:** MAOIs w/in 14 d; during AMI recovery phase **Disp:** Tabs 10, 25, 50, 75, 100, 150 mg; caps 25, 50 mg **SE:** Anticholinergic (blurred vision, urinary retention, xerostomia); orthostatic ↓ BP; ↑ QT interval, arrhythmias **Interactions:** ↑ Effects *W/* cimetidine, diltiazem, fluoxetine, indinavir, MAOIs, paroxetine, propoxyphene, quinidine, ritonavir ranitidine, EtOH, grapefruit juice; ↑ effects *OF* Li, sulfonylureas; ↓ effects *W/* barbiturates, carbamazepine rifampin, tobacco **NIPE:** Full effect of drug may take 4 wk; blue-green urine; risk of photosensitivity—use sunscreen

Desloratadine (Clarinex) [Antihistamine/Selective H₁-Receptor Antagonist] Uses: *Seasonal & perennial allergic rhinitis; chronic idiopathic urticaria* **Action:** Active metabolite of Claritin, H₁-antihistamine, blocks inflammatory mediators **Dose:** *Adults & Peds >12 y:* 5 mg PO daily; 5 mg PO qod w/ hepatic/renal impair **Caution:** [C, ?/–] RediTabs contain phenylalanine; safety not established for <12 y **Disp:** Tabs & RediTabs (rapid dissolving) 5 mg, syrup 0.5 mg/mL **SE:** Allergy, anaphylaxis, somnolence, HA, dizziness, fatigue, pharyngitis, xerostomia, N, dyspepsia, myalgia **Labs:** ↑ LFTs, bilirubin **NIPE:** Take w/o regard to food

Desmopressin (DDAVP, Stimate) [Antidiuretic/Hormone] Uses: *DI (intranasal & parenteral); bleeding due to uremia, hemophilia A, & type I von Willebrand Dz (parenteral), nocturnal enuresis* **Action:** Synthetic analog of vasopressin (human ADH); ↑ factor VIII **Dose:** *DI: Intranasal: Adults.* 0.1–0.4 mL (10–40 µg/d in 1–3 ÷ doses). *Peds 3 mo–12 y:* 0.05–0.3 mL/d in 1 or 2 doses. *Parenteral: Adults.* 0.5–1 mL (2–4 µg/d in 2 ÷ doses); converting from nasal to parenteral, use 1/10 nasal dose. *PO: Adults.* 0.05 mg bid; ↑ to max of 1.2 mg. *Hemophilia A & von Willebrand Dz (typeI): Adults & Peds >10 kg:* 0.3 µg/kg in 50 mL NS, inf over 15–30 min. *Peds <10 kg.* As above w/ dilution to 10 mL w/ NS. *Nocturnal enuresis: Peds >6 y:* 20 µg intranasally hs **Caution:** [B, M] Avoid overhydration **Contra:** Hemophilia B; CrCl <50 mL/min, severe classic von Willebrand Dz; pts w/ factor VIII antibodies **Disp:** Tabs 0.1, 0.2 mg; inj 4, 15 µg/mL; nasal soln 0.1, 1.5 mg/mL **SE:** Facial flushing, HA, dizziness, vulval pain, nasal congestion, pain at inj site, ↓ Na⁺, H₂O intox **Interactions:** ↑ Antidiuretic effects *W/* carbamazepine, chlorpropamide, clofibrate; ↑ effects *OF* vasopressors; ↓ antidiuretic effects *W/* demeclocycline, Li, norepinephrine **NIPE:** Monitor I&O; ⊘ EtOH, overhydration; in very young & old pts, ↓ fluid intake to avoid H₂O intox & ↓ Na⁺

Dexamethasone, Nasal (Dexacort Phosphate Turbinaire) [Anti-inflammatory, Immunosuppressant/Glucocorticoid] Uses: *Chronic nasal inflammation or allergic rhinitis* Action: Anti-inflammatory corticosteroid Dose: *Adult & Peds >12 y:* 2 sprays/nostril bid-tid, max 12 sprays/d. *Peds 6–12 y:* 1–2 sprays/nostril bid, max 8 sprays/d Caution: [C, ?] Contra: Untreated Infxn Disp: Aerosol, 84 μg/activation SE: Local irritation NIPE: Use decongestant nose gtt 1st if nasal congestion

Dexamethasone, Ophthalmic (AK-Dex Ophthalmic, Decadron Ophthalmic) [Anti-inflammatory, Immunosuppressant/ Glucocorticoid] Uses: *Inflammatory or allergic conjunctivitis* Action: Anti-inflammatory corticosteroid Dose: Instill 1–2 gtt tid-qid Caution: [C, ?/–] Contra: Active untreated bacterial, viral, & fungal eye Infxns Disp: Susp & soln 0.1%; oint 0.05% SE: Long-term use associated w/ cataracts NIPE: Eval intraocular pressure and lens if prolonged use

Dexamethasone Systemic, Topical (Decadron) [Anti-inflammatory, Immunosuppressant/Glucocorticoid] See Steroids, Systemic, & Tables 3 and 4; Interactions: ↑ Effects W/ cyclosporine, estrogens, OCPs, macrolides; ↑ effects OF cyclosporine; ↓ effects W/ aminoglutethimide, antacids, barbiturates, carbamazepine, cholestyramine, colestipol, phenytoin, phenobarbital, rifampin; ↓ effects OF anticoagulants, hypoglycemics, INH, toxoids, salicylates, vaccines Labs: False—allergy skin tests NIPE: ⊘ Vaccines, breast-feeding, use on broken skin

Dexpanthenol (Ilopan-Choline PO, Ilopan) [Cholinergic] Uses: *Minimize paralytic ileus, Rx postop distention* Action: Cholinergic agent Dose: *Adults. Relief of gas:* 2–3 tabs PO tid. *Prevent postop ileus:* 250–500 mg IM stat, repeat in 2 h, then q6h PRN. *Ileus:* 500 mg IM stat, repeat in 2 h, then q6h, PRN Caution: [C, ?] Contra: Hemophilia, mechanical bowel obst Disp: Inj 250 mg/mL; tabs 50 mg; cream 2% SE: GI cramps NIPE: Monitor BP during IV administration

Dexrazoxane (Zinecard) [Chelating Agent] Uses: *Prevent anthracycline-induced (eg, doxorubicin) cardiomyopathy* Action: Chelates heavy metals; binds intracellular iron & prevents anthracycline-induced free radicals Dose: 10:1 ratio dexrazoxane:doxorubicin 30 min prior to each dose, 5:1 ratio w/ CrCl <40 mL/min Caution: [C, ?] Contra: Component sensitivity Disp: Inj powder 250, 500 mg (10 mg/mL) SE: ↓ BM (esp. leukopenia), fever, Infxn, stomatitis, alopecia, N/V/D Interactions: ↑ Length of muscle relaxation W/ succinylcholine Labs: Mild ↑ transaminase; NIPE: inj site pain

Dextran 40 (Rheomacrodex, Gentran 40) [Plasma Volume Expander; Glucose Polymer] Uses: *Shock, prophylaxis of DVT & thromboembolism, adjunct in peripheral vascular surgery* Action: Expands plasma volume; ↓ blood viscosity Dose: *Shock:* 10 mL/kg inf rapidly; 20 mL/kg max 1st 24 h; beyond 24 h 10 mL/kg max; D/C after 5 d. *Prophylaxis of DVT & thromboembolism:* 10 mL/kg IV day of surgery, then 500 mL/d IV for 2–3 d, then

500 mL IV q2–3d based on risk for up to 2 wk **Caution:** [C, ?] **Inf Rxns:** w/ corticosteroids **Contra:** Major hemostatic defects; cardiac decompensation; renal Dz w/ severe oliguria/anuria **Disp:** 10% dextran 40 in 0.9% NaCl or 5% dextrose **SE:** Allergy/anaphylactoid Rxn (observe during 1st min of inf), arthralgia, cutaneous Rxns, ↓ BP, fever **Interactions:** ↑ Bleeding times W/ antiplt agents or anticoagulants **Labs:** Monitor Cr & lytes; ↑ ALT, AST **NIPE:** Draw blood before administration of drug; pt should be well hydrated prior to inf

Dextromethorphan (Mediquell, Benylin DM, PediaCare 1, Delsym, others) [OTC] [Antitussive]
Uses: *Control nonproductive cough* **Action:** Suppresses medullary cough center **Dose:** *Adults.* 10–30 mg PO q4h PRN (max 120 mg/24 h). *Peds. 2–6 y:* 2.5–7.5 mg q4–8h (max 30 mg/24 h). *7–12 y:* 5–10 mg q4–8h (max 60 mg/24/h) **Caution:** [C, ?/–] Not for persistent or chronic cough contra: (2 y) **Disp:** Caps 30 mg; lozenges 2.5, 5, 7.5, 15 mg; syrup 15 mg/15 mL, 10 mg/5 mL; Liq 10 mg/15 mL, 3.5, 7.5, 15 mg/5 mL; sustained-action Liq 30 mg/5 mL **SE:** GI disturbances **Interactions:** ↑ Effects W/ amiodarone, fluoxetine, quinidine, terbinafine; ↑ risk of serotonin syndrome W/ sibutramine, MAOIs; ↑ CNS depression W/ antihistamines, antidepressants, sedative, opioids, EtOH **NIPE:** ↑ Fluids, humidity to environment, stop MAOIs for 2 wk before administering drug; Found in combo OTC products w/ guaifenesin; deaths reported in <2 y; abuse potential; efficacy in children debated

Diazepam (Valium, Diastat) [C-IV] [Anxiolytic, Skeletal Muscle Relaxant, Anticonvulsant, Sedative/Hypnotic/Benzodiazepine]
Uses: *Anxiety, EtOH withdrawal, muscle spasm, status epilepticus, panic disorders, amnesia, preop sedation* **Action:** Benzodiazepine **Dose:** *Adults. Status epilepticus:* 5–10 mg q10–20min to 30 mg max in 8-h period. *Anxiety, muscle spasm:* 2–10 mg PO bid-qid or IM/IV q3–4h PRN. *Preop:* 5–10 mg PO or IM 20–30 min or IV just prior to procedure. *EtOH withdrawal:* Initial 2–5 mg IV, then 5–10 mg q5–10min, 100 mg in 1 h max. May require up to 1000 mg/24 h for severe withdrawal; titrate to agitation; avoid excessive sedation; may lead to aspiration or resp arrest. *Peds. Status epilepticus: <5 y:* 0.05–0.3 mg/kg/dose IV q15–30min up to a max of 5mg. *>5 y:* max of 10 mg. *Sedation, muscle relaxation:* 0.04–0.3 mg/kg/dose q2–4h IM or IV to max of 0.6 mg/kg in 8 h, or 0.12–0.8 mg/kg/24 h PO ÷ tid-qid; ↓ w/ hepatic impair **Caution:** [D, ?/–] **Contra:** Coma, CNS depression, resp depression, NAG, severe uncontrolled pain, PRG **Disp:** Tabs 2, 5, 10 mg; soln 1, 5mg/mL; inj 5 mg/mL; rectal gel 2.5, 5, 10, 20 mg/mL **SE:** Sedation, amnesia, bradycardia, ↓ BP, rash, ↓ resp rate **Notes:** 5 mg/min IV max in adults or 1–2 mg/min in peds (resp arrest possible) **Interactions:** ↑ Effects W/ antihistamines, azole antifungals, BBs, CNS depressants, cimetidine, ciprofloxin, disulfiram, INH, OCP, omeprazole, phenytoin, valproic acid, verapamil, EtOH, kava kava, valerian; ↑ effects OF digoxin, diuretics; ↓ effects W/ barbiturates, carbamazepine, theophylline, ranitidine, tobacco; ↓ effects OF haloperidol, levodopa **Labs:** Monitor LFTs, BUN, Cr, CBC w/ long-term drug use **NIPE:** Risk ↑ Sz activity; IM absorption erratic; avoid abrupt D/C

Diazoxide (Proglycem) [Antihypertensive/Peripheral Vasodilator] Uses: *Hypoglycemia due to hyperinsulinism (Proglycem); hypertensive crisis (Hyperstat)* Action: ↓ Pancreatic insulin release; antihypertensive Dose: Repeat in 5–15 min until BP controlled; repeat every 4–24 h; monitor BP closely. *Hypoglycemia:* **Adults & Peds.** 3–8 mg/kg/24 h PO ÷ q8–12h. **Neonates.** 8–15 mg/kg/24 h ÷ in 3 equal doses; maint 8–10 mg/kg/24 h PO in 2–3 equal doses Caution: [C, ?] ↓ Effect w/ phenytoin; ↑ effect w/ diuretics, warfarin Contra: Allergy to thiazides or other sulfonamide-containing products; HTN associated w/ aortic coarctation, AV shunt, or pheochromocytoma Disp: Caps 50 mg; PO susp 50 mg/mL SE: Hyperglycemia, ↓ BP, dizziness, Na⁺ & H₂O retention, N/V, weakness Interactions: ↑ Effects W/ carboplatin, cisplatin, diuretics, phenothiazines; ↑ effects **OF** anticoagulants; ↓ effects W/ sulfonylureas; ↓ effects **OF** phenytoin, sulfonylureas Labs: ↑ Serum uric acid, glucose, false—response to glucagon; ↓ neutrophil count, HMG, Hct, WBC NIPE: Daily weights, ↑ reversible body hair growth; can give false—insulin response to glucagons; Rx extrav w/ warm compress

Dibucaine (Nupercainal) [Topical Anesthetic] Uses: *Hemorrhoids & minor skin conditions* Action: Topical anesthetic Dose: Insert PR w/ applicator bid & after each bowel movement; apply sparingly to skin Caution: [C, ?] Contra: Component sensitivity Disp: 1% oint w/ rectal applicator; 0.5% cream SE: Local irritation, rash Interactions: None noted

Diclofenac (Cataflam, Felctor, Voltaren) [Antiarthritic, Antiinflammatory/NSAID] WARNING: May ↑ risk of cardiovascular events & GI bleeding Uses: *Arthritis & pain* Action: NSAID Dose: 50–75 mg PO bid; w/ food or milk; 1 patch to painful area BID Caution: [B (D 3rd tri or near delivery), ?] CHF, HTN, renal/hepatic dysfunction, & h/o PUD Contra: NSAID/ASA allergy; porphyria; perioperative pain following CABG Disp: Tabs 50 mg; tabs DR 25, 50, 75, 100 mg; XR tabs 100 mg; Flector Patch 10 × 14 cm, opht soln 0.1% SE: Abd cramps, heartburn, GI ulceration, rash, interstitial nephritis; patch: pruritus, dermatitis, burning, N, HA Interactions: ↑ Risk of bleeding W/ feverfew, garlic, ginger, ginkgo biloba; ↑ effects **OF** digoxin, MTX, cyclosporine, Li, insulin sulfonylureas, K-sparing diuretics, warfarin; ↓ effects W/ ASA; ↓ effects **OF** thiazide diuretics, furosemide, BBs Labs: ↑ LFTs, serum glucose & cortisol; ↑ serum uric acid; monitor LFTs, CBC, BUN, Cr NIPE: Risk of photosensitivity—use sunscreen; take w/ food; ⊘ crush tabs; do not apply patch to damaged skin or while bathing; watch for GI bleed

Dicloxacillin (Dynapen, Dycill) [Antibiotic/Penicillin] Uses: *Rx of pneumonia, skin, & soft tissue Infxns, & osteomyelitis caused by penicillinase-producing staphylococci* Action: Bactericidal; ↓ cell wall synth. Spectrum *S. aureus & Streptococcus* Dose: **Adults.** 250–500 mg qid **Peds <40 kg.** 12.5–100 mg/kg/d ÷ qid; take on empty stomach Caution: [B, ?] Contra: Component or PCN sensitivity Disp: Caps 125, 250, 500 mg; soln 62.5 mg/5 mL SE: N/D, abd pain Interactions: ↑ Effects W/ disulfiram, probenecid; ↑ effects **OF** MRX, ↓ effects W/

macrolides, tetracyclines, food; ↓ effects *OF* OCPs, warfarin **Labs:** False ↑ urine glucose; ↑ eosinophils; ↓ HMG, Hct, plts, WBC **NIPE:** Take w/ water; monitor PTT if pt on warfarin

Dicyclomine (Bentyl) [Antimuscarinic, GI Antispasmodic/Anticholinergic]
Uses: *Functional IBS* Action: Smooth-muscle relaxant **Dose: Adults.** 20 mg PO qid; ↑ to 160 mg/d max or 20 mg IM q6h, 80mg/d ÷ QID then ↑ to 160 mg/d, max 2 wk **Peds. Infants >6 mo:** 5mg/dose tid–qid **Children:** 10 mg/dose tid-qid **Caution:** [B, –] **Contra:** Infants <6 mo, NAG, MyG, severe UC, BOO **Disp:** Caps 10, 20 mg; tabs 20 mg; syrup 10 mg/5 mL; inj 10 mg/mL **SE:** Anticholinergic SEs may limit dose **Interactions:** ↑ Anticholinergic effects *W/* anticholinergics, antihistamines, amantadine, MAOIs, TCAs, phenothiazides; ↓ effects *OF* atenolol, digoxin; ↓ effects *W/* antacids; ↓ effects *OF* haloperidol, ketoconazole, levodopa, phenothiazines **NIPE:** Do not administer IV; ⊘ EtOH, CNS depressant; adequate hydration; take 30–60 min before meal

Didanosine [ddI] (Videx) [Antiretroviral, NRTI] WARNING:
Allergy manifested as fever, rash, fatigue, GI/resp Sxs reported; D/C drug immediately & do not rechallenge; lactic acidosis & hepatomegaly/steatosis reported Uses: *HIV Infxn in zidovudine-intolerant pts* Action: NRTI Dose: *Adults.* >60 *kg:* 400 mg/d PO or 200 mg PO bid. <*60 kg:* 250 mg/d PO or 125 mg PO bid; adults should take 2 tabs/administration. *Peds.* 2 wk to 8 mo age 100 mg/m², >8 mo 120 mg/m² PO BID; ↓ in renal impair **Caution:** [B, –] CDC recommends HIV-infected mothers not to breast-feed **Contra:** Component sensitivity **Disp:** Chew tabs 25, 50, 100, 150, 200 mg; powder packets 100, 167, 250, 375 mg; powder for soln 2, 4 g **SE:** Pancreatitis, peripheral neuropathy, D, HA **Interactions:** ↑ Effects *W/* allopurinol, ganciclovir; ↓ effects *W/* methadone, food; ↑ risk of pancreatitis *W/* thiazide diuretics, IV pentamidine, EtOH; ↓ effects *OF* azole antifungals, dapsone, delavirdine, ganciclovir, indinavir, quinoline, ranitidine, tetracycline **Labs:** ↑ LFTs, uric acid, amylase, lipase, triglycerides **NIPE:** May cause hyperglycemia; do not take w/ meals; thoroughly chew tablets, do not mix w/ fruit juice or acidic beverages; reconstitute powder w/ H₂O

Diflunisal (Dolobid) [Analgesic, Antipyretic, Anti-inflammatory/NSAID] WARNING: May ↑ risk of cardiovascular events & GI bleeding
Uses: *Mild–moderate pain; osteoarthritis* **Action:** NSAID **Dose:** *Pain:* 500 mg PO qid. *Osteoarthritis:* 500–1500 mg PO in 2–3 ÷ doses; ↓ in renal impair, take w/ food/milk **Caution:** [C (D 3rd tri or near delivery), ?] CHF, HTN, renal/hepatic dysfunction, & h/o PUD **Contra:** Allergy to NSAIDs or ASA, active GI bleed **Disp:** Tabs 250, 500 mg **SE:** May ↑ bleeding time; HA, abd cramps, heartburn, GI ulceration, rash, interstitial nephritis, fluid retention **Interactions:** ↑ Effects *W/* probenecid; ↑ effects *OF* acetaminophen, anticoagulants, digoxin, HCTZ, indomethacin, Li, MTX, phenytoin, sulfonamides, sulfonylureas; ↑ effects *W/* antacids, ASA; ↓ effects *OF* furosemide **NIPE:** Take w/ food, ⊘ chew or crush tabs

Digoxin (Lanoxin, Lanoxicaps, Digitek) [Antiarrhythmic/ Cardiac Glycoside] Uses: **CHF, AF & flutter, & PAT** Action: Positive inotrope; ↑ AV node refractory period **Dose:** *Adults. PO digitalization:* 0.5–0.75 mg PO, then 0.25 mg PO q6–8h to total 1–1.5 mg. *IV or IM digitalization:* 0.25–0.5 mg IM or IV, then 0.25 mg q4–6h to total 0.125–0.5 mg/d PO, IM, or IV (average daily dose 0.125–0.25 mg). *Peds. Preterm infants: Digitalization:* 30 μg/kg PO or 25 μg/kg IV; give 1/2 of dose initial, then 1/4 of dose at 8–12-h intervals for 2 doses. *Maint:* 5–7.5 μg/kg/24 h PO or 4–6 μg/ kg/24 h IV ÷ q12h. *Term infants. Digitalization:* 25–35 μg/kg PO or 20–30 μg/kg IV; give 1/2 the initial dose, then 1/3 of dose at 8–12 h. *Maint:* 6–10 μg/kg/24 h PO or 5–8 μg/kg/24 h ÷ q12h. *1 mo–2 y: Digitalization:* 35–60 μg/kg PO or 30–50 μg/kg IV; give 1/2 the initial dose, then 1/3 dose at 8–12-h intervals for 2 doses. *Maint:* 10–15 μg/kg/24 h PO or 7.5–15 μg/kg/24 h IV ÷ q12h. *2–10 y: Digitalization:* 30–40 μg/kg PO or 25 μg/kg IV; give 1/2 initial dose, then 1/3 of the dose at 8–12-h intervals for 2 doses. *Maint:* 8–10 μg/kg/24 h PO or 6–9 μg/kg/24 h IV ÷ q12h. *7–10 y:* Same as for adults; *↓ in* renal impair **Caution:** [C, +] **Contra:** AV block; idiopathic hypertrophic subaortic stenosis; constrictive pericarditis **Disp:** Caps 0.05, 0.1, 0.2 mg; tabs 0.125, 0.25, 0.5 mg; elixir 0.05 mg/mL; inj 0.1, 0.25 mg/mL **SE:** Can cause heart block; ↓ K⁺ potentiates tox; N/V, HA, fatigue, visual disturbances (yellow-green halos around lights), cardiac arrhythmias **Notes:** *Levels: Trough:* Just before next dose. *Thera peutic:* 0.8–2.0 ng/mL. *Toxic:* >2 ng/mL. *1/2 life:* 36 h **Interactions:** ↑ Effects *W/* alprazolam, amiodarone, azole antifungals, BBs, carvedilol, cyclosporine, corticos teroids, diltiazem, diuretics, erythromycin, NSAIDs, quinidine, spironolactone, tetracyclines, verapamil, goldenseal, hawthorn, licorice, quinine, Siberian ginseng ↓ effects *W/* charcoal, cholestyramine, cisapride, neomycin, rifampin, sucralfate, thyroid hormones, psyllium, St. John's wort **Labs:** Monitor serum electrolyte **NIPE:** Different bioavailability in various brands; IM inj painful, has erratic ab sorption & should not be used

Digoxin Immune Fab (Digibind, DigiFab) [Cardiac Glycoside Antidote/Antibody Fragment] Uses: **Life-threatening digoxin intox** Action: Antigen-binding fragments bind & inactivate digoxin **Dose:** *Adult. & Peds.* Based on serum level & pt's wt; see charts provided w/ drug **Caution:** [C, ?] **Contra:** Sheep product allergy **Disp:** Inj 38 mg/vial **SE:** Worsening of cardiac out put or CHF, ↓ K⁺, facial swelling, & redness **Notes:** Each vial binds ≈0.6 mg of digoxin **Interactions:** ↑ Effects *OF* cardiac glycosides; ↓ K⁺ level **NIPE:** Wil take up to 1 wk for accurate serum digoxin levels after use of Digibind; renal fail ure may require redosing in several days

Diltiazem (Cardizem, Cardizem CD, Cardizem SR, Cartia XT Dilacor XR, Diltia XT, Taztia XT, Tiamate, Tiazac) [Antianginal CCB] Uses: **Angina, prevention of reinfarction, HTN, AF or flutter, & PAT** Action: CCB Dose: *PO:* Initial, 30 mg PO qid; ↑ to 180–360 mg/d in 3–4 ÷ dose PRN. *SR:* 60–120 mg PO bid; ↑ to 360 mg/d max. *CD or XR:* 120–360 mg/d (ma

480 mg/d). *IV:* 0.25 mg/kg IV bolus over 2 min; may repeat in 15 min at 0.35 mg/kg; begin inf of 5–15 mg/h. *Acute rate control:* 15–20 mg (0.25 mg/kg) IV over 2 min, Repeat in 15 min at 20–25 mg (0.35 mg/kg) over 2 min (*ECC 2005*) **Caution:** [C, +] ↑ Effect W/ amiodarone, cimetidine, fentanyl, lithium, cyclosporine, digoxin, β-blockers, theophylline **Contra:** SSS, AV block, ↓ BP, AMI, pulm congestion **Disp:** *Cardizem CD:* Caps 120, 180, 240, 300, 360 mg; *Cardizem SR:* Caps 60, 90, 120 mg; *Cardizem:* Tabs 30, 60, 90, 120 mg; *Cartia XT:* Caps 120, 180, 240, 300 mg; *Dilacor XR:* Caps 180, 240 mg; *Diltia XT:* Caps 120, 180, 240 mg; *Tiazac:* Caps 120, 180, 240, 300, 360, 420 mg; *Tiamate (XR):* Tabs 120, 180, 240 mg; inj 5 mg/mL; *Taztia XT:* 120, 180, 240, 300, 360 mg **SE:** Gingival hyperplasia, bradycardia, AV block, ECG abnormalities, peripheral edema, dizziness, HA **Notes:** Cardizem CD, Dilacor XR, & Tiazac not interchangeable **Interactions:** ↑ Effects W/ α-blockers, azole antifungals, BBs, erythromycin, H₂-receptor antagonists, nitroprusside, quinidine, EtOH, grapefruit juice; ↑ effects *OF* carbamazepine, cyclosporine, digitalis glycosides, quinidine, phenytoin, prazosin, theophylline, TCAs; ↓ effects W/ NSAIDs, phenobarbital, rifampin **Labs:** ↑ LFTs **NIPE:** ⊘ Chew or crush SR or ER preps; risk of photosensitivity—use sunscreen

Dimenhydrinate (Dramamine, others) [Antiemetic/Antivertigo/Anticholinergic] **Uses:** *Prevention & Rx of N/V, dizziness, or vertigo of motion sickness* **Action:** Antiemetic **Dose:** *Adults.* 50–100 mg PO q4–6, max 400 mg/d; 50 mg IM/IV PRN. *Peds. 2–6 y:* 12.5–25 mg q6–8h max 75 mg/d. *6–12 y:* 25–50 mg q6–8h max 150 mg/d **Caution:** [B, ?] **Contra:** Component sensitivity **Disp:** Tabs 50 mg; chew tabs 50 mg; Liq 12.5 mg/4 mL, 12.5 mg/5 mL, 15.62 mg/5 mL **SE:** Anticholinergic side effects **Interactions:** ↑ Effects W/ CNS depressants, antihistamines, opioids, quinidine, TCAs, EtOH; prolonged anticholinergic effects W/ MAOIs **Labs:** False ↓ allergy skin tests **NIPE:** ⊘ Drug 72 h prior to allergy skin testing, take before motion sickness occurs

Dimethyl Sulfoxide [DMSO] (Rimso 50) [GU Agent] **Uses:** *Interstitial cystitis* **Action:** Unknown **Dose:** Intravesical, 50 mL, retain for 15 min; repeat q2wk until relief **Caution:** [C, ?] **Contra:** Component sensitivity **Disp:** 50% & 100% soln **SE:** Cystitis, eosinophilia, GI, & taste disturbance **Interactions:** ↓ Effects *OF* sulindac **Labs:** Monitor CBC, LFTs, BUN, Cr levels **NIPE:** ↑ Taste & smell of garlic

Dinoprostone (Cervidil Vaginal Insert, Prepidil Vaginal Gel, Prostin E2) [Prostaglandin/Abortifacient] **WARNING:** Should only be used by trained personnel in an appropriate hospital setting **Uses:** *Induce labor; terminate PRG (12–20 wk); evacuate uterus in missed abortion or fetal death* **Action:** Prostaglandin, changes consistency, dilatation, & effacement of the cervix; induces uterine contraction **Dose:** *Gel:* 0.5 mg; if no cervical/uterine response, repeat 0.5 mg q6h (max 24-h dose 1.5 mg). *Vaginal insert:* 1 insert (10 mg = 0.3 mg dinoprostone/h over 12 h); remove w/ onset of labor or 12 h after insertion. *Vaginal supp:* 20 mg repeated every 3–5 h; adjust PRN supp: 1 high in vagina, repeat at 3–5-h intervals until abortion (240 mg max) **Caution:** [X, ?] **Contra:** Ruptured membranes, allergy to prostaglandins, placenta previa or AUB, when oxytocic drugs contraindicated or if prolonged uterine contractions are inappropriate (h/o C-section, cephalopelvic disproportion, etc) **Disp:** *Endocervical gel:* 0.5 mg in 3-g syringes (w/ 10- & 20-mm shielded catheter) *Vaginal gel:* 0.5 mg/3 g *Vaginal supp:* 20 mg *Vaginal insert, CR:* 10 mg **SE:** N/V/D, dizziness, flushing, HA, fever, abnormal uterine contractions **Interactions:** ↑ Effects of oxytocics, ↓ effects W/ large amts ETOH **NIPE:** Pt supine after insertion of supp or gel up to 1/2 h

Diphenhydramine (Benadryl) [OTC] [Antihistamine/Antitussive/Antiemetic]   **Uses:** *Rx & prevent allergic Rxns, motion sickness, potentiate narcotics, sedation, cough suppression, & Rx of extrapyramidal Rxns* **Action:** Antihistamine, antiemetic **Dose:** *Adults.* 25–50 mg PO, IV, or IM bid–tid. *Peds.* > 2 y: 5 mg/kg/24 h PO or IM ÷ q6h (max 300 mg); ↑ dosing interval w/ moderate–severe renal insuff **Caution:** [B, –] **Contra:** acute asthma **Disp:** Tabs, caps 25, 50 mg; chew tabs 12.5 mg; elixir 12.5 mg/5 mL; syrup 12.5 mg/5 mL; Liq 6.25 mg/5 mL, 12.5 mg/5 mL; inj 50 mg/mL, cream 2% **SE:** Anticholinergic (xerostomia, urinary retention, sedation) **Interactions:** ↑ Effects W/ CNS depressants, antihistamines, opioids, MAOIs, TCAs, EtOH **Labs:** ↓ Response to allergy skin testing; ↓ HMG, Hct, plts **NIPE:** ↑ Risk of photosensitivity—use sunscreen; may cause drowsiness

Diphenoxylate + Atropine (Lomotil, Lonox) [C-V] [Opioid Antidiarrheal]   **Uses:** *D* **Action:** Constipating meperidine congener, ↓ GI motility **Dose:** *Adults.* Initial, 5 mg PO tid–qid until controlled, then 2.5–5 mg PO bid; 20 mg/d max *Peds >2 y:* 0.3–0.4 mg/kg/24 h (of diphenoxylate) bid–qid, 10 mg/d max **Caution:** [C, +] **Contra:** Obstructive jaundice, D due to bacterial Infxn; children <2 y **Disp:** Tabs 2.5 mg diphenoxylate/0.025 mg atropine; Liq 2.5 mg diphenoxylate/0.025 mg atropine/5 mL **SE:** Drowsiness, dizziness, xerostomia, blurred vision, urinary retention, constipation **Interactions:** ↑ Effects W/ CNS depressants, opioids, EtOH, ↑ risk HTN crisis W/ MAOIs **NIPE:** ↓ Effectiveness w/ diarrhea caused by antibiotics

Diphtheria, Tetanus Toxoids, & Acellular pertussis adsorbed, Hepatitis B (Recombinant), & Inactivated Poliovirus Vaccine [IPV] combined (Pediarix) [Vaccine, Inactivated]   **Uses:** *Vaccine against diphtheria, tetanus, pertussis, HBV, polio (types 1, 2, 3) as a 3-dose primary series in infants & children <7, born to HBsAg–mothers* **Actions:** Active immunization **Dose:** *Infants:* Three 0.5-mL doses IM, at 6–8-wk intervals, start at 2 mo; child given 1 dose of Hep B vaccine, same; previously vaccinated w/ one or more doses IPV, use to complete series **Caution:** [C, N/A] **Contra:** HbsAg+ mother, adults, children >7 y, immunosuppressed, allergy to yeast, neomycin, polymyxin B, or any component, encephalopathy, or progressive neurologic disorders; caution in bleeding disorders. **Disp:** Single-dose vials 0.5 mL **SE:** Drowsiness, restlessness, fever, fussiness, ↓ appetite, nodule redness, inj site pain/swelling **Interactions:** ↓ Effects *W/* immunosuppressants, corticosteroids **NIPE:** If IM use only preservative-free injection

Dipivefrin (Propine) [Alpha Adrenergic Agonist/Glaucoma Agent] Uses: *Open-angle glaucoma* **Action:** α-Adrenergic agonist **Dose:** 1 gtt in eye q12h **Caution:** [B, ?] **Contra:** NAG **Disp:** 0.1% soln **SE:** HA, local irritation, blurred vision, photophobia, HTN **Interactions:** ↑ Effects *W/* BBs, ophthalmic anhydrase inhibitors, osmotic drugs, sympathomimetics, ↑ risk of cardiac arrhythmias *W/* digoxin, TCAs **NIPE:** Discard discolored solutions

Dipyridamole (Persantine) [Coronary Vasodilator/Platelet Aggregation Inhibitor] Uses: *Prevent postop thromboembolic disorders, often in combo w/ ASA or warfarin (eg, CABG, vascular graft); w/ warfarin after artificial heart valve; chronic angina; w/ ASA to prevent coronary artery thrombosis; dipyridamole IV used in place of exercise stress test for CAD* **Action:** Antiplt activity; coronary vasodilator **Dose:** *Adults.* 75–100 mg PO tid–qid; stress test 0.14 mg/kg/min (max 60 mg over 4 min). *Peds >12 y.* 3–6 mg/kg/d ÷ tid (safety/efficacy not established) **Caution:** [B, ?/–] w/ other drugs that affect coagulation **Contra:** Component sensitivity **Disp:** Tabs 25, 50, 75 mg; inj 5 mg/mL **SE:** HA, ↓ BP, N, abd distress, flushing rash, dizziness, dyspnea **Interactions:** ↑ Effects *W/* anticoagulants, heparin, evening primrose oil, feverfew, garlic, ginger, ginkgo biloba, ginseng, grapeseed extract; ↑ effects *OF* adenosine; ↑ bradycardia *W/* BBs; ↓ effects *W/* aminophylline **NIPE:** IV use can worsen angina; ⊘ EtOH or tobacco because of vasoconstriction effects; + effects may take several mo

Dipyridamole & Aspirin (Aggrenox) [Platelet Aggregation Inhibitor] Uses: *↓ Reinfarction after MI; prevent occlusion after CABG; ↓ risk of stroke* **Action:** ↓ Plt aggregation (both agents) **Dose:** 1 cap PO bid **Caution:** [C, ?] **Contra:** Ulcers, bleeding diathesis **Disp:** Dipyridamole (XR) 200 mg/ASA 25 mg **SE:** ASA component: allergic Rxns, allergic Rxns, ulcers/GI bleed, bronchospasm; dipyridamole component: dizziness, HA, rash **Interactions:** ↑ Risk of GI bleed *W/* EtOH, NSAIDs; ↑ effects *OF* acetazolamide, adenosine, anticoagulants, methotrexate, oral hypoglycemics; ↓ effects *OF* ACEIs, BB, cholinesterase inhibitors, diuretics **NIPE:** Swallow capsule whole

Dirithromycin (Dynabac) [Antibiotic, Macrolide] Uses: *Bronchitis, community-acquired pneumonia, & skin & skin structure Infxns* **Action:** Macrolide antibiotic. *Spectrum:* M. catarrhalis, S. pneumoniae, Legionella, H. influenzae, S. pyogenes, S. aureus **Dose:** 500 mg/d PO; w/ food; swallow whole **Caution:** [C, M] **Contra:** w/ pimozide **Disp:** Tabs 250 mg **SE:** Abd discomfort, HA, rash, ↑ K⁺ **NIPE:** Eval for macrolide sensitivity; take with food and swallow tablet whole

Disopyramide (Norpace, Norpace CR, NAPamide, Rhythmodan) [Antarrhythmic/Pyridine Derivative] **WARNING:** Excessive mortality or nonfatal cardiac arrest rate with use in asymptomatic non-life-threatening ventricular arrhythmias with MI 6 d to 2 y prior. Restrict use to life-threatening arrhythmias only **Uses:** *Suppression & prevention of VT* **Action:** Class 1A antiarrhythmic; stabilizes membranes, depresses action potential **Dose:** *Adults.* 400–600 mg/d ÷ q6h or q12h for CR, max 1600 mg/d. *Peds. <1 y:* 10–30 mg/kg/24 h PO (÷ qid). *1–4 y:* 10–20 mg/kg/24 h PO (÷ qid). *4–12 y:* 10–15 mg/kg/24 h PO (÷ qid). *12–18 y:* 6–15 mg/kg/24 h PO (÷ qid); ↓ in renal/hepatic impair **Caution:** [C, +] **Contra:** AV block, cardiogenic shock,↓ BP, CHF **Disp:** Caps 100, 150 mg; CR caps 100, 150 mg **SE:** Anticholinergic SEs; negative inotrope, may induce CHF **Notes:** *Levels: Trough:* Just before next dose: *Therapeutic:* 2–5 μg/mL; *Toxic:* >5 μg/mL; *1/2 life:* 4–10 h **Interactions:** ↑ Effects *W/* cimetidine, clarithromycin, erythromycin, quinidine; ↑ effects *OF* digoxin, hypoglycemics, insulin, warfarin; ↑ risk of arrhythmias *W/* pimozide; ↓ effects *W/* barbiturates, phenytoin, phenobarbital, rifampin **Labs:** ↑ LFTs, lipids, BUN, Cr; ↓ serum glucose, HMG, Hct **NIPE:** Risk of photosensitivity—use sunscreen; daily wt

Dobutamine (Dobutrex) [Inotropic/Adrenergic, Beta-1-Agonist] **Uses:** *Short-term in cardiac decompensation secondary to depressed contractility* **Action:** Positive inotrope **Dose:** *Adults & Peds.* Cont IV inf of 2.5–15 μg/kg/min; rarely, 40 μg/kg/min needed; titrate; titrate 2–20 μg/kg/min; titrate to HR not >10% of baseline *(ECC 2005)* **Caution:** [C, ?] **Contra:** Sensitivity to sulfites, IHSS **Disp:** Inj 250 mg/20 mL, 12.5/mL **SE:** Chest pain, HTN, dyspnea **Interactions:** ↑ Effects *W/* furazolidone, methyldopa, MAOIs, TCAs; ↓ effects *W/* BBs, NaHCO₃; ↓ effects *OF* guanethidine **Labs:** ↓ K **NIPE:** Eval for adequate hydration; monitor I&O; monitor PWP & cardiac output if possible; monitor ECG for ↑ HR or ectopic activity, monitor BP

Docetaxel (Taxotere) [Antineoplastic/Antimitotic Agent] **WARNING:** Do not administer if neutrophil count <1500 cell/mm³; severe Rxns possible in hepatic dysfxn **Uses:** *Breast (anthracycline-resistant), ovarian, lung, & prostate CA* **Action:** Antimitotic agent; promotes microtubule aggregation; semisynthetic taxoid **Dose:** 100 mg/m² over 1 h IV q3wk (per protocols); dexamethasone 8 mg bid prior & continue for 3–4 d; ↓ dose w/ ↑ bilirubin levels **Caution:** [D, –] **Contra:** Sensitivity to meds w/polysorbate 80, component sensitivity **Disp:** Inj 20 mg/0.5 mL, 80 mg/2 mL **SE:** ↓ BM, neuropathy, N/V, alopecia, fluid retention synd; cumulative doses of 300–400 mg/m² w/o steroid prep & posttreatment & 600–800 mg/m² w/ steroid prep; allergy possible (rare w/ steroid prep) **Interactions:** ↑ Effects *W/* cyclosporine, ketoconazole, erythromycin, terfenidine **Labs:** ↑ AST, ALT, alkaline phosphatase, bilirubin; ↓ plts, WBCs; monitor CBC during therapy **NIPE:** ↑ Fluids to 2–3 L/d, ↑ risk of hair loss, ↑ susceptibility to Infxn; urine may become reddish-brown

Docusate Calcium (Surfak)/Docusate Potassium (Dialose)/Docusate Sodium (DOSS, Colace) [Emollient Laxative/Fecal Softener] **Uses:** *Constipation; adjunct to painful anorectal conditions (hemorrhoids)* **Action:** Stool softener **Dose:** *Adults.* 50–500 mg PO ÷ daily qid. *Peds. Infants–3 y:* 10–40 mg/24 h ÷ daily qid. *3–6 y:* 20–60 mg/24 h ÷ daily qid. *6–12 y:*

40–120 mg/24 h ÷ daily qid **Caution:** [C, ?] **Contra:** Use w/ mineral oil; intestinal obst, acute abd pain, N/V **Disp:** *Ca:* Caps 50, 240 mg. *K:* Caps 100, 240 mg. *Na:* Caps 50, 100 mg; syrup 50, 60 mg/15 mL; Liq 150 mg/15 mL; soln 50 mg/mL **SE:** Rare abd cramping, D **Interactions:** ↑ Absorption of mineral oil **NIPE:** Take w/ full glass of H$_2$O; no laxative action; do not use >1 wk; short-term use

Dofetilide (Tikosyn) [Antiarrhythmic] **WARNING:** To minimize the risk of induced arrhythmia, hospitalize for minimum of 3 d to provide calculations of CrCl, continuous ECG monitoring, & cardiac resuscitation **Uses:** *Maintain normal sinus rhythm in AF/A flutter after conversion* **Action:** Type III antiarrhythmic, prolongs action potential **Dose:** Based on CrCl & QTc; CrCl >60 mL/min 500 μg PO q12h, check QTc 2–3 h after, if QTc >15% over baseline or >500 msec, ↓ to 250 μg q12h, ✓ after each dose; if CrCl <60 mL/sec, see insert; D/C if QTc > 500 msec after dosing adjustments **Caution:** [C, –] **Contra:** Baseline QTc >440 ms, CrCl <20 mL/min; w/ verapamil, cimetidine, trimethoprim, ketoconazole, quinolones, ACE inhibitors/HCTZ combo **Disp:** Caps 125, 250, 500 μg **SE:** Vent arrhythmias, QT ↑, torsades de pointes, rash, HA, CP, dizziness **Notes:** Restricted to participating prescribers **Interactions:** ↑ Effects *W/* amiloride, amiodarone, azole antifungals, cimetidine, diltiazem, macrolides, metformin, megestrol, nefazodone, norfloxacin, SSRIs, TCAs, triamterene, trimethoprim, verapamil, zafirlukast, quinine, grapefruit juice **Labs:** Monitor LFTs, BUN, Cr **NIPE:** Take w/o regard to food; Avoid w/ other drugs that ↑ QT interval; hold class I/III antiarrhythmics for 3 half-lives prior to dosing; amiodarone level should be <0.3 mg/L before use, do not initiate if HR <60 BPM

Dolasetron (Anzemet) [Antiemetic/Selective Serotonin 5-HT$_3$ Receptor Antagonist] **Uses:** *Prevent chemo-associated N/V* **Action:** 5-HT$_3$ receptor antagonist **Dose:** *Adults & Peds. IV:* 1.8 mg/kg IV as single dose 30 min prior to chemo *Adults. PO:* 100 mg PO as a single dose 1 h prior to chemo *Peds. PO:* 1.8 mg/kg PO to max 100 mg as single dose **Caution:** [B, ?] **Contra:** Component sensitivity **Disp:** Tabs 50, 100 mg; inj 20 mg/mL **SE:** ↑ QT interval, D, HTN, HA, abd pain, urinary retention **Interactions:** ↑ Effects *W/* cimetidine; ↑ risk of arrhythmias *W/* diuretics; ↓ effects *W/* rifampin **Labs:** Transient ↑ LFTs **NIPE:** Monitor ECG for prolonged QT interval; frequently causes HA

Dopamine (Intropin) [Vasopressor/Adrenergic] **Uses:** *Short-term use in cardiac decompensation secondary to* ↓ *contractility;* ↑ *organ perfusion (at low dose)* **Action:** Positive inotropic agent w/ dose response: 1–10 μg/kg/min β-effects (↑ CO & renal perfusion); 10–20 μg/kg/min β-effects (peripheral vasoconstriction, pressor); >20 μg/kg/min peripheral & renal vasoconstriction **Dose:** *Adults & Peds.* 5 μg/kg/min by cont inf, ↑ by 5 μg/kg/min to 50 μg/kg/min max to effect *(ECC 2005)* **Caution:** [C, ?] **Contra:** Pheochromocytoma, VF, sulfite sensitivity **Disp:** Inj 40, 80, 160 mg/mL, premixed 0.8 , 1.6 , 3.2 mg/mL **SE:** Tachycardia, vasoconstriction, ↓ BP, HA, N/V, dyspnea **Notes:** >10 μg/kg/min ↓ renal perfusion **Interactions:** ↑ Effects *W/* α-blockers, diuretics, ergot alkaloids,

MAOIs, BBs, anesthetics, phenytoin; ↓ effects W/ guanethidine **Labs:**↑ Glucose, urea levels **NIPE:** Maintain adequate hydration; monitor urinary output & ECG for ↑ HR, BP, ectopy; monitor PCWP & cardiac output if possible; phentolamine used for extrav

Dornase Alfa (Pulmozyme, DNase) [Respiratory Inhalant/Enzyme]

Uses: *↓ Frequency of resp Infxns in CF* **Action:** Enzyme cleaves extracellular DNA, ↓ mucous viscosity **Dose:** *Adult:* Inhal 2.5 mg/d, bid nebulizer w/ FVC >85% w/ recommended nebulizer *Peds > 5 y:* Inhal 2.5 mg/d, bid if FVC >85% **Caution:** [B, ?] **Contra:** Chinese hamster product allergy **Disp:** Soln for inhal 1 mg/mL **SE:** Pharyngitis, voice alteration, CP, rash **NIPE:** Teach pt to use nebulizer

Dorzolamide (Trusopt) [Carbonic Anhydrase Inhibitor, Sulfonamide/Glaucoma Agent]

Uses: *Glaucoma* **Action:** Carbonic anhydrase inhibitor **Dose:** 1 gtt in eye(s) tid **Caution:** [C, ?] **Contra:** Component sensitivity **Disp:** 2% soln **SE:** Irritation, bitter taste, punctate keratitis, ocular allergic Rxn **Interactions:** ↑ Effects W/ oral carbonic anhydrase inhibitors, salicylates **NIPE:** ⊘ Wear soft contact lenses

Dorzolamide & Timolol (Cosopt) [Carbonic Anhydrase Inhibitor/Beta-Adrenergic Blocker]

Uses: *Glaucoma* **Action:** Carbonic anhydrase inhibitor w/ β-adrenergic blocker **Dose:** 1 gtt in eye(s) bid **Caution:** [C, ?] CrCl <30 **Contra:** Component sensitivity, asthma, severe COPD, sinus bradycardia **Disp:** Soln dorzolamide 2% & timolol 0.5% **SE:** Irritation, bitter taste, superficial keratitis, ocular allergic Rxn **NIPE:** ⊘ Wear soft contact lenses

Doxazosin (Cardura, Cardura XL) [Antihypertensive/Alpha-Blocker]

Uses: *HTN & symptomatic BPH* **Action:** α₁-Adrenergic blocker; relaxes bladder neck smooth muscle **Dose:** *HTN:* Initial 1 mg/d PO; may be ↑ to 16 mg/d PO. *BPH:* Initial 1 mg/d PO, may ↑ to 8 mg/d; XR 2–8mg qAM **Caution:** [B, ?] **Contra:** Component sensitivity **Disp:** Tabs 1, 2, 4, 8 mg; XR 4, 8 mg **SE:** Dizziness, HA, drowsiness, sexual dysfunction, doses >4 mg ↑ postural ↓ BP risk **Interactions:** ↑ Effects W/ nitrates, antihypertensives, EtOH; ↓ effects W/ NSAIDs, butcher's broom; ↓ effects OF clonidine **NIPE:** May be taken w/ food; 1st dose hs; syncope may occur w/in 90 min of initial dose

Doxepin (Adapin) [Antidepressant/TCA]

WARNING: Closely monitor for worsening depression or emergence of suicidality **Uses:** *Depression, anxiety, chronic pain* **Action:** TCA; ↑ synaptic CNS serotonin or norepinephrine **Dose:** 25–150 mg/d PO, usually hs but can ÷ doses; up to 300 mg/d for depression ↓ in hepatic impair **Caution:** [C, ?/–] **Contra:** NAG, urinary retention, MAOI use w/in 14 d, in recovery phase of MI **Disp:** Caps 10, 25, 50, 75, 100, 150 mg; PO conc 10 mg/mL **SE:** Anticholinergic SEs, ↓ BP, tachycardia, drowsiness, photosens **Interactions:** ↑ Effects W/ fluoxetine, MAOIs, albuterol, CNS depressants, anticholinergics, propoxyphene, quinidine, EtOH, grapefruit juice; ↑ effects OF carbamazepine, anticoagulants, amphetamines, thyroid drugs, sympathomimetics;

↓ effects *W/* ascorbic acid, cholestyramine, tobacco; ↓ effects *OF* bretylium, guanethidine, levodopa **Labs:** ↑ Serum bilirubin, alkaline phosphatase, glucose **NIPE:** Risk of photosensitivity—use sunscreen, urine may turn blue-green, may take 4–6 wk for full effect

Doxepin, Topical (Zonalon, Prudoxin) [Antipruritic]
Uses: *Short-term Rx pruritus (atopic dermatitis or lichen simplex chronicus)* **Action:** Antipruritic; H₁- & H₂-receptor antagonism **Dose:** Apply thin coating qid, 8 d max **Caution:** [C, ?/–] **Contra:** Component sensitivity **Disp:** 5% cream **SE:** ↓ BP, tachycardia, drowsiness **NIPE:** Limit application area to avoid systemic tox; photosensitivity—use sunscreen

Doxorubicin (Adriamycin, Rubex) [Antineoplastic/Anthracycline Antibiotic]
Uses: *Acute leukemias; Hodgkin Dz & NHLs; soft tissue, osteo & Ewing sarcoma; Wilms tumor; neuroblastoma; bladder, breast, ovarian, gastric, thyroid, & lung CA* **Action:** Intercalates DNA; ↓ DNA topoisomerases I & II **Dose:** 60–75 mg/m² q3wk; ↓ w/ hepatic impair; IV use only ↓ cardiotox w/ weekly (20 mg/m²/wk) or cont inf (60–90 mg/m² over 96 h); (per protocols) **Caution:** [D, ?] **Contra:** Severe CHF, cardiomyopathy, preexisting ↓ BM, previous Rx w/ total cumulative doses of doxorubicin, idarubicin, daunorubicin **Disp:** Inj 10, 20, 50, 75, 150, 200 mg **SE:** ↓ BM, venous streaking & phlebitis, N/V/D, mucositis, radiation recall phenomenon, cardiomyopathy rare(dose-related) **Notes:** Limit of 550 mg/m² cumulative dose (400 mg/m² w/ prior mediastinal irradiation); dexrazoxane may limit cardiac tox **Interactions:** ↑ Effects *W/* streptozocin, verapamil, green tea; ↑ BM depression *W/* antineoplastic drugs and radiation; ↓ effects *W/* phenobarbital; ↓ effects *OF* digoxin, phenytoin, live virus vaccines **Labs:** ↑ Bilirubin, glucose, urine, & plasma uric acid levels; ↓ Ca, HMG, Hct, plts, WBCs **NIPE:** ⊘ PRG, use contraception at least 4 mo after drug Rx; red/orange urine; tissue damage w/ extrav

Doxycycline (Adoxa, Periostat, Oracea, Vibramycin, Vibra-Tabs) [Antibiotic/Tetracycline]
Uses: *Broad-spectrum antibiotic* acne vulgaris, uncomplicated GC, *Chlamydia* sp, PID, Lyme disease, skin Infxns, anthrax, malaria prophylaxis **Action:** Tetracycline; bacteriostatic; ↓ protein synth. *Spectrum:* Some gram(+) and (–), *Rickettsia* sp, *Chlamydia* sp, *M. pneumoniae, B. Anthraxus* **Dose:** *Adults.* 100 mg PO q12h on 1st d, then 100 mg PO daily bid or 100 mg IV q12h; acne daily dosing, *Chlamydia* 7d, Lyme disease 14–21 d, PID 14 d *Peds >8 y:* 5 mg/kg/24 h PO, to a max of 200 mg/d ÷ daily–bid **Caution:** [D, +] Hepatic impair **Contra:** Children <8 y, severe hepatic dysfunction **Disp:** Tabs 20, 50, 75, 100, 150 mg; caps 50, 100 mg; Oracea 40 mg caps (30 mg timed release, 10 mg delayed release); syrup 50 mg/5 mL; susp 25 mg/5 mL; inj 100, 200 mg/vial **SE:** D, GI disturbance, photosens **Interactions:** ↑ Effects *OF* digoxin, warfarin; ↓ effects *W/* antacids, Fe, barbiturates, carbamazepine, phenytoins, food; ↓ effects *OF* penicillins **Labs:** ↑ LFTs, BUN, eosinophils; ↓ HMG, Hct, plts, neutrophils, WBC **NIPE:** ↑ Risk of super Infxn, ⊘ PRG, use barrier contraception; tetracycline of choice w/in renal impair; for inhalational anthrax use w/ 1–2 additional antibiotics, not for CNS anthrax

Dronabinol (Marinol) [C-II] [Antiemetic, Appetite Stimulant/ Antivertigo] Uses: *N/V associated w/ CA chemo; appetite stimulation* Action: Antiemetic; ↓ V center in the medulla Dose: *Adults & Peds. Antiemetic:* 5–15 mg/m²/dose q4–6h PRN. *Adults. Appetite stimulant:* 2.5 mg PO before lunch & dinner; max 20 mg/d Caution: [C, ?] Contra: h/o schizophrenia, sesame oil hypersensitivity Disp: Caps 2.5, 5, 10 mg SE: Drowsiness, dizziness, anxiety, mood change, hallucinations, depersonalization, orthostatic ↓ BP, tachycardia Interactions: ↑ Effects W/ anticholinergics, CNS depressants, EtOH; ↓ effects OF theophylline NIPE: Principal psychoactive substance present in marijuana

Droperidol (Inapsine) [General Anesthetic/Butyrophenone] Uses: *N/V; anesthetic premedication, AIDS-associated anorexia* Action: Tranquilizer, sedation, antiemetic Dose: *Adults. N:* initial max 2.5 mg IV/IM, may repeat 1.25 mg based on response; *Premed:* 2.5–10 mg IV, 30–60 min preop. *Peds. Premed:* 0.1–0.15 mg/kg/dose Caution: [C, ?] Contra: Component sensitivity Disp: Inj 2.5 mg/mL SE: Drowsiness, ↓ BP, occasional tachycardia & extrapyramidal Rxns, ↑ QT interval, arrhythmias Interactions: ↑ Effects W/ CNS depressants, fentanyl, EtOH; ↑ hypotension W/ antihypertensives, nitrates NIPE: Give IVP slowly over 2–5 min

Drospirenone/Estradiol (Angelia) [Estrogen & Progestin Supl] Uses: Women w/ uterus for moderate to severe vasomotor symp of menopause; symp of vulvar & vaginal atrophy d/t menopause Action: Estrogen & progestin supl; Dose: 1 tab PO OD Caution: [X, –] Contra: Genital bleeding of unknown cause, breast CA, estrogen-dependent tumors, thromboembolic disorders, thrombophlebitis, recent MI, hepatic impair, adrenal insuff, renal insuff Disp: Tabs drospirenone 0.5mg/estradiol 1 mg SE: HA, breast pain, irreg vaginal bleeding/spotting, abd cramps/bloating, N, V, hair loss, HTN, edema, yeast Infxn, fibroid enlargement Interactions: ↑ Risk of hyperkalemia W/ ACEIs, ARBs, aldosterone antagonists, heparin, NSAIDs, spirolactone, K⁺ sparing diuretics, K⁺ supl, Labs: ↑ Uptake OF T₃, ↓ T₄ sex hormone-binding globulin levels; ↑ lipids; ↑ Prothrombin & factors VII, VIII, IX, X, plt aggregability NIPE: Antialdosterone activity ↑ risk of hyperkalemia in high risk pts; in pts taking meds that ↑ K⁺ monitor serum K⁺ during 1st treatment cycle; no effected by food intake

Drospirenone/Ethinyl Estradiol (YAZ) [Estrogen & Progestin Supl] WARNING: Cigarette smoking & use of estrogen-based OCPs have ↑ risk of serious cardiovascular SEs; risk ↑ w/ age (esp.>35 y) and smoking >15 cig/d Uses: OCPs; premenstrual dysphoric disorder Action: Suppresses ovulation by imitating the feedback inhibition of endogenous estrogen and progesterone on the pituitary and hypothalamus Dose: 1 tab PO OD × 28 d, repeat Caution: [X, –], has antimineralocorticoid activity w/ potential hyperkalemia in renal, adrenal, & hepatic insuff Contra: Pts w/ renal insuff, hepatic impair, adrenal insuff, DVT, PE, CVD, CAD, estrogen-dependent neoplasms, abnormal uterine bleeding, pregnancy, heavy smokers >35 y Disp: Drospirenone (3 mg)/ethinyl estradiol (20 μg),

28 d pack has 24 active tabs & 4 inert tabs **SE:** Hyperkalemia, HTN, N, V, HA, breakthrough bleeding, amenorrhea, mastodynia, ↑ risk of gallbladder disease & thromboembolic disorders **Interactions:** ↑ Risk of hyperkalemia (w/ ACEIs, ARBs, aldosterone antagonists, heparin, NSAIDs, spironolactone, K⁺ sparing diuretics, K⁺ supplements, ↑ effects *OF* cyclosporine, prednisolone, theophylline; ↓ effects *W/* barbiturates, carbamazepine, griseofulvin, modafinil, phenobarbital, phenylbutazone, phenytoin, pioglitazone, rifabutin, rifampin, ritonavir, topiramate, St John's wort **Labs:** ↑ uptake *OF* T_3, ↓ T_4 sex hormone-binding globulin levels; triglycerides **NIPE:** Antimineralocorticoid activity comparable to spironolactone 25 mg; in pts taking meds that ↑ K⁺, monitor serum K⁺ during 1st treatment cycle; Sunday start regimen or postpartum use requires additional contraceptive methods during 1st cycle; use barrier contraception if taking anticonvulsants; may cause vision changes or ↓ contact lens tolerability; ⊘ protection against HIV or STDs; ⊘ smoke cigarettes

Drotrecogin Alfa (Xigris) [Antithrombotic/Activated Protein C (Recombinant)]

Uses: *↓ Mortality in adults w/ severe sepsis (w/ acute organ dysfunction) at high risk of death (eg, determined by APACHE II, www.ncemi.org)* **Action:** Recombinant human-activated protein C; antithrombotic and anti-inflammatory, unclear mechanism **Dose:** 24 μg/kg/h, total of 96 h **Caution:** [C, ?] **Contra:** Active bleeding, recent stroke/CNS surgery, head trauma/CNS lesion w/ herniation risk, trauma w/ ↑ bleeding risk, epidural catheter, mifepristone **Disp:** 5-, 20-mg vials **SE:** Bleeding **Notes:** Single organ dysfunction & recent surgery may not be at high risk of death irrespective of APACHE II score & therefore not indicated. *Percutaneous procedures:* Stop inf 2 h before & resume 1 h after; major surgery: stop inf 2 h before & resume 12 h after in absence of bleeding **Interactions:** ↑ Risk of bleeding *W/* plt inhibitors, anticoagulants **Labs:** ↑ aPTT **NIPE:** D/C drug 2 h before invasive procedures

Duloxetine (Cymbalta) [Antidepressant/SSNRI]

WARNING: Antidepressants may ↑ ↑ risk of suicidality; consider risks/benefits of use. Closely monitor for clinical worsening, suicidality, or behavior changes **Uses:** *Depression, DM peripheral neuropathic pain, GAD* **Action:** Selective serotonin & norepinephrine reuptake inhibitor (SSNRI) **Dose:** *Depression:* 40–60 mg/d PO ÷ bid. *DM neuropathy:* 60 mg/d PO. *GAD:* 30–60 mg/d max 120 mg/d **Caution:** [C, ?/–]; Use in 3rd tri; avoid if CrCl <30 mL/min, NAG, w/ fluvoxamine, inhibitors of CYP2D6 (Table 11), TCAs, phenothiazines, type 1C antiarrhythmics (Table 10) **Contra:** MAOI use w/in 14 d, w/ thioridazine, NAG, hepatic insuff **Disp:** Caps delayed-release 20, 30, 60 mg **SE:** N, dizziness, somnolence, fatigue, sweating, xerostomia, constipation, ↓ appetite, sexual dysfunction, urinary hesitancy, HTN **Interactions:** ↑ Effects *OF* flecainide, propafenone, phenothiazines, TCAs; ↑ effects *W/* cimetidine, fluvoxamine, quinolones; ↑ risk *OF* hypertensive crisis *W/* MAOIs within 14 d of taking duloxetine **Labs:**?↑ LFTs **NIPE:**↑ Risk of liver damage *W/* EtOH use; ⊘ D/C drug abruptly; swallow whole; monitor BP

Dutasteride (Avodart) [Androgen Hormone Inhibitor/BPH Agent] Uses: *Symptomatic BPH* Action: 5α-Reductase inhibitor; ↓ intracellular DHT Dose: 0.5 mg PO/d Caution: [X, –] Hepatic impair; pregnant women should not handle pills Contra: Women & children Disp: Caps 0.5 mg SE: ↑ testosterone, TSH ↑, ↓ PSA levels, impotence, ↓ libido, gynecomastia Interactions: ↑ Effects W/ cimetidine, ciprofloxacin, diltiazem, ketoconazole, ritonavir, verapamil Labs: ↓ PSA levels; new baseline PSA @ 6 mo; corrected PSA × 2 NIPE: ⊘ Handling by PRG women; take w/o regard to food; no blood donation until 6 mo after D/C

Echothiophate Iodine (Phospholine Ophthalmic) [Cholinesterase Inhibitor/Glaucoma Agent] Uses: *Glaucoma* Action: Cholinesterase inhibitor Dose: 1 gtt eye(s) bid w/ 1 dose hs Caution: [C, ?] Contra: Active uveal inflammation, inflammatory Dz of iris/ciliary body, glaucoma iridocyclitis Disp: Powder, reconstitute 1.5 mg/0.03%; 3 mg/0.06%; 6.25 mg/0.125%; 12.5 mg/0.25% SE: Local irritation, myopia, blurred vision, ↓ BP, bradycardia Interactions: ↑ Effects W/ cholinesterase inhibitors, pilocarpine, succinylcholine, carbamate or organophosphate insecticides; ↑ effects OF cocaine; ↓ effects W/ anticholinergics, atropine, cyclopentolate, ophthalmic adrenocorticoids NIPE: ⊘ Drug 2 wk before surgery if succinylcholine is to be administered; keep drug refrigerated; monitor for lens opacities

Econazole (Spectazole) [Topical Antifungal] Uses: *Tinea, cutaneous Candida & tinea versicolor Infxns* Action: Topical antifungal Dose: Apply to areas bid (daily for tinea versicolor) for 2–4 wk Caution: [C, ?] Contra: Component sensitivity Disp: Topical cream 1% SE: Local irritation, pruritus, erythema Interactions: ↓ Effects W/ corticosteroids NIPE: Topical use only; ⊘ eye area; early symptom/clinical improvement; complete course to avoid recurrence

Eculizumab (Soliris) [Complement Inhibitor] WARNING: ↑ Risk of meningococcal Infxns (give meningococcal vaccine 2 weeks prior to 1st dose and revaccinate per guidelines) Uses: *Rx paroxysmal nocturnal hemoglobinuria* Action: Complement inhibitor Dose: 600 mg IV q7d × 4 wk, then 900 mg IV 5th dose 7 d later, then 900 mg IV q14d Caution: [C, ?] Contra: Active N. meningitides Infxn; if not vaccinated against N. meningitides Disp: 300-mg vial SE: Meningococcal Infxn, HA, nasopharyngitis, N, back pain, Infxns, fatigue, severe hemolysis on D/C NIPE: IV over 35 min (2-h max inf time); monitor for 1 h for S/Sx of inf Rxn

Edrophonium (Tensilon, Enlon, Reversol) [Cholinergic Muscle Stimulant/Anticholinesterase] Uses: *Diagnosis of MyG; acute MyG crisis; curare antagonist, reverse of nondepolarizing neuromuscular blockers* Action: Anticholinesterase Dose: Adults. Test for MyG: 2 mg IV in 1 min; if tolerated, give 8 mg IV; (+) test is brief ↑ in strength. Peds. Test for MyG: Total dose 0.2 mg/kg; 0.04 mg/kg test dose; if no Rxn, give remainder in 1-mg increments to 10 mg max; ↓ in renal impair Caution: [C, ?] Contra: GI/GU obst; allergy to sulfite **Disp:** Inj 10 mg/mL **SE:** N/V/D, excessive salivation, stomach cramps, ↑ aminotransferases **Interactions:** ↑ Effects *W/* tacrine; ↑ cardiac effects *W/* digoxin; ↑ effects *OF* neostigmine, pyridostigmine, succinylcholine, jaborandi tree, pill-bearing spurge; ↓ effects *W/* corticosteroids, procainamide, quinidine **Labs:** ↑ AST, ALT, serum amylase **NIPE:** ↑ Risk uterine irritability & premature labor in PRG pts near term; can cause severe cholinergic effects; keep atropine available

Efalizumab (Raptiva) [Antipsoriatic/Immunosuppressant]
WARNING: Associated w/ serious Infxns, malignancy, thrombocytopenia **Uses:** Chronic moderate–severe plaque psoriasis **Action:** MoAb *Dose: Adults.* 0.7 mg/kg SQ conditioning dose, followed by 1 mg/kg/wk; single doses should not exceed 200 mg **Caution:** [C, +/–], chronic Infxn, elderly **Contra:** Admin of most vaccines **Disp:** 150-mg vial **SE:** 1st-dose Rxn, HA, worsening psoriasis, ↑ LFT, hemolytic anemia immunosuppressive-related Rxns (see Warning) **Interactions:** ↑ Risk of Infxn & malignancy *W/* immunosuppressive agents; ↓ immune response *W/* live virus vaccines; **Labs:** ↑ Lymphocytes; ✓ plts monthly then every 3 mo & w/ dose ↑; **NIPE:** Reconstituted soln must be stored for 8 h; monitor for bleeding gums & bruising; minimize 1st-dose Rxn by conditioning dose; pts may be trained in self-admin

Efavirenz (Sustiva) [Antiretroviral/NNRTI]
Action: Antiretroviral; nonnucleoside RTI *Dose: Adults.* 600 mg/d PO qhs. *Peds.* See insert; avoid high-fat meals **Caution:** [D, ?] CDC recommends HIV-infected mothers not breast-feed **Contra:** Component sensitivity **Disp:** Caps 50, 100, 200; 600 mg tab **SE:** Somnolence, vivid dreams, dizziness, rash, N/V/D **Interactions:** ↑ Effects *W/*ritonavir; ↑ effects *OF* CNS depressants, ergot derivatives, midazolam, ritonavir, simvastatin, triazolam, warfarin; ↓ effects *W/* carbamazepine, phenobarbital, rifabutin, rifampin, saquinavir, St. John's wort; ↓ effects *OF* amprenavir, carbamazepine, clarithromycin, indinavir, phenobarbital, saquinavir, warfarin; may alter effectiveness of OCPs **Labs:** ↑ LFTs, cholesterol; monitor LFT, cholesterol **NIPE:** ⊘ High—fat foods; use w/o regard to food; use barrier contraception

Efavirenz, Emtricitabine, Tenofovir (Atripla) [Combination Antiretroviral]
WARNING: Lactic acidosis and severe hepatomegaly with steatosis, including fatal cases, have been reported with the use of nucleoside analogs alone or in combination with other antiretrovirals **Uses:** *HIV Infxns* **Action:** Triple fixed-dose combination antiretroviral *Dose: Adults.* 1 tab daily on empty stomach; hs dose may ↓ CNS effects **Caution:** [D, ?] CDC recommends HIV-infected mothers not to breast-feed **Contra:** <18 y, component sensitivity, w/ astemizole, midazolam, triazolam or ergot derivatives (competition for CYP3A4 by efavirenz could result in serious and/or life-threatening SE) **Disp:** Tab containing efavirenz 600 mg/emtricitabine 200 mg/tenofovir/300 mg **SE:** Somnolence, vivid dreams, HA, dizziness, rash, N/V/D, ↓ bone mineral density **Interactions:** ↑ Effects *OF* ritonavir, tenofovir, ethinyl estradiol levels ↓ *W/* phenobarbital, rifampin, rifabutin, saquinavir, ↓ effects *OF* indinavir, amprenavir, clarithromycin,

methadone, rifabutin, sertraine, statins, saquinavir; monitor warfarin levels **Labs:** Monitor LFT, cholesterol **NIPE:** ⊘ EtOH; ⊘ PRG & breast-feeding; register pregnant patients exposed to this drug at (800) 258-4263; do not use in HIV and Hep B coinfection; see individual agents for additional info

Eletriptan (Relpax) [Analgesic/Antimigraine Agent]   Uses: *Acute Rx of migraine* **Action:** Selective serotonin receptor (5-HT$_1$B/$_1$D) agonist **Dose:** 20–40 mg PO, may repeat in 2 h; 80 mg/24 h max **Caution:** [C, +] **Contra:** h/o ischemic heart Dz, coronary artery spasm, stroke or TIA, peripheral vascular Dz, IBD, uncontrolled HTN, hemiplegic or basilar migraine, severe hepatic impair, w/in 24 h of another 5-HT$_1$ agonist or ergot; w/in 72 h of CYP3A4 inhibitors **Disp:** Tabs 20, 40 mg **SE:** Dizziness, somnolence, N, asthenia, xerostomia, paresthesias; pain, pressure, or tightness in chest, jaw or neck; serious cardiac events **Interactions:** ↑ Risk of serotonin syndrome *W/* SSRIs; ↑ risks of prolonged vasospasms *W/* ergot-containing medications **Labs:** None known **NIPE:** Not for migraine prevention; ⊘ EtOH; ⊘ use for more than 3 migraine attacks/mo

Emedastine (Emadine) [Antihistamine]   Uses: *Allergic conjunctivitis* **Action:** Antihistamine; selective H$_1$-antagonist **Dose:** 1 gtt in eye(s) up to qid **Caution:** [B, ?] **Contra:** Allergy to ingredients (preservatives benzalkonium, tromethamine) **Disp:** 0.05% soln **SE:** HA, blurred vision, burning/stinging, corneal infiltrates/staining, dry eyes, foreign body sensation, hyperemia, keratitis, tearing, pruritus, rhinitis, sinusitis, asthenia, bad taste, dermatitis, discomfort **NIPE:** ⊘ Wear soft contact lens for 15 min after use; do not use contact lenses if eyes are red

Emtricitabine (Emtriva) [Antiretroviral/NRTI]   **WARNING:** Class warning for lipodystrophy, lactic acidosis, & severe hepatomegaly **Uses:** *HIV-1 Infxn* **Action:** NRTI **Dose:** 200 mg cap or 240 mg sol PO daily; ↓ w/ renal impair **Caution:** [B, –] Risk of liver Dz **Contra:** Component sensitivity **Disp:** *Soln:* 10 mg/mL, 200 mg caps **SE:** HA, D, N, rash, rare hyperpigmentation of feet & hands, posttreatment exacerbation of hepatitis **Notes:** 1st one-daily NRTI; caps/sol not equivalent; not rec as monotherapy; screen for HepB, do not use in established HIV and Hep B coinfection **Interactions:** None noted *W/* additional NRTIs **Labs:** ↑ LFTs, bilirubin, triglycerides, glucose **NIPE:** Take w/o regard to food; causes redistribution and accumulation of body fat; take w/ other antiretrovirals; not a cure for HIV or prevention of opportunistic Infxns

Enalapril (Vasotec) [Antihypertensive/ACEI]   Uses: *HTN, CHF, LVD*, DN* **Action:** ACE inhibitor **Dose:** *Adults.* 2.5–40 mg/d PO; 1.25 mg IV q6h. *Peds.* 0.05–0.08 mg/kg/d PO q12–24h; ↓ w/ renal impair **Caution:** [C (1st tri; D 2nd & 3rd tri), +] D/C immediately once pregnancy detected w/ NSAIDs, K$^+$ supls **Contra:** Bilateral RAS, angioedema **Disp:** Tabs 2.5, 5, 10, 20 mg; IV 1.25 mg/mL (1, 2 mL) **SE:** ↓ BP w/ initial dose (especially w/ diuretics), ↑ K$^+$, nonproductive cough, angioedema **Notes:** Monitor Cr; D/C diuretic for 2–3 d prior to start **Interactions:** ↑ Effects *W/* loop diuretics; ↑ risk of cough *W/* capsaicin;

↑ effects *OF* α-blockers, insulin, Li; ↑ risk of hyperkalemia *W/* K supl, K-sparing diuretics, salt substitutes, trimethoprim; ↓ effects *W/* ASA, NSAIDs, rifampin **Labs:** May cause ↑ serum K^+, direct Coombs test, false + urine acetone **NIPE:** Several weeks needed for full hypotensive effect

Enfuvirtide (Fuzeon) [Antiretroviral/Fusion Inhibitor] WARNING: Rarely causes allergy; never rechallenge **Uses:** *w/ antiretroviral agents for HIV-1 Infxn in treatment-experienced pts with evidence of viral replication despite ongoing antiretroviral therapy* **Action:** Viral fusion inhibitor **Dose:** 90 mg (1 mL) SQ bid in upper arm, anterior thigh, or abdomen; rotate site **Caution:** [B, –] **Contra:** Previous allergy to drug **Disp:** 90 mg/mL reconstituted; pt kit w/ monthly supplies **SE:** Inj site Rxns (in most); pneumonia, D, N, fatigue, insomnia, peripheral neuropathy **Interactions:** None noted *W/* other antiretrovirals **Labs:** ↑ LFTs, triglycerides; ↓ HMG, Hct, eosinophils **NIPE:** Does not cure HIV; does not ↓ risk of transmission or prevent opportunistic Infxns; take w/o regard to food; Available only via restricted distribution system; use immediately on recons or refrigerate (24 h max)

Enoxaparin (Lovenox) [Anticoagulant/Low Molecular Weight Heparin Derivative] WARNING: Recent or anticipated epidural/ spinal anesthesia ↑ risk of spinal/epidural hematoma w/ subsequent paralysis **Uses:** *Prevention & Rx of DVT; Rx PE; unstable angina & non-Q-wave MI* **Action:** LMW heparin; inhibit thrombin by complexing w/ antithrombin III **Dose:** *Adults.* Prevention: 30 mg SQ bid or 40 mg SQ q24h. *DVT/PE Rx:* 1 mg/kg SQ q12h or 1.5 mg/kg SQ q24h. *Angina:* 1 mg/kg SQ q12h; *Ancillary to fibrinolysis in AMI:* 30 mg IV bolus, then 1 mg/kg SQ bid *(ECC 2005);* CrCl <30 mL ↓ to 1/mg/kg SQ daily *Peds.* Prevention: 0.5 mg/kg SQ q12h. *DVT/PE Rx:* 1 mg/kg SQ q12h; ↓ dose w/ CrCl <30 mL/min **Caution:** [B, ?] Not for prophylaxis in prosthetic heart valves **Contra:** Active bleeding, HIT Ab(+), Cr >2.5 mg/dL men, 2 g/dL women **Disp:** Inj 10 mg/0.1 mL (30-, 40-, 60-, 80-, 100-, 120-, 150-mg syringes) 300-mg/3mL multidose vial **SE:** Bleeding, hemorrhage, bruising, thrombocytopenia, fever, pain/hematoma at site, ↑ AST/ALT **Interactions:** ↑ Bleeding effects *W/* ASA, anticoagulants, cephalosporins, NSAIDs, penicillin, chamomile, garlic, ginger, ginkgo biloba, feverfew, horse chestnut **Labs:** ↑ AST, ALT; No effect on bleeding time, actin Fxn, PT, or aPTT; monitor plt for HIT; may monitor antifactor Xa **NIPE:** Admin deep SQ; ⊘ IM

Entacapone (Comtan) [Antiparkinsonian Agent/COMT Inhibitor] **Uses:** *Parkinson Dz* **Action:** Selective & reversible carboxymethyl transferase inhibitor **Dose:** 200 mg w/ each levodopa/carbidopa dose; max 1600 mg/d; ↓ levodopa/carbidopa dose 25% w/ levodopa dose >800 mg **Caution:** [C, ?] Hepatic impair **Contra:** Use w/ MAOI **Disp:** Tabs 200 mg **SE:** Dyskinesia, hyperkinesia, N, D, dizziness, hallucinations, orthostatic ↓ BP **Interactions:** ↑ Effects *W/* ampicillin, chloramphenicol cholestyramine, erythromycin, MAOIs, probenecid, rifampin; ↑ risk of arrhythmias & HTN **W/** bitolterol, dopamine, dobutamine, epinephrine, isoetharine, methyldopa, norepinephrine **Labs:** Monitor LFTs NPE: ⊘ D/C abruptly, breast-feed; brownish-orange urine

Ephedrine [Vasopressor/Decongestant/Bronchodilator] Uses: *Acute bronchospasm, bronchial asthma, nasal congestion,* ↓ BP, narcolepsy, enuresis, & MyG **Action:** Sympathomimetic; stimulates α- & β-receptors; bronchodilator **Dose: Adults.** *Congestion:* 25–50 mg PO q6h PRN; ↓*BP:* 25–50 mg IV q5–10min, 150 mg/d max. **Peds.** 0.2–0.3 mg/kg/dose IV q4–6h PRN **Caution:** [C, ?/–] **Contra:** Arrhythmias; NAG **Disp:** Nasal soln 0.48%, 0.5%, oral capsule: 25, 37.5, 50 mg Inj 50 mg/mL; nasal spray 0.25% **SE:** CNS stimulation (nervousness, anxiety, trembling), tachycardia, arrhythmia, HTN, xerostomia, dysuria **Interactions:** ↑ Effects **W/** acetazolamide, antacids, MAOIs, TCAs, urinary alkalinizers; ↑ effects **OF** sympathomimetics; ↓ response **W/** diuretics, methyldopa, reserpine, urinary acidifiers; ↓ effects **OF** antihypertensives, BBs, dexamethasone, guanethidine **Labs:** False ↑ urine amino acids; can cause false + amphetamine EMIT **NIPE:** ⊘ EtOH; store away from light/heat; Protect from light; monitor BP, HR, urinary output; take last dose 4–6 h before hs; abuse potential, OTC sales mostly banned/restricted

Epinephrine (Adrenalin, Sus-Phrine, EpiPen, EpiPen Jr, others) (EpiPen Jr, others) [Vasopressor/Bronchodilator/Cardiac Stimulant, Local Anesthetic] Uses: *Cardiac arrest, anaphylactic Rxn, bronchospasm, open-angle glaucoma* **Action:** β-Adrenergic agonist, some a-effects **Dose: Adults.** 1.0 mg IV push, repeat q3–5min; (0.2 mg/kg max) if 1 mg dose fails. **Inf:** 30 mg (30 mL of 1:1000 soln) in 250 mL NS or D₅W, at 100 mL/h, titrate. **ET:** 2.0–2.5 mg in 20 mL NS. *Profound bradycardia/hypotension:* 2–10 μg/min (1 mg of 1:1000 in 500 mL NS, inf 1–5 mL/min) *(ECC 2005); Anaphylaxis:* 0.3–0.5 mL SQ of 1:1000 dilution, repeat PRN q5–15min to max 1 mg/dose & 5 mg/d. *Asthma:* 0.1–0.5 mL SQ of 1:1000 dilution, repeat q20-min to 4-h or 1 inhal (met-dose) repeat in 1–2 min or susp 0.1–0.3 mL SQ for extended effect. **Peds.** ACLS: 1st dose 0.1 mL/kg IV of 1:10,000 dilution, then 0.1 mL/kg IV of 1:1000 dilution q3–5min to response. *Anaphylaxis:* 0.15–0.3 mg IM depending on wt <30 kg 0.01 mg/kg *Asthma:* 0.01 mL/kg SQ of 1:1000 dilution q8–12h. **Caution:** [C, ?] ↓ Bronchodilation with β-blockers **Contra:** Cardiac arrhythmias, NAG **Disp:** Inj 1:1000, 1:2000, 1:10,000, 1:100,000; susp for inj 1:200; aerosol 220 μg/spray; 1% inhal soln; EpiPen AutoInjector 1 dose 0.30 mg; EpiPen Jr 0.15 mg **SE:** CV (tachycardia, HTN, vasoconstriction), CNS stimulation (nervousness, anxiety, trembling), ↓renal blood flow **Interactions:** ↑ HTN effects **W/** α-blockers, BBs, ergot alkaloids, furazolidone, MAOIs; ↑ cardiac effects **W/** antihistamines, cardiac glycosides, levodopa, thyroid hormones, TCAs; ↑ effects **OF** sympathomimetics; ↓ effects **OF** diuretics, guanethidine, hypoglycemics, methyldopa **Labs:** ↑ BUN, glucose, & lactic acid with prolonged use **NIPE:** ⊘ OTC inhalation drugs; can give via ET tube if no central line (use 2–2.5 × IV dose); EpiPen for pt self-use (www.EpiPen.com

Epinastine (Elestat) [Antihistamine] Uses: Itching w/ allergic conjunctivitis **Action:** Antihistamine **Dose:** 1 gtt bid **Caution:** [C, ?/–] **Disp:** Soln 0.05% **SE:** Burning, folliculosis, hyperemia, pruritus, URI, HA, rhinitis, sinusitis, cough, pharyngitis **NIPE:** Remove contacts before, reinsert in 10 min if eye not red; caution in pregnancy & lactation

Epirubicin (Ellence) [Antineoplastic/Anthracycline] **WARNING:** Do not give IM or SQ. Potential cardiotox; severe myelosupp Uses: *Adjuvant therapy for + axillary nodes after resection of primary breast CA*, **Actions:** Anthracycline cytotoxic agent **Dose:** Per protocols; ↓ dose w/ hepatic impair **Caution:** [D, –] **Contra:** Baseline neutrophil count <1500 cells/mm³, severe myocardial insuff, recent MI, severe arrhythmias, severe hepatic dysfunction, previous anthracyclines Rx to max cumulative dose **Disp:** Inj 50 mg/25 mL, 200 mg/100 mL **SE:** Mucositis, N/V/D, alopecia, ↓ BM, cardiotox, secondary AML, tissue necrosis w/ extrav, lethargy **Interactions:** ↑ Effects *W/* cimetidine; ↑ effects *OF* cytotoxic drugs, radiation therapy; ↑ risk of HF *W/* CCBs, trastuzumab; incompatible chemically *W/* fluorouracil, heparin **Labs:** ↓ HMG, Hct, neutrophils, plts, WBC **NIPE:** ⊘ Handle if PRG breast-feeding; urine reddish up to 2 d after treatment, use contraception during treatment, burning at inj site indicates infiltration, menstruation may cease permanently

Eplerenone (Inspra) [Antihypertensive/Selective Aldosterone Receptor Antagonist] Uses: *HTN* **Action:** Selective aldosterone antagonist **Dose:** *Adults:* 50 mg PO daily–bid, doses >100 mg/d no benefit w/ ↑ K⁺; ↓ to 25 mg PO daily if giving w/ CYP3A4 inhibitors **Caution:** [B, +/–] w/ CYP3A4 inhibitors (Table 11); monitor K⁺ with ACE inhibitor, ARBs, NSAIDs, K⁺-sparing diuretics; grapefruit juice, St. John's wort **Contra:** K⁺ >5.5 mEq/L; NIDDM w/ microalbuminuria; SCr >2 mg/dL (males), >1.8 mg/dL (females); CrCl <50 mL/min; w/ K⁺ supls/K⁺-sparing diuretics, ketoconazole **Disp:** Tabs 25, 50, 100 mg **SE:** HA, dizziness, gynecomastia, D, orthostatic ↓ BP **Interactions:** ↑ Risk hyperkalemia *W/* ACEIs; ↑ risk of toxic effects *W/* azole antifungals, erythromycin, saquinavir, verapamil, ↑ effects *OF* Li; ↓ effects *W/* NSAIDs **Labs:** ↑ K⁺, cholesterol, triglycerides **NIPE:** ⊘ High-K foods; may cause reversible breast pain or enlargement w/ use; may take 4 wk for full effect

Epoetin Alfa [Erythropoietin, EPO] (Epogen, Procrit) [Recombinant Human Erythropoietin] **WARNING:** Use lowest dose possible; may be associated with ↑ CV, thromboembolic events and/or mortality; D/C if Hgb >12 g/dL Uses: *CRF associated anemia* zidovudine Rx in HIV-infected pts, CA chemo; ↓ transfusions associated w/ surgery **Action:** Induces erythropoiesis **Dose:** *Adults & Peds.* 50–150 units/kg IV/SQ 3×/wk; adjust dose q4–6wk PRN. *Surgery:* 300 units/kg/d × 10 d before to 4 d after; ↓ dose if Hct 36% or Hgb, ↑ > ≅12 g/dL or Hgb >1 g/dL in 2-wk period; hold dose if Hgb >12 g/dL **Caution:** [C, +] **Contra:** Uncontrolled HTN **Disp:** Inj 2000,

3000, 4000, 10,000, 20,000, 40,000 units/mL **SE:** HTN, HA, fatigue, fever, tachycardia, N/V **Interactions:** None noted **Labs:** ↑ WBCs, plts; monitor baseline & post-treatment Hct/Hgb, BP, ferritin **NIPE:** Monitor for access line clotting, ⊘ shake vial; refrigerate

Epoprostenol (Flolan) [Antihypertensive] **Uses:** *Pulm HTN* **Action:** Dilates pulm/systemic arterial vascular beds; ↓ plt aggregation **Dose:** Initial 2 ng/kg/min; ↑ by 2 ng/kg/min q15min until dose-limiting SE (CP, dizziness, N/V, HA, ↓ BP, flushing); IV cont inf 4 ng/kg/min < maximum-tolerated rate; adjust based on response; see package insert **Caution:** [B, ?] ↑ Tox w/ diuretics, vasodilators, acetate in dialysis fluids, anticoagulants **Contra:** Chronic use in CHF 2nd-deg, if pt develops pulm edema w/ dose initiation, severe LVSD **Disp:** Inj 0.5, 1.5 mg **SE:** Flushing, tachycardia, CHF, fever, chills, nervousness, HA, N/V/D, jaw pain, flulike Sxs **Interactions:** ↑ Risk of bleeding w/ anticoagulants, antiplts; ↑ effects *OF* digoxin; ↓ BP w/ antihypertensives, diuretics, vasodilators **NIPE:** ⊘ Mix or administer w/ other drugs; Abrupt D/C can cause rebound pulm HTN; monitor bleeding w/ other antiplt/anticoagulants; watch ↓ BP w/ other vasodilators/diuretics

Eprosartan (Teveten) [Antihypertensive/ARB] **Uses:** *HTN*, DN, CHF **Action:** ARB **Dose:** 400–800 mg/d single dose or bid **Caution:** [C (1st tri); D (2nd & 3rd tri), D/C immediately when pregnancy detected] w/ Lithium, ↑ K+ with K+-sparing diuretics/supls/high-dose trimethoprim **Contra:** Bilateral RAS, 1st-deg aldosteronism **Disp:** Tabs 400, 600 mg **SE:** Fatigue, depression, URI, UTI, abd pain, rhinitis/pharyngitis/cough, hypertriglyceridemia **Interactions:** ↑ Risk of hyperkalemia *W/* K-sparing diuretics, K supls, trimethoprim; ↑ effects *OF* Li **Labs:** ↑ BUN, triglycerides; ↓ HMG, Hct, neutrophils **NIPE:** Monitor CBC & differential, renal Fxn; ⊘ PRG, breast-feeding

Eptifibatide (Integrilin) [Antiplatelet Agent] **Uses:** *ACS, PCI* **Action:** Glycoprotein IIb/IIIa inhibitor **Dose:** 180 µg/kg IV bolus, then 2 µg/kg/min cont inf; ↓ in renal impair (SCr >2 mg/dL, <4 mg/dL): 135 µg/kg bolus & 0.5 µg/kg/min inf); ACS: 180 µg/kg IV bolus then 2 µg/kg/min. PCI: 135 µg/kg IV bolus then 0.5 µg/kg/min; bolus again in 10 min *(ECC 2005)* **Caution:** [B, ?] Monitor bleeding w/ other anticoagulants **Contra:** Other GPIIb/IIIa inhibitors, h/o abnormal bleeding, hemorrhagic stroke (within 30 d), severe HTN, major surgery (within 6 wk), plt count <100,000 cells/mm³, renal dialysis **Disp:** Inj 0.75, 2 mg/mL **SE:** Bleeding, ↓ BP, inj site Rxn, thrombocytopenia; **Interactions:** ↑ Bleeding *W/* ASA, cephalosporins, clopidogrel, heparin, NSAIDs, thrombolytics, ticlopidine, warfarin, evening primrose oil, feverfew, garlic, ginger, ginkgo biloba, ginseng, **Labs:** ↓ Plts; Monitor bleeding, coags, plts, SCr, activated coagulation time (ACT) with prothrombin consumption index (keep ACT 200–300 sec)

Erlotinib (Tarceva) [Antineoplastic] **Uses:** *NSCLC after 1 chemo agent fails* **Action:** HER2/EGFR tyrosine kinase inhibitor **Dose:** 150 mg/d PO 1 h ac or 2 h pc; ↓ (in 50-mg decrements) w/ severe Rxn or w/ CYP3A4 inhibitors

(Table 11); per protocols **Caution:** [D, ?/–]; w/ CYP3A4 (Table 11) inhibitors **Disp:** Tabs 25, 100, 150 mg **SE:** Rash, N/V/D, anorexia, abd pain, fatigue, cough, dyspnea, edema, stomatitis, conjunctivitis, pruritus, dry skin, Infxn, interstitial lung disease **Interactions:** ↑ Drug plasma levels *W*/ CYP3A4 inhibitors (clarithromycin, ritonavir, ketoconazole); ↓ drug plasma levels *W*/ CYP3A4 inducers (carbamazepine, phenytoin, phenobarbital, St John's wort); ↑ risk of bleeding *W*/ anticoagulants, NSAIDs; **Labs:** Monitor LFTs, PT, INR; may ↑ INR w/ warfarin **NIPE:** ⊘ PRG or lactation; use adequate contraception; ↑ drug metabolism in smokers

Ertapenem (Invanz) [Anti-infective/Carbapenem] Uses: *Complicated intra-abd, acute pelvic, & skin Infxns, pyelonephritis, community-acquired pneumonia* **Action:** A carbapenem; β-lactam antibiotic, ↓ cell wall synth. *Spectrum:* Good gram (+/–) & anaerobic coverage, not *Pseudomonas* sp, PCN-resistant pneumococci, MRSA, *Enterococcus* sp, β-lactamase (+) *H. influenza, Mycoplasma* sp, *Chlamydia* sp **Dose:** *Adults.* 1 g IM/IV daily; 500 mg/d in CrCl <30 mL/min **Peds:** *3 mo–12 y:* 15 mg/kg bid IM/IV, max 1 g/d **Caution:** [C, ?/–] seizure h/o, CNS disorders, β-lactam & multiple allergies, Probenecid ↓ renal clearance **Contra:** component hypersensitivity or amide anesthetics **Disp:** Inj 1 g/vial **SE:** HA, N/V/D, inj site Rxns, thrombocytosis,; **Notes:** Can give IM × 7 d, IV × 14 d; 137 mg Na⁺ (6 mEq)/g ertapenem **Interactions:** ↑ Effects *W*/ probenecid **Labs:** ↑ LFTs, glucose, K⁺, Cr, PT, PTT, RBCs, urine WBCs **NIPE:** Monitor for super Infxn

Erythromycin (E-Mycin, E.E.S., Ery-Tab, EryPed, Ilotycin) [Antibiotic/Macrolide] Uses: *Bacterial Infxns; bowel prep*; ↑ GI motility *(prokinetic)*; *acne vulgaris* **Action:** Bacteriostatic; interferes w/ protein synth. *Spectrum:* Group A streptococci (*S. pyogenes*), *S. pneumoniae, N. meningitidis, N. gonorrhea* (if PCN-allergic), *Legionella* sp, *M. pneumoniae* **Dose:** *Adults.* Base 250–500 mg PO q6–12h or ethylsuccinate 400–800 mg q6–12h; 500 mg–1 g IV q6h. *Prokinetic:* 250 mg PO tid 30 min ac. *Peds.* 30–50 mg/kg/d PO ÷ q6–8h or 20–40 mg/kg/d IV ÷ q6h, max 2 g/d **Caution:** [B, +] ↑ tox of carbamazepine, cyclosporine, digoxin, methylprednisolone, theophylline, felodipine, warfarin, simvastatin/lovastatin; ↓ sildenafil dose w/ use **Contra:** Hepatic impair, preexisting liver Dz (estolate), use with pimozide **Disp:** *Lactobionate (Ilotycin): Powder for inj:* 500 mg, 1 g. *Base:* Tabs 250, 333, 500 mg; caps 250 mg. *Estolate (Ilosone):* Susp 125, 250 mg/5 mL. *Stearate (Erythrocin):* Tabs 250, 500 mg. *Ethylsuccinate (EES, EryPed):* Chew tabs 200 mg; tabs 400 mg; susp 200, 400 mg/5 mL **SE:** HA, abd pain, N/V/D; [QT prolongation, torsades de pointes, ventricular arrhythmias/tachycardias (rarely)]; cholestatic jaundice (estolate) **Notes:** 400 mg ethylsuccinate = 250 mg base/estolate; lactobionate contains benzyl alcohol (caution in neonates) **Interactions:** ↑ Effects *W*/ amprenavir, indinavir, ritonavir, saquinavir, grapefruit juice; ↑ effects *OF* alprazolam, benzodiazepines, buspirone, carbamazepine, clozapine, colchicines, cyclosporine, digoxin, felodipine, lovastatin, midazolam, quinidine, sildenafil, simvastatin, tacrolimus, theophylline, triazolam, valproic acid; ↑ QT *W*/ astemizole, cisapride; ↓ effects *OF* penicillin, zafirlukast **Labs:** ↑ LFTs, eosiniophils, neutrophils, plts; ↓ bicarbonate levels **NIPE:** Take w/ food if GI upset, monitor for super Infxn & ototox

Erythromycin & Benzoyl Peroxide (Benzamycin) [Anti-infective, Macrolide/Keratolytic] **Uses:** *Topical for acne vulgaris* **Action:** Macrolide antibiotic w/ keratolytic **Dose:** Apply bid (AM & PM) **Caution:** [C, ?] **Contra:** Component sensitivity **Disp:** Gel erythromycin 30 mg/benzoyl peroxide 50 mg/g **SE:** Local irritation, dryness

Erythromycin & Sulfisoxazole (Eryzole, Pediazole) [Anti-infective, Macrolide/Sulfonamide] **Uses:** *Upper & lower resp tract; bacterial Infxns; H. influenzae otitis media in children*; Infxns in PCN-allergic pts **Action:** Macrolide antibiotic w/ sulfonamide **Dose:** *Adults.* Based on erythromycin content; 400 mg erythromycin/1200 mg sulfisoxazole PO q6h. *Peds > 2 mo.* 40–50 mg/kg/d erythromycin & 150 mg/kg/d sulfisoxazole PO ÷ q6h; max 2 g/d erythromycin or 6 g/d sulfisoxazole × 10 d; ↓ in renal impair **Caution:** [C (D if near term), +] w/ PO anticoagulants, MRX, hypoglycemics, phenytoin, cyclosporine **Contra:** Infants <2 mo **Disp:** Susp erythromycin ethylsuccinate 200 mg/sulfisoxazole 600 mg/5 mL (100, 150, 200 mL) **SE:** GI upset **Additional Interactions:** ↑ Effects of sulfonamides W/ ASA, diuretics, NSAIDs, probenecid **Labs:** False + urine protein **NIPE:** ↑ Risk of photosensitivity—use sunscreen, ↑ fluid intake

Erythromycin, Ophthalmic (Ilotycin Ophthalmic) [Anti-infective, Macrolide, Opthalmic agent] **Uses:** *Conjunctival/corneal Infxns* **Action:** Macrolide antibiotic **Dose:** 1/2 in. 2–6 × /d **Caution:** [B, +] **Contra:** Erythromycin hypersensitivity **Disp:** 0.5% oint **SE:** Local irritation **NIPE:** May cause burning, stinging, blurred vision

Erythromycin, Topical (A/T/S, Eryderm, Erycette, T-Stat) [Topical Anti-infective, Macrolide] **Uses:** *Acne vulgaris* **Action:** Macrolide antibiotic **Dose:** Wash & dry area, apply 2% product over area bid **Caution:** [B, +] **Contra:** Component sensitivity **Disp:** Soln 1.5%, 2%; gel 2%; pads & swabs 2% **SE:** Local irritation

Escitalopram (Lexapro) [Antidepressant/SSRI] WARNING: Closely monitor for worsening depression or emergence of suicidality, particularly in ped pts **Uses:** Depression, anxiety **Action:** SSRI **Dose:** *Adults.* 10–20 mg PO daily; 10 mg/d in elderly & hepatic impair **Caution:** [C, +/–] Serotonin synd (Table 12) **Contra:** w/ or w/in 14 d of MAOI **Disp:** Tabs 5, 10, 20 mg; soln 1 mg/mL **SE:** N/V/D, sweating, insomnia, dizziness, xerostomia, sexual dysfunction **Interactions:** ↑ Risk of serotonin syndrome W/ linezolid; ↑ risk of bleeding W/ anticoagulants, ASA, NSAIDs; may ↑ CNS effects W/ CNS depressants **NIPE:** ⊘ D/C abruptly; may take up to 2–4 wk for full effects; take w/o regard to food; may cause ↑ appetite & wt gain

Esmolol (Brevibloc) [Antiarrhythmic/BB] **Uses:** *SVT & noncompensatory sinus tachycardia, AF/flutter* **Action:** β₁-Adrenergic blocker; class II antiarrhythmic **Dose:** *Adults & Peds.* Initial 500 µg/kg load over 1 min, then

50 µg/kg/min × 4 min; if inadequate response, repeat load & maint inf of 100 µg/kg/min × 4 min; titrate by repeating load, then incremental ↑ in the maint dose of 50 µg/kg/min for 4 min until desired HR reached or ↓ BP; average dose 100 µg/kg/min; 0.5 mg/kg over 1 min, then 0.05 mg/kg/min *(ECC 2005)* **Caution:** [C (1st tri; D 2nd or 3rd tri), ?] **Contra:** Sinus bradycardia, heart block, uncompensated CHF, cardiogenic shock, ↓ BP **Disp:** Inj 10, 20, 250 mg/mL; premix inf 10 mg/mL **SE:** ↓ BP; bradycardia, diaphoresis, dizziness **Interaction:** ↑ Effects W/ verapamil; ↑ effects *OF* digoxin, antihypertensives, nitrates; ↓ HTN W/ amphetamines, cocaine, ephedrine, epinephrine, MAOIs, norepinephrine, phenylephrine, pseudoephedrine; ↓ effects *OF* glucagons, insulin, hypoglycemics, theophylline; ↓ effects W/ NSAIDs, thyroid hormones **Labs:** ↑ Glucose, cholesterol **NIPE:** Monitor BS of pts w/ DM; pain on inj.; hemodynamic effects back to baseline w/in 30 min after D/C of

Esomeprazole (Nexium) [Gastric Acid Inhibitor/Proton Pump Inhibitor]

Uses: *Short-term (4–8 wk) for erosive esophagitis/GERD; H. pylori Infxn in combo with antibiotics* **Action:** Proton pump inhibitor, ↓ gastric acid **Dose:** *Adults. GERD/erosive gastritis:* 20–40 mg/d PO × 4–8 wk; 20–40 mg IV 10–30 min inf or >3 min IV push, 10 d max; *Maint:* 20 mg/d PO. *H. pylori Infxn:* 40 mg/d PO, plus clarithromycin 500 mg PO bid & amoxicillin 1000 mg bid for 10 d **Caution:** [B, ?/–] **Contra:** Component sensitivity **Disp:** Caps 20, 40 mg; IV 20, 40 mg **SE:** HA, D, abd pain **Notes:** Do not chew; may open capsule & sprinkle on applesauce **Interactions:** ↑ Effects W/ amoxicillin, clarithromycin; ↑ effects *OF* benzodiazepines, warfarin ; ↓ effects *OF* digoxin, ketoconazole, iron salts **Labs:** ↑ SCr, uric acid, LFTs, HMG, WBCs, plts, K⁺, thyroxine levels **NIPE:** Take drug 1 h before food; ⊘ EtOH

Estazolam (Prosom) [C-IV] [Hypnotic/Benzodiazepine]

Uses: *Short-term management of insomnia* **Action:** Benzodiazepine **Dose:** 1–2 mg PO qhs PRN; ↓ in hepatic impair/elderly/debilitated **Caution:** [X, –] ↑ effects w/ CNS depressants **Contra:** PRG **Disp:** Tabs 1, 2 mg **SE:** Somnolence, weakness, palpitations, anaphylaxis, angioedema, amnesia **Interactions:** ↑ Effects W/ amoxicillin, clarithromycin; ↑ effects *OF* diazepam, phenytoin, warfarin; ↓ effects W/ food; ↓ effects *OF* azole antifungals, digoxin **Labs:** ↑ LFTs, **NIPE:** Take at least 1 h ac; May cause psychological/physical dependence; avoid abrupt D/C after prolonged use

Esterified Estrogens (Estratab, Menest) [Estrogen Supplement]

WARNING: Do not use in the prevention of CV Dz or dementia; ↑ risk of endometrial CA **Uses:** *Vasomotor Sxs or vulvar/vaginal atrophy w/ menopause*; *female hypogonadism, Pca, prevent osteoporosis* **Action:** Estrogen supl **Dose:** *Menopausal vasomotor Sx:* 0.3–1.25 mg/d, cyclically 3 wk on, 1 wk off; add progestin 10–14 d w/ 28-d cycle w/ uterus intact; *Vulvovaginal atrophy:* Same regimen except use 0.3–1.25 mg; *Hypogonadism:* 2.5–7.5 mg/d PO × 20 d, off × 10 d; add progestin 10–14 d w/ 28-d cycle w/ uterus intact **Caution:** [X, –] **Contra:** Undiagnosed genital bleeding, breast CA, estrogen-dependent tumors, thromboembolic disorders, thrombophlebitis, recent MI, PRG, severe hepatic Dz **Disp:** Tabs 0.3, 0.625, 1.25, 2.5 mg **SE:** N, HA, bloating, breast enlargement/tenderness, edema, venous thromboembolism, hypertriglyceridemia, gallbladder Dz **Notes:** Use lowest dose for shortest time (see WHI data www.whi.org) **Interactions:** ↑ Effects OF corticosteroids, cyclosporine, TCAs, theophylline, caffeine, tobacco; ↓ effects W/ barbiturates, phenytoin, rifampin; ↓ effects *OF* anticoagulants, hypoglycemics, insulin, tamoxifen **Labs:** ↑ Prothrombin & factors VII, VIII, IX, X, plt aggregation, thyroid-binding globulin, T₄, triglycerides; ↓ antithrombin III, folate **NIPE:** ⊘ PRG, breast-feeding

Esterified Estrogens + Methyltestosterone (Estratest, Estratest HS, Syntest DS, HS) [Estrogen & Androgen Supplement] WARNING:
↑ Risk of dementia in postmenopausal women, unopposed estrogens may ↑ risk of endometrial carcinoma in postmenopausal women **Uses:** *Vasomotor Sxs*; postpartum breast engorgement **Action:** Estrogen & androgen supl **Dose:** 1 tab/d × 3 wk, 1 wk off **Caution:** [X, –] **Contra:** Genital bleeding of unknown cause, breast CA, estrogen-dependent tumors, thromboembolic disorders, thrombophlebitis, recent MI, PRG **Disp:** Tabs (estrogen/methyltestosterone) 0.625 mg/1.25 mg, 1.25 mg/2.5 mg **SE:** N, HA, bloating, breast enlargement/tenderness, edema, ↑ triglycerides, venous thromboembolism, gallbladder Dz **Notes:** Use lowest dose for shortest time; (see WHI data www.whi.org) **Additional Interactions:** ↑ Effects OF insulin; ↓ effects OF oral anticoagulants

Estradiol (Estrace, others) [Estrogen Supplement]
Uses: *Atrophic vaginitis, vasomotor Sxs associated w/ menopause, osteoporosis* **Action:** Estrogen supl **Dose:** *PO:* 1–2 mg/d, adjust PRN to control Sxs. *Vaginal cream:* 2–4 g/d × 2 wk, then 1 g 1–3 ×/wk **Caution:** [X, –] **Contra:** Genital bleeding of unknown cause, breast CA, porphyria, estrogen-dependent tumors, thromboembolic disorders, thrombophlebitis; recent MI; hepatic impair **Disp:** Ring, 0.05, 0.1, 2 mg; gel 0.061%; tabs 0.5, 1, 2 mg; vaginal cream 0.1 mg/g **SE:** N, HA, bloating, breast enlargement/tenderness, edema, ↑ triglycerides, venous thromboembolism, gallbladder Dz **Interactions:** ↑ Effects W/ grapefruit juice; ↑ effects OF corticosteroids, cyclosporine, TCAs, theophylline, caffeine, tobacco; ↓ effects W/ barbiturates, carbamazepine, phenytoin, primidone, rifampin; ↓ effects OF clofibrate, hypoglycemics, insulin, tamoxifen, warfarin **Labs:** ↑ Prothrombin & factors VII, VIII, IX, X, plt aggregation, thyroid-binding globulin, T₄, triglycerides; ↓ antithrombin III, folate **NIPE:** ⊘ PRG, breast-feeding

Estradiol gel (Elestrin) [Estrogen Supplement] WARNING:
Do not use in the prevention of CV Dz or dementia; ↑ risk of endometrial CA **Uses:** *Postmenopausal vasomotor symptoms* **Action:** Estrogenic **Dose:** Apply 0.87–1.7 g to skin daily; add progestin × 10–14 d/28-d cycle w/ intact uterus; use lowest effective estrogen dose **Caution:** [C, ?] **Contra:** breast CA, estrogen-dependent

tumors, thromboembolic disorders, recent MI, PRG, severe hepatic Dz **Disp:** 0.87 g gel = 0.52 mg estradiol/pump **SE:** Thromboembolic events, MI, stroke, ↑ BP, breast/ovarian/endometrial CA, site Rxns, vag spotting, breast changes, abd bloating, cramps, HA, fluid retention **NIPE:** Apply to upper arm, wait >25 min before sunscreen; avoid concomitant use for >7 d; ✓ BP, breast exams

Estradiol Cypionate & Medroxyprogesterone Acetate (Lunelle) [Estrogen & Progestin Supplement] **WARNING:** Cigarette smoking ↑ risk of serious CV side effects from contraceptives containing estrogen. This risk ↑ with age & with heavy smoking (>15 cig/d) & is quite marked in women >35 y. Women who use Lunelle should be strongly advised not to smoke **Uses:** *Contraceptive* **Action:** Estrogen & progestin **Dose:** 0.5 mL IM (deltoid, ant thigh, buttock) monthly, do not exceed 33 d **Caution:** [X, M] HTN, gallbladder Dz, ↑ lipids, migraines, sudden HA, valvular heart Dz with comps **Contra:** PRG, heavy smokers >35 y, DVT, PE, cerebro/CV Dz, estrogen-dependent neoplasm, undiagnosed AUB, porphyria, hepatic tumors, cholestatic jaundice **Disp:** Estradiol cypionate (5 mg), medroxyprogesterone acetate (25 mg) single-dose vial or syringe (0.5 mL) **SE:** Arterial thromboembolism, HTN, cerebral hemorrhage, MI, amenorrhea, acne, breast tenderness; see Estradiol **Additional Interactions:** ↓ Effects W/ aminoglutethimide **NIPE:** Start w/in 5 d of menstruation

Estradiol, Transdermal (Estraderm, Climara, Vivelle, Vivelle Dot) [Estrogen Supplement] **WARNING:** Do not use in the prevention of CV Dz or dementia; ↑ risk of endometrial CA **Uses:** *Severe menopausal vasomotor Sxs; female hypogonadism* **Action:** Estrogen supl **Dose:** Start 0.0375–0.05 mg/d patch–2 × wk based on product; adjust PRN to control Sxs; w/ intact uterus cycle 3 wk on 1 wk off or use cyclic progestin 10–14 d **Caution:** [X, –] See estradiol **Contra:** PRG, AUB, porphyria, breast CA, estrogen-dependent tumors, h/o thrombophlebitis, thrombosis **Disp:** TD patches (mg/24 h) 0.025, 0.0375, 0.05, 0.06, 0.075, 0.1 **SE:** N, bloating, breast enlargement/tenderness, edema, HA, hypertriglyceridemia, gallbladder Dz; see Estradiol **Additional NIPE:** Rotate application sites; do not apply to breasts, place on trunk

Estradiol/Levonorgestrel transdermal (Climara Pro) [Estrogen & Progesterone Supplement] **WARNING:** Do not use in the prevention of CV Dz or dementia **Uses:** *Menopausal vasomotor Sx; prevent postmenopausal osteoporosis* **Action:** Estrogen and progesterone **Dose:** 1 patch 1 ×/wk **Caution:** [X, –] w/ ↓ thyroid **Contra:** AUB, estrogen sens tumors, h/o thromboembolism, liver impair, PRG, hysterectomy **Disp:** *Pro* 0.045 mg/0.015/mg d patch **SE:** Site Rxn, vag bleed/spotting, breast changes, abd bloating/cramps, HA, retention fluid, edema, ↑ BP **NIPE:** Apply lower abd; for osteoporosis give Ca^{+2}/vitamin D supl; follow breast exams

Estradiol/Norethindrone Acetate (Femhrt, Activella) [Estrogen & Progesterone Supplement] **WARNING:** Estrogens & progestins should not be used for the prevention of CV Dz or dementia; the WHI study reported ↑ risks of MI, breast CA, & DVT in postmenopausal women during 5 y of treatment with estrogens combined with medroxyprogesterone acetate relative to placebo **Uses:** *Vasomotor Sxs associated w/ menopause; prevent osteoporosis* **Action:** Estrogen/progestin hormone replacement; plant derived **Dose:** 1 tab/d start w/ lowest dose combo **Caution:** [X, –] w/ ↓ Ca⁺²/thyroid **Contra:** PRG; h/o breast CA; estrogen-dependent tumor; abnormal genital bleeding; h/o DVT, PE, or related disorders; recent (w/in past year) arterial thromboembolic Dz (CVA, MI) **Disp:** Femhrt tabs 2.5/0.5, 5 μg/1 mg; Activella tabs 1.0/0.5, 0.5 mg/0.1 mg **SE:** Thrombosis, dizziness, HA, libido changes, insomnia, emotional stability, breast pain **NIPE:** Use in women w/ intact uterus; caution in heavy smokers

Estramustine Phosphate (Estracyt, Emcyt) [Antimicrotubule Agent]
Uses: *Advanced PCa* **Action:** Antimicrotubule agent; weak estrogenic & antiandrogenic activity **Dose:** 14 mg/kg/d in 3–4 ÷ doses; on empty stomach, no dairy products **Caution:** [Not used in females] **Contra:** Active thrombophlebitis or thromboembolic disorders **Disp:** Caps 140 mg **SE:** N/V, exacerbation of preexisting CHF, edema, hepatic disturbances, thrombophlebitis, MI, PE, gynecomastia in 20–100% **Interactions:** ↓ Effects *W/* antacids, Ca supls, Ca-containing foods; ↓ effects *OF* anticoagulants **NIPE:** Take on empty stomach, several wk may be needed for full effects, store in refrigerator

Estrogen, Conjugated (Premarin) [Estrogen/Hormone]
WARNING: Should not be used for the prevention of CV Dz or dementia. The WHI reported ↑ risk of MI, stroke, breast CA, PE, & DVT when combined with methoxyprogesterone over 5 y of Rx; ↑ risk of endometrial CA, unopposed estrogens, ↑ risk of dementia in premenopausal women **Uses:** *Moderate–severe menopausal vasomotor Sxs; atrophic vaginitis; palliative advanced CAP; prevent & Tx of estrogen-deficiency osteoporosis* **Action:** Estrogen hormonal replacement **Dose:** 0.3–1.25 mg/d PO cyclically; prostatic CA 1.25–2.5 mg PO tid; **Caution:** [X, –] **Contra:** Severe hepatic impair, genital bleeding of unknown cause, breast CA, estrogen-dependent tumors, thromboembolic disorders, thrombosis, thrombophlebitis, recent MI **Disp:** Tabs 0.3, 0.625, 0.9, 1.25, 2.5 mg; inj 25 mg/mL, vag cream 0.625 mg/g **SE:** ↑ Risk of endometrial CA, gallbladder Dz, thromboembolism, HA, & possibly breast CA; generic products not equivalent **Interactions:** ↑ Effects *OF* corticosteroids, cyclosporine, TCAs, theophylline, tobacco; ↓ effects *OF* anticoagulants, clofibrate; ↓ effects *W/* barbiturates, carbamazepine, phenytoin, rifampin **Labs:** ↑ Prothrombin & factors VII, VIII, IX, X, plt aggregation, thyroid-binding globulin, T₄, triglycerides; ↓ antithrombin III, folate **NIPE:** ⊘ PRG, breast-feeding

Estrogen, Conjugated Synthetic (Cenestin, Enjuvia) [Estrogen/Hormone]
WARNING: Do not use in the prevention of CV Dz or dementia; ↑ risk of endometrial CA **Uses:** *Vasomotor menopausal Sxs, vulvovaginal atrophy, prevent postmenopausal osteoporosis* **Action:** Multiple estrogen hormonal replacement **Dose:** For all w/ intact uterus progestin × 10–14 d/28-d cycle;

Vasomotor 0.3–1.25 mg (Enjuvia) 0.625–1.25 mg (*Cenestin*) PO daily; *Vaginal atrophy* 0.3 mg/d; *osteoporosis* (*Cenestin*) 0.625 mg/d **Caution:** [X, –] **Contra:** See estrogen, conjugated **Disp:** Tabs *Cenestin* 0.3, 0.45, 0.625, 0.9 mg; *Enjuvia* ER 0.3, 0.45, 0.625, 1.25 mg **SE:** ↑ risk endometrial/breast CA, gallbladder Dz, thromboembolism; see Estrogen, Conjugated

Estrogen, Conjugated + Medroxyprogesterone (Prempro, Premphase) [Estrogen/Progestin Hormones] WARNING: Should not be used for the prevention of CV Dz or dementia; ↑ risk of dementia in premenopausal women; the WHI study reported ↑ risk of MI, stroke, breast CA, PE, & DVT over 5 y of Rx **Uses:** *Moderate–severe menopausal vasomotor Sxs; atrophic vaginitis; prevent postmenopausal osteoporosis* **Action:** Hormonal replacement **Dose:** Prempro 1 tab PO daily; premphase 1 tab PO daily **Caution:** [X, –] **Contra:** Severe hepatic impair, genital bleeding of unknown cause, breast CA, estrogen-dependent tumors, thromboembolic disorders, thrombosis, thrombophlebitis **Disp:** (As estrogen/medroxyprogesterone) *Prempro:* Tabs 0.625/2.5, 0.625/5 mg; *Premphase:* Tabs 0.625/0 (d 1–14) & 0.625/5 mg (d 15–28) **SE:** Gallbladder Dz, thromboembolism, HA, breast tenderness **Notes:** See WHI www.whi.org; see Estrogen, Conjugated **Additional Interactions:** ↓ Effects W/ aminoglutethimide

Estrogen, Conjugated + Methylprogesterone (Premarin + Methylprogesterone) [Estrogen & Androgen Hormones] WARNING: Do not use in the prevention of CV Dz or dementia; ↑ risk of endometrial CA **Uses:** *Menopausal vasomotor Sxs; osteoporosis* **Action:** Estrogen & androgen combo **Dose:** 1 tab/d **Caution:** [X, –] **Contra:** Severe hepatic impair, AUB, breast CA, estrogen-dependent tumors, thromboembolic disorders, thrombosis, thrombophlebitis **Disp:** Tabs 0.625 mg estrogen, conjugated, & 2.5 or 5 mg of methylprogesterone **SE:** N, bloating, breast enlargement/tenderness, edema, HA, hypertriglyceridemia, gallbladder Dz; see Estrogen, Conjugated

Estrogen, Conjugated + Methyltestosterone (Premarin + Methyltestosterone) [Estrogen & Androgen Hormones] WARNING: Do not use in the prevention of CV Dz or dementia; ↑ risk of endometrial CA **Uses:** *Moderate–severe menopausal vasomotor Sxs*; postpartum breast engorgement **Action:** Estrogen & androgen combo **Dose:** 1 tab/d × 3 wk, then 1 wk off **Caution:** [X, –] **Contra:** Severe hepatic impair, genital bleeding of unknown cause, breast CA, estrogen-dependent tumors, thromboembolic disorders, thrombophlebitis **Disp:** Tabs (estrogen/ methyltestosterone) 0.625 mg/5 mg, 1.25 mg/10 mg **SE:** N, bloating, breast enlargement/tenderness, edema, HA, hypertriglyceridemia, gallbladder Dz; see Estrogen, Conjugated **Additional Interactions:** ↑ Effects *OF* insulin

Eszopiclone (Lunesta) [C-IV] [Hypnotic/Nonbenzodiazepine] **Uses:** *Insomnia* **Action:** Nonbenzodiazepine hypnotic **Dose:** 2–3 mg/d hs *Elderly:* 1–2 mg/d hs; w/ hepatic impair/use w/ CYP3A4 inhibitor (Table 11): 1 mg/d hs **Caution:**

[C, ?/–] **Disp:** Tabs 1, 2, 3 mg **SE:** HA, xerostomia, dizziness, somnolence, hallucinations, rash, Infxn, unpleasant taste, anaphylaxis, angioedema **Interactions:** ↑ Effects W/ itraconazole, ketoconazole, ritonavir; ↑ CNS effects W/ CNS depressants; ↓ effects W/ rifampin **NIPE:** High-fat meals ↓ absorption

Etanercept (Enbrel) [Antirheumatic/TNF Blocker] Uses: *Reduces Sxs of RA in pts who fail other DMARD*, Crohn Dz **Action:** Binds TNF **Dose: Adults.** RA 50 mg sc weekly or 25 mg sc 2×/wk (separated by at least 72–96 h). **Peds 4–17 y.** 0.8 mg/kg/wk (max 50 mg/wk) or 0.4 mg/kg (max 25 mg/dose) twice weekly 72–96 h apart **Caution:** [B, ?] w/ predisposition to Infxn (ie, DM) **Contra:** Active Infxn; **Disp:** Inj 25 mg/vial, 50 mg/mL **SE:** HA, rhinitis, inj site Rxn, URI **Interactions:** ↓ Response to live virus vaccine **NIPE:** Rotate inj sites; ⊘ live vaccines

Ethambutol (Myambutol) [Antitubercular Agent] Uses: *Pulm TB* & other mycobacterial Infxns, MAC **Action:** ↓ RNA synth **Dose: Adults & Peds >12 y.** 15–25 mg/kg/d PO single dose; ↓ in renal impair, take w/ food, avoid antacids **Caution:** [B, +] **Contra:** Unconscious patients, optic neuritis **Disp:** Tabs 100, 400 mg **SE:** HA, hyperuricemia, acute gout, abd pain, ↑ LFTs, optic neuritis, GI upset **Interactions:** ↑ Neurotox W/ neurotoxic drugs; ↓ effects W/ Al salts **NIPE:** Monitor visual acuity

Ethinyl Estradiol (Estinyl, Feminone) [Estrogen Supplement] Uses: *Menopausal vasomotor Sxs; female hypogonadism* **Action:** Estrogen supl **Dose:** 0.02–1.5 mg/d ÷ daily–tid **Caution:** [X, –] **Contra:** Severe hepatic impair; genital bleeding of unknown cause, breast CA, estrogen-dependent tumors, thromboembolic disorders, thrombophlebitis **Disp:** Tabs 0.02, 0.05, 0.5 mg **SE:** N, bloating, breast enlargement/tenderness, edema, HA, hypertriglyceridemia, gallbladder Dz **Interactions:** ↑ Effects OF corticosteroids; ↓ effects W/ barbiturates, carbamazepine, hypoglycemics, insulin, phenytoin, primidone, rifampin, ↓ effects OF anticoagulants, tamoxifen **Labs:** ↑ Prothrombin & factors VII, VIII, IX, X, plt aggregation, thyroid-binding globulin, T_4, triglycerides; ↓ antithrombin III, folate **NIPE:** ⊘ PRG, breast-feeding

Ethinyl Estradiol & Drospirenone (YAZ) [Estrogen & Progestin Supplement] WARNING: Cigarette smoking & use of estrogen-based OCPs have ↑ risk of serious cardiovascular side effects; risk ↑ w/ age (esp >35 y) and smoking >15 cig/d Uses: *Oral contraception; premenstrual dysphoric disorder* **Action:** Suppresses ovulation by imitating the feedback inhibition of endogenous estrogen and progesterone on the pituitary and hypothalamus **Dose:** 1 tab PO OD × 28 d, repeat **Caution:** [X, –], has antimineralocorticotic activity w/ potential hyperkalemia in renal insuff, adrenal insuff, hepatic insuff **Contra:** Pts w/ renal insuff, hepatic impair, adrenal insuff, DVT, PE, CVD, CAD, estrogen-dependent neoplasms, abnormal uterine bleeding, PRG, heavy smokers >35 y **Disp:** Ethinyl estradiol (20 μg), drospirenone (3 mg) 28-d pack has 24 active tabs & 4 inert tabs **SE:** Hyperkalemia, HTN, N, V, HA, breakthrough bleeding, amenorrhea, mastodynia,

↑ risk of gallbladder Dz & thromboembolic disorders **Interactions:** ↑ Risk **OF** hyperkalemia **W/** ACEIs, ARBs, aldosterone antagonists, heparin, NSAIDs, spironolactone, K⁺ sparing diuretics, K⁺ supplements, ↑ effects **OF** cyclosporine, prednisolone, theophylline; ↓ effects **W/** barbiturates, carbamazepine, griseofulvin, modafinil, phenobarbital, phenylbutazone, phenytoin, pioglitazone, rifabutin, rifampin, ritonavir, topiramate, St John's wort **Labs:** ↑ Uptake **OF** T_3, ↓ T_4 sex hormone-binding globulin levels; triglycerides **NIPE:** Antimineralocorticoid activity comparable to spironolactone 25 mg; in pts taking meds that ↑ K⁺ monitor serum K⁺during 1st Rx cycle; Sunday start regimen or postpartum use requires additional contraceptive methods during 1st cycle; use barrier contraception if taking anticonvulsants; may cause vision changes or ↓ contact lens tolerability; ⊘ protection against HIV or STDs; ⊘ smoke cigarettes

Ethinyl Estradiol & Levonorgestrel (Preven) [Estrogen & Progestin Supplements]
Uses: *Emergency contraceptive* ("morning-after pill"); prevent PRG (contraceptive failure, unprotected intercourse) **Actions:** Estrogen & progestin; interferes with implantation **Dose:** 4 tabs, take 2 tabs q12h × 2 (w/in 72 h of intercourse) **Caution:** [X, M] **Contra:** Known/suspected PRG, AUB, h/o or current DVT/PE, stroke, MI CVD, CAD; severe HTN; severe HA with focal neurological Sx; breast or endometrial CA; estrogen-dependent neoplasms; undiagnosed abnormal genital bleeding; hepatic dysfn; jaundice; major surgery with prolonged immobilization; heavy smoking if >35 y **Disp:** *Kit:* Ethinyl estradiol (0.05), levonorgestrel (0.25) blister pack with 4 pills & urine PRG test **SE:** Peripheral edema, N/V/D, bloating, abd pain, fatigue, HA, & menstrual changes; see Ethinyl Estradiol **Additional Interactions:** ↑ Effects **OF** ASA, benzodiazepines, metoprolol, TCAs **NIPE:** Monitor for vision changes or ↓ tolerance of contact lens; will not induce abortion; may ↑ risk of ectopic PRG

Ethinyl Estradiol/Levonorgestrel (Seasonale) [Estrogen & Progestin Supplement]
WARNING: Cigarette smoking & use of estrogen-based OCPs have ↑ risk of serious cardiovascular side effects; risk ↑ w/ age (esp>35 y) and smoking >15 cig/d **Uses:** Oral contraceptive **Action:** Suppresses ovulation by imitating the feedback inhibition of endogenous estrogen and progesterone on the pituitary and hypothalamus **Dose:** 1 tab PO OD for 91 d; repeat. Use Sunday start for 1st cycle **Caution:** [X, –]; **Contra:** Pts w/ DVT, PE, CVD, CAD, estrogen-dependent neoplasms, abnormal uterine bleeding, PRG, hepatic impair **Disp:** Tabs levonorgestrel 0.15 mg and ethinyl estradiol 30 μg; 91-d pack has 84 active tabs & 7 inert tabs **SE:** HTN, N, V, HA, breakthrough bleeding, amenorrhea, mastodynia, ↑ risk of gallbladder Dz & thromboembolic disorders **Interactions:** ↓ Effects **W/** barbiturates, carbamazepine, griseofulvin, modafinil, phenobarbital, phenytoin, pioglitazone, rifabutin, rifampin, ritonavir, topiramate, St John's wort **Labs:** ↑ Uptake **OF** T_3, ↓ T_4 sex hormone-binding globulin levels **NIPE:** Sunday start regimen requires additional contraceptive methods during 1st cycle; use barrier contraception if taking

anticonvulsants; may cause vision changes or ↓ contact lens tolerability; ⊘ protection against HIV or STDs; ⊘ smoke cigarettes

Ethinyl Estradiol & Norelgestromin (Ortho Evra [Estrogen & Progestin Hormones]) Uses: *Contraceptive patch* Action: Estrogen & progestin Dose: Apply patch to abdomen, buttocks, upper torso (not breasts), or upper outer arm at the beginning of the menstrual cycle; new patch is applied weekly for 3 wk; week 4 is patch-free Caution: [X, M] Contra: PRG, h/o or current DVT/PE, stroke, MI, CVD, CAD; severe HTN; severe HA w/ focal neurologic Sx; breast/endometrial CA; estrogen-dependent neoplasms; hepatic dysfn; jaundice; major surgery w/ prolonged immobilization; heavy smoking if >35 y Disp: 20 cm² patch (6 mg norelgestromin [active metabolite norgestimate] & 0.75 mg of ethinyl estradiol) SE: Breast discomfort, HA, site Rxns, N, menstrual cramps; thrombosis risks similar to OCP; see Ethinyl Estradiol Additional Labs: ↑ Serum amylase, Na, Ca, protein NIPE: Less effective in women >90 kg; instruct patient that drug does not protect against STD/HIV

Ethosuximide (Zarontin) [Anticonvulsant] Uses: *Absence (petit mal) Szs* Action: ↓ Sz threshold Dose: Adults. Initial, 250 mg PO ÷ bid; ↑ by 250 mg/d q4–7d PRN (max 1500 mg/d) usual maint 20–30 mg/kg. Peds 3–6 y. Initial: 15 mg/kg/d PO ÷ bid. Maint: 15–40 mg/kg/d ÷ bid, max 1500 mg/d Caution: [C, +] in renal/hepatic impair Contra: Component sensitivity Disp: Caps 250 mg; syrup 250 mg/5 mL SE: Blood dyscrasias, GI upset, drowsiness, dizziness, irritability Notes: Levels: Trough: Just before next dose; Therapeutic: Peak: 40–100 μg/mL; Toxic Trough: >100 μg/mL; 1/2 life: 30–60 h Interactions: ↑ Effects W/ INH, phenobarbital, EtOH; ↑ effects OF CNS depressants, phenytoin; ↓ effects W/ carbamazepine, valproic acid, ginkgo biloba; ↓ effects OF phenobarbital NIPE: Take w/ food, ⊘ EtOH

Etidronate Disodium (Didronel) [Hormone/Bisphosphonates] Uses: *↑ Ca²⁺ of malignancy, Paget Dz, & heterotopic ossification* Action: ↓ nl & abnormal bone resorption Dose: Paget Dz: 5–10 mg/kg/d PO ÷ doses (for 3–6 mo). ↑ Ca²⁺: 7.5 mg/kg/d IV inf over 2 h × 3 d, then 20 mg/kg/d PO on last day of inf × 1–3 mo Caution: [B PO (C parenteral), ?] Contra: Overt osteomalacia, SCr >5 mg/dL Disp: Tabs 200, 400 mg; inj 50 mg/mL SE: GI intolerance (↓ by ÷ daily doses); hypophosphatemia, hypomagnesemia, bone pain, abnormal taste, fever, convulsions, nephrotox Interactions: ↓ Effects W/ antacids, foods that contain Ca NIPE: ⊘ Take w/ food d/t < drug absorption; take PO on empty stomach 2 h before any meal

Etodolac [Antiarthritic/NSAID] WARNING: May ↑ risk of cardiovascular events & GI bleeding Uses: *Osteoarthritis & pain,* RA Action: NSAID Dose: 200–400 mg PO bid–qid (max 1200 mg/d) Caution: [C (D 3rd tri), ?] ↑ bleeding risk w/ ASA, warfarin; ↑ nephrotox w/ cyclosporine; h/o CHF, HTN, renal/hepatic impair, PUD Contra: Active GI ulcer Disp: Tabs 400, 500 mg; ER tabs 400, 500, 600 mg; caps 200, 300 mg SE: N/V/D, gastritis, abd cramps, dizziness, HA,

depression, edema, renal impair **Interactions:** ↑ Risk of bleeding *W/* anticoagulants, antiplts; ↑ effects *OF* Li, MTX, digoxin, cyclosporine; ↓ effects *W/* ASA; ↓ effects *OF* antihypertensives **Labs:**↑ LFTs, BUN, Cr; ↓ HMG, Hct, plts, WBC, uric acid **NIPE:** Take w/ food; do not crush tabs

Etonogestrel/Ethinyl Estradiol (NuvaRing) [Estrogen & Progestin Hormones] Uses: *Contraceptive* **Action:** Estrogen & progestin combo **Dose:** Rule out PRG 1st; insert ring vaginally for 3 wk, remove for 1 wk; insert new ring 7 d after last removed (even if bleeding) at same time of day ring removed. 1st day of menses is day 1, insert before day 5 even if bleeding. Use other contraception for 1st 7 d of starting therapy. See insert if converting from other contraceptive; after delivery or 2nd tri abortion, insert 4 wk postpartum (if not breast-feeding) **Caution:** [X, ?/–] HTN, gallbladder Dz, ↑ lipids, migraines, sudden HA **Contra:** PRG, heavy smokers >35 y, DVT, PE, cerebro-/CV Dz, estrogen-dependent neoplasm, undiagnosed abnormal genital bleeding, hepatic tumors, cholestatic jaundice **Disp:** *Intravaginal ring:* Ethinyl estradiol 0.015 mg/d & etonogestrel 0.12 mg/d; *see* Ethinyl Estradiol; if ring removed, rinse w/ cool/lukewarm H_2O (not hot) & reinsert ASAP; if not reinserted w/in 3 h, effectiveness ↓; do not use with diaphragm

Etonogestrel subdermal implant (Implanon) [Hormone] Uses: *Contraception* **Action:** Transforms endometrium from proliferative to secretory **Dose:** 1 implant subdermally q3y **Caution:** [X, +] exclude pregnancy before implant **Contra:** PRG, hormonally responsive tumors, Breast CA, AUB, hepatic tumor, active liver Dz, h/o thromboembolic Dz **Disp:** 68-mg implant **SE:** Spotting, irregular periods, amenorrhea, dysmenorrhea, HA, tender breasts, N, wt gain, acne, ectopic PRG, PE, ovarian cysts, stroke, ↑ BP **NIPE:** 99% effective; remove implant and replace; restricted distribution; health care provider must register and train; does not protect against STDs

Etoposide [VP-16] (VePesid, Toposar) [Antineoplastic] Uses: *Testicular, non-small-cell lung CA, Hodgkin Dz & NHLs, peds ALL, & allogeneic/autologous BMT in high doses* **Action:** Topoisomerase II inhibitor **Dose:** 50 mg/m²/d IV for 3–5 d; 50 mg/m²/d PO for 21 d (PO availability = 50% of IV); 2–6 g/m² or 25–70 mg/kg in BMT (per protocols); ↓ in renal/hepatic impair **Caution:** [D, –] **Contra:** IT administration **Disp:** Caps 50 mg; inj 20 mg/mL **SE:** N/V (emesis in 10–30%), ↓ BM, alopecia, ↓ BP w/ rapid IV, anorexia, anemia, leukopenia, ↑ risk secondary leukemias **Interactions:** ↑ Bleeding *W/* ASA, NSAIDs, warfarin; ↑ BM suppression *W/* antineoplastics & radiation; ↑ effects *OF* cisplatin; ↓ effects *OF* live vaccines **Labs:** ↑ Uric acid; ↓ HMG, Hct, plts, RBC, WBC **NIPE:** ⊘ EtOH, immunizations, PRG, breast-feeding; use contraception, 2–3 L/d fluids

Exemestane (Aromasin) [Antineoplastic] Uses: *Advanced breast CA in postmenopausal women w/ progression after tamoxifen* **Action:** Irreversible, steroidal aromatase inhibitor; ↓ estrogens **Dose:** 25 mg PO daily after a meal **Caution:** [D, ?/–] **Contra:** PRG, Component sensitivity **Disp:** Tabs 25 mg **SE:** Hot flashes, N, fatigue **Interactions:** ↓ Effects W/ erythromycin, ketoconazole, pheno-barbital, rifampin, other drugs that inhibit P4503A4, St John's wort, black cohosh, dong quai **Labs:** ↑ Alkaline phosphatase, bilirubin, alk phos **NIPE:** ⊘ PRG, breast-feeding; take pc and same time each day; monitor BP

Exenatide (Byetta) [Hypoglycemic/Incretin] Uses: Type 2 DM combined w/ metformin &/or sulfonylurea **Action:** An incretin mimetic: ↑ insulin release, ↓ glucagon secretion, ↓ gastric emptying, promotes satiety **Dose:** 5 µg SQ bid w/in 60 min before AM & PM meals; ↑ to 10 µg SQ bid after 1 mo PRN; do not give pc **Caution:** [C, ?/–] May ↓ absorption of other drugs (take antibiotics/contra-ceptives 1 h before) **Contra:** CrCl <30 mL/min **Disp:** Soln 5, 10 µg/dose in pre-filled pen **SE:** Hypoglycemia, N/V/D, dizziness, HA, dyspepsia, ↓ appetite, jittery **NIPE:** Consider ↓ sulfonylurea to ↓ risk of hypoglycemia; discard pen 30 d after 1st use

Ezetimibe (Zetia) [Antilipemic/Selective Cholesterol Absorp-tion Inhibitor] Uses: *Hypercholesterolemia alone or w/ a HMG-CoA re-ductase inhibitor* **Action:** ↓ Cholesterol & phytosterol absorption **Dose:** *Adults & Peds >10 y.* 10 mg/d PO **Caution:** [C, +/–] Bile acid sequestrants ↓ bioavailability **Contra:** Hepatic impair **Disp:** Tabs 10 mg **SE:** HA, D, abd pain, ↑ transaminases w/ HMG-CoA reductase inhibitor **Interactions:** ↑ Effects W/ cyclosporine; ↓ effects W/ cholestyramine, fenofibrate, gemfibrozil **Labs:** ↑ LFTs **NIPE:** If used w/ fibrates ↑ risk of cholethiasis

Ezetimibe/Simvastatin (Vytorin) [Antilipemic/HMG-CoA Re-ductase Inhibitor] Uses: *Hypercholesterolemia* **Action:** ↓ Absorption of cholesterol & phytosterol w/ HMG-CoA-reductase inhibitor **Dose:** 10/10–10/80 mg/d PO; w/ cyclosporine or danazol: 10/10 mg/d max; w/ amiodarone or vera-pamil: 10/20 mg/d max; ↓ w/ severe renal insuff **Caution:** [X, –]; w/ CYP3A4 in-hibitors (Table 11), gemfibrozil, niacin >1g/d, danazol, amiodarone, verapamil **Contra:** PRG/lactation; liver Dz, ↑ LFTs **Disp:** Tabs (ezetimibe/simvastatin) 10/10, 10/20, 10/40, 10/80 mg **SE:** HA, GI upset, myalgia, myopathy (muscle pain, weakness, or tenderness w/ CK 10 × ULN, rhabdomyolysis), hepatitis, Infxn **Interactions:** ↑ Risk of myopathy W/ clarithromycin, erythromycin, itra-conazole, ketoconazole **Labs:** Monitor LFTs **NIPE:** ⊘ PRGor lactation; use adequate contraception; ⊘ EtOH

Famciclovir (Famvir) [Antiviral/Synthetic Nucleoside] Uses: *Acute herpes zoster (shingles) & genital herpes* **Action:** ↓ viral DNA synth **Dose:** *Zoster:* 500 mg PO q8h ×7 d. *Simplex:* 125–250 mg PO bid; ↓ w/ renal im-pair **Caution:** [B, –] **Contra:** Component sensitivity **Disp:** Tabs 125, 250, 500 mg **SE:** Fatigue, dizziness, HA, pruritus, N/D **Interactions:** ↑ Effects W/ cimetidine, probenecid, theophylline; ↑ effects OF digoxin **NIPE:** Not affected by food, ther-apy most effective if taken w/in 72 h of initial sympt

Famotidine (Pepcid, Pepcid AC) [OTC] [Antisecretory/H₂-Receptor Antagonist] Uses: *Short-term Tx of duodenal ulcer & benign*

gastric ulcer; maint for duodenal ulcer, hypersecretory conditions, GERD, & heartburn* **Action:** H₂-Antagonist; ↓ gastric acid **Dose: Adults. Ulcer:** 20 mg IV q12h or 20–40 mg PO qhs × 4–8 wk. **Hypersecretion:** 20–160 mg PO q6h. **GERD:** 20 mg PO bid × 6 wk; maint: 20 mg PO hs. **Heartburn:** 10 mg PO PRN q12h. **Peds.** 0.5–1 mg/kg/d; ↓ in severe renal insuff **Caution:** [B, M] **Contra:** Component sensitivity **Disp:** Tabs 10, 20, 40 mg; chew tabs 10 mg; susp 40 mg/5mL; gelatin cap 10 mg, inj 10 mg/2 mL **SE:** Dizziness, HA, constipation, D, thrombocytopenia **Interactions:** ↑ GI irritation **W/** caffeinated foods, EtOH, nicotine **Labs:** ↑ BUN, Cr, LFTs **NIPE:** ⊘ ASA, EtOH, tobacco, caffeine; take hs; chew tabs contain phenylalanine

Felodipine (Plendil) [Antihypertensive/CCB]

Uses: *HTN & CHF* **Action:** CCB **Dose:** 2.5–10 mg PO daily; swallow whole; ↓ in hepatic impair **Caution:** [C, ?] ↑ Effect with azole antifungals, erythromycin, grapefruit juice **Contra:** Component sensitivity **Disp:** ER tabs 2.5, 5, 10 mg **SE:** Peripheral edema, flushing, tachycardia, HA, gingival hyperplasia **Interactions:** ↑ Effects **W/** azole antifungals, cimetidine, cyclosporine, ranitidine, propranolol, EtOH, grapefruit juice; ↓ effects **OF** digoxin, erythromycin; ↑ effects **W/** barbiturates, carbamazepine, nafcillin, NSIDS, oxcarbazepine, phenytoin; rifampin; ↓ effects **OF** theophylline **NIPE:** ⊘ D/C abruptly; follow BP in elderly & w/ hepatic impair

Fenofibrate (Tricor, Anatra, Lofibra, Lipofen, Triglide) [Antilipemic/Fibric Acid Derivative]

Uses: *Hypertriglyceridemia, hypercholesteremia* **Action:** ↓ Triglyceride synth **Dose:** 48–145 mg daily; ↓ in renal impair, take w/ meals **Caution:** [C, ?] **Contra:** Hepatic/severe renal insuff, primary biliary cirrhosis, unexplained ↑ LFTs, gallbladder Dz **Disp:** Caps 50, 100, 150 mg, *Cap (micronized):* (Lofibra) 67, 134, 200 mg (Antara) 43, 130 mg; Tabs 54, 160 mg **SE:** GI disturbances, cholecystitis, arthralgia, myalgia, dizziness, ↑ LFTs **Interactions:** ↑ Effects **OF** anticoagulants; ↑ risk of rhabdomyolysis & ARF **W/** statins; ↑ risk of renal dysfunction **W/** immunosuppressants, nephrotoxic agents; ↓ effects **W/** bile acid sequestrants **Labs:** ↑ LFTs, BUN, Cr; ↓ Hgb, Hct, WBCs, uric acid **NIPE:** food ↑ drug absorption; EtOH ↑ triglycerides; may take up to 2 mo to modify lipids

Fenoldopam (Corlopam) [Antihypertensive/Vasodilator]

Uses: *Hypertensive emergency* **Action:** Rapid vasodilator **Dose:** Initial 0.03–0.1 μg/kg/min IV inf, titrate q15min by 1.6 μg/kg/min to max 0.05–0.1 μg/kg/min **Caution:** [B, ?] ↓ BP w/ β-blockers **Contra:** Allergy to sulfites **Disp:** Inj 10 mg/mL **SE:** ↓ BP, edema, facial flushing, N/V/D, atrial flutter/fibrillation, ↑ IOP **Interactions:** ↑ Effects **W/** acetaminophen; ↓ hypotension **W/** BBs; ↓ effects **W/** dopamine antagonists, metoclopramide **Labs:** ↓ Serum urea nitrogen, Cr, LFTs, LDH, K⁺ **NIPE:** Avoid concurrent β-blockers; asthmatics have ↑ risk of sulfite sensitivity

Fenoprofen (Nalfon) [Analgesic/NSAID]

WARNING: May ↑ risk of cardiovascular events & GI bleeding **Uses:** *Arthritis & pain* **Action:** NSAID **Dose:** 200–600 mg q4–8h, to 3200 mg/d max; w/ food **Caution:** [B (D 3rd tri), +/–]

CHF, HTN, renal/hepatic impair, h/o PUD **Contra:** NSAID sensitivity **Disp:** Caps 200, 300, 600 mg **SE:** GI disturbance, dizziness, HA, rash, edema, renal impair, hepatitis **Interactions:** ↑ Effects *W/* ASA, anticoagulants; ↑ hyperkalemia *W/* K-sparing diuretics; ↑ effects *OF* anticoagulants, MTX; ↓ effects *W/* phenobarbital; ↓ effects *OF* antihypertensives **Labs:** False ↑ free and total T_3 levels **NIPE:** ⊘ ASA, EtOH, OTC drugs; swallow whole

Fentanyl (Sublimaze) [C-II] [Opioid Analgesic] Uses: *Short-acting analgesic* in anesthesia & PCA **Action:** Narcotic analgesic **Dose:** *Adults.* 25–100 µg/kg/dose IV/IM titrated; *Anesthesia:* 5–15 µg/kg; *Pain:* 200 µg over 15 min, titrate to effect **Peds.** 1–2 µg/kg IV/IM q1–4h titrate; ↓ in renal impair **Caution:** [B, +] **Contra:** Paralytic ileus ↑ ICP, resp depression, severe renal/hepatic impair **Disp:** Inj 0.05 mg/mL **SE:** Sedation, ↓ BP, bradycardia, constipation, N, resp depression, miosis **Interactions:** ↑ Effects *W/* CNS depressants, cimetidine, erythromycin, ketoconazole, phenothiazine, ritonavir, TCAs, EtOH, grapefruit juice; ↑ risks of HTN crisis *W/* MAOIs; ↑ risk of CNS & resp depression *W/* Protease Inhibitors; ↓ effects *W/* buprenorphine, dezocine, nalbuphine, pentazocine **Labs:** ↑ Serum amylase, lipase; ↓ HMG, Hct, plts, WBCs **NIPE:** 0.1 mg fentanyl = 10 mg morphine IM

Fentanyl Iontophoretic Transdermal System (Ionsys) [Opioid Analgesic] WARNING: May only be used for the treatment of hospitalized patients, D/C on discharge; fentanyl may result in potentially life-threatening respiratory depression and death **Uses:** *Short-term in hospital analgesia* **Action:** Opioid narcotic, transdermal administration **Dose:** 40 µg/activation by patient; dose given over 10 min; max over 24 h 3.2 mg (80 doses) **Caution:** [C, –] **Contra:** See Fentanyl **Disp:** Battery-operated self-contained iontophoretic transdermal system, 40 µg/activation, 80 doses **SE:** See Fentanyl, site Rxn **Interactions:** ↑ Effects *W/* CNS depressants, cimetidine, erythromycin, ketoconazole, phenothiazine, ritonavir, TCAs, EtOH, grapefruit juice; ↑ risks of HTN crisis *W/* MAOIs; ↑ risk of CNS & resp depression *W/* protease inhibitors; ↓ effects *W/* buprenorphine, dezocine, nalbuphine, pentazocine **Labs:** ↑ Serum amylase, lipase; ↓ HMG, Hct, plts, WBCs **NIPE:** Choose normal skin site chest or upper outer arm; titrate to comfort, patients must have access to supplemental analgesia; instruct in device use; dispose properly at discharge

Fentanyl, Transdermal (Duragesic) [C-II] [Opioid Analgesic] WARNING: Potential for abuse and fatal overdose **Uses:** *Persistent moderate-severe chronic pain in patients already tolerant to opioids* **Action:** Narcotic **Dose:** Apply patch to upper torso q72h; dose based on narcotic requirements in previous 24 h; start 25 µg/h patch q72h; ↓ in renal impair **Caution:** [B, +] w/ CYP3A4 inhibitors (Table 11) may ↑ fentanyl effect, w/ h/o substance abuse **Contra:** Not opioid tolerant, short-term pain management, postop pain in outpatient surgery, mild pain, PRN use ↑ ICP, resp depression, severe renal/hepatic impair, peds <2 y **Disp:** Patches 12.5, 25, 50, 75, 100 µg/h **SE:** Resp depression (fatal), sedation, ↓ BP, bradycardia, constipation, N, miosis **Interactions:** ↑ Effects W/ CNS depressants, cimetidine, erythromycin, ketoconazole, phenothiazine, ritonavir, TCAs, EtOH, grapefruit juice; ↑ risks OF HTN crisis W/ MAOIs; ↑ risk of CNS & resp depression W/ protease inhibitors; ↓ effects W/ buprenorphine, dezocine, nalbuphine, pentazocine **Labs:** ↑ Serum amylase, lipase; ↓ HMG, Hct, plts, WBCs **NIPE:** 0.1 mg fentanyl = 10 mg morphine IM; do not cut patch; peak level 24–72 h; ↑ risk of ↑ absorption w/ elevated temperature; cleanse skin only w/ water, ∅ soap, lotions, or EtOH because they may ↑ absorption; ∅ use in children <110 lb

Fentanyl, Transmucosal System (Actiq, Fentora) [C-II] [Opioid Analgesic] **WARNING:** Potential for abuse and fatal overdose; use only in CA patients with chronic pain who are opioid tolerant; buccal formulation ↑ bioavailability over trans mucosal; do not substitute on a μg/μg basis; use w/ strong CYP3A4 inhibitors may ↑ fentanyl levels **Uses:** *Breakthrough CA pain* **Action:** Narcotic analgesic, trans mucosal absorption **Dose:** Start 100 μg buccal (Fentora) ×1, may repeat ×1 in 30 min, 4 tabs/dose max; titrate; start 200 μg PO (Actiq) ×1, may repeat ×1 after 30 min; titrate **Caution:** [B, +] **Contra:** ↑ ICP, resp depression, severe renal/hepatic impair, management of postop or awake pain **Disp:** (Actiq) Lozenges on stick 200, 400, 600, 800, 1200, 1600 μg; (Fentora) Buccal Tabs 100, 200, 300, 400, 600, 800 μg **SE:** Sedation, ↓ BP, bradycardia, constipation, N, resp depression, miosis **Interactions:** ↑ Effects W/ CNS depressants, cimetidine, erythromycin, ketoconazole, phenothiazine, ritonavir, TCAs, EtOH, grapefruit juice; ↑ risks OF HTN crisis W/ MAOIs; ↑ risk of CNS & resp depression W/ protease inhibitors; ↓ effects W/ buprenorphine, dezocine, nalbuphine, pentazocine **Labs:** ↑ Serum amylase, lipase; ↓ HMG, Hct, plts, WBCs; 0.1 mg fentanyl = 10 mg IM morphine; for use in patients already tolerant to opioid therapy; ∅ use within 14 d of MAOI

Ferrous Gluconate (Fergon) [Oral Iron Supplement] **Uses:** *Iron deficiency anemia* & Fe supl **Action:** Dietary supl **Dose:** *Adults.* 100–200 mg of elem Fe/d ÷ doses. *Peds.* 4–6 mg/kg/d ÷ doses; on empty stomach (OK w/ meals if GI upset occurs); avoid antacids **Caution:** [A, ?] **Contra:** Hemochromatosis, hemolytic anemia **Disp:** Tabs 246 mg (2.8 mg elem), 240 mg (27 mg elem), 300 (34 mg Fe), 325 mg (36 mg Fe) **SE:** GI upset, constipation, dark stools, discoloration of urine, may stain teeth **Notes:** 12% elem Fe; false + stool guaiac; keep away from children; severe tox in overdose **Interactions:** ↑ Effects W/ chloramphenicol, citrus fruits or juices, vitamin C; ↓ effects W/ antacids, levodopa, black cohosh, chamomile, feverfew, gossypol, hawthorn, nettle, plantain, St. John's wort, whole-grain breads, cheese, eggs, milk, coffee, tea, yogurt; ↓ effects OF fluoroquinolones, tetracycline **Labs:** False + stool guaiac test **NIPE:** ∅ Antacids, tetracyclines, take Liq form in Liq and through a straw to prevent teeth staining; 12% elem Fe; keep away from children; severe tox in overdose

Ferrous Gluconate Complex (Ferrlecit) [Iron Supplement] **Uses:** *Iron deficiency anemia or supl to erythropoietin therapy* **Action:** Fe Supl

Dose: *Test dose:* 2 mL (25 mg Fe) IV over 1 h, if OK, 125 mg (10 mL) IV over 1 h. Usual cumulative dose 1 g Fe over 8 sessions (until favorable Hct) **Caution:** [B, ?] **Contra:** Non-Fe-deficiency anemia; CHF; Fe overload **Disp:** Inj 12.5 mg/mL Fe **SE:** ↓ BP, serious allergic Rxns, GI disturbance, inj site Rxn **Interactions:** ↑ Effects *W/* chloramphenicol, citrus fruits or juices, vitamin C; ↓ effects *W/* antacids, levodopa, black cohosh, chamomile, feverfew, gossypol, hawthorn, nettle, plantain, St. John's wort, whole-grain breads, cheese, eggs, milk, coffee, tea, yogurt; ↓ effects *OF* fluoroquinolones, tetracycline **Labs:** False + stool guaiac test **NIPE:** Dose expressed as mg Fe; may infuse during dialysis

Ferrous Sulfate (OTC) [Iron Supplement]   **Uses:** *Fe deficiency anemia & Fe supl* **Action:** Dietary supl **Dose:** *Adults.* 100–200 mg elem Fe/d in ÷ doses. *Peds.* 1–6 mg/kg/d ÷ daily–tid; on empty stomach (OK w/ meals if GI upset occurs); avoid antacids **Caution:** [A, ?] ↑ Absorption w/ vitamin C; ↓ absorption w/ tetracycline, fluoroquinolones, antacids, H₂-blockers, proton pump inhibitors **Contra:** Hemochromatosis, hemolytic anemia **Disp:** Tabs 187 (60 mg Fe), 200 (65 mg Fe), 324 (65 mg Fe), 325 (65 mg Fe); SR caplets & tabs 160 mg (50 mg Fe), 200 mg (65 mg Fe); gtt 75 mg/0.6 mL (15 mg Fe/0.6 mL); elixir 220 mg/5 mL (44 mg Fe/5 mL); syrup 90 mg/5 mL (18 mg Fe/5 mL) **SE:** GI upset, constipation, dark stools, discolored urine **Interactions:** ↑ Effects *W/* chloramphenicol, citrus fruits or juices, vitamin C; ↓ effects *W/* antacids, levodopa, black cohosh, chamomile, feverfew, gossypol, hawthorn, nettle, plantain, St. John's wort, whole-grain breads, cheese, eggs, milk, coffee, tea, yogurt; ↓ effects *OF* fluoroquinolones, tetracycline **Labs:** False + stool guaiac test **NIPE:** Take w/ meals if GI upset

Fexofenadine (Allegra, Allegra-D) [Antihistamine/H₁-Receptor Antagonist]   **Uses:** *Allergic rhinitis* **Action:** Selective antihistamine, antagonizes H₁-receptors **Dose:** *Adults & Peds >12 y.* 60 mg PO bid or 180 mg/d; ↓ in renal impair **Contra:** Component sensitivity **Disp:** Caps 60 mg; tabs 30, 60, 180 mg; Susp 6 mg/mL; Allegra-D (60 mg fexofenadine/120 mg pseudoephedrine) **SE:** Drowsiness (rare), HA **Interactions:** ↑ Effects *W/* erythromycin, ketoconazole; ↓ absorption & effects *W/* antacids, apples, oranges, grapefruit juice **NIPE:** ⊘ EtOH or CNS depressants

Filgrastim [G-CSF] (Neupogen) [Hematopoietic/Colony-Stimulating Factor]   **Uses:** *↓ Incidence of Infxn in febrile neutropenic pts; Rx chronic neutropenia* **Action:** Recombinant G-CSF **Dose:** *Adults & Peds.* 5 µg/kg/d SQ or IV single daily dose; D/C when ANC >10,000 **Caution:** [C, ?] w/ drugs that potentiate release of neutrophils (eg, lithium) **Contra:** Allergy to *E. coli*-derived proteins or G-CSF **Disp:** Inj 300, 600 µg/mL **SE:** Fever, alopecia, N/V/D, splenomegaly, bone pain, HA, rash **Interactions:** ↑ Interference *W/* cytotoxic drugs; ↑ release of neutrophils *W/* Li **Labs:** Monitor CBC & plts **NIPE:** Monitor for cardiac events; no benefit w/ ANC >10,000/mm³

Finasteride (Proscar, Propecia) [Androgen Hormone Inhibitor/Steroid]   **Uses:** *BPH & androgenetic alopecia* **Action:** ↓ 5α-Reductase **Dose:**

BPH: 5 mg/d PO. *Alopecia:* 1 mg/d PO; food may ↓ absorption **Caution:** [X, –] Hepatic impair **Contra:** Pregnant women should avoid handling pills, teratogen to male fetus **Disp:** Tabs 1 mg (*Propecia*), 5 mg (*Proscar*) **SE:** ↓ Libido, volume ejaculate, ED, gynecomastia **Interactions:** ↑ Effects *W/* saw palmetto; ↓ effects *W/* anticholinergics, adrenergic bronchodilators, theophylline; **Labs:** ↓ PSA by 50%; reestablish PSA baseline 6 mo (double PSA for "true" reading) **NIPE:** 3–6 mo for effect on urinary Sxs; continue to maintain new hair, not for use in women

Flavoxate (Urispas) [Antispasmodic] Uses: *Relief of Sx of dysuria, urgency, nocturia, suprapubic pain, urinary frequency, incontinence* **Action:** Antispasmodic **Dose:** 100–200 mg PO tid–qid **Caution:** [B, ?] **Contra:** GI obst, GI hemorrhage, ileus, achalasia, BPH **Disp:** Tabs 100 mg **SE:** Drowsiness, blurred vision, xerostomia **Interactions:** ↑ Effects *OF* CNS depressants **NIPE:** ↑ Risk of heat stroke w/ exercise and in hot weather

Flecainide (Tambocor) [Antiarrhythmic/Benzamide Anesthetic] **WARNING:** ↑ Mortality in patients with ventricular arrhythmias and recent MI; pulmonary effects reported; pro-ventricular effects seen in atrial arrhythmias **Uses:** Prevent AF/flutter & PSVT, *prevent/suppress life-threatening ventricular arrhythmias* **Action:** Class 1C antiarrhythmic **Dose:** *Adults.* 100 mg PO q12h; ↑ by 50 mg q12h q4d to max 400 mg/d. *Peds.* 3–6 mg/kg/d in 3 ÷ doses; ↓ w/ renal impair. **Caution:** [C, +] Monitor w/ hepatic impair, ↑ conc with amiodarone, digoxin, quinidine, ritonavir/amprenavir, BB, verapamil; may worsen arrhythmias **Contra:** 2nd-/3rd-degree AV block, RBBB w/ bifascicular or trifascicular block, cardiogenic shock, CAD, ritonavir/amprenavir, alkalinizing agents **Disp:** Tabs 50, 100, 150 mg **SE:** Dizziness, visual disturbances, dyspnea, palpitations, edema, chest pain, tachycardia, CHF, HA, fatigue, rash, N **Notes:** *Levels: Trough:* Just before next dose; *Therapeutic:* 0.2–1 μg/mL; *Toxic:* >1 μg/mL; *1/2 life:* 11–14 h **Interactions:** ↑ Effects *W/* alkalinizing drugs, amiodarone, cimetidine, propranolol, quinidine; ↑ effects *OF* digoxin; ↑ risk of arrhythmias *W/* CCBs, antiarrhythmics, disopyramide; ↓ effects *W/* acidifying drugs, tobacco **Labs:** ↑ Alkaline phosphatase **NIPE:** Initiate Rx in hospital; dose q8h if pt is intolerant/uncontrolled at q12h; full effects may take 3–5 d

Floxuridine (FUDR) [Pyrimidine Antimetabolite] **WARNING:** Administration by experienced physician only; patients should be hospitalized for 1st course due to risk for severe Rxn **Uses:** *GI adenoma, liver, renal cancers*; colon & pancreatic CAs **Action:** Converted to 5-FU; inhibits thymidylate synthase; ↓ DNA synth (S-phase specific) **Dose:** 0.1–0.6 mg/kg/d for 1–6 wk (per protocols) usually intra-arterial for liver mets **Caution:** [D, –] Interaction w/ vaccines **Contra:** BM suppression, poor nutritional status, potentially serious Infxn **Disp:** Inj 500 mg **SE:** ↓ BM, anorexia, abd cramps, N/V/D, mucositis, alopecia, skin rash, & hyperpigmentation; rare neurotox (blurred vision, depression, nystagmus, vertigo, & lethargy); intra-arterial catheter-related problems (ischemia, thrombosis, bleeding, & Infxn) **Interactions:** ↑ Effects *W/* metronidazole **Labs:** ↑ LFTs, 5-HIAA urine excretion; ↓ plasma albumin **NIPE:** Need effective birth control; palliative Rx for inoperable/incurable pts; ↑ risk of photosensitivity—use sunscreen

Fluconazole (Diflucan) [Antifungal/Synthetic Azole] Uses: *Candidiasis (esophageal, oropharyngeal, urinary tract, vaginal, prophylaxis); cryptococcal meningitis* **Action:** Antifungal; ↓ cytochrome P-450 sterol demethylation. *Spectrum:* All *Candida* sp except *C. krusei* **Dose:** *Adults.* 100–400 mg/d PO or IV. *Vaginitis:* 150 mg PO daily. *Crypto:* doses up to 800 mg/d reported: 400 mg day 1, then 200 mg × 10–12 wk after CSF (−). *Peds.* 3–6 mg/kg/d PO or IV; 12 mg/kg/d/systemic Infxn; ↓ in renal impair **Caution:** [C, −] **Contra:** None **Disp:** Tabs 50, 100, 150, 200 mg; susp 10, 40 mg/mL; inj 2 mg/mL **SE:** HA, rash, GI upset **Interactions:** ↑ Effects W/ HCTZ, anticoagulants; ↑ effects *OF* amitriptyline, benzodiazepines, carbamazepine, cyclosporine, hypoglycemics, losartan, methadone, phenytoin, quinidine, tacrolimus, TCAs, theophylline, caffeine, zidovudine; ↓ effects W/ cimetidine, rifampin **Labs:** ↑ LFTs; ↓ K⁺ **NIPE:** PO (preferred) = IV levels

Fludarabine Phosphate (Flamp, Fludara) [Antineoplastic] Uses: *Autoimmune hemolytic anemia, CLL, cold agglutinin hemolysis*, low-grade lymphoma, mycosis fungoides **Action:** ↓ Ribonucleotide reductase; blocks DNA polymerase-induced DNA repair **Dose:** 18–30 mg/m²/d for 5 d, as a 30-min inf (per protocols) **Caution:** [D, −] Give cytarabine before fludarabine (↓ its metabolism) **Contra:** w/ pentostatin, severe Infxns, CrCl <30 mL/min, hemolytic anemia **Disp:** Inj 50 mg **SE:** ↓ BM, N/V/D, edema, CHF, fever, chills, fatigue, dyspnea, nonproductive cough, pneumonitis, severe CNS tox rare in leukemia, autoimmune hemolytic anemia **Interactions:** ↑ Effects W/ other myelosuppressive drugs; ↑ risk of pulmonary effects W/ pentostatin **Labs:?** ↑ LFT **NIPE:** May take several weeks for full effect, use barrier contraception

Fludrocortisone Acetate (Florinef) [Steroid/Mineralocorticoid] Uses: *Adrenocortical insuff, Addison Dz, salt-wasting synd* **Action:** Mineralocorticoid **Dose:** *Adults.* 0.1–0.2 mg/d PO. *Peds.* 0.05–0.1 mg/d PO **Caution:** [C, ?] **Contra:** Systemic fungal Infxns; known allergy **Disp:** Tabs 0.1 mg **SE:** HTN, edema, CHF, HA, dizziness, convulsions, acne, rash, bruising, hyperglycemia, HPA suppression, cataracts **Interactions:** ↑ Risk of hypokalemia W/ amphotericin B, thiazide diuretics, loop diuretics; ↑ effects W/ rifampin, barbiturates, hydantoins; ↓ effects *OF* ASA, INH **Labs:** ↓ Serum K⁺ **NIPE:** Eval for fluid retention; For adrenal insuff, use w/ glucocorticoid; dose changes based on plasma renin activity

Flumazenil (Romazicon) [Antidote/Benzodiazepine] Uses: *Reverse sedative effects of benzodiazepines & general anesthesia* **Action:** Benzodiazepine receptor antagonist **Dose:** *Adults.* 0.2 mg IV over 15 s; repeat PRN; to 1 mg max (3 mg max in benzodiazepine OD). *Peds.* 0.01 mg/kg (0.2 mg/dose max) IV over 15 s; repeat 0.005 mg/kg at 1-min intervals to max 1 mg total; ↓ in hepatic impair **Caution:** [C, ?] **Contra:** TCA OD; if pts given benzodiazepines to control life-threatening conditions (ICP/status epilepticus) **Disp:** Inj 0.1 mg/mL **SE:** N/V, palpitations, HA, anxiety, nervousness, hot flashes, tremor, blurred vision, dyspnea, hyperventilation, withdrawal synd **Interactions:** ↑ Risk of Szs and arrhythmias when benzodiazepine action is reduced **NIPE:** Food given during IV administration will reduce drug serum level; does not reverse narcotic Sx or amnesia; use associated w/ Sz

Flunisolide (AeroBid, Aerospan, Nasarel) [Corticosteroid]
Uses: *Asthma in pts requiring chronic steroid therapy; relieve seasonal/perennial allergic rhinitis* **Action:** Topical steroid **Dose:** *Adults.* Met-dose inhal: 2 inhal bid (max 8/d). *Nasal:* 2 sprays/nostril bid (max 8/d). *Peds >6 y.* Met-dose inhal: 2 inhal bid (max 4/d). *Nasal:* 1–2 sprays/nostril bid (max 4/d) **Caution:** [C, ?] w/ adrenal insuff **Contra:** Status asthmaticus, viral, TB, fungal, bacterial Infxn; **Disp:** Aerobid 0.25 mg/Inh; Nasarel 29 µg/spray; Aerospan 80 µg/Inh (CFC-Free) **SE:** Tachycardia, bitter taste, local effects, oral candidiasis **NIPE:** Shake well before use; not for acute asthma

Fluorouracil [5-FU] (Adrucil) [Antineoplastic/Antimetabolite] **WARNING:** Administration by experienced physician only; patients should be hospitalized for 1st course due to risk for severe Rxn **Uses:** *Colorectal, gastric, pancreatic, breast, basal cell*, head, neck, bladder, CAs **Action:** Inhibitor of thymidylate synthetase (interferes with DNA synth, S-phase specific) **Dose:** 370–1000 mg/m²/d for 1–5 d IV push to 24-h cont inf; protracted venous inf of 200–300 mg/m²/d (per protocol); 800 mg/d max **Caution:** [D, ?] ↑ Tox w/ allopurinol; do not give MRX before 5-FU **Contra:** Poor nutritional status, depressed BM Fxn, thrombocytopenia, major surgery w/in past mo, G6PD enzyme deficiency, PRG, serious Infxn, bilirubin >5 mg/dL **Disp:** Inj 50 mg/mL **SE:** Stomatitis, esophagopharyngitis, N/V/D, anorexia, ↓ BM, rash/dry skin/photosens, tingling in hands/feet w/ pain (palmar–plantar erythrodysesthesia), phlebitis/discoloration at inj sites **Interactions:** ↑ Effects **W/** leucovorin Ca **Labs:** ↑ LFTs **NIPE:** ↑ Thiamine intake; ⊘ EtOH, ↑ risk of photosensitivity—use sunscreen, ↑ fluids 2–3 L/d, use barrier contraception

Fluorouracil, Topical [5-FU] (Efudex) [Antineoplastic/Antimetabolite] **Uses:** *Basal cell carcinoma; actinic/solar keratosis* **Action:** Inhibits thymidylate synthetase (↓ DNA synth, S-phase specific) **Dose:** 5% cream bid ×2–6 wk **Caution:** [D, ?] Irritant chemo **Contra:** Component sensitivity **Disp:** Cream 0.5, 1, 5%; soln 1, 2, 5% **SE:** Rash, dry skin, photosens; see Fluorouracil **Additional NIPE:** Healing may not be evident for 1–2 mo; ⊘ use occlusive dressing; wash hands immediately after; do not overuse application

Fluoxetine (Prozac, Sarafem) [Antidepressant/SSRI] **WARNING:** Closely monitor for worsening depression or emergence of suicidality, particularly in ped pts **Uses:** *Depression, OCD, panic disorder, bulimia (Prozac) PMDD (Sarafem)* **Action:** SSRI **Dose:** 20 mg/d PO (max 80 mg/d ÷ dose); weekly 90 mg/wk after 1–2 wk of standard dose. *Bulimia:* 60 mg q AM. *Panic disorder:* 20 mg/d.

OCD: 20–80 mg/d. *PMDD:* 20 mg/d or 20 mg intermittently, start 14 d prior to menses, repeat with each cycle; ↓ in hepatic failure **Caution:** [B, ?/–] Serotonin synd with MAOI, SSRI, serotonin agonists, linezolid; QT prolongation w/ phenothiazine **Contra:** MAOI/thioridazine (wait 5 wk after D/C before MAOI) **Disp:** *Prozac:* Caps 10, 20, 40 mg; scored tabs 10 mg; SR cap 90 mg; soln 20 mg/5 mL. *Sarafem:* Caps 10, 20 mg **SE:** N, nervousness, wt loss, HA, insomnia **Interactions:** ↑ Effects **W/** CNS depressants, MAOIs, EtOH, St. John's wort; ↑ effects **OF** alprazolam, BBs, carbamazepine, clozapine, cardiac glycosides, diazepam, dextromethorphan, loop diuretics, haloperidol, phenytoin, Li, ritonavir, thioridazine, tryptophan, warfarin, sympathomimetic drugs; ↓ effects **W/** cyproheptadine; ↓ effects **OF** buspirone, statins **Labs:** ↑ LFTs, BUN, Cr, urine albumin; **NIPE:** ↑ risk of serotonin synd **W/** St. John's wort; may take >4 wk for full effects;

Fluoxymesterone (Halotestin, Androxy) [Hormone] Uses: Androgen-responsive met *breast CA, hypogonadism* **Action:** ↓ Secretion of LH & FSH (feedback inhibition) **Dose:** *Breast CA:* 10–40 mg/d ÷ × 1–3 mo. *Hypogonadism:* 5–20 mg/d **Caution:** [X, ?/–] ↑ effect w/ anticoagulants, cyclosporine, insulin, lithium, narcotics **Contra:** Serious cardiac, liver, or kidney Dz; PRG **Disp:** Tabs 2, 5, 10 mg **SE:** Priapism, edema, virilization, amenorrhea & menstrual irregularities, hirsutism, alopecia, acne, N, cholestasis; suppression of factors II, V, VII, & X & polycythemia; ↑ libido, HA, anxiety **Interactions:** ↑ Effects **W/** narcotics, EtOH, echinacea; ↑ effects **OF** anticoagulants, cyclosporine, insulin, hypoglycemics, tacrolimus; ↓ effects **W/** anticholinergics, barbiturates **Labs:** ↑ Cr, CrCl; ↓ thyroxine-binding globulin, serum total T_4 **NIPE:** Radiographic studies of skeletal maturation (hand/wrist) q6mo in prepubertal children; monitor fluid retention

Fluphenazine (Prolixin, Permitil) [Antipsychotic/Phenothiazine] Uses: *Schizophrenia* **Action:** Phenothiazine antipsychotic; blocks postsynaptic mesolimbic dopaminergic brain receptors **Dose:** 0.5–10 mg/d in ÷ doses PO q6–8h, average maint 5 mg/d; or 1.25 mg IM, then 2.5–10 mg/d in ÷ doses q6–8h PRN; ↓ in elderly **Caution:** [C, ?/–] **Contra:** Severe CNS depression, coma, subcortical brain damage, blood dyscrasias, hepatic Dz, w/ caffeine, tannic acid, or pectin-containing products **Disp:** Tabs 1, 2.5, 5, 10 mg; elixir 2.5 mg/5 mL; inj 2.5 mg/mL; depot inj 25 mg/mL **SE:** Drowsiness, extrapyramidal effects **Interactions:** ↑ Effects **W/** antimalarials, BBs, CNS depressants, EtOH, kava kava; ↑ effects **OF** anticholinergics, BBs, nitrates; ↓ effects **W/** antacids, caffeine, tobacco; ↓ effects **OF** anticonvulsants, guanethidine, levodopa, sympathomimetics **Labs:** ↑ LFTs, ↓ HMG, Hct, plts, WBC **NIPE:** Photosensitivity—use sunscreen; urine may turn pink or red, ↑ risk of heatstroke in hot weather; less sedative/hypotensive than chlorpromazine

Flurazepam (Dalmane) [C-IV] [Sedative/Hypnotic/Benzodiazepine] Uses: *Insomnia* **Action:** Benzodiazepine **Dose:** *Adults & Peds >15 y.* 15–30 mg PO qhs PRN; ↓ in elderly **Caution:** [X, ?/–] Elderly, low albumin, hepatic impair **Contra:** NAG; PRG **Disp:** Caps 15, 30 mg **SE:** "Hangover" due to accumulation of metabolites, apnea, anaphylaxis, angioedema, amnesia **Interactions:** ↑ CNS depression W/ antidepressants, antihistamines, opioids, EtOH; ↑ effects **OF** digoxin, phenytoin; ↑ effects W/ cimetidine, disulfiram, fluoxetine, isoniazid, ketoconazole, metoprolol, OCPs, propranolol, SSRIs, valproic acid, chamomile, kava, passion flower, valerian; ↓ effects **OF** levodopa; ↓ effects W/ barbiturates, rifampin, theophylline, nicotine **Labs:** ↑ LFTs **NIPE:** ⊘ In PRG or lactation; use adequate contraception; ⊘ EtOH; ⊘ D/C abruptly with long-term use; may cause dependency

Flurbiprofen (Ansaid, Ocufen) [Analgesic/NSAID] WARNING: May ↑ risk of cardiovascular events and GI bleeding Uses: *Arthritis, ocular surgery* Action: NSAID Dose: 50–300 mg/d ÷ bid–qid, max 300 mg/d w/ food, ocular 1 gtt q30min × 4, beginning 2 h preop Caution: [B (D in 3rd tri), +] Contra: PRG (3rd tri); ASA allergy Disp: Tabs 50, 100 mg SE: GI upset, peptic ulcer Dz, ocular irritation Interactions: ↑ Effects W/ amprenavir, anticonvulsants, azole antifungals, BBs, CNS depressants, cimetidine, ciprofloxin, clozapine, digoxin, disulfiram, diltiazem, INH, levodopa, macrolides, OCPs, rifampin, ritonavir, SSRIs, valproic acid, verapamil, EtOH, grapefruit juice, kava kava, valerian; ↓ effects W/ aminophylline, carbamazepine, rifampin, rifabutin, theophylline; ↓ effects OF levodopa Labs: ↑ LFTs NIPE: ⊘ PRG, breast-feeding; take with food to ↓ GI upset

Flutamide (Eulexin) [Antineoplastic/Antiandrogen] WARNING: Liver failure & death reported. Measure LFT before, monthly, & periodically after; D/C immediately if ALT 2 × upper limits of nl or jaundice develops Uses: Advanced *PCa* (w/ LHRH agonists, eg, leuprolide or goserelin); w/ radiation & GnRH for localized CAP Action: Nonsteroidal antiandrogen Dose: 250 mg PO tid (750 mg total) Caution: [D, ?] Contra: Severe hepatic impair Disp: Caps 125 mg SE: Hot flashes, loss of libido, impotence, N/V/D, gynecomastia, hepatic failure Interactions: ↑ Effects W/ anticoagulants Labs: ↑ LFTs (monitor) NIPE: ⊘ EtOH; urine amber/yellow-green in color

Fluticasone, Nasal (Flonase) [Anti-inflammatory/Corticosteroid] Uses: *Seasonal allergic rhinitis* Action: Topical steroid Dose: Adults & Peds >12 y: 2 sprays/nostril/d. Peds 4–11 y: 1–2 sprays/nostril/d Caution: [C, M] Contra: Primary Rx of status asthmaticus Disp: Nasal spray 50 μg/activation SE: HA, dysphonia, oral candidiasis Interactions: ↑ Effects W/ ketoconazole Labs: ↑ glucose NIPE: Clear nares of exudate before use

Fluticasone, Oral (Flovent, Flovent Rotadisk) [Anti-inflammatory/Corticosteroid] Uses: Chronic *asthma* Action: Topical steroid Dose: Adults & Adolescents. 2–4 puffs bid. Peds 4–11 y. 50 μg bid Caution: [C, M] Contra: Primary Rx of status asthmaticus Disp: Rotadisk dry powder: 50, 100, 250 μg/activation SE: HA, dysphonia, oral candidiasis Interactions: ↑ Effects W/ ketoconazole Labs: ↑ Cholesterol NIPE: Risk of thrush, rinse mouth after use; counsel on use of device; ⊘ & report exposure to measles & chickenpox

Fluticasone Propionate & Salmeterol Xinafoate (Advair Diskus, Advair HFA, 45/21, 115/21, 230/21 Inhaled Aerosol) [Anti-inflammatory/Corticosteroid] WARNING: Increased risk of worsening wheezing or asthma-related death with long acting β_2-adrenergic agonists Uses: *Maint therapy for asthma* Action: Corticosteroid w/ LA bronchodilator β_2-agonist Dose: *Adults & Peds >12 y.* 1 inhal bid q12h; titrate to lowest effective dose (4 inhal or 920/84 μg/d max) Caution: [C, M] Contra: Acute asthma attack; conversion from PO steroids; w/ phenothiazines Disp: Diskus = met-dose inhal powder (fluticasone/salmeterol in μg) 100/50, 250/50, 500/50; HFA = aerosol 45/21, 115/21, 230/21 mg SE: Upper resp Infxn, pharyngitis, HA Interactions: ↑ Bronchospasm W/ BBs; ↑ hypokalemia W/ loop and thiazide diuretics; ↑ effects W/ ketoconazole, MAOIs, TCAs Labs: ↑ Cholesterol NIPE: Combo of Flovent & Serevent; do not wash mouthpiece, do not exhale into device; ADVAIR HFA for patients not controlled on other medications (eg, low-medium dose inhal steroids) or whose disease severity warrants 2 maint therapies; ⊘ & report exposure to measles & chickenpox, rinse mouth after use

Fluvastatin (Lescol) [Antilipemic/HMG-CoA Reductase Inhibitor] Uses: *Atherosclerosis, primary hypercholesterolemia, heterozygous familial hypercholesterolemia hypertriglyceridemia* Action: HMG-CoA reductase inhibitor Dose: 20–40 mg bid PO or XL 80 d ↓ w/ hepatic impair Caution: [X, –] Contra: Active liver Dz, ↑ LFTs, PRG, breast-feeding Disp: Caps 20, 40 mg; XL 80 mg SE: HA, dyspepsia, N/D, abd pain Interactions: ↑ Effects W/ azole antifungals, cimetidine, danazol, glyburide, macrolides, phenytoin, ritonavir, EtOH, grapefruit juice; ↑ effects OF diclofenac, glyburide, phenytoin, warfarin; ↓ effects W/ cholestyramine, colestipol, isradipine, rifampin Labs: ↑ LFTs, (monitor) NIPE: Dose no longer limited to hs; ↑ photosensitivity—use sunscreen

Fluvoxamine (Luvox) [Antidepressant/SSRI] WARNING: Closely monitor for worsening depression or emergence of suicidality, particularly in ped pts Uses: *OCD* Action: SSRI Dose: Initial 50-mg single qhs dose, ↑ to 300 mg/d in ÷ doses; ↓ in elderly/hepatic impair, titrate slowly; ÷ doses >100 mg Caution: [C, ?/-] Interactions (MAOIs, phenothiazines, SSRIs, serotonin agonists, others) Contra: MAOI w/in 14 d Disp: Tabs 25, 50, 100 mg SE: HA, N/D, somnolence, insomnia Interactions: ↑ Effects W/ melatonin, MAOIs; ↑ effects OF BBs, benzodiazepines, methadone, carbamazepine, haloperidol, Li, phenytoin, TCAs, theophylline, warfarin, St. John's wort; ↑ risks of serotonin synd W/ buspirone, dexfenfluramine, fenfluramine, tramadol, nefazodone, sibutramine, tryptophan; ↓ effects W/ buspirone, cyproheptadine, tobacco; ↓ effects OF buspirone, HMG-CoA reductase inhibitors NIPE: ⊘ MAOIs for 14 d before start of drug; ⊘ EtOH

Folic Acid [Vitamin Supplement] Uses: *Megaloblastic anemia; folate deficiency* Action: Dietary supl Dose: **Adults.** *Supl:* 0.4 mg/d PO. *PRG:* 0.8 mg/d PO. *Folate deficiency:* 1 mg PO daily–tid. **Peds.** *Supl:* 0.04–0.4 mg/24 h PO, IM, IV, or SQ. *Folate deficiency:* 0.5–1 mg/24 h PO, IM, IV, or SQ Caution: [A, +]

Contra: Pernicious, aplastic, normocytic anemias **Disp:** Tabs 0.4, 0.8, 1 mg; inj 5 mg/mL **SE:** Well tolerated **Interactions:** ↓ Effects W/ anticonvulsants, sulfasalazine, aminosalicylic acid, chloramphenicol, MTX, OCPs, pyrimethamine, triamterene, trimethoprim; ↓ effects OF phenobarbital, phenytoin **NIPE:** OK for all women of child-bearing age; ↓ fetal neural tube defects by 50%; no effect on normocytic anemias

Fondaparinux (Arixtra) [Anticoagulant/Factor X Inhibitor]

WARNING: When epidural/spinal anesthesia or spinal puncture is used, pts anticoagulated or scheduled to be anticoagulated with LMW heparins, heparinoids, or fondaparinux are at risk for epidural or spinal hematoma, which can result in long-term or permanent paralysis **Uses:** *DVT prophylaxis* w/ hip fracture or replacement, knee replacement, abd surgery; w/ DVT or PE in combo w/ warfarin **Action:** Synthetic inhibitor of activated factor X; a LMW heparin **Dose:** 2.5 mg SQ daily, up to 5–9 d; start at least 6 h postop **Caution:** [B, ?] ↑ Bleeding risk w/ anticoagulants, antiplts, drotrecogin alfa, NSAIDs **Contra:** Wt <50 kg, CrCl <30 mL/min, active bleeding, SBE, ↓ plt w/ antiplt Ab **Disp:** Prefilled syringes w/ 27 gauge needle: 2.5 /0.5, 5/0.4, 7.5 /0.6, 10/0.8, mg/mL **SE:** Thrombocytopenia, anemia, fever, N **Interactions:** ↑ Effects W/ anticoagulants, cephalosporins, NSAIDs, penicillins, salicylates **Labs:** ↑ LFTs; ↓ HMG, Hct, plts **NIPE:** D/C if plts <100,000 mm³; only give SQ; may monitor antifactor Xa levels

Formoterol (Foradil Aerolizer) [Bronchodilator/Beta2-Adrenergic Agonist]

WARNING: Increased risk of worsening wheezing or asthma-related death with long-acting β₂-adrenergic agonists **Uses:** Maint Rx of *asthma & prevent bronchospasm* w/ reversible obst airway Dz; exercise-induced bronchospasm **Action:** LA β₂-adrenergic agonist, bronchodilator **Dose:** *Adults & Peds >5y. Asthma:* Inhale one 12-μg cap q12h w/ aerolizer, 24 μg/d max. *Adults & Peds > 12y. Exercise-induced bronchospasm:* 1 inhal 12-μg cap 15 min before exercise **Caution:** [C, ?] **Contra:** Acute asthma, phenothiazines **Disp:** 12-μg powder for inhal (as caps) for use in Aerolizer **SE:** Paradoxical bronchospasm, URI, pharyngitis, back pain; **Interactions:** ↑ Effects W/ adrenergics; ↑ effects OF BBs; ↑ risk of hypokalemia W/ corticosteroids, diuretics, xanthines; ↑ risk of arrhythmias W/ MAOIs, TCAs **Labs:** ↑ Glucose; ↓ K⁺ **NIPE:** Do not swallow caps; only use w/ inhaler; do not start w/ worsening or acutely deteriorating asthma

Fosamprenavir (Lexiva) [Antiretroviral/Protease Inhibitor]

WARNING: Do not use with severe liver dysfunction, reduce dose with mild–moderate liver impair (fosamprenavir 700 mg bid w/o ritonavir) **Uses:** HIV Infxn **Action:** Protease inhibitor **Dose:** 1400 mg bid w/o ritonavir; w/ ritonavir, fosamprenavir 1400 mg + ritonavir 200 mg daily or fosamprenavir 700 mg + ritonavir 100 mg bid; w/ efavirenz & ritonavir: fosamprenavir 1400 mg + ritonavir 300 mg daily **Caution:** [C, ?/–]; **Contra:** w/ ergot alkaloids, midazolam, triazolam, or pimozide; sulfa allergy **Disp:** Tabs 700 mg **SE:** N/V/D, HA, fatigue, rash **Interactions:** ↑ Effects W/ indinavir, nelfinavir; ↑ effects OF antiarrhythmics, amitriptyline, atorvastatin, benzodiazepine, bepridil, CCBs, cyclosporine, ergotamine, ethinyl estradiol, imipramine, itraconazole, ketoconazole, midazolam, norethindrone, rapamycin, rifabutin, sildenafil, tacrolimus, TCA, vardenafil, warfarin; ↓ effects *W/* antacids, carbamazepine, dexamethasone, didanosine, efavirenz, H_2-receptor antagonists, nevirapine, phenobarbital, phenytoin, proton pump inhibitors, rifampin St. John's wort; ↓ effects *OF* methadone **Labs:** ↑ LFTs; triglycerides, lipase; ↓ neutrophils **NIPE:** Take w/o regard to food; use barrier contraception; monitor for opportunistic Infxn; inform about fat redistribution/accumulation

Foscarnet (Foscavir) [Antiviral] Uses: **CMV retinitis*; acyclovir-resistant *herpes Infxns** **Action:** ↓ Viral DNA polymerase & RT **Dose:** *CMV retinitis: Induction:* 60 mg/kg IV q8h or 100 mg/kg q12h × 14–21 d. *Maint:* 90–120 mg/kg/d IV (Monday–Friday). *Acyclovir-resistant HSV: Induction:* 40 mg/kg IV q8–12h × 14–21 d; use central line; ↓ with renal impair **Caution:** [C, –] ↑ Sz potential w/ fluoroquinolones; avoid nephrotoxic Rx (cyclosporine, aminoglycosides, ampho B, protease inhibitors) **Contra:** CrCl <0.4 mL/min/kg **Disp:** Inj 24 mg/mL **SE:** Nephrotox, electrolyte abnormalities **Interactions:** ↑ Risks of Sz *W/* quinolones; ↑ risks of nephrotox *W/* aminoglycosides, amphotericin B, didanosine, pentamidine, vancomycin **Labs:** ↑ LFTs, BUN, SCr; ↓ HMG, Hct, Ca^{2+}, Mg^{2+}, K^+, P; monitor ionized Ca^{2+} **NIPE:** ↑ Fluids; perioral tingling, extremity numbness & paresthesia indicates electrolyte imbalance; Na loading (500 mL 0.9% NaCl) before & after helps minimize nephrotox

Fosfomycin (Monurol) [Antibiotic] Uses: **Uncomplicated UTI** **Action:** ↓ cell wall synth. *Spectrum:* Gram(+) (staphylococci, pneumococci); gram(–) (*E. coli, Enterococcus* sp, *Salmonella* sp, *Shigella* sp, *H. influenzae, Neisseria,* indole-negative *Proteus* sp, *Providencia* sp); *B. fragilis* & anaerobic gram(–) cocci are resistant **Dose:** 3 g PO in 90–120 mL of H_2O single dose; ↓ in renal impair **Caution:** [B, ?] ↓ absorption w/ antacids/Ca salts **Contra:** Component sensitivity **Disp:** Granule packets 3 g **SE:** HA, GI upset **Interactions:** ↓ Effects *W/* antacids, metoclopramide **Labs:** ↑ LFTs; ↓ HMG, Hct **NIPE:** May take w/o regard to food; may take 2–3 d for Sxs to improve

Fosinopril (Monopril) [Antihypertensive/ACEI] Uses: **HTN,* CHF*, DN **Action:** ACE inhibitor **Dose:** 10 mg/d PO initial; max 40 mg/d PO; ↓ in elderly; ↓ in renal impair **Caution:** [D, +] ↑ K^+ w/ K^+ supls, ARBs, K^+-sparing diuretics; ↑ renal AE w/ NSAIDs, diuretics, hypovolemia **Contra:** Hereditary/ idiopathic angioedema or angioedema w/ ACE inhibitor, bilateral RAS **Disp:** Tabs 10, 20, 40 mg **SE:** Cough, dizziness, angioedema, ↑ K^+ **Interactions:** ↑ Effects *W/* antihypertensives, diuretics; ↑ effects *OF* Li; ↑ risk of hyperkalemia *W/*K-sparing diuretics, salt substitutes; ↑ cough *W/* capsaicin; ↓ effects *W/* antacids, ASA, NSAIDs **Labs:** ↑ LFTs, K^+; ↓ HMG, Hct **NIPE:** ⊘ PRG, breast-feeding

Fosphenytoin (Cerebyx) [Anticonvulsant/Hydantoin] Uses: **Status epilepticus** **Action:** ↓ Sz spread in motor cortex **Dose:** As phenytoin equivalents (PE). *Load:* 15–20 mg PE/kg. *Maint:* 4–6 mg PE/kg/d; ↓ dosage, monitor levels in hepatic impair **Caution:** [D, +] May ↑ phenobarbital **Contra:** Sinus bradycardia, SA block, 2nd-/3rd-degree AV block, Adams–Stokes synd, rash during Rx **Disp:** Inj 75 mg/mL **SE:** ↓ BP, dizziness, ataxia, pruritus, nystagmus **Interactions:** ↑ Effects W/ amiodarone, chloramphenicol, cimetidine, diazepam, disulfiram, estrogens, INH, omeprazole, phenothiazine, salicylates, sulfonamides, tolbutamide; ↓ effects W/ TCAs, antituberculosis drugs, carbamazepine, EtOH, nutritional supls, ginkgo biloba; ↓ effects **OF** anticoagulants, corticosteroids, digitoxin, doxycycline, OCPs, folic acid, Ca, vitamin D, rifampin, quinidine, theophylline **Labs:** ↑ Serum glucose, alkaline phosphatase; ↓ serum thyroxine, Ca **NIPE:** Breast-feeding, for short-term use; 15 min to convert fosphenytoin to phenytoin; admin <150 mg PE/min to prevent ↓ BP; administer with BP monitoring

Frovatriptan (Frova) [Migraine Suppressant/5-HT Agonist]
Uses: *Rx acute migraine* Action: Vascular serotonin receptor agonist Dose: 2.5 mg PO repeat in 2 h PRN, 7.5 mg/d max PO dose; max 7.5 mg/d Caution: [C, ?/–] Contra: Angina, ischemic heart Dz, coronary artery vasospasm, hemiplegic or basilar migraine, uncontrolled HTN, ergot use, MAOI w/in 14 d Supplied: Tabs 2.5 mg SE: N, V, dizziness, hot flashes, paresthesias, dyspepsia, dry mouth, hot/cold sensation, chest pain, skeletal pain, flushing, weakness, numbness, coronary vasospasm, HTN Interactions: ↑ Vasoactive reaction W/ ergot drugs; serotonin 5-HT₁ agonists; ↑ effects W/ hormonal contraceptives, propranolol; ↑ risk of serotonin synd W/ SSRIs NIPE: Risk of photosensitivity

Fulvestrant (Faslodex) [Antineoplastic/Antiestrogen]
Uses: *HR(+) met breast CA in postmenopausal women w/ progression following antiestrogen therapy* Action: Estrogen receptor antagonist Dose: 250 mg IM monthly, as single 5-mL inj or two concurrent 2.5-mL IM inj in buttocks Caution: [X, ?/–] ↑ Effects w/ CYP3A4 inhibitors (Table 11); w/ hepatic impair Contra: PRG Disp: Prefilled syringes 50 mg/mL (single 5 mL, dual 2.5 mL) SE: N/V/D, constipation, abd pain, HA, back pain, hot flushes, pharyngitis, inj site Rxns Interactions: ↑ Risk of bleeding W/ anticoagulants NIPE: ⊘ PRG, breast-feeding; use barrier contraception; only use IM

Furosemide (Lasix) [Antihypertensive/Loop Diuretic]
Uses: *CHF, HTN, edema*, ascites Action: Loop diuretic; ↓ Na & Cl reabsorption in ascending loop of Henle & distal tubule Dose: *Adults* 20–80 mg PO or IV bid. *Peds.* 1 mg/kg/dose IV q6–12h; 2 mg/kg/dose PO q12–24h (max 6 mg/kg/dose) Caution: [C, +] ↓ K+, ↑ risk of digoxin tox; ↑ risk of ototox w/ aminoglycosides, cisplatin (esp in renal dysfunction) Contra: Allergy to sulfonylureas; anuria; hepatic coma; electrolyte depletion Disp: Tabs 20, 40, 80 mg; soln 10 mg/mL, 40 mg/5 mL; inj 10 mg/mL SE: ↓ BP, hyperglycemia, ↓ K+ Interactions: ↑ Nephrotoxic effects W/ cephalosporins; ↑ ototox W/ aminoglycosides, cisplatin; ↑ risk of hypokalemia W/ antihypertensives, carbenoxolone, corticosteroids, digitalis glycosides,

terbutaline; ↓ effects W/ barbiturates, cholestyramine, colestipol, NSAIDs, phenytoin, dandelion, ginseng; ↓ effects OF hypoglycemics **Labs:** ↑ BUN, Cr; cholesterol, glucose, uric acid, ↓ serum K⁺, Na⁺, Ca²⁺, Mg²⁺, monitor electrolytes, renal fxn; **NIPE:** Risk of photosensitivity—use sunscreen; high doses IV may cause ototox

Gabapentin (Neurontin) [Anticonvulsant] **Uses:** Adjunct in *partial Szs; postherpetic neuralgia (PHN)*; chronic pain synds **Action:** Anticonvulsant **Dose:** *Anticonvulsant:* 300–1200 mg PO tid (max 3600 mg/d). *PHN:* 300 mg day 1, 300 mg bid day 2, 300 mg tid day 3, titrate (1800–3600 mg/d); ↓ in renal impair **Caution:** [C, ?] **Contra:** Component sensitivity **Disp:** Caps 100, 300, 400, soln 250 mg/5 mL; tab 600, 800 mg **SE:** Somnolence, dizziness, ataxia, fatigue **Notes:** Not necessary to monitor levels **Interactions:** ↑ Effects W/ CNS depressants; ↓ effects W/ antacids, ginkgo biloba **Labs:** ↓ WBCs **NIPE:** Take w/o regard to food

Galantamine (Razadyne) [Cholinesterase Inhibitor] **Uses:** *Alzheimer Dz* **Action:** Acetylcholinesterase inhibitor **Dose:** 4 mg PO bid, ↑ to 8 mg bid after 4 wk; may ↑ to 12 mg bid in 4 wk **Caution:** [B, ?] ↑ Effect w/ succinylcholine, amiodarone, diltiazem, verapamil, NSAIDs, digoxin; ↓ effect w/ anticholinergics, ↑ risk of death vs placebo **Contra:** Severe renal/hepatic impair **Disp:** Tabs 4, 8, 12 mg; soln 4 mg/mL **SE:** GI disturbances, wt loss, sleep disturbances, dizziness, HA **Interactions:** ↑ Effects W/ amitriptyline, cimetidine, erythromycin, fluoxetine, fluvoxamine, ketoconazole, paroxetine, quinidine **Labs:** ↓ HMG, Hct; **NIPE:** ↑ Dosage q4wk, if D/C several days then restart at lowest dose; take w/ food and maintain adequate fluid intake; Caution w/ urinary outflow obst, Parkinson Dz, severe asthma/COPD, severe heart Dz or ↓ BP

Gallium Nitrate (Ganite) [Hormone] **Uses:** *↑ Ca²⁺ of malignancy*; bladder CA **Action:** ↓ bone resorption of Ca²⁺ **Dose:** ↑ *Ca²⁺* 200 mg/m²/d × 5 d. *CA:* 350 mg/m² cont inf × 5 d to 700 mg/m² rapid IV inf q2wk in antineoplastic settings (per protocols) **Caution:** [C, ?] Do not give w/ live or rotavirus vaccine **Contra:** SCr >2.5 mg/dL **Disp:** Inj 25 mg/mL **SE:** Renal insuff, ↓ Ca²⁺, hypophosphatemia, ↓ bicarb, <1% acute optic neuritis **Interactions:** ↑ Risks of nephrotox W/ amphotericin B, aminoglycosides, vancomycin **NIPE:** Monitor SCr, adequate fluids; bladder CA, use in combo w/ vinblastine & ifosfamide

Ganciclovir (Cytovene, Vitrasert) [Antiviral/Synthetic Nucleoside] **Uses:** *Rx & prevent CMV retinitis, prevent CMV Dz* in transplant recipients **Action:** ↓ Viral DNA synth **Dose:** Adults & Peds. *IV:* 5 mg/kg IV q12h for 14–21 d, then maint 5 mg/kg/d IV × 7 d/wk or 6 mg/kg/d IV × 5 d/wk. *Ocular implant:* One implant q5–8mo. *Adults. PO:* Following induction, 1000 mg PO tid. *Prevention:* 1000 mg PO tid; with food; ↓ in renal impair **Caution:** [C, –] ↑ Effect w/ immunosuppressives, imipenem/cilastatin, zidovudine, didanosine, other nephrotoxic Rx **Contra:** ANC <500, plt <25,000, intravitreal implant **Disp:** Caps 250, 500 mg; inj 500 mg, ocular implant 4.5 mg **SE:** Granulocytopenia &

thrombocytopenia, fever, rash, GI upset **Interactions:** ↑ Effects *W*/ cytotoxic drugs, immunosuppressive drugs, probenecid; ↑ risks of nephrotox *W*/ amphotericin B, cyclosporine; ↑ effects *W*/ didanosine **Labs:** ↑ LFTs; ↓ blood glucose **NIPE:** Take w/ food; ⊘ PRG, breast-feeding, EtOH, NSAIDs; photosensitivity—use sunscreen; not a cure for CMV; handle inj w/ cytotox cautions; no systemic benefit w/implant

Gefitinib (Iressa) [Antineoplastic] Uses: *Rx locally advanced or met NSCLC after platinum-based & docetaxel chemo fails* Action: ↓ Phosphorylation of tyrosine kinases; inhibits intracellular domain of EGFR **Dose:** 250 mg/d PO **Caution:** [D, –] **Disp:** Tabs 250 mg **SE:** D, rash, acne, dry skin, N/V, interstitial lung Dz, ↑ transaminases **Interactions:** ↑ Effects *W*/ ketoconazole, itraconazole, and other CYP3A4 inhibitors; ↑ risk of bleeding *W*/ warfarin; ↓ effects *W*/ cimetidine, ranitidine and other H₂ receptor antagonists, phenytoin, rifampin, and other CYP3A4 inducers **Labs:** ↑ LFTs (monitor) **NIPE:** ⊘ PRG or breast-feeding; take w/o regard to food; ↑ risk of corneal erosion/ulcer; only give to patients who have already received drug—no new patients because it has not been shown to increase survival

Gemcitabine (Gemzar) [Antineoplastic/Nucleoside Analog] Uses: *Pancreatic CA, brain mets, NSCLC*, gastric CA **Action:** Antimetabolite; ↓ ribonucleotide reductase; produces false nucleotide base-inhibiting DNA synth **Dose:** 1000 mg/m² over 30 min–1 h IV inf/wk × 3–4 wk or 6–8 wk; modify dose based on hematologic Fxn (per protocol) **Caution:** [D, ?/–] **Contra:** PRG **Disp:** Inj 200 mg, 1 g **SE:** ↓ BM, N/V/D, drug fever, skin rash **Interactions:** ↑ BM depression *W*/ radiation therapy, antineoplastic drugs; ↓ live virus vaccines **Labs:** ↑ LFTs, BUN, SCr (monitor) **NIPE:** ⊘ EtOH, NSAIDs, immunizations, PRG; Reconstituted soln 38 mg/mL

Gemfibrozil (Lopid) [Antilipemic/Fibric Acid Derivative] Uses: *Hypertriglyceridemia, coronary heart Dz* **Action:** Fibric acid **Dose:** 1200 mg/d PO ÷ bid 30 min ac AM & PM **Caution:** [C, ?] ↑ warfarin effect, sulfonylureas; ↑ risk of myopathy w/ HMG-CoA reductase inhibitors; ↓ effects w/ cyclosporine **Contra:** Renal/hepatic impair (SCr >2.0 mg/dL), gallbladder Dz, primary biliary cirrhosis **Disp:** Tabs 600 mg **SE:** Cholelithiasis, GI upset **Interactions:** ↑ Effects *OF* anticoagulants, sulfonylureas; ↑ risk of rhabdomyolysis *W*/ HMG-CoA reductase inhibitors; ↑ effects *W*/ rifampin; ↓ effects *OF* cyclosporine **Labs:** ↑ LFTs, ↓ HMG, Hct, WBCs; ✓ LFTs & serum lipids; **NIPE:** Avoid w/ HMG-CoA reductase inhibitor

Gemifloxacin (Factive) [Antibiotic/Fluoroquinolone] Uses: *CAP, acute exacerbation of chronic bronchitis* **Action:** ↓ DNA gyrase & topoisomerase IV; *Spectrum:* S. pneumoniae (including MDR strains), H. influenzae, H. parainfluenzae, M. catarrhalis, M. pneumoniae, C. pneumoniae, K. pneumoniae **Dose:** 320 mg PO daily; CrCl <40 mL/min: 160 mg PO daily **Caution:** [C, ?/–]; children <18 y; h/o of ↑ QTc interval, electrolyte disorders, w/ Class IA/III antiarrhythmics, erythromycin, TCAs, antipsychotics, ↑ INR and bleed risk w/ warfarin

Contra: Fluoroquinolone allergy **Disp:** Tab 320 mg **SE:** Rash, N/V/D, abd pain, dizziness, xerostomia, arthralgia, allergy/anaphylactic Rxns, peripheral neuropathy, tendon rupture **Interactions:** ↑ Risk of prolonged QT interval W/ amiodarone, antipsychotics, erythromycin, procainamide, quinidine, sotalol, TCAs; ↑ effect *OF* warfarin; ↑ effects W/ probenecid; ↓ effects W/ antacids, didanosine, iron, sucalfrate **Labs:** ↑ LFTs **NIPE:** ↑ Fluid intake; D/C if c/o tenderness/pain in muscles/tendons; ⊘ excessive sunlight exposure—use sunscreen; take 3 h before or 2 h after Al/Mg antacids, Fe, Z, or other metal meds

Gemtuzumab Ozogamicin (Mylotarg) [Chemotherapeutic Agent/Monoclonal Antibody] WARNING: Can cause severe allergic Rxns & other inf-related Rxns including severe pulm events; hepatotox, including severe hepatic venoocclusive Dz (VOD) reported Uses: *Relapsed CD33+ AML in pts >60 who are poor candidates for chemo* Action: MoAb linked to calicheamicin; selective for myeloid cells Dose: Per protocol Caution: [D,?/–] Contra: Component sensitivity Disp: 5 mg/20 mL vial SE: ↓ BM, allergy, anaphylaxis, chills, fever, N/V, HA, pulm events, hepatotox Interactions: ↑ Risk for allergic or hypersensitive reaction and thrombocytopenia W/ abciximab; ↓ effects W/ abciximab Labs: Monitor before & after therapy CBC, ALT, AST, electrolytes NIPE: Monitor for bleeding, myelosuppression, BP; ⊘ ASA, PRG, breast-feeding; single-agent use only, not in combo; premedicate w/ diphenhydramine & acetaminophen

Gentamicin (Garamycin, G-Mycitin, others) [Antibiotic/Aminoglycoside] Uses: *Serious Infxns* due to *Pseudomonas, Proteus, E. coli, Klebsiella, Enterobacter, & Serratia* & initial Rx gram(–) sepsis Action: Bactericidal; ↓ protein synth Spectrum: gram(–) (not *Neisseria, Legionella, Acinetobacter*); synergy w/ PCNs Dose: Adults. 3–7 mg/kg/24h IV ÷ q8–24h. Synergy: 1 mg/kg q8h Peds. Infants <7 d <1200 g: 2.5 mg/kg/dose q18–24h. Infants >1200 g: 2.5 mg/kg/dose q12–18h. Infants >7 d: 2.5 mg/kg/dose IV q8–12h. Children: 2.5 mg/kg/d IV q8h; ↓ w/ renal insuff Caution: [C, +/–] Avoid other nephrotoxics Contra: Aminoglycoside sensitivity Disp: Premixed infus 40, 60, 70, 80, 90, 100, 120 mg; ADD-Vantage inj vials 10 mg/mL; inj 40 mg/mL; IT preservative-free 2 mg/mL SE: Nephro/oto/neurotoxicity Notes: Levels: Peak: 30 min after inf; Trough < 0.5 h before next dose; Therapeutic: Peak 5–8 mcg/mL, Trough < 2 mcg/mL; Toxic Peak > 12 mcg/mL; 1/2 life: 2h; Interactions: ↑ Ototoxicity, neurotoxicity, nephrotoxicity W/ aminoglycosides, amphotericin B, cephalosporins, loop diuretics, penicillins; ↑ effects W/ NSAIDs; ↓ effects W/ carbenicillin; Labs: ↑ LFTs, BUN, crea; ↓ hmg, hct, platelets, WBC; NIPE: Photosensitivity—use sunscreen; Follow CrCl, SCr & serum conc for dose adjustments; daily dosing popular; use IBW to dose (use adjusted if obese > 30% IBW);

Gentamicin & Prednisolone, Ophthalmic (Pred-G Ophthalmic) [Antibiotic/Anti-inflammatory] Uses: *Steroid-responsive ocular & conjunctival Infxns* sensitive to gentamicin Action: Bactericidal; ↓ protein synth w/ anti-inflammatory. Spectrum: Staphylococcus sp, E. coli, H. influenzae, Klebsiella

sp, *Neisseria* sp, *Pseudomonas* sp, *Proteus* sp, & *Serratia* sp **Dose:** *Oint:* 1/2 in. in conjunctival sac daily–tid. *Susp:* 1 gtt bid–qid, up to 1 gtt/h for severe Infxns **Contra:** Aminoglycoside sensitivity **Caution:** [C, ?] **Disp:** *Oint, ophth:* Prednisolone acetate 0.6% & gentamicin sulfate 0.3% (3.5 g). *Susp, ophth:* Prednisolone acetate 1% & gentamicin sulfate 0.3% (2, 5, 10 mL) **SE:** Local irritation; see Gentamicin **Additional NIPE:** Systemic effects **W/** long-term use

Gentamicin, Ophthalmic (Garamycin, Genoptic, Gentacidin, Gentak, others) [Antibiotic] Uses: *Conjunctival Infxns* Action: Bactericidal; ↓ protein synth **Dose:** Apply 1/2 in. bid–tid. *Soln:* 1–2 gtt q2–4h, up to 2 gtt/h for severe Infxn **Caution:** [C, ?] **Contra:** Aminoglycoside sensitivity **Disp:** Soln & oint 0.1% and 0.3% **SE:** Local irritation; see Gentamicin **NIPE:** ⊘ Other eye drops for 10 min after administering this drug; do not touch dropper to eye

Gentamicin, Topical (Garamycin, G-Mycitin) [Antibiotic] Uses: *Skin Infxns* caused by susceptible organisms Action: Bactericidal; ↓ protein synth **Dose:** *Adults & Peds >1 y.* Apply tid–qid **Caution:** [C, ?] **Contra:** Aminoglycoside sensitivity **Disp:** Cream & oint 0.1% **SE:** Irritation; see Gentamicin **NIPE:** ⊘ Apply to large denuded areas

Glimepiride (Amaryl) [Hypoglycemic/Sulfonylurea] Uses: *Type 2 DM* **Action:** Sulfonylurea; ↑ pancreatic insulin release; ↑ peripheral insulin sensitivity; ↓ hepatic glucose output/production **Dose:** 1–4 mg/d, max 8 mg **Caution:** [C, –] **Contra:** DKA **Disp:** Tabs 1, 2, 4 mg **SE:** HA, N, hypoglycemia **Interactions:** ↑ Effects **W/** ACEIs, adrenergic antagonists, BBs, chloramphenicol, MAOIs, NSAIDs, probenecid, salicylates, sulfonamides, warfarin, ginseng, garlic; ↓ effects **W/** corticosteroids, estrogens, INH, OCPs, nicotinic acid, phenytoin, sympathomimetics, thiazide diuretics, thyroid hormones **Labs:** ↑ LFTs, BUN, Cr; ↓ HMG, Hct, plts, WBC, RBC, glucose **NIPE:** Antabuse-like effect **W/** EtOH; Give **W/** 1st meal of day

Glimepiride/pioglitazone (Duetact) [Hypoglycemic/Sulfonylurea/Thiazolidinedione] Uses: *Adjunct to exercise type 2 DM not controlled by single agent* **Action:** Sulfonylurea (↓ glucose) w/ agent that ↑ insulin sens & ↓ gluconeogenesis **Dose:** initial 30 mg/2 mg PO qAM; 45 mg pioglitazone/8 mg glimepiride/d max; w/ food **Caution:** [C, ?/–] w/ liver impair, elderly **Contra:** Component hypersensitivity, DKA **Disp:** Tabs 30/2, 30 mg/4 mg **SE:** Hct, ↑ ALT, ↓ glucose, URI, ↑ wt, edema, HA, N/D, may ↑ CV mortality **Interactions:** ↑ Effects **W/** ACEIs, adrenergic antagonists, BBs, chloramphenicol, MAOIs, NSAIDs, probenecid, salicylates, sulfonamides, warfarin, ginseng, garlic; ↓ effects **W/** corticosteroids, estrogens, INH, OCPs, nicotinic acid, phenytoin, sympathomimetics, thiazide diuretics, thyroid hormones **Labs:** ↑ LFTs, BUN, Cr; ↓ HMG, Hct, plts, WBC, RBC, glucose; monitor CBC, ALT, Cr **NIPE:** Monitor wt

Glipizide (Glucotrol, Glucotrol XL) [Hypoglycemic/Sulfonylurea] Uses: *Type 2 DM* **Action:** Sulfonylurea; ↑ pancreatic insulin release;

↑ peripheral insulin sensitivity; ↓ hepatic glucose output/production; ↓ intestinal glucose absorption **Dose:** 5 mg initial, ↑ by 2.5–5 mg/d, max 40 mg/d; XL max 20 mg; 30 min ac; hold if NPO **Caution:** [C, ?/–] Severe liver Dz **Contra:** DKA, Type 1 DM, sulfonamide sensitivity **Disp:** Tabs 5, 10 mg; XR tabs 2.5, 5, 10 mg **SE:** HA, anorexia, N/V/D, constipation, fullness, rash, urticaria, photosens **Interactions:** ↑ Effects W/ azole antifungals, anabolic steroids, chloramphenicol, cimetidine, clofibrate, MAOIs, NSAIDs, probenecid, salicylates, sulfonamides, TCAs, warfarin, celery, coriander, dandelion root, fenugreek, ginseng, garlic, juniper berries; ↓ effects W/ amphetamines, corticosteroids, epinephrine, estrogens, glucocorticoids, OCPs, phenytoin, rifampin, sympathomimetics, thiazide diuretics, thyroid hormones, tobacco **LABS:** ↑ BUN, Cr, AST, lipids; ↓ glucose, HMG, WBC, plts **NIPE:** Antabuse-like effect w/ EtOH; give 30 min before meal; hold dose if pt NPO; counsel about DM management; wait several days before adjusting dose; monitor glucose

Glucagon [Antihypoglycemic/Hormone] Uses: Severe *hypoglycemic* Rxns in DM with sufficient liver glycogen stores; β-blocker OD **Action:** Accelerates liver gluconeogenesis **Dose:** *Adults.* 0.5–1 mg SQ, IM, or IV; repeat in 20 min PRN. β-*blocker OD:* 3–10 mg IV; repeat in 10 min PRN; may give cont inf 1–5 mg/h *(ECC 2005).* *Peds. Neonates:* 0.3 mg/kg/dose SQ, IM, or IV q4h PRN. *Children:* 0.025–0.1 mg/kg/dose SQ, IM, or IV; repeat in 20 min PRN **Caution:** [B, M] **Contra:** Pheochromocytoma **Disp:** Inj 1 mg **SE:** N/V, ↓ BP **Interactions:** ↑ Effect W/ epinephrine, phenytoin; ↑ effects *OF* anticoagulants **Labs:** ↓ Serum K⁺ **NIPE:** Response w/in 20 min after inj; administration of glucose IV necessary; ineffective in starvation, adrenal insuff, or chronic hypoglycemia

Glyburide (DiaBeta, Micronase, Glynase) [Hypoglycemic/Sulfonylurea] Uses: *Type 2 DM* Action: Sulfonylurea; ↑ pancreatic insulin release; ↑ peripheral insulin sensitivity; ↓ hepatic glucose output/production; ↓ intestinal glucose absorption **Dose:** 1.25–10 mg daily–bid, max 20 mg/d. *Micronized:* 0.75–6 mg daily–bid, max 12 mg/d **Caution:** [C, ?] Renal impair **Contra:** DKA, Type I DM **Disp:** Tabs 1.25, 2.5, 5 mg; micronized tabs 1.5, 3, 6 mg **SE:** HA, hypoglycemia **Interactions:** ↑ Effects W/ anticoagulants, anabolic steroids, BBs, chloramphenicol, cimetidine, clofibrate, MAOIs, NSAIDs, probenecid, salicylates, sulfonamides, TCAs, EtOH, celery, coriander, dandelion root, fenugreek, ginseng, garlic, juniper berries; ↓ effects W/ amphetamines, corticosteroids, baclofen, epinephrine, glucocorticoids, OCPs, phenytoin, rifampin, sympathomimetics, thiazide diuretics, thyroid hormones, tobacco **Labs:** ↑ LFTs, BUN; ↓ glucose, HMG, Hct, plts, WBC **NIPE:** Antabuse-like effect w/ EtOH; not OK for CrCl <50 mL/min; hold dose if NPO

Glyburide/Metformin (Glucovance) [Hypoglycemic/Sulfonylurea & Biguanide] Uses: *Type 2 DM* Action: *Sulfonylurea:* ↑ Pancreatic insulin release. *Metformin:* Peripheral insulin sensitivity; ↓ hepatic glucose output/production; ↓ intestinal glucose absorption **Dose:** 1st line (naive pts), 1.25/250 mg PO daily–bid; 2nd line, 2.5/500 mg or 5/500 mg bid (max 20/2000 mg);

take w/ meals, slowly ↑ dose; hold before & 48 h after ionic contrast media **Caution:** [C, –] **Contra:** SCr >1.4 in females or >1.5 in males; hypoxemic conditions (sepsis, recent MI); alcoholism; metabolic acidosis; liver Dz **Disp:** Tabs 1.25/250 mg, 2.5/500 mg, 5/500 mg **SE:** HA, hypoglycemia, lactic acidosis, anorexia, N/V, rash **Notes:** See Glyburide **Additional Interactions:** ↑ Effects W/ amiloride, ciprofloxacin cimetidine, digoxin, miconazole, morphine, nifedipine, procainamide, quinidine, quinine, ranitidine, triamterene, trimethoprim, vancomycin; ↓ effects W/ CCBs, INH, phenothiazines **Labs:** Monitor folate levels (megaloblastic anemia) **NIPE:** Avoid EtOH; hold dose if NPO

Glycerin Suppository [Laxative] Uses: *Constipation* Action: Hyperosmolar laxative Dose: *Adults.* 1 adult supp PR PRN. *Peds.* 1 infant supp PR daily–bid PRN Caution: [C, ?] Disp: Supp (adult, infant); Liq 4 mL/applicatorful SE: D Interactions: ↑ Effects W/ diuretics Labs: ↑ Serum triglycerides, phosphatidylglycerol in amniotic fluid; ↓ serum Ca NIPE: Insert and retain for 15 min

Gonadorelin (Lutrepulse) [Gonadotropin-Releasing Hormone] Uses: *Primary hypothalamic amenorrhea* Action: Stimulates pituitary release of LH & FSH Dose: 5 µg IV q90min × 21 d using pump kit Caution: [B, M] ↑ Levels w/ androgens, estrogens, progestins, glucocorticoids, spironolactone, levodopa; ↓ levels w/ OCP, digoxin, dopamine antagonists Contra: Condition exacerbated by PRG or reproductive hormones, ovarian cysts, causes of anovulation other than hypothalamic, hormonally dependent tumor Disp: Inj 100 µg SE: Multiple PRG risk Interactions: ↑ Effects W/ androgens, estrogens, glucocorticoids, levodopa, progestins, spironolactone; ↓ effects W/ digoxin, dopamine antagonists, OCPs, phenothiazines Labs: Monitor LH, FSH NIPE: Inj site pain

Goserelin (Zoladex) [Antineoplastic/Gonadotropin-Releasing Hormone] Uses: Advanced *CA Prostate* & radiation for localized high-risk Dz, *endometriosis, breast CA* Action: LHRH agonist, transient ↑ then ↓ in LH, w/ ↓ testosterone Dose: 3.6 mg SQ (implant) q28d or 10.8 mg SQ q3mo; usually lower abd wall Caution: [X, –] Contra: PRG, breast-feeding, 10.8-mg implant not for women Disp: SQ implant 3.6 (1 mo), 10.8 mg (3 mo) SE: Hot flashes, ↓ libido, gynecomastia, & transient exacerbation of CA-related bone pain ("flare Rxn") 7–10 d after 1st dose) Interactions: None noted Labs: ↑ LFTs, cholesterol, triglycerides; initial ↑ then ↓ after 1–2 wk FSH, LH, testosterone NIPE: Inj SQ into fat in abd wall; do not aspirate; females must use contraception

Granisetron (Kytril) [Antiemetic/5-HT₃ Antagonist] Uses: *Prevention of N/V* Action: Serotonin receptor antagonist Dose: *Adults & Peds.* 10 µg/kg/dose IV 30 min prior to chemo *Adults.* Inj 0.1, 1 mg/mL 2 mg PO 1 h prior to chemo, then 12 h later. *Postop N/V:* 1 mg IV before end of OR case Caution: [B, +/–] St. John's wort ↓ levels Contra: Liver Dz, children <2 y Disp: Tabs 1 mg; inj 0.1, 1 mg/mL; soln 2 mg/10 mL SE: HA, constipation Interactions: ↑ Serotonergic effects W/ horehound; ↑ extrapyramidal Rxns W/ drugs causing these effects Labs: ↑ ALT, AST; ↓ HMG, Hct, plts, WBC NIPE: May cause anaphylactic Rxn

Guaifenesin (Robitussin, Others) [Expectorant/Propanediol Derivative] Uses: *Relief of dry, nonproductive cough* Action: Expectorant Dose: *Adults.* 200–400 mg (10–20 mL) PO q4h SR 600–1200 mg PO BID, (max 2.4 g/d). *Peds. <2 y:* 12 mg/kg/d in 6 ÷ doses. *2–5 y:* 50–100 mg (2.5–5 mL) PO q4h (max 600 mg/d). *6–11 y:* 100–200 mg (5–10 mL) PO q4h (max 1.2 g/d) Caution: [C, ?] Disp: Tabs 100, 200; SR tabs 600, 1200 mg; caps 200 mg; SR caps 300 mg; Liq 100 mg/5 mL SE: GI upset Interactions: ↑ Bleeding W/ heparin Labs: ↓ serum uric acid level, HMG, plts, WBCs NIPE: Give w/ large amount of H₂O; some dosage forms contain EtOH

Guaifenesin & Codeine (Robitussin AC, Brontex, Others) [C-V] [Expectorant/Analgesic/Antitussive] Uses: *Relief of dry cough* Action: Antitussive w/ expectorant Dose: *Adults.* 5–10 mL or 1 tab PO q6–8h (max 60 mL/24 h). *Peds. 2–6 y:* 1–1.5 mg/kg codeine/d ÷ dose q4–6h (max 30 mg/24 h). *6–12 y:* 5 mL q4h (max 30 mL/24 h) Caution: [C, +] Disp: Brontex tab 10 mg codeine/300 mg guaifenesin; Liq 2.5 mg codeine/75 mg guaifenesin 5 mL; others 10 mg codeine/100 mg guaifenesin/5 mL SE: Somnolence Interactions: ↑ CNS depression W/ barbiturates, antihistamines, glutethimide, methocarbamol, cimetidine, EtOH; ↓ effects W/ quinidine Labs: ↑ Urine morphine; ↓ serum uric acid level, HMG, plts, WBCs NIPE: Take w/ food

Guaifenesin & Dextromethorphan (Many OTC Brands) [Expectorant/Antitussive] Uses: *Cough* due to upper resp tract irritation Action: Antitussive w/ expectorant Dose: *Adults & Peds >12 y.* 10 mL PO q6–8h (max 40 mL/24 h). *Peds. 2–6 y:* Dextromethorphan 1–2 mg/kg/24 h ÷ 3–4 × d (max 10 mL/d). *6–12 y:* 5 mL q6–8h (max 20 mL/d) Caution: [C, +] Interactions: Administration w/ MAOI Disp: Many OTC formulations SE: Somnolence Interactions: ↑ Effects W/ quinidine, terbinafine; ↑ effects OF isocarboxazid, MAOIs, phenelzine; ↑ risk of serotonin synd W/ sibutramine Labs: ↓ Serum uric acid level, HMG, plts, WBCs NIPE: Give with plenty of fluids

Haemophilus B Conjugate Vaccine (ActHIB, HibTITER, Ped-vaxHIB, Prohibit, Others) [Vaccine/Inactivated] Uses: Routine *immunization* of children against *H. influenzae* type B Dzs Action: Active immunization against *Haemophilus* type B Dose: *Peds.* 0.5 mL (25 mg) IM in deltoid or vastus lateralis Caution: [C, +] Contra: Febrile illness, immunosuppression, allergy to thimerosal Disp: Inj 7.5, 10, 15, 25 µg/0.5 mL SE: Observe for anaphylaxis; edema, ↑ risk of *Haemophilus* type B Infxn the week after vaccination Interactions: ↓ Effects W/ immunosuppressives, steroids NIPE: Booster not required; report SAE to VAERS: 1-800-822-7967

Haloperidol (Haldol) [Antipsychotic/Butyrophenone] Uses: *Psychotic disorders, agitation, Tourette disorders, hyperactivity in children* Action: Antipsychotic, neuroleptic Dose: *Adults. Moderate Sxs:* 0.5–2 mg PO bid–tid. *Severe Sxs/agitation:* 3–5 mg PO bid–tid or 1–5 mg IM q4h PRN (max 100 mg/d).

Peds. 3–6 y: 0.01–0.03 mg/kg/24 h PO daily. *6–12 y:* Initial, 0.5–1.5 mg/24 h PO; ↑ by 0.5 mg/24 h to maint of 2–4 mg/24 h (0.05–0.1 mg/kg/24 h) or 1–3 mg/dose IM q4–8h to 0.1 mg/kg/24 h max; Tourette Dz may require up to 15 mg/24 h PO; ↓ in elderly **Caution:** [C, ?] ↑ Effects w/ SSRIs, CNS depressants, TCA, in- domethacin, metoclopramide; avoid levodopa (↓ antiparkinsonian effects) **Contra:** NAG, severe CNS depression, coma, Parkinson Dz, BM suppression, severe car- diac/hepatic Dz **Disp:** Tabs 0.5, 1, 2, 5, 10, 20 mg; conc Liq 2 mg/mL; inj 5 mg/mL; decanoate inj 50, 100 mg/mL **SE:** Extrapyramidal Sxs (EPS), ↓ BP, anxiety, dysto- nias **Interactions:** ↑ Effects *W/* CNS depressants, quinidine, EtOH; ↑ hypotension *W/* antihypertensives, nitrates; ↑ anticholinergic effects *W/* antihistamines, antide- pressants, atropine, phenothiazines, quinidine, disopyramide; ↓ effects *W/* antacids, carbamazepine, Li, nutmeg, tobacco; ↓ effects *OF* anticoagulants, levodopa, guanethidine **Labs:** ↑ LFTs **NIPE:** ↑ Risk of photosensitivity—use sunscreen; do not give decanoate IV; dilute PO conc Liq w/ H₂O/juice; monitor for EPS

Heparin [Aticoagulant/Antithrombotic] Uses:
Rx & prevention of DVT & PE, unstable angina, AF w/ emboli, & acute arterial occlusion **Action:** Acts w/ antithrombin III to inactivate thrombin & ↓ thromboplastin formation **Dose:** *Adults. Prophylaxis:* 3000–5000 units SQ q8–12h. *Thrombosis Rx:* Load 50–80 units/kg IV, then 10–20 units/kg IV qh (adjust based on PTT); bolus 60 IU/kg (max 4000 IU); then 12 IU/kg/h (max 1000 IU/h for patients >70 kg) round to nearest 50 IU; keep PTT 1.5–2.0 (control 48 h or until angiography *(ECC 2005)* *Peds. Infants:* Load 50 units/kg IV bolus, then 20 units/kg/h IV by cont inf. *Chil- dren:* Load 50 units/kg IV, then 15–25 units/kg cont inf or 100 units/kg/dose q4h IV intermittent bolus (adjust based on PTT) **Caution:** [B, +] ↑ Risk of hemorrhage w/ anticoagulants, ASA, antiplts, cephalosporins w/ MTT side chain **Contra:** Un- controlled bleeding, severe thrombocytopenia, suspected ICH **Disp:** Inj 10, 100, 1000, 2000, 2500, 5000, 7500, 10,000, 20,000, 40,000 units/mL **SE:** Bruising, bleeding, thrombocytopenia **Interactions:** ↑ Effects *W/* anticoagulants, antihista- mines, ASA, clopidogrel, cardiac glycosides, cephalosporins, pyridamole, NSAIDs, quinine, tetracycline, ticlopidine, feverfew, ginkgo biloba, ginger, valer- ian; ↓ effects *W/* nitroglycerine, ginseng, goldenseal, ↓ effects *OF* insulin **Labs:** ↑ LFTs; follow PTT, thrombin time, or activated clotting time; little PT effect; thera- peutic PTT 1.5–2 × control for most conditions; monitor for HIT w/ plt counts

Hepatitis A Vaccine (Havrix, Vaqta) [Vaccine/Inactivated] Uses:
Prevent Hep A in high-risk individuals (eg, travelers, certain professions, or high- risk behaviors) **Action:** Active immunity **Dose:** (Expressed as ELISA units [E.L.U.]) *Havrix: Adults.* 1440 E.L.U. single IM dose. *Peds >2 y.* 720 E.L.U. single IM dose. *Vaqta: Adults.* 50 units single IM dose. *Peds.* 25 units single IM dose **Caution:** [C, +] **Contra:** Component allergy **Disp:** Inj 720 E.L.U./0.5 mL, 1440 E.L.U./1 mL; 50 units/mL **SE:** Fever, fatigue, HA, inj site pain **Interactions:** None noted **NIPE:** ⊘ if pt febrile; booster OK 6–12 mo after primary; report SAE to VAERS: 1-800-822-7969

Hepatitis A (Inactivated) & Hepatitis B (Recombinant) Vaccine (Twinrix) [Vaccine/Inactivated] Uses: *Active immunization against Hep A/B* **Action:** Active immunity **Dose:** 1 mL IM at 0, 1, & 6 mo **Caution:** [C, +] **Contra:** Component sensitivity **Disp:** Single-dose vials, syringes **SE:** Fever, fatigue, pain at site, HA; **Interactions:** ↓ Immune response W/ corticosteroids, immunosuppressants **NIPE:** ↑ Response if inj in deltoid vs gluteus; booster OK 6–12 mo after vaccination; report SAE to VAERS: 1-800-822-7967

Hepatitis B Immune Globulin (HyperHep, H-BIG) [Hepatitis B Prophylaxis/Immunoglobuline] Uses: *Exposure to HBsAg(+) material* (eg, blood, plasma, or serum, accidental needlestick, mucous membrane contact, PO) **Action:** Passive immunization **Dose:** *Adults & Peds.* 0.06 mL/kg IM 5 mL max; w/in 24 h of exposure; w/in 14 d of sexual contact; repeat 1 mo if nonresponder or refused initial after exposure **Caution:** [C, ?] **Contra:** Allergies to γ-globulin or anti-immunoglobulin Ab; allergies to thimerosal; IgA deficiency **Disp:** Inj **SE:** Inj site pain, dizziness **Interactions:** ↓ Immune response if given W/ live virus vaccines; IM in gluteal or deltoid; w/ continued exposure, give Hep B vaccine

Hepatitis B Vaccine (Engerix-B, Recombivax HB) [Vaccine/Inactivated] Uses: *Prevent Hep B* **Action:** Active immunization; recombinant DNA **Dose:** *Adults.* 3 IM doses 1 mL each; 1st 2 doses 1 mo apart; the 3rd 6 mo after the 1st. *Peds.* 0.5 mL IM adult schedule **Caution:** [C, +] w/ immunosuppressives **Contra:** Yeast allergy **Disp:** *Engerix-B:* Inj 20 μg/mL; peds inj 10 μg/0.5 mL. *Recombivax HB:* Inj 10 & 40 μg/mL; peds inj 5 μg/0.5 mL **SE:** Fever, inj site pain **Interactions:** ↓ Immune response W/ corticosteroids, immunosuppressants **NIPE:** ↑ Response inj in deltoid vs gluteus; deltoid IM inj adults/older peds; younger peds, use anterolateral thigh

Hetastarch (Hespan) [Plasma Volume Expander] Uses: *Plasma volume expansion* adjunct in shock & leukapheresis **Action:** Synthetic colloid; acts similar to albumin **Dose:** *Volume expansion:* 500–1000 mL (1500 mL/d max) IV (20 mL/kg/h max rate). *Leukapheresis:* 250–700 mL; ↓ in renal failure **Caution:** [C, +] **Contra:** Severe bleeding disorders, CHF, oliguric/anuric renal failure **Disp:** Inj 6 g/100 mL **SE:** Bleeding (↑ PT, PTT, bleed time) **Labs:** Monitor CBC, PT, PTT **NIPE:** Observe for anaphylactic Rxns; not blood or plasma substitute

Human Papillomavirus (Types 6,11,16,18) Recombinant Vaccine (Gardasil) [Vaccine] Uses: *Prevent cervical CA, precancerous genital lesions, and genital warts due to HPV types 6, 11, 16, 18 in females 9–26 y* **Action:** Recombinant vaccine, passive humoral immunity **Dose:** 0.5 mL IM initial, then 2 and 6 mo **Caution:** [B, ?/–] **Disp:** Single-dose vial and prefilled syringe: 0.5 mL **SE:** Site Rxn (pain, erythema, swelling, pruritus), fever **Interactions:** w/ immunosuppressants, may get decreased response **NIPE:** Give IM in deltoid or upper thigh; 1st approved CA vaccine; report adverse events to VAERS 1-800-822-7967; register PRG patients exposed to drug (800) 986-8999

Hydralazine (Apresoline, Others) [Antihypertensive/Vasodilator] Uses: *Moderate–severe HTN; CHF* (w/ Isordil) Action: Peripheral vasodilator Dose: *Adults.* Initial 10 mg PO qid, ↑ to 25 mg qid 300 mg/d max. Peds. 0.75–3 mg/kg/24 h PO ÷ q6–12h; ↓ in renal impair; ✓ CBC & ANA before Caution: [C, +] ↓ Hepatic Fxn & CAD; ↑ tox w/ MAOI, indomethacin, β-blockers Contra: Dissecting aortic aneurysm, mitral valve/rheumatic heart Dz Disp: Tabs 10, 25, 50, 100 mg; inj 20 mg/mL SE: SLE-like synd w/ chronic high doses; SVT following IM route, peripheral neuropathy Interactions: ↑ Effects W/ antihypertensives, diazoxide, diuretics, MAOIs, nitrates, EtOH; ↓ pressor response W/ epinephrine; ↓ effects W/ NSAIDs; NIPE: Take w/ food; compensatory sinus tachycardia eliminated w/ β-blocker

Hydrochlorothiazide (HydroDIURIL, Esidrix, Others) [Antihypertensive/Thiazide Diuretic] Uses: *Edema, HTN* Action: Thiazide diuretic; ↓ distal tubule Na reabsorption Dose: *Adults.* 25–100 mg/d PO single or ÷ doses. Peds. *<6 mo:* 2–3 mg/kg/d in 2 ÷ doses. *>6 mo:* 2 mg/kg/d in 2 ÷ doses Caution: [D, +] Contra: Anuria, sulfonamide allergy, renal insuff Disp: Tabs 25, 50, mg; caps 12.5 mg; PO soln 50 mg/5 mL SE: ↓ K⁺, hyperglycemia, hyperuricemia, ↓ Na⁺ Interactions: ↑ Hypotension W/ ACEIs, antihypertensives, carbenoxolone, ↑ hypokalemia W/ carbenoxolone, corticosteroids; ↑ hypergylcemia W/ BBs, diazoxide, hypoglycemic drugs; ↑ effects OF Li, MRX; ↓ effects W/ amphetamines, cholestyramine, colestipol, NSAIDs, quinidine, dandelion Labs: ↑ Glucose, cholesterol, Ca, uric acid levels; ↓ K⁺, Na⁺, HMG, Hct, plts, WBCs NIPE: Take w/ food; ↑ risk of photosensitivity—use sunscreen

Hydrochlorothiazide & Amiloride (Moduretic) [Antihypertensive/Thiazide & K⁺ Sparing Diuretic] Uses: *HTN* Action: Combined thiazide & K⁺-sparing diuretic Dose: 1–2 tabs/d PO Caution: [D, ?] Contra: Renal failure, sulfonamide allergy Disp: Tabs (amiloride/HCTZ) 5 mg/50 mg SE: ↑ BP, photosens, ↑ K⁺/↓ K⁺, hyperglycemia, ↑ Na⁺, hyperlipidemia, hyperuricemia Interactions: ↑ Hypotension W/ACEIs, antihypertensives, carbenoxolone, ↑ hypokalemia W/ amphotericin B, carbenoxolone, corticosteroids, licorice; ↑ risk of hyperkalemia W/ ACE-I, K-sparing diuretics, NSAIDs, & K salt substitutes; ↑ hypergylcemia W/ BBs, diazoxide, hypoglycemic drugs; ↑ effects OF amantadine, antihypertensives, digoxin, Li, MTX; ↑ effects W/ CNS depressants; ↓ effects W/ amphetamines, cholestyramine, colestipol, NSAIDs, quinidine, dandelion Labs: ↑ Glucose, cholesterol,Ca, uric acid levels; ↑ Na⁺, HMG, Hct, plts, WBCs; ↑ K⁺/↓ K⁺; interferes W/ glucose tolerance test; monitor electrolytes, LFTs, uric acid NIPE: Take w/ food, I&O, daily wt, ⊘ salt substitutes, bananas, & oranges ↑ risk of photosensitivity—use sunscreen

Hydrochlorothiazide & Spironolactone (Aldactazide) [Antihypertensive/Thiazide & K⁺ Sparing Diuretic] Uses: *Edema, HTN* Action: Thiazide & K⁺-sparing diuretic Dose: 25–200 mg each component/d, ÷ doses Caution: [D, +] Contra: Sulfonamide allergy Disp: Tabs (HCTZ/spironolactone) 25 mg/25 mg, 50 mg/50 mg SE: Photosens, ↓ BP, ↑ or ↓ K⁺, ↑ Na⁺, hyperglycemia, hyperlipidemia, hyperuricemia **Additional Interactions** ↑ Risk of hyperkalemia W/ ACEIs, K-sparing diuretics, K supls, salt substitutes; ↓ effects *OF* digoxin **NIPE:** DC drug 3 d before glucose tolerance test

Hydrochlorothiazide & Triamterene (Dyazide, Maxzide) [Antihypertensive/Thiazide & K⁺ sparing Diuretic] Uses: *Edema & HTN* **Action:** Combo thiazide & K⁺-sparing diuretic **Dose:** *Dyazide:* 1–2 caps PO daily–bid. *Maxzide:* 1 tab/d PO **Caution:** [D, +/–] **Contra:** Sulfonamide allergy **Disp:** (Triamterene/HCTZ) 37.5 mg/25 mg, 75 mg/50 mg **SE:** Photosens, ↓ BP, ↑ or ↓ K⁺, ↑ Na⁺, hyperglycemia, hyperlipidemia, hyperuricemia; See Hydrochlorothiazide. **Additional Interactions:** ↑ Risk of hyperkalemia W/ ACEIs, K-sparing diuretics, K supls, salt substitutes; ↑ effects W/ cimetidine, licorice root, ↓ effects *OF* digoxin **Labs:** ↑ Serum glucose, BUN, Cr, K⁺, Mg²⁺, uric acid, urinary Ca²⁺; interference W/ assay of quinidine & lactic dehydrogenase **NIPE:** Urine may turn blue; HCTZ component in Maxzide more bioavailable than in Dyazide

Hydrocodone & Acetaminophen (Lorcet, Vicodin, Hycet, Others) [C-III] [Narcotic Analgesic/Antitussive] Uses: *Moderate–severe pain*; **Action:** Narcotic analgesic w/ nonnarcotic analgesic **Dose:** *Adult:* 1–2 caps or tabs PO q4–6h PRN; soln 15 mL q4–6h **Peds:** Soln (Hycet) 0.27 mL/kg q4–6h **Caution:** [C, M] **Contra:** CNS depression, severe resp depression **Disp:** Many formulations; specify hydrocodone/APAP dose; caps 5/500; tabs 2.5/500, 5/325, 5/400, 5/500, 7.5/325, 7.5/400, 7.5/500, 7.5/650, 7.5/750, 10/325, 10/400, 10/500, 10/650, 10/660, 10/750; soln *Hycet* (fruit punch) (7.5 mg hydrocodone/325 mg acetaminophen /15 mL **SE:** GI upset, sedation, fatigue; **Interactions:** ↑ Effects W/ antihistamines, cimetidine, CNS depressants, dextroamphetamines, glutethimide, MAOIs, protease inhibitors, TCAs, EtOH, St. John's wort; ↑ effects *OF* warfarin; ↓ effects W/ phenothiazines **Labs:** False ↑ amylase, lipase **NIPE:** Take w/ food, ↑ fluid intake; do not exceed >4 g APAP/d

Hydrocodone & Aspirin (Lortab ASA, others) [C-III] [Narcotic Analgesic] Uses: *Moderate–severe pain* **Action:** Narcotic analgesic with NSAID **Dose:** 1–2 PO q4–6h PRN, w/ food/milk **Caution:** [C, M] ↑ Renal Fxn, gastritis/PUD, **Contra:** Component sensitivity; children w/ chickenpox (Reye synd) **Disp:** 5 mg hydrocodone/500 mg ASA/tab **SE:** GI upset, sedation, fatigue **Notes:** Monitor for GI bleed; see Hydrocodone and Acetaminophen

Hydrocodone & Guaifenesin (Hycotuss Expectorant, others) [C-III] [Narcotic/Expectorant] Uses: *Nonproductive cough* associated with resp Infxn **Action:** Expectorant w/ cough suppressant **Dose:** *Adults & Peds >12 y.* 5 mL q4h pc & hs. *Peds. <2 y:* 0.3 mg/kg/d ÷ qid. *2–12 y:* 2.5 mL q4h pc & hs **Caution:** [C, M] **Contra:** Component sensitivity **Disp:** Hydrocodone 5 mg/guaifenesin 100 mg/5 mL **SE:** GI upset, sedation, fatigue see Hydrocodone and Acetaminophen **Additional Interactions:** ↑ Bleeding W/ heparin

Hydrocodone & Homatropine (Hycodan, Hydromet, others) [C-III] [Narcotic Analgesic/Antitussive] Uses: *Relief of cough*

Action: Combo antitussive **Dose:** (Based on hydrocodone) *Adults.* 5–10 mg q4–6h. *Peds.* 0.6 mg/kg/d ÷ tid–qid **Caution:** [C, M] **Contra:** NAG, ↑ ICP, depressed ventilation **Disp:** Syrup 5 mg hydrocodone/5 mL; tabs 5 mg hydrocodone **SE:** Sedation, fatigue, GI upset; see Hydrocodone and Acetaminophen **Additional Labs:** ↑ ALT, AST **NIPE:** Do not give < q4h

Hydrocodone & Ibuprofen (Vicoprofen) [C-III] [Narcotic Analgesic/NSAID]

Uses: *Moderate–severe pain (<10 d)* **Action:** Narcotic w/ NSAID **Dose:** 1–2 tabs q4–6h PRN **Caution:** [C, M] Renal insuff; ↓ effect w/ ACE inhibitors & diuretics; ↑ effect w/ CNS depressants, EtOH, MAOI, ASA, TCA, anticoagulants **Contra:** Component sensitivity **Disp:** Tabs 7.5 mg hydrocodone/200 mg ibuprofen, **SE:** Sedation, fatigue, GI upset; see Hydrocodone and Acetaminophen **Additional Interactions:** ↓ Effects *OF* ACEIs, diuretics

Hydrocodone & Pseudoephedrine (Detussin, Histussin-D, others) [C-III] [Antitussive/Decongestant]

Uses: *Cough & nasal congestion* **Action:** Narcotic cough suppressant with decongestant **Dose:** 5 mL qid, PRN **Caution:** [C, M] **Contra:** MAOIs **Disp:** Hydrocodone/pseudoephedrine 5 mg /60 mg, 3 mg/15 mg 5 mL; tab 5 mg/60 mg **SE:** ↑ BP, GI upset, sedation, fatigue; see Hydrocodone and Acetaminophen **Additional Interactions:** ↑ Effects *W/* sympathomimetics

Hydrocodone, Chlorpheniramine, Phenylephrine, Acetaminophen, & Caffeine (Hycomine Compound) [C-III] [Narcotic Analgesic/Antitussive/Antihistamine]

Uses: *Cough & Sxs of URI* **Action:** Narcotic cough suppressant w/ decongestant & analgesic **Dose:** 1 tab PO q4h PRN **Caution:** [C, M] **Contra:** NAG **Disp:** Hydrocodone 5 mg/chlorpheniramine 2 mg/phenylephrine 10 mg/APAP 250 mg/caffeine 30 mg/tab **SE:** ↑ BP, GI upset, sedation, fatigue; see Hydrocodone and Acetaminophen

Hydrocortisone, Rectal (Anusol-HC Suppository, Cortifoam Rectal, Proctocort, others) [Corticosteroid]

Uses: *Painful anorectal conditions*, radiation proctitis, ulcerative colitis **Action:** Anti-inflammatory steroid **Dose:** *Adults.* Ulcerative colitis: 10–100 mg PR daily-bid for 2–3 wk **Caution:** [B, ?/–] **Contra:** Component sensitivity **Disp:** *Hydrocortisone acetate:* Rectal aerosol 90 mg/applicator; supp 25 mg. *Hydrocortisone base:* Rectal 0.5%, 1%, 2.5%; rectal susp 100 mg/60 mL **SE:** Minimal systemic effect **NIPE:** Administer after BM, insert supp blunt end 1st, admin enema *W/* pt lying on side and retain for 1 h

Hydrocortisone, Topical & Systemic (Cortef, Solu-Cortef) [Corticosteroid]

See Steroids and Tables 3 & 4 **Caution:** [B, –] **Contra:** Viral, fungal, or tubercular skin lesions; serious Infxns (except septic shock or TB meningitis) **SE:** Systemic: ↑ appetite, insomnia, hyperglycemia, bruising **Notes:** May cause HPA axis suppression **Interactions:** ↑ Effects *W/* cyclosporine, estrogens; ↑ effects *OF* cardiac glycosides, cyclosporine; ↑ risk of GI bleed *W/* NSAIDs; ↓ effects *W/* aminoglutethimide, antacids, barbiturates, cholestyramine, colestipol, ephedrine, phenobarbital, phenytoin, rifampin; ↓ effects *OF* anticoagulants, hypoglycemics, insulin, INH, salicylates **Labs:** ↑ Glucose, cholesterol; ↓ K⁺, Ca⁺ **NIPE:** ⊘ EtOH, live virus vaccines, abrupt D/C of drug; take w/ food; may mask S/Sxs Infxn

Hydromorphone (Dilaudid) [C–II] [Narcotic Analgesic]   **Uses:** *Moderate/severe pain* **Action:** Narcotic analgesic **Dose:** 1–4 mg PO, IM, IV, or PR q4–6h PRN; 3 mg PR q6–8h PRN; ↓ w/ hepatic failure **Caution:** [B (D if prolonged use or high doses near term), ?] ↑ respiratory depression and CNS effects CNS depressants, phenothiazines, TCA **Contra:** Component sensitivity **Disp:** Tabs 2, 4, 8 mg; Liq 5 mg/5 mL or 1 mg/mL; inj 1, 2, 4, 10 mg/mL; supp 3 mg **SE:** Sedation, dizziness, GI upset **Interactions:** ↑ Effects W/ CNS depressants, phenothiazines, TCAs, EtOH, St. John's wort; ↓ effects W/ nalbuphine, pentazocine **Labs:** ↑ Serum amylase, lipase **NIPE:** Take w/ food; ↑ fluids & fiber to prevent constipation; morphine 10 mg IM = hydromorphone 1.5 mg IM

Hydroxocobalamin (Cyanokit) [Antidote]   **Uses:** *Cyanide poisoning* **Action:** Binds cyanide to form nontoxic cyanocobalamin excreted in urine **Dose:** 70 mg/kg IV ×1, repeat X1 PRN max 5-g single dose; inf over 7.5 min **Caution:** [C, ?] **Contra:** None known **Disp:** Kit 2 2.5 g vials w/ inf set **SE:** ↑ BP (can be severe) anaphylaxis, chest tightness, edema, urticaria, rash, chromaturia, N, HA **NIPE:** Inj site Rxns

Hydroxyurea (Hydrea, Droxia) [Antineoplastic/Antimetabolite]   **Uses:** *CML, head & neck, ovarian & colon CA, melanoma, ALL, sickle cell anemia, polycythemia vera, HIV* **Action:** Ribonucleotide reductase **Dose:** (per protocol) 50–75 mg/kg for WBC >100,000 cells/mL; 20–30 mg/kg in refractory CML. *HIV:* 1000–1500 mg/d in single or ÷ doses; ↓ in renal insuff **Caution:** [D, –] ↑ Effects w/ zidovudine, zalcitabine, didanosine, stavudine, fluorouracil **Contra:** Severe anemia, BM suppression, WBC <2500 or plt <100,000, PRG **Disp:** Caps 200, 300, 400, 500 mg, tabs 1000 mg **SE:** ↓ BM (mostly leukopenia), N/V, rashes, facial erythema, radiation recall Rxns, renal impair **Interactions:** ↑ Risk of pancreatitis W/ didanosine, indinavir, stavudine; ↑ BM depression W/ antineoplastic drugs or radiation therapy **Labs:** ↑ Serum uric acid, BUN, Cr **NIPE:** Fluids 10–12 glasses/d, use barrier contraception, ↑ risk *OF* infertility; empty caps into H₂O

Hydroxyzine (Atarax, Vistaril) [Antipsychotic, Sedative/ Hypnotic/Antihistamine]   **Uses:** *Anxiety, sedation, itching* **Action:** Antihistamine, antianxiety **Dose:** *Adults. Anxiety/sedation:* 50–100 mg PO or IM qid or PRN (max 600 mg/d). *Itching:* 25–50 mg PO or IM tid–qid. *Peds.* 0.5–1.0 mg/kg/24 h PO or IM q6h; ↓ w/ hepatic impair **Caution:** [C, +/–] ↑ Effects w/ CNS depressants, anticholinergics, EtOH **Contra:** Component sensitivity **Disp:** Tabs 10, 25, 50 mg; caps 25, 50 mg; syrup 10 mg/5 mL; susp 25 mg/5 mL; inj 25, 50 mg/mL **SE:** Drowsiness, anticholinergic effects **Interactions:** ↑ Effects W/

antihistamines, anticholinergics, CNS depressants, EtOH **Labs:** False—skin allergy tests; false ↑ in urinary 17-hydroxycorticosteroid levels **NIPE:** Used to potentiate narcotic effects; not for IV/SQ (thrombosis & digital gangrene possible)

Hyoscyamine (Anaspaz, Cystospaz, Levsin, others) [Antispasmodic/Anticholinergic] Uses: *Spasm w/ GI & bladder disorders* **Action:** Anticholinergic **Dose:** *Adults.* 0.125–0.25 mg (1–2 tabs) SL/PO tid–qid, ac & hs; 1 SR cap q12h **Caution:** [C, +] ↑ effects w/ amantadine, antihistamines, antimuscarinics, haloperidol, phenothiazines, TCA, MAOI **Contra:** BOO, GI obst, NAG, MyG, paralytic ileus, ulcerative colitis, MI **Disp:** (Cystospaz-M, Levsinex): time release caps 0.375 mg; elixir (EtOH); soln 0.125 mg/5 mL; inj 0.5 mg/mL; tab 0.125 mg; tab (Cystospaz) 0.15 mg; XR tab (Levbid): 0.375 mg; SL (Levsin SL) 0.125 mg **SE:** Dry skin, xerostomia, constipation, anticholinergic SE, heat prostration w/ hot weather **Interactions:** ↑ Effects W/ amantadine, antimuscarinics, haloperidol, phenothiazines, quinidine, TCAs, MAOIs; ↓ effects W/ antacids, antidiarrheals; ↓ effects OF levodopa **NIPE:** ↑ Risk of heat intolerance; photophobia; administer tabs before meals/food

Hyoscyamine, Atropine, Scopolamine, & Phenobarbital (Donnatal, others)[Antispasmodic Anticholinergic Uses: *Irritable bowel, spastic colitis, peptic ulcer, spastic bladder* **Action:** Anticholinergic, antispasmodic **Dose:** 0.125–0.25 mg (1–2 tabs) tid–qid, 1 cap q12h (SR), 5–10 mL elixir tid–qid or q8h **Caution:** [D, M] **Contra:** NAG **Disp:** Many combos/manufacturers; *Cap* (Donnatal, others): Hyosc. 0.1037 mg/atropine 0.0194 mg/scop 0.0065 mg/phenobarbital 16.2 mg. *Tabs* (Donnatal, others): Hyosc. 0.1037 mg/atropine 0.0194 mg/scop 0.0065 mg/phenobarbital 16.2 mg. *LA* (Donnatal): Hyosc. 0.311 mg/atropine 0.0582 mg/scop 0.0195 mg/phenobarbital 48.6 mg. *Elixirs* (Donnatal, others): Hyosc. 0.1037 mg/atropine 0.0194 mg/scop 0.0065 mg/phenobarbital 16.2 mg/5 mL **SE:** Sedation, xerostomia, constipation **Interactions:** ↑ Anticholinergic effects W/ amantadine, antihistamines, disopyramide; merperidine, procainamide, quinidine, TCA; ↑ effects OF/ atenolol; ↓ effects W/ antacids **NIPE:** Take drug without food

Ibandronate (Boniva) [Bone Resorption Inhibitor/Bisphosphonate] Uses: *Rx & prevent osteoporosis in postmenopausal women* **Action:** Bisphosphonate, ↓ osteoclast-mediated bone-resorption **Dose:** 2.5 mg PO daily or 150 mg once/mo on same day (do not lie down for 60 min after); 3 mg IV over 15–30 sec q3mo **Caution:** [C, ?/–] Avoid w/ CrCl <30 mL/min **Contra:** Uncorrected ↓ Ca²⁺; inability to stand/sit upright for 60 min (PO) **Disp:** Tabs 2.5, 150 mg, inj IV 3 mg/3 mL **SE:** Jaw osteonecrosis (avoid extensive dental procedures) N/D, HA, dizziness, asthenia, HTN, Infxn, dysphagia, esophagitis, esophageal/gastric ulcer, musculoskeletal pain **Interactions:** ↑ GI upset W/ ASA, NSAIDs; ↓ absorption W/ antacids, vitamins, supl or other drugs containing Ca⁺, Mg⁺, Fe; EtOH, food, milk **Labs:** ↑ Cholesterol; ↓ alk phos **NIPE:** ↑ Risk OF photophobia, constipation, urinary hesitancy; take 1st thing in AM w/ H$_2$O (6–8 oz) >60 min before 1st food/beverage & any meds w/ multivalent cations; give adequate Ca^{2+} & vitamin D supls

Ibuprofen (Motrin, Rufen, Advil, Others) [OTC] [Anti-inflammatory, Antipyretic, Analgesic/NSAID] **WARNING:** May ↑ risk of cardiovascular events & GI bleeding **Uses:** *Arthritis, pain, fever* **Action:** NSAID **Dose:** *Adults.* 200–800 mg PO bid–qid (max 2.4 g/d); *Peds.* 30–40 mg/kg/d in 3–4 ÷ doses (max 40 mg/kg/d); w/ food **Caution:** May interfere w/ ASA's antiplt effect if given <8 hr before ASA [B, +] **Contra:** 3rd tri PRG, severe hepatic impair, allergy, use w/ other NSAIDs, UGI bleed, ulcers **Disp:** Tabs 100, 200, 400, 600, 800 mg; chew tabs 50, 100 mg; caps 200 mg; susp 100 mg/2.5 mL, 100 mg/5 mL, 40 mg/mL (200 mg OTC form) **SE:** Dizziness, peptic ulcer, plt inhibition, worsening of renal insuff **Interactions:** ↑ Effects *W/* ASA, corticosteroids, probenecid, EtOH; ↑ effects *OF* aminoglycosides, anticoagulants, digoxin, hypoglycemics, Li, MTX; ↑ risks of bleeding *W/* abciximab, cefotetan, valproic acid, thrombolytic drugs, warfarin, ticlopidine, garlic, ginger, ginkgo biloba; ↓ effects *W/* feverfew; ↓ effects *OF* antihypertensives **Labs:** ↑ BUN, Cr, LFTs; ↓ HMG, Hct, BS, plts, WBCs **NIPE:** Take w/ food

Ibutilide (Corvert) [Antiarrhythmic/Ibutilide Derivative] **Uses:** *Rapid conversion of AF/flutter* **Action:** Class III antiarrhythmic **Dose:** *Adults* >60 kg 0.01 mg/kg (max 1 mg) IV inf over 10 min; may repeat × 1; <60 kg use 0.01 mg/kg (*ECC 2005*; D/C cardioversion preferred) **Caution:** [C, –] **Contra:** w/ class I/III antiarrhythmics (Table 10); QTc >440 ms **Disp:** Inj 0.1 mg/mL **SE:** Arrhythmias, HA **Interactions:** ↑ Refractory effects *W/* amiodarone, disopyramide, procainamide, quinidine, sotalol; ↑ QT interval *W/* antihistamines, antidepressants, erythromycin, phenothiazines, TCAs **NIPE:** Give w/ ECG monitoring

Idarubicin (Idamycin) [Antineoplastic/Anthracycline] **WARNING:** Administer only under supervision of a health care provider experienced in leukemia and in an institution with resources to maintain a patient compromised by drug tox **Uses:** *Acute leukemias* (AML, ALL, ANLL), *CML in blast crisis, breast CA* **Action:** DNA intercalating agent; ↓ DNA topoisomerases I & II **Dose:** (per protocol) 10–12 mg/m^2/d for 3–4 d; ↓ in renal/hepatic impairment **Caution:** [D, –] **Contra:** Bilirubin >5 mg/dL, PRG **Disp:** Inj (5, 10, 20 mg vials) **SE:** ↓ BM, cardiotox, N/V, mucositis, alopecia, & IV site Rxns, rarely ↑ renal/hepatic Fxn **Interactions:** ↑ Myelosuppression *W/* antineoplastic drugs and radiation therapy; ↓ effects *OF* live virus vaccines **Labs:** ↑ BUN, Cr, uric acid, LFTs; ↓ HMG, Hct, plts, RBCs, WBCs **NIPE:** ↑ Fluids to 2–3 L/d; Avoid extrav, potent vesicant; IV only

Ifosfamide (Ifex, Holoxan) [Antineoplastic/Alkylating Agent] **Uses:** *Lung, breast, pancreatic & gastric CA, HL/NHL, soft tissue sarcoma* **Action:** Alkylating agent **Dose:** (per protocol) 1.2 g/m^2/d for 5 d bolus or cont inf; 2.4 g/m^2/d for 3 d; w/ Mesna uroprotection; ↓ in renal/hepatic impair **Caution:**

[D, M] ↑ Effect w/ phenobarbital, carbamazepine, phenytoin; St. John's wort may ↓ levels **Contra:** ↓ BM Fxn, PRG **Disp:** Inj 1, 3 g **SE:** Hemorrhagic cystitis, nephrotox, N/V, mild–moderate leukopenia, lethargy & confusion, alopecia, ↑ hepatic enzyme **Interactions:** ↑ Risk of bleeding W/ anticoagulants, ASA, NSAIDs; ↑ effects W/ barbiturates, chloral hydrate, phenytoin; ↑ myelosuppression W/ antineoplastic drugs and radiation therapy; ↓ effects OF live virus vaccines; ↓ effects W/ corticosteroids **Labs:** ↑ LFTs, uric acid; ↓ plts, WBCs **NIPE:** ↑ Fluids to 2–3 L/d; administer w/ mesna to prevent hemorrhagic cystitis

Iloprost (Ventavis) [Prostaglandin Analog] WARNING: Associated with syncope; may require dosage adjustment Uses: NYHA Class III/IV pulm arterial HTN* Action: Prostaglandin analog Dose: Initial 2.5 µg; if tolerated, ↑ to 5 µg inh 6–9 ×/d (at least 2 h apart) while awake Caution: [C, ?/–] Antiplt effects, ↑ bleeding risk w/ anticoagulants; ↓ additive hypotensive effects Contra: SBP <85 mm Hg Disp: Inh soln 10 µg/mL SE: Syncope, ↓ BP, vasodilation, cough, HA, trismus Interactions: ↑ Effects OF anticoagulants, antihypertensives, antiplts Labs: ↑ Alk phos NIPE: Instruct pt of syncope risk; monitor BP; requires Pro-Dose AAD or I-neb ADD system nebulizer; counsel on syncope risk

Imatinib (Gleevec) [Antineoplastic/Tyrosin Kinase Inhibitor]
Uses: *Rx CML Ph+, CML blast crisis, ALL Ph+, myelodysplastic/myeloproliferative Dz, aggressive systemic mastocytosis, chronic eosinophilic leukemia, GIST, dermatofibrosarcoma protuberans* **Action:** ↓ BCL-ABL tyrosine kinase (signal transduction) **Dose: Adult:** *Typical dose:* 400–600 mg PO daily; w/ meal. **Peds:** CML Ph+ newly diagnosed 340 mg/m²/d, 600 mg/d max; recurrent 260 mg/m²/d PO ÷ daily–bid, to 340 mg/m²/d max **Caution:** [D, ?/–] w/ CYP3A4 meds (Table 11), warfarin **Contra:** Component sensitivity **Disp:** Tab 100, 400 mg **SE:** GI upset, fluid retention, muscle cramps, musculoskeletal pain, arthralgia, rash, HA, neutropenia, thrombocytopenia **Additional Interactions:** ↑ Effects OF cyclosporine, CCB, HMG-CoA reductase inhibitiros, triazolobenzodiazepines, erythromycine, itraconazole, ketoconazole; ↑ risk of liver tox W/ acetaminophen; ↓ effects W/ carbamazepine, dexamethasone, phenobarbital, phenytoin, rifampin, St. John's wort **Labs:** ↑ LFTs; ↓ HMG, Hct, neutrophils, plts; follow CBCs & LFTs baseline and monthly **NIPE:** Take w/ food & ↑ fluids to decrease GI irritation, use barrier contraception

Imipenem–Cilastatin (Primaxin) [Antibiotic/Carbapenem]
Uses: *Serious Infxns* due to susceptible bacteria **Action:** Bactericidal; ↓ cell wall synth. *Spectrum:* Gram(+) (S. aureus, group A & B streptococci), gram(–) (not Legionella sp), anaerobes **Dose: Adults.** 250–1000 mg (imipenem) IV q6–8h, 500–750 mg IM 1/2 h. **Peds.** 60–100 mg/kg/24 h IV ÷ q6h; ↓ if CrCl is <70 mL/min **Caution:** [C, +/–] Probenecid ↑ tox **Contra:** Ped pts w/ CNS Infxn (↑ Sz risk) & <30 kg w/ renal impair **Disp:** Inj (imipenem/cilastatin) 250/250 mg, 500/500 mg **SE:** Szs if drug accumulates, GI upset, thrombocytopenia **Interactions:** ↑ Risks of Szs W/ cyclosporine, ganciclovir; ↑ effects W/ probenicid **Labs:** ↑ LFTs, BUN, Cr; ↓ HMG, Hct, plts, WBCs **NIPE:** Eval for super Infxn

Imipramine (Tofranil) [Antidepressant/TCA]   WARNING: Close observation for suicidal thinking or unusual changes in behavior **Uses:** *Depression, enuresis*, panic attack, chronic pain **Action:** TCA; ↑ CNS synaptic serotonin or norepinephrine **Dose:** *Adults. Hospitalized:* Initial 100 mg/24 h PO in ÷ doses; ↑ over several wk 300 mg/d max. *Outpatient:* Maint 50–150 mg PO hs, 300 mg/24 h max. *Peds. Antidepressant:* 1.5–5 mg/kg/24 h ÷ daily–qid. *Enuresis:* >6 y: 10–25 mg PO qhs; ↑ by 10–25 mg at 1–2-wk intervals (max 50 mg for 6–12 y, 75 mg for >12 y); Rx for 2–3 mo, then taper **Caution:** [D, ?/–] **Contra:** Use with MAOIs, NAG, acute recovery from MI, PRG, CHF, angina, CVD, arrhythmias **Disp:** Tabs 10, 25, 50 mg; caps 75, 100, 125, 150 mg **SE:** CV Sxs, dizziness, xerostomia, discolored urine **Interactions:** ↑ Effects W/ amiodarone, anticholinergics, BBs, cimetidine, diltiazem, Li, OCPs, quinidine, phenothiazines, ritonavir, verapamil, EtOH, evening primrose oil; ↑ effects OF CNS depressants, hypoglycemics, warfarin; ↑ risk of serotonin synd W/ MAOIs; ↓ effects W/ tobacco; ↓ effects OF clonidine **Labs:** ↑ Serum glucose, LFTs **NIPE:** D/C 48 h before surgery; D/C MAOIs 2 wk before admin this drug; 4–6 wk for full effects; take w/ food; less sedation than amitriptyline

Imiquimod Cream, 5% (Aldara) [Topical Immunomodulator]
Uses: *Anogenital warts, HPV, condylomata acuminata* **Action:** Unknown; ? cytokine induction **Dose:** Apply 3 ×/wk, leave on 6–10 h & wash off w/ soap & water, continue 16 wk max **Caution:** [B, ?] **Contra:** Component sensitivity **Disp:** Single-dose packets 5% (250 mg cream) **SE:** Local skin Rxns **NIPE:** Condoms & vag diaphragms may be weakened—⊘ contact; wash hands before & after use; not a cure

Immune Globulin, IV (Gamimune N, Sandoglobulin, Gammar IV) [Immune Serum/Immunologic Agent] **Uses:** *IgG Ab deficiency Dz states, (eg, congenital agammaglobulinemia, CVH, & BMT), HIV, Hep A prophylaxis, ITP* **Action:** IgG supl **Dose:** *Adults & Peds. Immunodeficiency:* 100–200 mg/kg/mo IV at 0.01–0.04 mL/kg/min to 400 mg/kg/dose max. *ITP:* 400 mg/kg IV daily × 5 d. *BMT:* 500 mg/kg/wk; ↓ in renal insuff **Caution:** [C, ?] Separate administration of live vaccines by 3 mo **Contra:** IgA deficiency w/ Abs to IgA, severe thrombocytopenia or coagulation disorders **Disp:** Inj **SE:** Associated mostly w/ inf rate; GI upset **Interactions:** ↓ Effects OF live virus vaccines **Labs:** ↑ BUN, Cr **NIPE:** Give live virus vaccines 3 mo after this drug; rapid inf can cause anaphylactoid Rxn

Immune Globulin, Subcutaneous (Vivaglobin) [Immune Serum] **Uses:** *Primary immunodeficiency* **Action:** IgG supl **Dose:** 100–200 mg/kg BW subq weekly abdomen, thighs, upper arms, or lateral hip **Caution:** [C, ?] **Contra:** h/o anaphylaxis to immune globulin; some IGA deficiency **Disp:** 10- & 20-mL vials w/ 160 mg/IgG/mL **SE:** Inj site Rxns, HA, GI complaint, fever, N, D, rash, sore throat **NIPE:** May instruct in home administration; keep refrigerated; discard unused drug

Inamrinone [Amrinone] (Inocor) [Inotropic/Vasodilator]
Uses: *Acute CHF, ischemic cardiomyopathy* **Action:** Inotrope w/ vasodilator **Dose:** IV bolus 0.75 mg/kg over 2–3 min; maint 5–10 µg/kg/min, 10 mg/kg/d max; ↓ if ClCr <10 mL/min **Caution:** [C, ?] **Contra:** Bisulfite allergy **Disp:** Inj 5 mg/mL **SE:** Monitor fluid, electrolyte, & renal changes **Interactions:** Diuretics cause significant hypovolemia; ↑ effects *OF* cardiac glycosides **Labs:** Monitor LFTs **NIPE:** Monitor I&O, daily wt, BP, pulse; incompatible w/ dextrose solns; observe for arrhythmias

Indapamide (Lozol) [Antihypertensive/Thiazide Diuretic]
Uses: *HTN, edema, CHF* **Action:** Thiazide diuretic; ↑ Na, Cl, & H_2O excretion in distal tubule **Dose:** 1.25–5 mg/d PO **Caution:** [D, ?] ↑ Effect w/ loop diuretics, ACE inhibitors, cyclosporine, digoxin, Li **Contra:** Anuria, thiazide/sulfonamide allergy, renal insuff, PRG **Disp:** Tabs 1.25, 2.5 mg **SE:** ↓ BP, dizziness, photosens **Interactions:** ↑ Effects *W/* antihypertensives, diazoxide, nitrates, EtOH; ↑ effects *OF* ACEIs, Li; ↑ risk of hypokalemia *W/* amphotericin B, corticosteroids, mezlocillin, piperacillin, ticarcillin; ↓ effects *W/* cholestyramine, colestipol, NSAIDs **Labs:** ↑ Serum glucose, cholesterol, uric acid, ↓ K$^+$, Na, Cl **NIPE:** ↑ Risk photosensitivity—use sunscreen; take w/ food; no additional effects w/ doses >5 mg; take early to avoid nocturia

Indinavir (Crixivan) [Antiretroviral/Protease Inhibitor]
Uses: *HIV Infxn* **Action:** Protease inhibitor; ↓ maturation of noninfectious virions to mature infectious virus **Dose:** 800 mg PO q8h; in combo w/ other antiretrovirals; on empty stomach; ↓ w/ hepatic impair **Caution:** [C, ?] Numerous drug interactions **Contra:** w/ triazolam, midazolam, pimozide, ergot alkaloids, simvastatin, lovastatin, sildenafil, St. John's wort, amiodarone **Disp:** Caps 100, 200, 333, 400 mg **SE:** Nephrolithiasis, dyslipidemia, lipodystrophy, GI effects **Interactions:** ↑ Effects *W/* azole antifungals, clarithromycin, delavirdine, interleukins, quinidine, zidovudine; ↑ effects *OF* amiodarone, cisapride, clarithromycin, ergot alkaloids, fentanyl, HMG-CoA reductase inhibitors, INH, OCPs, phenytoin, rifabutin, ritonavir, sildenafil, stavudine, zidovudine; ↓ effects *W/* efavirenz, fluconazole, phenytoin, rifampin, St. John's wort, high-fat/protein foods, grapefruit juice; ↓ effects *OF* midazolam, triazolam **Labs:** ↑ Serum glucose, LFTs, ↓ HMG, plts, neutrophils **NIPE:** ↑ Fluids 1–2 L/d, caps moisture sensitive—keep dessicant in container

Indomethacin (Indocin) [Analgesic, Anti-inflammatory, Antipyretic/NSAID] **WARNING:** May ↑ risk of cardiovascular events & GI bleeding **Uses:** *Arthritis; close ductus arteriosus; ankylosing spondylitis* **Action:** ↓ Prostaglandins **Dose:** *Adults.* 25–50 mg PO bid–tid, max 200 mg/d. *Infants:* 0.2–0.25 mg/kg/dose IV; may repeat in 12–24 h up to 3 doses; w/ food **Caution:** [B, +] **Contra:** ASA/NSAID sensitivity, peptic ulcer/active GI bleed, precipitation of asthma/urticaria/rhinitis by NSAIDs/ASA, premature neonates w/ NEC, ↓ renal Fxn, active bleeding, thrombocytopenia, 3rd tri PRG **Disp:** Inj 1 mg/vial; caps 25, 50 mg; SR caps 75 mg; susp 25 mg/5 mL **SE:** GI bleeding or upset, dizziness, edema **Interactions:** ↑ Effects *W/* acetaminophen, anti-inflammatories, gold compounds, diflunisal, probenicid; ↑ effects *OF* aminoglycosides, anticoagulants, digoxin, hypoglycemics, Li, MTX, nifedipine, phenytoin, penicillinamine, verapamil; ↓ effects *W/* ASA; ↓ effects *OF* antihypertensives **Labs:** ↑ LFTs, serum K⁺, BUN, Cr, ↓ HMG, Hct, leukocytes, plts **NIPE:** Take w/ food

Infliximab (Remicade) [Anti-inflammatory/Monoclonal Antibody] **WARNING:** TB, invasive fungal Infxns, & other opportunistic Infxns reported, some fatal; perform TB skin testing prior to use; possible association with rare lymphoma **Uses:** *Moderate–severe Crohn Dz; fistulizing Crohn Dz; ulcerative colitis; RA (w/ MTX) psoriasis, ankylosing spondylitis* **Action:** IgG1K neutralizes TNF-a **Dose:** *Adult: Crohn Dz: Induction:* 5 mg/kg IV inf, w/ doses 2 & 6 wk after. *Maint:* 5 mg/kg IV inf q8wk. *RA:* 3 mg/kg IV inf at 0, 2, 6 wk, then q8wk. *Peds >6 y:* 5 mg/kg IV q8wk **Caution:** [B, ?/–] Active Infxn, hepatic impairment, h/o or risk of TB, Hep B **Contra:** Murine allergy, moderate–severe CHF, live w/ live vaccines (eg, smallpox) **Disp:** 100 mg Inj **SE:** Allergic Rxns; HA, fatigue, GI upset, inf Rxns; hepatotox; reactivation Hep B, pneumonia, BM suppression, systemic vasculitis, pericardial effusion **Interactions:** May ↓ effects *OF* live virus vaccines **Labs:** Monitor LFTs; PPD at baseline; monitor Hep B carrier; **NIPE:** ↑ Susceptibility to Infxn; skin exam for malignancy w/ psoriasis

Influenza Vaccine (Fluarix, Flulaval, Fluzone, Fluvirin) [Antiviral/Vaccine] **Uses:** *Prevent influenza* in adults >50 y, children 6–23 mo, PRG women (2nd/3rd tri during flu season), nursing home residents, chronic Dzs, health care workers, household contacts of high-risk pts, children <9 y receiving vaccine for the 1st time **Action:** Active immunization **Dose:** *Adults and Peds >9 y.* 0.5 mL/dose IM annually *Peds.6 mo >3 y:* 0.25 mL IM annually; 0.25 mL IM × 2 doses >4 wk apart 1st vaccination; give 2 doses in 2nd vaccination year if only 1 dose given in 1st year–; *3–8 y:* 0.5 mL IM annually, start 0.5 mL IM × 2 doses 4> wk >in 1st vaccination year **Caution:** [C, +] **Contra:** Egg, gentamicin, or thimerosal allergy, Infxn at site, acute resp or febrile illness, h/o Guillain–Barré synd, immunocompromised, children 5–17 y on ASA **Disp:** Based on manufacturer, 0.25- & 0.5-mL prefilled syringes **SE:** Inj site soreness, fever, myalgia, malaise, Guillain–Barré synd (controversial) **Interactions:** ↑ Effects *OF* theophylline, warfarin; ↓ effects *W/* corticosteroids, immunosuppressants; ↓ effects *OF* aminopyrine, phenytoin **NIPE:** Fluvarix not labelled for peds; Optimal in US Oct–Nov, protection begins 1–2 wk after, lasts up to 6 mo; each y, vaccines based on predictions of flu active in flu season (Dec–spring in US); whole or split virus for adults; peds <13 y split virus or purified surface antigen to ↓ febrile Rxns; www.cdc.gov/flu for more info

Influenza Virus Vaccine Live, Intranasal (FluMist) [Antiviral/Vaccine] **Uses:** *Prevent influenza* **Action:** Live-attenuated vaccine **Dose:** *Adults 18–49 y:* 1 0.1 mL each nostril × 1 annually *Peds 5–8 yo:* 0.1 mL each nostril × 1 annually; Initial 0.1 mL each nostril × 2 doses >6 wk apart in

1st vaccination year *Peds >9 y*: See adult dose **Caution:** [C,?/–] **Contra:** Egg allergy, PRG, h/o Guillain–Barré synd, known/suspected immune deficiency, asthma or reactive airway Dz, acute febrile illness, 5–17 y on ASA **Disp:** Prefilled, single-use, intranasal sprayer; shipped frozen, store 35–46°F; new refrigerated shipping form for 2008 **SE:** Runny nose, nasal congestion, HA, cough **NIPE:** ⊘ Take **W/** antivirals, ASA, NSAIDs, immunosuppressants, corticosteroids, radiation therapy; do not give w/ other vaccines; avoid contact w/ immunocompromised individuals for 21 d

Insulin, Injectable [Hypoglycemic/Hormone] (See Table 5)

Uses: *Type 1 or type 2 DM refractory to diet or PO hypoglycemic agents; acute life-threatening ↑ K^+* **Action:** Insulin supl **Dose:** Based on serum glucose; usually SQ; can give IV (only regular)/IM; type 1 typical start dose 0.5–1 units/kg/d; type 2 0.3–0.4 units/kg/d; renal failure ↓ insulin needs **Caution:** [B, +] **Contra:** Hypoglycemia **Disp:** See Table 5 **SE:** Highly purified insulins ↑ free insulin; monitor for several wk when changing doses/agents **Interactions:** ↑ Hypoglycemic effects **W/** α-blockers, anabolic steroids, BBs, clofibrate, fenfluramine, guanethidine, MAOIs, NSAIDs, pentamidine, phenylbutazone, salicylates, sulfinpyrazone, tetracyclines, EtOH, celery, coriander, dandelion root, fenugreek, ginseng, garlic, juniper berries; ↓ hypoglycemic effects **W/** corticosteroids, dextrothyroxine, diltiazem, dobutamine, epinephrine, niacin, OCPs, protease inhibitor antiretrovirals, rifampin, thiazide diuretics, thyroid preps, marijuana, tobacco **NIPE:** If mixing insulins, draw up short-acting preps 1st in syringe

Withdrawn from US market

Insulin Human Inhalation Powder (Exubera) [Hypoglycemic/Hormone]

Uses: *Type 1 DM in adults combo w/ LA insulin; Type 2 DM monotherapy or w/ other agents* **Action:** Regulates glucose metabolism **Dose:** Premeal (mg) = BW(kg) × 0.05 mg/kg; round down to nearest whole mg; give w/in 10 min pc; titrate based on glucose; 1 mg blister = 3 IU of SC regular human insulin; 3 mg blister = 9 IU of SC regular human insulin **Caution:** [C, M] **Contra:** Smoker/or D/C smoking <6 mo before start; D/C if smoking resumes; unstable or poorly controlled lung disease **Disp:** Unit dose blisters: 1, 3 mg w/ Exubera Inhaler **SE:** Hypoglycemia, dry mouth, chest pain, otitis media, cough, dyspnea, pharyngitis, rhinitis, sinusitis, epistaxis, ↑ sputum **Interactions:** ↑ Effects **W/** albuterol w/in 30 min; salicylates, MAOIs, sulfonamides, ACEIs, active cigarette smoke; ↓ abortion **W/** bronchodilators and other inhaled agents; ↓ effects **W/** corticosteroids, thiazides, phenothiazines, sympathomimetics, and passive cigarette smoke; **Labs:** ✓ Pulm Fxn before Tx and 6–12 mo **NIPE:** Assess pulmonary Fxn before Tx and 6–12 mo; store blisters at room temperature

Interferon Alfa (Roferon-A, Intron-A) [Antineoplastic/Immunomodulator]

WARNING: Can cause or aggravate fatal or life-threatening neuropsychiatric, autoimmune, ischemic, and infectious disorders. Monitor patients closely **Uses:** *Hairy cell leukemia, Kaposi sarcoma, melanoma,*

CML, chronic Hep B & C, follicular NHL, condylomata acuminata* **Action:** Antiproliferative; modulates host immune response; ↓ viral replication in infected cells **Dose: *Adults.*** *Hairy cell leukemia: Alfa-2a (Roferon-A):* 3 M units/d for 16–24 wk SQ/IM then 3 M units 3 ×/wk × 6–24 mo; *Alfa-2b (Intron A):* 2 M units/m² IM/ SQ 3 ×/wk for 2–6 mo *Chronic Hep B: Alfa-2b (Intron A):* 3 M units/m² SQ 3 ×/wk × 1 wk, then 6 M units/m² 3 ×/wk (max 10 M units 3 ×/wk, total duration 16–24 wks). *Follicular NHL:* (Intron A) 5 M units SQ 3 ×/wk for 18 mo; *Melanoma:* (Intron A) 20 M units m² IV × 5 d/wk × 4 wk, then 10 M units/m² SQ 3 ×/wk × 48 wks; *Kaposi sarcoma:* (Intron A) 30 M units/m IM/SQ 3 ×/wk × 10–12 wk, then 36 M units IM/SQ 3 ×/wk; *Chronic hep C:* (Intron A) 3 m units 3 ×/wk × 16 wk (continue 18–24 mo if response) *Roferon A:* 3 M units 3 ×/wk for 12 mo SQ/IM; *Condyloma:* (Intron A) 1 M units/lesion (max 5 lesions) 3 ×/wk for 3 wk. **Peds.** *CML: Alfa-2a (Roferon-A):* 2.5–5 M units/m² IM daily. **Contra:** Benzyl alcohol sens, decompensated liver Dz, autoimmune Dz, immunosuppressed, neonates, infants **Disp:** Inj forms (see also PEG interferon) **SE:** Flu-like Sxs, fatigue, anorexia, neurotox at high doses; up to 40% neutralizing Ab w/ therapy **Interactions:** ↑ Effects *OF* antineoplastics, CNS depressants, doxorubicin, theophylline; ↓ effects *OF* live virus vaccine **Labs:** ↑ LFTs, BUN, SCr, glucose, phosphorus, ↓ HMG, Hct, Ca **NIPE:** ASA & EtOH use may cause GI bleed, ↑ fluids to 2–3 L/d

Interferon Alfa-2b & Ribavirin Combo (Rebetron) [Antineoplastic/Immunomodulator]

WARNING: Can cause or aggravate fatal or life-threatening neuropsychiatric, autoimmune, ischemic, and infectious disorders. Monitor patients closely. Contraindicated in PRG females & their male partners. **Uses:** *Chronic Hep C in pts w/ compensated liver Dz who relapse after α-interferon therapy* **Action:** Combo antiviral agents (see individual agents) **Dose:** 3 M units Intron A SQ 3 ×/wk w/ 1000–1200 mg of Rebetron PO ÷ bid dose for 24 wk. *Pts <75 kg:* 1000 mg of Rebetron/d **Caution:** [X, ?] **Contra:** PRG, males w/ PRG female partner, autoimmune hepatitis, CrCl <50 mL/min **Disp:** *Pts <75 kg:* Combo packs: 6 vials Intron A (3 M units/0.5 mL) w/ 6 syringes & EtOH swabs, 70 Rebetol caps; one 18-M unit multidose vial of Intron A inj (22.8 M units/3.8 mL; 3 M units/0.5 mL) & 6 syringes & swabs, 70 Rebetol caps; one 18 M units Intron A inj multidose pen (22.5 M units/1.5 mL; 3 M units/0.2 mL, 4 M needles & swabs, 70 Rebetol caps. *Pts >75 kg:* Identical except 84 Rebetol caps/pack **SE:** See Warning, flu-like Sxs, HA, anemia **NIPE:** Monthly PRG test; instruct in self-administration of SQ Intron A

Interferon Alfacon-1 (Infergen) [Immunomodulator]

WARNING: Can cause or aggravate fatal or life-threatening neuropsychiatric, autoimmune, ischemic, and infectious disorders. Monitor patients closely **Uses:** *Chronic Hep C* **Action:** Biologic response modifier **Dose:** 9 μg SQ 3 ×/wk × 24 wk **Caution:** [C, M] **Contra:** *E. coli* product allergy **Disp:** Inj 9, 15 μg **SE:** Flulike Sxs, depression, blood dyscrasias, colitis, pancreatitis, hepatic decompensation, ↑ SCr, eye disorders, ↓ thyroid **Interactions:** ↑ Effects *OF* theophylline

Labs: ↑ Triglycerides, TSH; ↓ HMG, Hct; monitor CBC, plt, SCr, TFT **NIPE:** Refrigerate; ⊘ shake; use barrier contraception; allow >48 h between inj

Interferon Beta-1a (Rebif) [Immunomodulator] WARNING: Can cause or aggravate fatal or life-threatening neuropsychiatric, autoimmune, ischemic, and infectious disorders. Monitor patients closely **Uses:** *MS, relapsing* **Action:** Biologic response modifier **Dose:** 44 μg SC 3 ×/wk; start 8.8 μg SC 3 ×/wk × 2 wk, then 22 μg SC 3 ×/wk × 2 wk **Caution:** [C, ?] w/ hepatic impair, depression, Sz disorder, thyroid Dz **Contra:** Human albumin allergy **Disp:** 0.5 mL prefilled syringes w/ 29 gauge needle titrate pak 8.8 and 22 μg; 22 or 44 μg **SE:** Inj site Rxn, HA, flu-like Sx, malaise, fatigue, rigors, myalgia, depression w/ suicidal ideation, hepatotox, ↓ BM **Interactions:** Caution with other hepatotoxic drugs **Labs:** Monitor CBC 1, 3, 6 mo; TFTs q6mo w/ h/o thyroid Dz **NIPE:** Dose >48 h apart; D/C if jaundice occurs; may have abortifacient effects

Interferon Beta-1b (Betaseron) [Immunomodulator] **Uses:** *MS, relapsing/remitting/secondary progressive* **Action:** Biologic response modifier **Dose:** 0.25 mg SQ qod **Caution:** [C, ?] **Contra:** Human albumin allergy **Disp:** Powder for inj 0.3 mg (32 M units inf) **SE:** Flu-like Sxs, depression, blood dyscrasias, inj site necrosis, anaphylaxis **Interactions:** ↑ Effects *OF* theophylline, zidovudine **Labs:** ↑ LFTs, BUN, urine protein; monitor LFTs, CBC 1, 3, 6 mo, TFT q6mo **NIPE:** ↑ Risk *OF* photosensitivity—use sunscreen, abortion; ↑ fluid intake, use barrier contraception; pt self inj, rotate sites

Interferon Gamma-1b (Actimmune) [Immunomodulator] **Uses:** *↓ Incidence of serious Infxns in chronic granulomatous Dz (CGD), osteoporosis* **Action:** Biologic response modifier **Dose:** *Adults. CGD:* 50 μg/m² SQ (1.5 M units/m²) BSA >0.5 m²; if BSA <0.5 m², give 1.5 μg/kg/dose; given 3 × wk. **Caution:** [C, ?] **Contra:** Allergy to *E. coli*-derived products **Disp:** Inj 100 μg (2 M units) **SE:** Flulike Sxs, depression, blood dyscrasias, dizziness, altered mental status, gait disturbance, hepatic tox **Interactions:** ↑ Myelosuppression *W/* myelosuppresive drugs **Labs:** ↑ LFTs; ↓ neutrophils, plts **NIPE:** small freq meals may decrease GI upset; rotate inj sites

Ipecac Syrup [OTC] [Antidote] **Uses:** *Drug OD, certain cases of poisoning* **NOTE:** Usage is falling out of favor & is no longer recommended by some groups **Action:** Irritation of the GI mucosa; stimulation of the chemoreceptor trigger zone **Dose:** *Adults.* 15–30 mL PO, followed by 200–300 mL of H₂O; if no emesis in 20 min, repeat once. *Peds. 6–12 y:* 5–10 mL PO, followed by 10–20 mL/kg of H₂O; if no emesis in 20 min, repeat once. *1–12 y:* 15 mL PO followed by 10–20 mL/kg of H₂O; if no emesis in 20 min, repeat once **Caution:** [C, ?] **Contra:** Ingestion of petroleum distillates, strong acid, base, or other caustic agents; comatose/unconscious **Disp:** Syrup 15, 30 mL **SE:** Lethargy, D, cardiotox, protracted V **Interactions:** ↑ Effects *OF* myelosuppressives, theophylline, zidovudine **NIPE:** ↑ Fluids to 2–3 L/d, ⊘ EtOH, CNS depressants; activated charcoal considered more effective; caution in CNS depressant OD (www.clintox.org/PosStatements/Ipecac.html)

Ipratropium (Atrovent HFA, Atrovent Nasal) [Bronchodilator/ Anticholinergic] Uses: *Bronchospasm w/ COPD, rhinitis, rhinorrhea* **Action:** Synthetic anticholinergic similar to atropine; antagonizes acetylcholine receptors, inhibits mucous gland secretions **Dose:** *Adults & Peds >12 y.* 2–4 puffs qid, max 12 inh/d Nasal: 2 sprays/nostril bid–tid; *Nebulization:* 500 µg 3–4 times/d **Caution:** [B, +/–] w/ inhal insulin **Contra:** Allergy to soya lecithin/related foods **Disp:** HFA Met-dose inhal 18 µg/dose; inhal soln 0.02%; nasal spray 0.03, 0.06% **SE:** Nervousness, dizziness, HA, cough, bitter taste, nasal dryness, URI, epistaxis **Interactions:** ↑ Effects W/ albuterol; ↑ effects OF anticholinergics, antimuscarinics; ↓ effects W/ jaborandi tree, pill-bearing spurge **NIPE:** Adequate fluids; separate inhalation of other drugs by 5 min; not for acute bronchospasm

Irbesartan (Avapro) [Antihypertensive/ARB] Uses: *HTN, DN*, CHF **Action:** Angiotensin II receptor antagonist **Dose:** 150 mg/d PO, may ↑ to 300 mg/d **Caution:** [C (1st tri; D 2nd/3rd tri), ?/–] **Disp:** Tabs 75, 150, 300 mg **SE:** Fatigue, ↓ BP ↑ K **Interactions:** ↑ Risk of hyperkalemia W/ K-sparing diuretics, trimethoprim, K supls; ↑ effects OF Li **Labs:** ↑ K+ (monitor) **NIPE:** ⊘ PRG, breast-feeding

Irinotecan (Camptosar) [Antineoplastic] WARNING: D and myelosuppression Uses: *Colorectal* & lung CA **Action:** Topoisomerase I inhibitor; ↓ DNA synth **Dose:** Per protocol; 125–350 mg/m^2 qwk–q3wk (↓ hepatic dysfunction, as tolerated per tox) **Caution:** [D, –] **Contra:** Allergy to component **Disp:** Inj 20 mg/mL **SE:** ↓ BM, N/V/D, abd cramping, alopecia; D is dose limiting; Rx acute D w/ atropine; Rx subacute D w/ loperamide **Interactions:** ↑ Effects OF antineoplastics; ↑ risk OF akathisia W/ prochlorperazine **Labs:** ↑ LFTs **NIPE:** Use barrier contraception; ⊘ exposure to Infxn; D correlated to levels of metabolite SN-38

Iron Dextran (Dexferrum, INFeD) [Iron Supplement] WARNING: Anaphylactic Rxns with use; use only if oral Fe not possible; administer where resuscitation techniques available Uses: *Fe deficiency when cannot supplement PO* **Action:** Fe supl **Dose:** *Adults. Iron defic anemia:* Estimate Fe deficiency, give 25–100 mg IM/IV day until total dose met; total dose (mL) = [–.0442 × (desired Hgb – observed Hgb) × LBW] + (0.26 × LBW); *Iron replacement, blood loss:* total dose (mg) = blood loss (mL) × Hct (as decimal fraction) max 100 mg/d; *Peds >4 mo.* As above; max: 0.5 mL (wt <5 kg), 1 mL (5–10 kg), 2 mL (>10 kg) per dose IM or direct IV **Caution:** [C, M] **Contra:** Anemia w/o Fe deficiency. **Disp:** Inj 50 mg (Fe)/mL **SE:** Anaphylaxis, flushing, dizziness, inj site & inf Rxns, metallic taste **Interactions:** ↓ Effects W/ chloramphenicol, ↓ absorption OF oral Fe **Labs:** False ↓ serum Ca; false + guaiac test **NIPE:** ⊘ Take oral Fe; give IM w/ "Z-track" technique; IV preferred; give test dose >1 h before

Iron Sucrose (Venofer) [Iron Supplement] Uses: *Fe deficiency anemia w/ chronic HD in those receiving erythropoietin* **Actions:** Fe replacement. **Dose:** 5 mL (100 mg) IV on dialysis, 1 mL (20 mg)/min max **Caution:** [C, M] **Contra:** Anemia w/o Fe deficiency **Disp:** 20 mg elemental Fe/mL, 5-mL vials.

SE: Anaphylaxis, ↓ BP, cramps, N/V/D, HA **Interactions:** ↓ Absorption *OF* oral Fe supls **Labs:** Monitor ferritin, HMG, Hct, transferrin saturation; obtain Fe levels 48 h > IV dose; ↑ LFTs **NIPE:** ⊘ use oral & IV supls together; most pts require cumulative doses of 1000 mg; give slowly

Isoniazid (INH) [Antitubercular]
Uses: *Rx & prophylaxis of TB* **Action:** Bactericidal; interferes w/ mycolic acid synth, disrupts cell wall **Dose:** *Adults.* *Active TB:* 5 mg/kg/24 h PO or IM (usually 300 mg/d) or DOT: 15mg/kg (max 900 mg) 3 ×/wk. *Prophylaxis:* 300 mg/d PO for 6–12 mo or 900 mg 2 ×/wk. *Peds.* *Active TB:* 10–15 mg/kg/d daily–bid PO or IM 300 mg/d max. *Prophylaxis:* 10 mg/kg/24 h PO; ↓ in hepatic/renal dysfunction **Caution:** [C, +] Liver Dz, dialysis; avoid EtOH **Contra:** Acute liver Dz, h/o INH hepatitis **Disp:** Tabs 100, 300 mg; syrup 50 mg/5 mL; inj 100 mg/mL **SE:** Hepatitis, peripheral neuropathy, GI upset, anorexia, dizziness, skin Rxn **Interactions:** ↑ Effects *OF* acetaminophen, anticoagulants, carbamazepine, cycloserine, diazepam, meperidine, hydantoins, theophylline, valproic acid, EtOH; ↑ effects *W/* rifampin; ↓ effects *W/* Al salts; ↓ effects *OF* anticoagulants, ketoconazole **Labs:** ↑ LFTs, glucose; ↓ HMG, plts, WBCs **NIPE:** Only take w/ food if GI upset; use w/ 2–3 other drugs for active TB, based on INH resistance patterns when TB acquired & sensitivity results; prophylaxis usually w/ INH alone. IM rarely used. ↓ peripheral neuropathy w/ pyridoxine 50–100 mg/d. ✓ CDC guidelines (*MMWR*) for current recommendations

Isoproterenol (Isuprel) [Bronchodilator/Sympathomimetic]
Uses: *Shock, cardiac arrest, AV nodal block* **Action:** β_1- & β_2-receptor stimulant **Dose:** *Adults.* 2–10 µg/min IV inf; titrate; 2–10 µg/min titrate (*ECC 2005*) *Peds.* 0.2–2 µg/kg/min IV inf; titrate. **Caution:** [C, ?] **Contra:** Angina, tachyarrhythmias (digitalis-induced or others) **Disp:** 0.02 mg/mL, 0.2 mg/mL **SE:** Insomnia, arrhythmias, HA, trembling, dizziness **Interactions:** ↑ Effects *W/* albuterol, guanethidine, oxytocic drugs, sympathomimetics, TCAs; ↑ risk of arrhythmias *W/* amitriptyline, bretylium, cardiac glycosides, K-depleting drugs, theophylline; ↓ effects *W/* BBs **Labs:** False ↑ serum AST, bilirubin, glucose **NIPE:** Saliva may turn pink in color, ↑ fluids to 2–3 L/d; more specific β_2-agonists preferred d/t excessive β_1 cardiac stimulation of drug; drug induces ischemia & dysrhythmias; pulse >130 bpm may induce arrhythmias

Isosorbide Dinitrate (Isordil, Sorbitrate, Dilatrate-SR) [Antianginal/Nitrate]
Uses: *Rx & prevent angina*, CHF (w/ hydralazine) **Action:** Relaxes vascular smooth muscle **Dose:** *Acute angina:* 5–10 mg PO (chew tabs) q2–3h or 2.5–10 mg SL PRN q5–10 min; do not give >3 doses in a 15–30-min period. *Angina prophylaxis:* 5–40 mg PO q6h; do not give nitrates on a chronic q6h or qid basis >7–10 d; tolerance may develop; provide 10–12-h drug-free intervals **Caution:** [C, ?] **Contra:** Severe anemia, NAG, postural ↓ BP, cerebral hemorrhage, head trauma (can ↑ ICP), w/ sildenafil, tadalafil, vardenafil **Disp:** Tabs 5, 10, 20, 30; SR tabs 40 mg; SL tabs 2.5, 5, mg; SR caps 40 mg **SE:** HA, ↓ BP, flushing, tachycardia, dizziness **Interactions:** ↑ Hypotension *W/* antihypertensives,

ASA, CCBs, phenothiazines, sildenafil, EtOH **Labs:** False ↓ serum cholesterol **NIPE:** ⊘ Nitrates for an 8–12-h period/d to avoid tolerance; higher PO dose needed for same results as SL forms

Isosorbide Dinitrate & Hydralazine HCL (BiDil) [Antianginal, Antihypertensive/Vasodilator, Nitrate]

Uses: HF in AA pts; improve survival & functional status, prolong time between hospitalizations for HF **Action:** Relaxes vascular smooth muscle; peripheral vasodilator **Dose:** Initially. 1 tab tid PO (if not tolerated reduce to 1/2 tab tid), titrate >3–5 d as tolerated. Max: 2 tabs tid **Caution:** [C, ?/–] recent MI, syncope, hypovolemia, hepatic impair **Contra:** ⊘ For children, concomitant use w/ PDE5 inhibitors (sildenafil) **Disp:** Isosorbide dinitrate 20 mg/hydralazine HCL 37.5 mg tabs **SE:** HA, dizziness, orthostatic hypotension, sinusitis, GI distress, tachycardia, paresthesia, amblyopia **Interactions:** ↑ Risk of severe hypotension W/ antihypertensives, ASA, CCBs, MAOIs, phenothiazines, sidenafil, tadalafil, vardenafil, ETOH; ↓ pressor response W/ epinephrine; ↓ effects W/ NSAIDs **Labs:** False ↓ serum cholesterol **NIPE:** ⊘ Nitrates for an 8–12-h period/d to avoid tolerance; take w/food

Isosorbide Mononitrate (Ismo, Imdur) [Antianginal/Nitrate]

Uses: *Prevention/Rx of angina pectoris* **Action:** Relaxes vascular smooth muscle **Dose:** 5–10 mg PO bid, w/ the 2 doses 7 h apart or XR (Imdur) 30–60 mg/d PO, max 240 mg **Caution:** [C, ?] **Contra:** Head trauma/cerebral hemorrhage (can ↑ ICP), w/ sildenafil, tadalafil, vardenafil **Disp:** Tabs 10, 20 mg; XR 30, 60, 120 mg **SE:** HA, dizziness, ↓ BP; **Interactions:** ↑ Hypotension w/ ASA, CCB, nitrates, sildenafil, EtOH **Labs:** False ↓ serum cholesterol

Isotretinoin [13-*cis* Retinoic Acid] (Accutane, Amnesteem, Claravis, Sotret) [Anti-acne Agent]

WARNING: Must not be used by PRG females; can induce severe birth defects; pt must be capable of complying w/ mandatory contraceptive measures; prescribed according to product-specific risk management system. Because of teratogenicity, Accutane is approved for marketing only under a special restricted distribution FDA program called iPLEDGE **Uses:** *Refractory severe acne* **Action:** Retinoic acid derivative **Dose:** 0.5–2 mg/kg/d PO ÷ bid; ↓ in hepatic Dz, take w/ food **Caution:** [X, –] Avoid tetracyclines **Contra:** Retinoid sensitivity, PRG **Disp:** Caps 10, 20, 30, 40 mg **SE:** Rare: Depression, psychosis, suicidal thoughts; derm sensitivity, xerostomia, photosens, LFTs, triglycerides; **Interactions:** ↑ Effects W/ corticosteroids, phenytoin, vitamin A; ↑ risk of pseudotumor cerebri w/ tetracyclines; ↑ triglyceride levels w/ EtOH; ↑ effects of carbamazepine **Labs:** ↑ LFTs, triglycerides; **NIPE:** ↑ Risk of photosensitivity—use sunscreen, take w/ food, ⊘ PRG; low dose progesterone only hormonal contraceptives may not be adequate birth control alone; Risk management program requires 2 (–) PRG tests before Rx & use of 2 forms of contraception 1 mo before, during, & 1 mo after therapy; to prescribe isotretinoin, the prescriber must access the iPLEDGE system via the Internet (www.ipledgeprogram.com): monitor LFTs & lipids

Isradipine (DynaCirc) [Antihypertensive/CCB] Uses: **HTN** **Action:** CCB **Dose:** *Adults.* 2.5–5 mg PO bid. **Caution:** [C, ?] **Contra:** Severe heart block, sinus bradycardia, CHF, dosing w/in several hours of IV β-blockers **Disp:** Caps 2.5, 5 mg; tabs CR 5, 10 mg **SE:** HA, edema, flushing, fatigue, dizziness, palpitations **Interactions:** ↑Effects W/ azole antifungals, BBs, cimetidine; ↑ effects *OF* carbamazepine, cyclosporine, digitalis glycosides, prazosin, quinidine; ↓ effects W/ Ca, rifampin; ↓ effect OF lovastatin **Labs:** ↑ LFTs **NIPE:** ⊘ D/C abruptly

Itraconazole (Sporanox) [Antifungal] WARNING: Potential for negative inotropic effects on the heart; if signs or Sxs of CHF occur during administration, continued use should be assessed Uses: **Fungal Infxns (aspergillosis, blastomycosis, histoplasmosis, candidiasis)** **Action:** ↓ Ergosterol synth **Dose:** 200 mg PO or IV daily–bid (capsule w/ meals or cola/grapefruit juice); PO soln on empty stomach; avoid antacids **Caution:** [C, ?] Numerous interactions **Contra:** Inj. if CrCl <30 mL/min, h/o CHF or ventricular dysfunction, w/ H₂-antagonist, omeprazole **Disp:** Caps 100 mg; soln 10 mg/mL; inj 10 mg/mL **SE:** N, rash, hepatitis, ↓ K⁺, CHF (mostly w/ IV use) **Interactions:** ↑ Effects W/ clarithromycin, erythromycin; ↑ effects *OF* alprazolam, anticoagulants, atevirdine, atorvastatin, buspirone, cerivastatin, chlordiazepoxide, cyclosporine, diazepam, digoxin, felodipine, fluvastatin, indinavir, lovastatin, methadone, methylprednisolone, midazolam, nelfinavir, pravastatin, ritonavir, saquinavir, simvastatin, tacrolimus, tolbutamide, triazolam, warfarin; ↑ QT prolongation W/ astemizole, cisapride, pimozide, quinidine, terfenadine; ↓ effects W/ antacids, Ca, cimetidine, didanosine, famotidine, lansoprazole, Mg, nizatidine, omeprazole, phenytoin, rifampin, sucralfate, grapefruit juice **Labs:** ↑ LFTs, BUN, SCr **NIPE:** Take capsule w/ food & soln w/o food, ⊘ PRG or breast-feeding, ↑ risk of disulfiram-like response w/ EtOH; PO soln & caps not interchangeable; useful in pts who cannot take ampho B, can cause ↑ QTc in combo w/ other drugs

Kaolin-Pectin (Kaodene, Kao-Spen, Kapectolin) [Antidiarrheal/Absorbent] [OTC] Uses: **D** **Action:** Absorbent demulcent **Dose:** *Adults.* 60–120 mL PO after each loose stool or q3–4h PRN. *Peds. 3–6 y:* 15–30 mL/dose PO PRN. *6–12 y:* 30–60 mL/dose PO PRN **Caution:** [C, +] **Contra:** D due to pseudomembranous colitis **Disp:** Multiple OTC forms; also available w/ opium (Parepectolin [CII]) **SE:** Constipation, dehydration **Interaction:** ↓ Effects *OF* ciprofloxacin, clindamycin, digoxin, lincomycin, lovastatin, penicillamine, quinidine, tetracycline **NIPE:** Take other meds 2–3 h before or after this drug

Ketoconazole (Nizoral, Nizoral AD Shampoo) [Shampoo–OTC] [Antifungal/Imidazole] Uses: **Systemic fungal Infxns; topical for local fungal Infxns due to dermatophytes & yeast; shampoo for dandruff,** PCa when rapid ↓ testosterone needed (ie, cord compression) **Action:** ↓ Fungal cell wall synth **Dose:** *Adults.* PO: 200 mg PO daily; ↑ to 400 mg PO daily for serious Infxn; PCa 400 mg PO tid (short-term). *Topical:* Apply daily (cream/shampoo). *Peds >2 y.* 5–10 mg/kg/24 h PO ÷ q12–24h (↓ in hepatic Dz) **Caution:** [C, +/–]

Any agent that ↑ gastric pH prevents absorption; may enhance anticoagulants; w/ EtOH (disulfiram-like Rxn) numerous interactions **Contra:** CNS fungal Infxns (poor CNS penetration), w/ astemizole, topical use on broken/inflamed skin **Disp:** Tabs 200 mg; topical cream 2%; gel 2%; shampoo 1% and 2% **SE:** N **Interactions:** ↑ Effects *OF* alprazolam, anticoagulants, atevirdine, atorvastatin, buspirone, chlordiazepoxide, cyclosporine, diazepam, felodipine, fluvastatin, indinavir, lovastatin, methadone, methylprednisolone, midazolam, nelfinavir, pravastatin, ritonavir, saquinavir, simvastatin, tacrolimus, tolbutamide, triazolam, warfarin; ↑ QT prolongation *W/* astemizole, cisapride, quinidine, terfenadine; ↓ effects *W/* antacids, Ca, cimetidine, didanosine, famotidine, lansoprazole, Mg, nizatidine, omeprazole, phenytoin, rifampin, sucralfate **Labs:** ↑ LFTs; monitor LFTs w/ systemic use **NIPE:** Take tabs w/ citrus juice, take w/ food; shampoo wet hair 1 min, rinse, repeat for 3 min; ⊘ PRG or breast-feeding;

Ketoprofen (Orudis, Oruvail) [Analgesic/NSAID] WARNING: May ↑ risk of cardiovascular events & GI bleeding Uses: *Arthritis, pain* Action: NSAID; ↓ prostaglandins Dose: 25–75 mg PO tid–qid, 300 mg/d/max; w/ food Caution: [B (D 3rd tri), ?] Contra: NSAID/ASA sensitivity Disp: Caps 25, 50, 75 mg; caps, SR 100, 150, 200 mg SE: GI upset, peptic ulcers, dizziness, edema, rash Interactions: ↑ Effects *W/* ASA, corticosteroids, NSAIDs, probenicid, EtOH; ↑ effects *OF* antineoplastics, hypoglycemics, insulin, Li, MTX; ↑ risk of nephrotox *W/* aminoglycosides, cyclosporines; ↑ risk of bleeding *W/* anticoagulants, defamandole, cefotetan, cefoperazone, clopidogrel, eptifibatide, plicamycin, thrombolytics, tirofiban, valproic acid, dong quai, feverfew, garlic, ginkgo biloba, ginger, horse chestnut, red clover; ↓ effects *OF* antihypertensives, diuretics Labs: ↑ LFTs, BUN, Cr, PT; ↓ plts, WBCs NIPE: ↑ Risk of photosensitivity—use sunscreen, take w/ food

Ketorolac (Toradol) [Analgesic/NSAID] WARNING: Indicated for short-term (=5 d) Rx of moderate–severe acute pain that requires opioid analgesia levels Uses: *Pain* Action: NSAID; ↓ prostaglandins Dose: 15–30 mg IV/IM q6h or 10 mg PO qid; max IV/IM 120 mg/d, max PO 40 mg/d; do not use for >5 d; ↓ for age & renal dysfunction and <50 kg Caution: [B (D 3rd tri), –] Contra: Peptic ulcer Dz, NSAID sensitivity, advanced renal Dz, CNS bleeding, anticipated major surgery, labor & delivery, nursing mothers Disp: Tabs 10 mg; inj 15 mg/mL, 30 mg/mL SE: Bleeding, peptic ulcer Dz, renal failure, Cr, edema, dizziness, allergy Interactions: ↑ Effects *W/* ASA, corticosteroids, NSAIDs, probenicid, EtOH; ↑ effects *OF* antineoplastics, hypoglycemics, insulin, Li, MTX; ↑ risk of nephrotox *W/* aminoglycosides, cyclosporines; ↑ risk of bleeding *W/* anticoagulants, defamandole, cefotetan, cefoperazone, clopidogrel, eptifibatide, plicamycin, thrombolytics, tirofiban, valproic acid, dong quai, feverfew, garlic, ginkgo biloba, ginger, horse chestnut, red clover; ↓ effects *OF* antihypertensives, diuretics Labs: ↑ LFTs, PT; ↓ HMG, Hct NIPE: 30-mg dose equals comparative analgesia of meperidine 100 mg or morphine 12 mg; PO only as continuation of IM/IV therapy

Ketorolac Ophthalmic (Acular, Acular LS, Acular PF) [Analgesic, Anti-inflammatory/NSAID] Uses: *Ocular itching w/ seasonal allergies*; inflammation w/ cataract extraction; pain/photophobia w/ incisional refractive surgery (Acular PF); pain w/ corneal refractive surgery (Acular LS) **Action:** NSAID **Dose:** 1 gtt qid **Caution:** [C, +] **Disp:** Acular LS: 0.4%; Acular, Acular PF Soln 0.5% **SE:** Local irritation **NIPE:** Teach use of eye drops

Ketotifen (Zaditor) [Ophthalmic Antihistamine/Histamine Antagonist & Mast Cell Stabilizer] Uses: *Allergic conjunctivitis* **Action:** H_1-receptor antagonist, mast cell stabilizer **Dose:** *Adults & Peds.* 1 gtt in eye(s) q8–12h **Caution:** [C,?/–] **Disp:** Soln 0.025%/5 mL **SE:** Local irritation, HA, rhinitis **NIPE:** Insert soft contact lenses 10 min after drug use; ⊘ wear contact lenses if eyes red

Kunecatechins (Veregen) [Botanical] Uses: *External genital/perianal warts* **Action:** Unknown **Dose:** Apply 0.5 cm ribbon to each wart 3 ×/d until all warts clear; not >16 wk **Caution:** [C; ?] **Disp:** Oint 15% **SE:** Local Rxns (erythema, pruritus, burning, pain, erosion/ulceration, edema, induration, rash) **NIPE:** Wash hands before/after use; not necessary to wipe off prior to next use; ⊘ internal or mucous membrane warts or on broken skin; ⊘ condoms or diaphragm—ointment may weaken rubber

Labetalol (Trandate) [Antihypertensive/Alpha & Beta-Blocker] Uses: *HTN* & hypertensive emergencies (IV) **Action:** α- & β-Adrenergic blocker **Dose:** *Adults. HTN:* Initial, 100 mg PO bid, then 200–400 mg PO bid. *Hypertensive emergency:* 20–80 mg IV bolus, then 2 mg/min IV inf, titrate up to 300 mg; 10 mg IV over 1–2 min; repeat or double dose q10min (150 mg max); or initial bolus, then 2–8 mg/min *(ECC 2005)* *Peds.* PO: 3–20 mg/kg/d in ÷ doses. *Hypertensive emergency:* 0.4–1.5 mg/kg/h IV cont inf **Caution:** [C (D in 2nd or 3rd tri), +] **Contra:** Asthma/COPD, cardiogenic shock, uncompensated CHF, heart block **Disp:** Tabs 100, 200, 300 mg; inj 5 mg/mL **SE:** Dizziness, N, ↓ BP, fatigue, CV effects **Interactions:** ↑ Effects *W/* cimetidine, diltiazem, nitroglycerine, quinidine, paroxetine, verapamil; ↑ tremors *W/* TCAs; ↓ effects *W/* glutethimide, NSAIDs, salicylates; ↓ effects *OF* antihypertensives, β-adrenergic bronchodilators, sulfonylureas **Labs:** False + amphetamines in urine drug screen; ↑ LFTS **NIPE:** May have transient tingling of scalp

Lactic Acid & Ammonium Hydroxide [Ammonium Lactate] (Lac-Hydrin) [Emollient] Uses: *Severe xerosis & ichthyosis* **Action:** Emollient moisturizer **Dose:** Apply bid **Caution:** [B, ?] **Disp:** Cream, lotion, lactic acid 12% w/ ammonium hydroxide **SE:** Local irritation **NIPE:** ⊘ Children <2 y; ↓ sun exposure—use sunscreen; risk of hyperpigmentation

Lactobacillus (Lactinex Granules) [Antidiarrheal] [OTC] Uses: *Control of D*, especially after antibiotic therapy **Action:** Replaces nl ntestinal flora **Dose:** *Adults & Peds >3 y.* 1 packet, 1–2 caps, or 4 tabs daily–qid **Caution:** [A, +] **Contra:** Milk/lactose allergy **Disp:** Tabs; caps; EC caps; powder n packets (all OTC) **SE:** Flatulence

Lactulose (Constulose, Generlac, Enulose, others) [Laxative/Osmotic] Uses: *Hepatic encephalopathy; constipation* Action: Acidifies the colon, allows ammonia to diffuse into colon Dose: *Acute hepatic encephalopathy:* 30–45 mL PO q1h until soft stools, then tid–qid. *Chronic laxative therapy:* 30–45 mL PO tid–qid; adjust q1–2d to produce 2–3 soft stools/d. *Rectally:* 200 g in 700 mL of H$_2$O PR. **Peds.** *Infants:* 2.5–10 mL/24 h ÷ tid–qid. Other Peds *Peds.* 40–90 mL/24 h ÷ tid–qid Caution: [B, ?] Contra: Galactosemia Disp: Syrup 10 g/15 mL, soln 10 g/15 mL, 10, 20 g/packet SE: Severe D, flatulence; life-threatening electrolyte disturbances Interactions: ↓ Effects W/ antacids, antibiotics, neomycin Labs: ↓ Serum ammonia NIPE: May take 24–48 h for results

Lamivudine (Epivir, Epivir-HBV) [Antiretroviral/NRTI] WARNING: Lactic acidosis & severe hepatomegaly w/ steatosis reported w/ nucleoside analogs Uses: *HIV Infxn, chronic Hep B* Action: NRTI, ↓ HIV RT & Hep B viral polymerase, causes viral DNA chain termination Dose: *HIV: Adults & Peds >16 y.* 150 mg PO bid or 300 mg PO daily. *Peds <16 y.* 4 mg/kg PO bid. *HBV: Adults.* 100 mg/d PO. *Peds 2–17 y.* 3 mg/kg/d PO, 100 mg max; ↓ w/ renal impair Caution: [C, –] Disp: Tabs 100 mg (HBV) 150 mg, 300 mg; soln 5 mg/mL (HBV), 10 mg/mL SE: HA, pancreatitis, GI upset, lactic acidosis, peripheral neuropathy Interactions: ↑ Effects W/ cotrimoxazole, trimethoprim/sulfamethoxazole; ↑ risk of lactic acidosis W/ antiretrovirals, reverse transcriptase inhibitors Labs: ↑ LFTs; ↓ HMG, Hct, plts NIPE: Take w/ food to < GI upset

Lamotrigine (Lamictal) [Anticonvulsant/Phenyltriazine] WARNING: Serious rashes requiring hospitalization & D/C of Rx reported; rash less frequent in adults Uses: *Partial Szs, tonic-clonic Szs, bipolar disorder Lennox–Gastaut synd* Action: Phenyltriazine antiepileptic, ↓ glutamate, stabilize neuronal membrane Dose: *Adults. Szs:* Initial 50 mg/d PO, then 50 mg PO bid for 2 wk, maint 300–500 mg/d in 2 ÷ doses. *Bipolar:* Initial 25 mg/d PO, 50 mg PO daily for 2 wk, 100 mg PO daily for 1 wk, maint 200 mg/d. **Peds.** 0.6 mg/kg in 2 ÷ doses for wk 1 & 2, then 1.2 mg/kg for wk 3 & 4, maint 15 mg/kg/d (max 400 mg/d) 1–2 ÷ doses; ↓ in hepatic Dz or w/ enzyme inducers or valproic acid Caution: [C, –] Interactions w/ other antiepileptics Disp: Tabs 25, 100, 150, 200 mg; chew tabs 2, 5, 25 mg SE: Photosens, HA, GI upset, dizziness, ataxia, rash (potentially life-threatening in children > adults) Notes: ? value of therapeutic monitoring Interactions: ↑ Effects *OF* valproic acid; ↑ effects *OF* carbamazepine; ↓ effects W/ acetaminophen, OCPs, phenobarbital, phenytoin, primidone NIPE: ↑ Risk of photosensitivity—use sunscreen

Lansoprazole (Prevacid, Prevacid IV) [Antisecretory/Proton-Pump Inhibitor] Uses: *Duodenal ulcers, prevent & Rx NSAID gastric ulcers, IV alternative for = 7 d w/ erosive esophagitis.* H. pylori Infxn, erosive esophagitis, & hypersecretory conditions, GERD Action: Proton pump inhibitor Dose: 15–30 mg/d PO; NSAID ulcer prevention 15 mg PO = 12 wk, NSAID ulcers 30 mg PO, × 8 wk; 30 mg IV daily = 7 d change to PO for 6–8 wk; ↓ in severe hepatic impair **Caution:** [B, ?/–] **Disp:** Caps 15, 30 mg; granules for susp 15, 30 mg, IV 30 mg; OD tabs 15, 30 mg **SE:** HA, fatigue **Interactions:** ↓ Effects *W/* sucralfate; ↓ effects *OF* ampicillin, digoxin, iron, ketoconazole **NIPE:** Take ac; for IV provided in-line filter must be used

Lanthanum Carbonate (Fosrenol) [Renal & GU Agent/Phosphate Binder] **Uses:** *Hyperphosphatemia in renal disease* **Action:** Phosphate binder **Dose:** 750–1500 mg PO daily ÷ doses, w/ or immediately after meal; titrate every 2–3 wk based on PO_4^{-2} levels **Caution:** [C, ?/–] No data in GI disease **Disp:** Chew tabs 250, 500, 750, 1000 mg **SE:** N/V, graft occlusion, HA ↓ BP **Labs:** ↑ Serum Ca level; monitor serum phosphate levels **NIPE:** Use cautiously *W/* GI disease; monitor for bone pain or deformity; chew tabs before swallowing; separate from meds that interact with antacids by 2 h

Lapatinib (Tykerb) [Tyrosine Kinase Inhibitor] **Uses:** *Advanced breast CA w/ capecitabine w/ tumors that overexpress HER2 and have failed therapy w/ anthracycline, taxane, and trastuzumab* **Action:** Tyrosine kinase inhibitor **Dose:** Per protocol, 1250 mg PO days 1–21 w/ capecitabine 2000 mg/m²/d divided 2 doses/d day 1–14 **Caution:** [D; ?] avoid CYP3A4 inhibitors **Contra:** w/ phenothiazines **Disp:** Tabs 250 mg **SE:** N/V/D, anemia, ↓ plt, neutropenia, hand-foot synd, rash, ↓ LVEF; **Interactions:** ↑ Effects *W/* potent CYP3A4 inhibitors (eg, ketoconazole), grapefruit; ↓ effects *W/* potent CYP3A4 inducers (eg, carbamazepine) **Labs:**↑ LFTs **NIPE:** Consider baseline LVEF and periodic ECG; take 1 h before or 1 h after a meal

Latanoprost (Xalatan) [Glaucoma Agent] **Uses:** *Open angle glaucoma, ocular HTN* **Action:** Prostaglandin, ↑ outflow of aqueous humor **Dose:** 1 gtt eye(s) hs **Caution:** [C, ?] **Disp:** 0.005% soln **SE:** May darken light irides; blurred vision, ocular stinging, & itching **Interactions:** ↑ Risk *OF* precipitation if mixed w/ eye drops w/ thimerosal

Leflunomide (Arava) [Antirheumatic DMARDs/Immunomodulator] **WARNING:** PRG must be excluded prior to start of Rx **Uses:** *Active RA* **Action:** ↓ Pyrimidine synth **Dose:** Initial 100 mg/d PO for 3 d, then 10–20 mg/d **Caution:** [X, –] **Contra:** PRG **Disp:** Tabs 10, 20, 100 mg **SE:** D, infxn, HTN, alopecia, rash, N, joint pain, hepatitis **Interactions:** ↑ Effects *W/* rifampin; ↑ risk of hepatotox *W/* hepatotoxic drugs, MRX; ↓ effects *OF* NSAIDs; ↓ effects *W/* activated charcoal, cholestyramine **Labs:** ↑ LFTs; monitor LFTs during initial therapy **NIPE:** ⊘ PRG, breast-feeding, live virus vaccines

Lenalidomide (Revlimid) [Immunomodulator] **WARNING:** Significant teratogen; patient must be enrolled in RevAssist risk reduction program **Uses:** *MDS* multiple myeloma **Action:** Thalidomide analog, immune modulator **Dose:** *Adults.* 10 mg PO daily; swallow whole w/ water **Caution:** [X, –] w/ renal impair **Disp:** Caps 5, 10, 15, 25 mg **SE:** D, pruritus, rash, fatigue, ↓ BM, thromboembolism, ↑ LFT **Interactions:** Monitor digoxin **Labs:** Monitor CBC; routine PRG tests required; ↑ LFTs, monitor for myelosuppression, thromboembolism, hepatotox **NIPE:** Routine PRG tests required; Rx only in 1-mo increments; limited distribution network; males must use condom and not donate sperm; use contraception at least 4 wk beyond D/C

Lepirudin (Refludan) [Anticoagulant/Thrombin Inhibitor]

Uses: *HIT* **Action:** Direct thrombin inhibitor **Dose:** Bolus 0.4 mg/kg IV, then 0.15 mg/kg/h inf (↓ dose & inf rate if CrCl <60 mL/min) **Caution:** [B, ?/–] Hemorrhagic event or severe HTN **Contra:** Active bleeding **Disp:** Inj 50 mg **SE:** Bleeding, anemia, hematoma **Interactions:** ↑ Risk of bleeding W/ antiplt drugs, cephalosporins, NSAIDs, thrombolytics, salicylates, feverfew, ginkgo biloba, ginger, valerian **Labs:** Adjust based on aPTT ratio, maintain aPTT 1.5–2.0

Letrozole (Femara) [Antineoplastic/Aromatase Inhibitor]

Uses: *Advanced breast CA in postmenopausal* **Action:** Nonsteroidal aromatase inhibitor **Dose:** 2.5 mg/d PO **Caution:** [D, ?] **Contra:** PRG **Disp:** Tabs 2.5 mg **SE:** Anemia, N, hot flashes, arthralgia **Interactions:** ↑ Risk of interference W/ action of drug W/ estrogens and OCPs **Labs:** ↑ LFTs, cholesterol; monitor CBC, thyroid Fxn, lytes, LFT, & SCr

Leucovorin (Wellcovorin) [Folic Acid Derivative/Vitamin]

Uses: *OD of folic acid antagonist; megaloblastic anemia, augment 5-FU impaired MTX elimination* **Action:** Reduced folate source; circumvents action of reductase inhibitors (eg, MTX) **Dose:** *Leucovorin rescue:* 10 mg/m² PO/IM/IV q6h start w/in 24 h after dose or 15 mg PO/IM/IV q6h, 25 mg/dose max PO; *Folate antagonist overdose (eg pemetrexed)* 100 mg/m² IM/IV ×1 then 50 mg/m² IM/IV q6h × 8 d 100 mg/m² ×1; *5-FU adjuvant Tx, colon CA per protocol; low dose:* 20 mg/m²/d IV × 5 d w/ 5-FU 425 mg/m²/d IV × 5 d, repeat q4–5wk × 6; *high dose:* 500 mg/m² IV qwk × 6, w/ 5-FU 500 mg/m² IV qwk × 6 wk, repeat after 2 wk off × 4; *Megaloblastic anemia:* 1 mg/IV daily **Caution:** [C, ?/–] **Contra:** Pernicious anemia **Disp:** Tabs 5, 10, 15, 25 mg; inj 50, 100, 200, 350, 500 **SE:** Allergic Rxn, N/V/D, fatigue **Interactions:** ↑ Effects *OF* fluorouracil; ↓ effects *OF* MTX, phenobarbital, phenytoin, primidone, trimethoprim/sulfamethoxazole **Labs:** Monitor Cr, methotrexate levels q24h w/ leucovorin rescue **NIPE:** ↑ Fluids to 3 L/d; do not use intrathecally/intraventricularly

Leuprolide (Lupron, Lupron DEPOT, Lupron DEPOT-Ped, Viadur, Eligard) [Antineoplastic/GnRH Analog]

Uses: *Advanced prostatic CA (all products except Depot-Ped), endometriosis (Lupron) uterine fibroids (Lupron), & precocious puberty (Lupron-Ped)* **Action:** LHRH agonist; paradoxically ↑ release of gonadotropin, resulting in ↓ pituitary gonadotropins (↓ LH); in men ↓ testosterone **Dose:** *Adults. PCa: Lupron DEPOT* 7.5 mg IM q28d or 22.5 mg IM q3mo or 30 mg IM q4mo; *Eligard:* 7.5 mg IM/SQ q28d or 22.5 mg IM q3mo or 30 mg IM/SQ q4mo; Eligard 45 mg SQ 6 mo; Viadur implant (PCa only): insert in inner upper arm w/ local anesthesia, replace q12mo *Endometriosis (Lupron DEPOT):* 3.75 mg IM qmo × 6. *Fibroids:* 3.75 mg IM qmo × 3. *Peds.* CPP (Lupron-Ped): 50 μg/kg/d SQ inj; ↑ by 10 μg/kg/d until total down-regulation achieved. *DEPOT: <25 kg:* 7.5 mg IM q4wk. *>25–37.5 kg*

11.25 mg IM q4wk. >*37.5 kg:* 15 mg IM q4wk **Caution:** [X, ?] w/ impending cord compression in PCa **Contra:** AUB, implant in women/peds; PRG **Disp:** Inj 5 mg/mL; Lupron DEPOT 3.75 (1 mo for fibroids, endometriosis); *Lupron DEPOT for PCa:* 7.5 mg (1 mo), 11.25 mg (3 mo), 22.5 (3 mo), 30 mg (4 mo); *Eligard DEPOT for PCa:* 7.5 mg (1 mo); 22.5 mg (3 mo), 30 mg (4 mo), 45 mg (6 mo); Viadur 65 mg 12-mo SQ implant, Lupron-Ped 7.5, 11.25, 15 mg **SE:** Hot flashes, gynecomastia, N/V, alopecia, anorexia, dizziness, HA, insomnia, paresthesias, depression exacerbation, peripheral edema, & bone pain (transient "flare Rxn" at 7–14 d after the 1st dose [LH/testosterone surge before suppression]) **Interactions:** ↓ Effects W/ androgens, estrogens **Labs:** ↑ LFTs, BUN, Cr, uric acid, lipids, WBC; ↓ PT, PTT, plts **NIPE:** Nonsteroidal antiandrogen (eg, bicalutamide) may block flare in men W/ PCa

Levalbuterol (Xopenex, Xopenex HFA) [Bronchodilator/Beta₂-Agonist]

$Beta_2$-Agonist **Uses:** *Asthma (Rx & prevention of bronchospasm)* **Action:** Sympathomimetic bronchodilator; *R*-isomer of albuterol **Dose:** *Adult.* HFA 2 puffs q4–6h, 12 puffs/d max; 0.63–1.25 mg neb q6–8h prn; *Peds >4 y.* HFA 2 puffs q4–6h, 12 puffs/d max; *Peds 6–11> y.* 0.31–0.63 mg neb q6–8h; *Peds > 11 y.* 0.63–1.25 mg neb q6–8h **Caution:** [C, ?] CAD, HTN, arrhythmias **Contra:** w/ phenothiazines, MAOI w/in 14 d **Disp:** Multidose inhaler (HFA) 45 μg/puff (15 g); Soln neb inhal 0.31, 0.63, 1.25 mg/3 mL **SE:** paradox bronchospasm, anaphylaxis, angioedema, tachycardia, nervousness,V **Interactions:** ↑ Effects W/ MAOIs, TCAs; ↑ risk of hypokalemia W/ loop & thiazide diuretics; ↓ effects W/ BBs; ↓ effects *OF* digoxin **Labs:** ↑ Serum glucose, ↓ serum K⁺ **NIPE:** May ↓ CV side effects compared w/ albuterol; do not mix w/ other nebs or dilute; use other inhalants 5 min after this drug

Levetiracetam (Keppra) [Anticonvulsant/ Pyrrolidine Agent]

Uses: *Partial onset Szs* **Action:** Unknown **Dose:** *Adults and >16 y.* 500 mg PO bid, may ↑ 3000 mg/d max; *Peds.* 4–15 y: 10–20 mg/kg/d ÷ in 2 doses, 60 mg/kg/d max (↓ in renal insuff) **Caution:** [C, ?/–] Elderly, w/ renal impair, psych disorders **Contra:** Component allergy **Disp:** Tabs 250, 500, 750, 1000 mg, Sol 100 mg/mL **SE:** Dizziness, somnolence, HA, hostility, aggression, myelosupp, impaired coordination **Interactions:** ↑ Effects W/ antihistamines, TCAs, benzodiazepines, narcotics, phenytoin, EtOH **NIPE:** May take w/ food; do not D/C abruptly

Levobunolol (A-K Beta, Betagan) [Glaucoma Agent/Beta-Adrenergic Blocker]

Uses: *Glaucoma* **Action:** β-Adrenergic blocker **Dose:** 1 gtt daily–bid **Caution:** [C, ?] **Disp:** Soln 0.25, 0.5% **SE:** Ocular stinging or burning **Interactions:** ↑ Effects W/ BBs; ↑ risk of hypotension & bradycardia W/ quinidine, verapamil; ↓ intraocular pressure W/ carbonic anhydrase inhibitors, epinephrine, pilocarpine **NIPE:** Night vision and acuity may be decreased; possible systemic effects if absorbed

Levocabastine (Livostin) [Antihistamine]

Uses: *Allergic seasonal conjunctivitis* **Action:** Antihistamine **Dose:** 1 gtt in eye(s) qid = 2 wk **Caution:** [C,+/–] **Disp:** 0.05% gtt **SE:** Ocular discomfort **NIPE:** ⊘ Insert soft contact lenses

Levofloxacin (Levaquin, Quixin & Iquix Ophthalmic) [Antibiotic/Fluoroquinolone] Uses: *Lower resp tract Infxns, sinusitis, chronic bact prostatitis, pyelonephritis, UTI uncomp; skin Infxns; anthrax; topical for bacterial conjunctivitis* **Action:** Quinolone, ↓ DNA gyrase. **Spectrum:** Excellent gram(+) except MRSA & *E. faecium*; excellent gram(−) except *S. maltophilia* & *Acinetobacter* sp; poor anaerobic **Dose:** Usual 250–750 mg/d PO or IV; *Sinusitis* 750 mg PO/IV × 5 d; *Prostatitis* 500 mg PO/IV × 28 d; *Uncomp UTI female* 250 mg PO/IV × 3 d, if complicated × 10 d; *CAP* 750 mg/d for 5 d; *Anthrax acute* 500 mg PO/d × 60, start IV w/ other antibiotics; postexposure 500 mg PO daily × 60; *ophth* 1–2 gtt in eye(s) q2h while awake for 2 d, then q4h while awake for 5 d; ↓ in renal impair, avoid antacids if PO; oral sol 1 h before, 2 h after meals **Caution:** [C, −] w/ cation-containing products (eg, antacids) **Contra:** Quinolone sensitivity **Disp:** Tabs 250, 500, 750 mg; premixed IV 250, 500, 750 mg, inj 25 mg/mL; Leva-Pak 750 mg × 5 d; Sol: 25 mg/mL ophth soln 0.5% (Quixin), 1.5% (Iquix) **SE:** N/D, dizziness, rash, GI upset, photosens **Interactions:** ↑ Effects *OF* cyclosporine, digoxin, theophylline, warfarin, caffeine; ↑ risk of Szs *W/* foscarnet, NSAIDs; ↑ risk of hyper- or hypoglycemia *W/* hypoglycemic drugs; ↓ effects *W/* antacids, antineoplastics, Ca, cimetidine, didanosine, famotidine, Fe, lansoprazole, Mg, nizatidine, omeprazole, phenytoin, ranitidine, NaHCO$_3$, sucralfate, Zn **NIPE:** Risk of tendon rupture & tendonitis—D/C if pain or inflammation; ↑ fluids, use sunscreen, antacids 2 h before or after this drug

Levonorgestrel (Plan B) [Progestin/Hormone] Uses: *Emergency contraceptive ("morning-after pill")*; prevents PRG if taken <72 h after unprotected sex/contraceptive fails **Action:** Progestin, alters tubal transport, and endometrium **Dose:** *Adult and Peds (post menarche females):* 0.75 mg q12h × 2 **Caution:** [X, M] **Contra:** Known/suspected PRG, AUB **Disp:** Tab, 0.75 mg, 2 blister pack **SE:** N/V, abd pain, fatigue, HA, menstrual changes **Interactions:** ↓ Effects *W/* barbiturates, carbamazepine, modafinil, phenobarbital, phenytoin, pioglitazone, rifabutin, rifampin, ritonavir, topiramate **NIPE:** Will not induce abortion; ↑ risk of ectopic PRG; OTC if >18 y, Rx if <18 y varies by state

Levonorgestrel IUD (Mirena) [Progestin/Hormone] Uses: *Contraception, long-term* **Action:** ?, May alter endometrium, thicken cervical mucus, interfere w/ sperm survival or capacitation **Dose:** Up to 5 y, insert w/in 7 d menses onset or immediately after 1st tri ab; wait 6 wk if postpartum; replace any time during menstrual cycle **Caution:** [C, ?] **Contra: Disp:** 52 mg IUD **SE:** Failed insertion, ectopic PRG, sepsis, PID, infertility, PRG comps w/ IUD left in place, abortion, embedment, ovarian cysts, perforation uterus/cervix, intestinal obst/perf, peritonitis **NIPE:** Counsel patient does not protect against STD/HIV; see insert for instructions

Levorphanol (Levo-Dromoran) [C-II] [Narcotic Analgesic] Uses: *Moderate–severe pain; chronic pain* **Action:** Narcotic analgesic **Dose:** 2–4 mg PO PRN q6–8h; 1–2 mg IM/SQ PRN q6–8h; ↓ in hepatic impair **Caution:** [B/D (prolonged use/high doses at term), ?] **Contra:** Component allergy **Disp:** Tabs 2 mg inj 2 mg/mL **SE:** Tachycardia, ↓ BP, drowsiness, GI upset, constipation, resp depression, pruritus **Interactions:** ↑ CNS effects **W/** antihistamines, cimetidine, CNS depressants, glutethimide, methocarbamol, EtOH, St. John's wort **Labs:**↑ Amylase, lipase **NIPE:** ↑ Fluids & fiber, take w/ food

Levothyroxine (Synthroid, Levoxyl, Others) [Thyroid Hormone] **Uses:** *Hypothyroidism, myxedema coma* **Action:** Supplement L-thyroxine **Dose:** *Adults. Hypothyroid* Initial, 12.5–50 μg/d PO; ↑ by 25–50 μg/d every mo; usual 100–200 μg/d. *Myxedema:* 200–500 μg IV, then 100–300 μg/d *Peds. Hypothyroid: 0–3 mo:* 10–15 μg/kg/24 h PO; *3–6 mo:* 8–10 μg/kg/d PO; *6–12 mo:* 6–8 μg/kg/d PO; *1–5 y:* 5–6 μg/kg/d PO; *6–12 y:* 4–5 μg/kd/d PO; *>12 y:* 2–3 μg/kg/d PO. Reduce dose by 50% if IV; titrate based on response & thyroid tests; dose can ↑ rapidly in young/middle-aged **Caution:** [A, +] **Contra:** Recent MI, uncorrected adrenal insuff **Disp:** Tabs 25, 50, 75, 88, 100, 112, 125, 137, 150, 175, 200, 300 μg; inj 200, 500 μg. **SE:** Insomnia, wt loss, alopecia, arrhythmia **Interactions:** ↑ Effects **OF** anticoagulants, sympathomimetics, TCAs, warfarin; ↓ effects **W/** antacids, BBs, carbamazepine, cholestyramine, estrogens, Fe salts, phenytoin, phenobarbital, rifampin, simethicone, sucralfate, ↓ effects **OF** digoxin, hypoglycemics, theophylline **Labs:** ↓ Thyroid function tests; drug alters thyroid uptake of radioactive I—D/C drug 4 wk before studies **NIPE:** ⊘ Switch brands due to different bioavailabilities; take w/ full glass of water (prevents choking)

Lidocaine (Anestacon Topical, Xylocaine, others) [Antiarrhythmic/Local Anesthetic] **Uses:** *Local anesthetic; Rx cardiac arrhythmias* **Action:** Anesthetic; class IB antiarrhythmic **Dose:** *Adults. Antiarrhythmic, ET:* 5 mg/kg; follow w/ 0.5 mg/kg in 10 min if effective. *IV load:* 1 mg/kg/dose bolus over 2–3 min; repeat in 5–10 min; 200–300 mg/h max; cont inf 20–50 μg/kg/min or 1–4 mg/min; *Cardiac arrest from VF/VT:* Initial: 1.0–1.5 mg/kg IV. *Refractory VF:* Additional 0.5–0.75 mg/kg IV push, repeat in 5–10 min, max total 3 mg/kg. ET: 2–4 mg/kg. *Perfusing stable VT, wide complex tachycardia or ectopy:* 1.0–1.5 mg/kg IV push; repeat 0.5–0.75 mg/kg q5–10min; max total 3 mg/kg; maint 1–4 mg/min (30–50 μg/min) *(ECC 2005) Peds. Antiarrhythmic, ET, load:* 1 mg/kg; repeat in 10–15 min 5 mg/kg max total, then IV inf 20–50 μg/kg/min. *Topical:* Apply max 3 mg/kg/dose. *Local inj anesthetic:* Max 4.5 mg/kg (Table 2) **Caution:** [C, +] **Contra:** Do not use lidocaine w/ epi on digits, ears, or nose (risk of vasoconstriction & necrosis); heart block **Disp:** *Inj local:* 0.5, 1, 1.5, 2, 4, 10, 20%. *Inj IV:* 1% (10 mg/mL), 2% (20 mg/mL); admixture 4, 10, 20%. *IV inf:* 0.2%, 0.4%; cream 2%; gel 2, 2.5%; oint 2.5, 5%; Liq 2.5%; soln 2, 4%; viscous 2% **SE:** Dizziness, paresthesias, & convulsions associated w/ tox **Notes:** Systemic levels: steady state 6–12h: *Therapeutic:* 1.2–5 μg/mL; *Toxic:* >6 μg/mL; *1/2 life:* 1.5 h **Interactions:** ↑ Effects **W/** amprenavir, BBs, cimetidine; ↑ neuromuscular blockade **W/** aminoglycosides, tubocuraine, pareira; ↑ cardiac depression **W/** procainamide, phenytoin, propranolol, quinidine, tocainide; ↓ effects **OF** succinylcholine **Labs:** ↑ SCr, ↑ CPK for 48 h after IM inj **NIPE:** Oral spray/soln may impair swallowing; 2nd line to amiodarone in ECC; dilute ET dose 1–2 mL w/ NS; epi may be added for local anesthesia to ↑ effect & ↓ bleeding; for IV forms, ↓ **W/** liver Dz or CHF

Lidocaine/Prilocaine (EMLA, LMX) [Topical Anesthetic] Uses: *Topical anesthetic*; adjunct to phlebotomy or dermal procedures **Action:** Topical anesthetic **Dose:** *Adults. EMLA cream, anesthetic disc (1 g/10 cm^2):* Thick layer 2–2.5 g to intact skin, cover w/ occlusive dressing (eg, Tegaderm) for at least 1 h. *Anesthetic disc:* 1 g/10 cm^2 for at least 1 h. *Peds. Max dose:* <3 mo or <5 kg: 1 g/10 cm^2 for 1 h. *3–12 mo & >5 kg:* 2 g/20 cm^2 for 4 h. *1–6 y & >10 kg:* 10 g/100 cm^2 for 4 h. *7–12 y & >20 kg:* 20 g/200 cm^2 for 4 h **Caution:** [B, +] Methemoglobinemia **Contra:** Use on mucous membranes, broken skin, eyes; allergy to amide-type anesthetics **Disp:** Cream 2.5% lidocaine/2.5% prilocaine; anesthetic disc (1 g) **SE:** Burning, stinging, methemoglobinemia; see Lidocaine **NIPE:** Low risk of systemic adverse effects; longer contact time ↑ effect

Lidocaine/Tetracaine Transdermal (Synera) [Topical Anesthetic] Uses: topical anesthetic; adjunct to phlebotomy or dermal procedures; **Action:** topical anesthetic; **Dose:** *Adults & Children >3 yrs. Phlebotomy:* apply to intact skin 20–30 min prior to venipuncture; *Dermal procedures:* apply to intact skin 30 min prior to procedure; **Caution:** (B, ±); **Contra:** pts w/ allergy to lidocaine/ tetracaine/ amide & ester type anesthetics; use on mucous membranes, broken skin, eyes; pts w/ PABA hypersensitivity; **Disp:** TD patch lidocaine 70 mg / tetracaine 70 mg; **SE:** erythema,blanching, edema, rash, burning, dizziness, HA, paresthesias; **Notes:** ⊘ use multiple patches simultaneously or sequentially; **Interactions:** ↑ systemic effects of Class I antiarrhythmic drugs (tocainide, mexiletine); ↑ systemic effects with other local anesthetics; **NIPI:** ⊘ cut patch/remove top cover-may cause thermal injury; low risk of systemic adverse effects.

Lindane (Kwell) [OTC] [Scabicide/Pediculicide] Uses: *Head lice, crab lice, scabies* **Action:** Ectoparasiticide & ovicide **Dose:** *Adults & Peds. Cream or lotion:* Thin layer after bathing, leave for 8–12 h, pour on laundry. *Shampoo:* Apply 30 mL, develop a lather w/ warm water for 4 min, comb out nits **Caution:** [C, +/–] **Contra:** Open wounds, Sz disorder **Disp:** Lotion 1%; shampoo 1% **SE:** Arrhythmias, Szs, local irritation, GI upset **Interactions:** Oil-based hair creams ↑ drug absorption **NIPE:** Apply to dry hair/dry, cool skin; caution w/ overuse (may be absorbed); may repeat Rx in 7 d

Linezolid (Zyvox) [Antibiotic/Oxazolidinones] Uses: *Infxns caused by gram(+) bacteria (including vancomycin-resistant Enterococcus, VRE), pneumonia, skin Infxns* **Action:** Unique, binds ribosomal bacterial RNA; bactericidal for streptococci, bacteriostatic for enterococci & staphylococci. *Spectrum:* Excellent gram(+) including VRE & MRSA **Dose:** *Adults.* 400–600 mg IV or PO q12h. *Peds.* 10 mg/kg IV or PO q8h (q12h in preterm neonates) **Caution:** [C, ?/–] w/ reversible MAOI, avoid foods w/ tyramine & cough/cold products w/ pseudoephedrine; w/ ↓ BM **Disp:** Inj 2 mg/mL; tabs 600 mg; susp 100 mg/5 mL **SE:** HTN, N/D, HA, insomnia, GI upset, ↓ BM, tongue discoloration **Interactions:** ↑ Risk of serotonin synd **W/** SSRIs, sibutramine, trazodone, venlafaxine; ↑ HTN **W/** amphetamines, dextromethorphan, dopamine, epinephrine, levodopa, MAOIs, meperidine, metaraminol, phenylephrine, phenylpropanolamine, pseudoephedrine, tyramine, ginseng, ephedra, ma huang, tyramine-containing foods; ↑ risk of bleeding W/ antiplts **Labs:** Follow weekly CBC **NIPE:** Take w/o regard to food, ⊘ tyramine-containing foods

Liothyronine (Cytomel) [Thyroid Hormone]

Uses: *Hypothyroidism, goiter, myxedema coma, thyroid suppression therapy* T₃ replacement **Dose:** *Adults.* Initial 25 μg/24 h, titrate q1–2wk to response & TFT; maint of 25–100 μg/d PO. *Myxedema coma:* 25–50 μg IV. *Peds.* Initial 5 μg/24 h, titrate by 5-μg/24-h increments at 1–2-wk intervals; maint 20–75 μg/24 h PO daily; ↓ in elderly **Caution:** [A, +] **Contra:** Recent MI, uncorrected adrenal insuff, uncontrolled HTN **Disp:** Tabs 5, 25, 50 μg; inj 10 μg/mL **SE:** Alopecia, arrhythmias, CP, HA, sweating **Interactions:** ↑ Effects OF anticoagulants; ↓ effects W/ bile acid sequestrants, carbamazepine, estrogens, phenytoin, rifampin; ↓ effects OF hypoglycemics, theophylline **Labs:** Monitor TFT **NIPE:** Monitor cardiac status, take in AM

Lisdexamfetamine (Vyvanse) [Stimulant]

WARNING: Amphetamines have high abuse potential. Long-term use may cause dependency **Uses:** *ADHD* **Action:** Prodrug of dextroamfetamine **Dose:** *Peds 6–12 y.* 30 mg PO qAM, ↑ 20 mg/d each wk, max 70 mg/d **Caution:** [C, –] ↑ Sudden cardiac death, may exacerbate preexisting psych disorders **Contra:** Severe CV Dz, ↑ thyroid, BP, NAG, h/o drug abuse, w/in 14 d of MOI **Disp:** Caps 30, 50, 70 mg **SE:** N/V, dry mouth, pyrexia, ↓ appetite & wt, dizziness, HA, irritability, insomnia, rash **Interactions:** Risk of HTN crisis W/ MAOIs, furazolidone; ↑ effects W/ TCA, propoxyphene; ↑ effects OF meperidine, norepinephrine, phenobarbital, phenobarbital, TCA; ↓ effects W/ haloperidol, chlorpromazine, Li; ↓ effects OF adrenergic blockers, antihistamines, antihypertensives **Labs:** Monitor phenytoin levels; may interfere W/ urinary steroid tests **NIPE:** Adult approval pending; OK to open and dissolve in H₂O

Lisinopril (Prinivil, Zestril) [Antihypertensive/ACEI]

Uses: *HTN, CHF, prevent DN & AMI* **Action:** ACE inhibitor **Dose:** 5–40 mg/24 h PO daily–bid. *AMI:* 5 mg w/in 24 h of MI, then 5 mg after 24 h, 10 mg after 48 h, then 10 mg/d; ↓ in renal insuff **Caution:** [D, –] **Contra:** ACE inhibitor sensitivity **Disp:** Tabs 2.5, 5, 10, 20, 30, 40 mg **SE:** Dizziness, HA, cough, ↓ BP, angioedema, ↑ K⁺ **Interactions:** ↑ Effects W/ α-blockers, diuretics ↑ risk of hyperkalemia W/ K⁺-sparing diuretics, trimethoprim, salt substitutes; ↑ risk of cough W/ capsaicin; ↑ effects OF insulin, Li; ↓ effects W/ ASA, indomethacin, NSAIDs **Labs:** ↑ LFTs, serum K⁺, Cr, BUN **NIPE:** Maximum effect may take several weeks; To prevent DN, start when urinary microalbuminemia begins

Lithium Carbonate (Eskalith, Lithobid, others) [Antipsychotic]

Uses: *Manic episodes of bipolar Dz* **Action:** Effects shift toward intraneuronal metabolism of catecholamines **Dose:** *Adults.* Bipolar, acute mania: 1800 mg/d PO in 3 ÷ doses in desired serum CNS. 1–15 mg/L. *Bipolar maintenance:* 900–1200/d PO in 2–3 ÷ dose *Peds 2–12 y.* 15–60 mg/kg/d in 3–4 ÷ doses;

must titrate; ↓ in renal insuff, elderly **Caution:** [D, –] Many drug interactions **Contra:** Severe renal impair or CV Dz, lactation **Disp:** Caps 150, 300, 600 mg; tabs 300 mg; SR tabs 300, CR tabs 450 mg; syrup 300 mg/5 mL **SE:** Polyuria, polydipsia, nephrogenic DI, tremor; Na retention or diuretic use may ↑ tox; arrhythmias, dizziness **Notes:** *Levels:* Trough: Just before next dose: *Therapeutic:* 0.8–1.2 mEq/mL; *Toxic:* >2 mEq/mL; *1/2 life:* 18–20h **Interactions:** ↑ Effects *OF* TCA; ↑ effects *W/* ACEIs, bumetanide, carbamazepine, ethacrynic acid, fluoxetine, furosemide, methyldopa, NSAIDs, phenytoin, phenothiazines, probenecid, tetracyclines, thiazide diuretics, dandelion, juniper; ↓ effects *W/* acetazolamide, antacids, mannitol, theophylline, urea, verapamil, caffeine **Labs:** ↑ Serum glucose, I-131 uptake, WBC; ↓ uric acid, T_3, T_4 **NIPE:** Several wk before full effects of med, ↑ fluid intake to 2–3 L/d

Lodoxamide (Alomide) [Antihistamine]

Uses: *Vernal conjunctivitis/keratitis* **Action:** Stabilizes mast cells **Dose:** *Adults & Peds >2 y.* 1–2 gtt in eye(s) qid × 3 mo **Caution:** [B, ?] **Disp:** Soln 0.1% **SE:** Ocular burning, stinging, HA **NIPE:** ⊘ children <2 y; ⊘ wear contact lens *W/* drug

Lomefloxacin (Maxaquin) [Antibiotic/Fluoroquinolone]

Uses: *UTI, acute exacerbation of chronic bronchitis; prophylaxis in transurethral procedures* **Action:** Quinolone antibiotic; ↓ DNA gyrase. **Spectrum:** Good gram(–) including *H. influenzae* except *S. maltophilia, Acinetobacter* sp, & *P. aeruginosa* **Dose:** 400 mg/d PO; ↓ w/ renal insuff, avoid antacids **Caution:** [C, –] Interactions w/ cation-containing products **Contra:** Quinolone allergy, children <18 y, ↑ QT interval, ↓K^+ **Disp:** Tabs 400 mg **SE:** N/V/D, abd pain, photosens, Szs, HA, dizziness, tendon rupture, peripheral neuropathy, pseudomembranous colitis, anaphylaxis **Interactions:** ↑ Effects *W/* cimetidine, probenecid; ↑ effects *OF* cyclosporine, warfarin, caffeine; ↓ effects *W/* antacids **Labs:** ↑ LFTs, ↓ K^+ **NIPE:** ↑ Risk of photosensitivity—use sunscreen, ↓ fluids to 2 L/d

Loperamide (Imodium) [OTC] [Antidiarrheal]

Uses: *D* **Action:** Slows intestinal motility **Dose:** *Adults.* Initial 4 mg PO, then 2 mg after each loose stool, up to 16 mg/d. *Peds. 2–5 y, 13–20 kg:* 1 mg PO tid. *6–8 y, 20–30 kg:* 2 mg PO tid. *8–12 y, >30 kg:* 2 mg PO tid **Caution:** [B, +] Not for acute D caused by *Salmonella* sp, *Shigella* sp, or *C. difficile* **Contra:** Pseudomembranous colitis, bloody D **Disp:** Caps 2 mg; tabs 2 mg; Liq 1 mg/5 mL (OTC) **SE:** Constipation, sedation, dizziness **Interactions:** ↑ Effects *W/* antihistamines, CNS depressants, phenothiazines, TCAs, EtOH

Lopinavir/Ritonavir (Kaletra) [Antiretroviral/Protease Inhibitor]

Uses: *HIV Infxn* **Action:** Protease inhibitor **Dose:** *Adults. Tx naïve:* 2 tab PO daily or 1 tab PO bid; *Tx experienced pt:* 1 tab PO bid (↑ dose if w/ amprenavir, efavirenz, fosamprenavir, nelfinavir, nevirapine). *Peds. 7–15 kg:* 12/3 mg/kg PO bid. *15–40 kg:* 10/2.5 mg/kg PO bid. *>40 kg:* Adult dose; w/ food **Caution:** [C, ?/–] Numerous interactions **Contra:** w/ drugs dependent on CYP3A/CYP2D6 (Table 11) **Disp:** (mg lopinavir/ritonavir) Tab 200/50, soln 400/100/5 mL **SE:** Avoid disulfiram (soln has EtOH), metronidazole; GI upset, asthenia, ↑ cholesterol/triglycerides, pancreatitis; protease metabolic synd; **Interactions:** ↑ Effects *W/* clarithromycin, erythromycin; ↑ effects *OF* amiodarone, amprenavir, azole antifungals, bepridil, cisapride, cyclosporine, CCBs, ergot alkaloids, flecainide, flurazepam, HMG-CoA reductase inhibitors, indinavir, lidocaine, meperidine, midazolam, pimozide, propafenone, propoxyphene, quinidine, rifabutin, saquinavir, sildenafil, tacrolimus, terfenadine, triazolam, zolpidem; ↓ effects *W/* barbiturates, carbamazepine, dexamethasone, didanosine, efavirenz, nevirapine, phenytoin, rifabutin, rifampin, St. John's wort; ↓ effects *OF* OCPs, warfarin **Labs:** ↑ LFTs, cholesterol, triglycerides **NIPE:** Take w/ food, use barrier contraception

Loracarbef (Lorabid) [Antibiotic/Cephalosporin-2nd Generation] Uses: *Upper & lower resp tract, skin, urinary tract* **Action:** 2nd-gen cephalosporin; ↓ cell wall synth. *Spectrum:* Weaker than 1st-gen against gram(+), enhanced gram(−) **Dose:** *Adults.* 200–400 mg PO daily–bid. *Peds.* 7.5–15 mg/kg/d PO ÷ bid; on empty stomach; ↓ in severe renal insuff **Caution:** [B, +] **Disp:** Caps 200, 400 mg; susp 100, 200 mg/5 mL **SE:** D **Interactions:** ↑ Effects *W/* probenecid; ↓ effects *OF* warfarin; ↑ nephrotox *W/* aminoglycosides, furosemide **NIPE:** Take w/o food

Loratadine (Claritin, Alavert) [Antihistamine] Uses: *Allergic rhinitis, chronic idiopathic urticaria* **Action:** Nonsedating antihistamine **Dose:** *Adults.* 10 mg/d PO **Peds.** 2–5 y: 5 mg PO daily. >6 y: Adult dose; on empty stomach; ↓ in hepatic insuff **Caution:** [B, +/−] **Contra:** Component allergy **Disp:** Tabs 10 mg (OTC); rapidly disintegrating Reditabs 10 mg; syrup 1 mg/mL **SE:** HA, somnolence, xerostomia **Interactions:** ↑ Effects *W/* CNS depressants, erythromycin, ketoconazole, MAOIs, protease inhibitors, procarbazine, EtOH **NIPE:** Take w/o food

Lorazepam (Ativan, Others) [C-IV] [Anxiolytic, Sedative/Hypnotic/Benzodiazepine] Uses: *Anxiety & anxiety w/ depression; preop sedation; control status epilepticus*; EtOH withdrawal; antiemetic **Action:** Benzodiazepine; antianxiety agent **Dose:** *Adults. Anxiety:* 1–10 mg/d PO in 2–3 ÷ doses. *Preop:* 0.05 mg/kg to 4 mg max IM 2 h before surgery. *Insomnia:* 2–4 mg PO hs. *Status epilepticus:* 4 mg/dose IV PRN q10–15min; usual total dose 8 mg. *Antiemetic:* 0.5–2 mg IV or PO q4–6h PRN. *EtOH withdrawal:* 2–5 mg IV or 1–2 mg PO initial depending on severity; titrate **Peds.** *Status epilepticus:* 0.05 mg/kg/dose IV, repeat at 1–20 min intervals × 2 PRN. *Antiemetic, 2–15 y:* 0.05 mg/kg (to 2 mg/dose) prechemo; ↓ in elderly; do not administer IV >2 mg/min or 0.05 mg/kg/min **Caution:** [D, ?/−] **Contra:** Severe pain, severe ↓ BP, sleep apnea, NAG, allergy to propylene glycol or benzyl alcohol **Disp:** Tabs 0.5, 1, 2 mg; soln, PO conc 2 mg/mL; inj 2, 4 mg/mL **SE:** Sedation, ataxia, tachycardia, constipation, resp depression **Interactions:** ↑ Effects *W/* cimetidine, disulfiram, probenecid, calendula, catnip, hops, lady's slipper, passionflower, kava kava, valerian; ↑ effects *OF* phenytoin; ↑ CNS depression *W/* anticonvulsants, antihistamines, CNS depressants, MAOIs, scopolamine, EtOH; ↓ effects *W/* caffeine, tobacco; ↓ effects *OF* levodopa **Labs:** ↑ LFTs **NIPE:** ⊘ D/C abruptly; =10 min for effect if IV

Losartan (Cozaar) [Antihypertensive/ARB] Uses: *HTN*, CHF, DN **Action:** Angiotensin II antagonist **Dose:** 25–50 mg PO daily–bid, max 100 mg; ↓ in elderly/hepatic impair **Caution:** [C (1st tri, D 2nd & 3rd tri), ?/–] **Disp:** Tabs 25, 50, 100 mg **SE:** ↓ BP in pts on diuretics; GI upset, angioedema **Interactions:** ↑ Risk of hyperkalemia **W/** K-sparing diuretics, K supls, trimethoprim; ↑ effects **OF** Li; ↓ effects **W/** diltiazem, fluconazole, phenobarbital, rifampin **NIPE:** ⊘ PRG, breast-feeding

Lovastatin (Mevacor, Altocor) [Antilipemic/HMG-CoA Reductase Inhibitor] Uses: *Hypercholesterolemia* **Action:** HMG-CoA reductase inhibitor **Dose:** 20 mg/d PO w/ PM meal; may ↑ at 4-wk intervals to 80 mg/d max or 60 mg ER tab; take w/ meals **Caution:** [X, –] Avoid w/ grapefruit juice, gemfibrozil. **Contra:** Active liver Dz **Disp:** Tabs 10, 20, 40 mg; ER tabs 10, 20, 40, 60 mg **SE:** HA & GI intolerance common; promptly report any unexplained muscle pain, tenderness, or weakness (myopathy) **Interactions:** ↑ Effects **W/** grapefruit juice; ↑ risk of severe myopathy **W/** azole antifungals, cyclosporine, erythromycin, gemfibrozil, HMG-CoA inhibitors, niacin; ↑ effects **OF** warfarin; ↓ effects **W/** isradipine, pectin **Labs:** ↑ LFTs; monitor LFT q12wk × 1 y, then q6mo **NIPE:** ⊘ PRG, take drug PM, periodic eye exams; maintain cholesterol-lowering diet

Lubiprostone (Amitiza) [Laxative] Uses: *Chronic idiopathic constipation in adults* **Action:** Selective Cl channel activator **Dose:** *Adults.* 24 µg PO bid w/ food **Contra:** Mechanical GI obst **Caution:** [C,?/–] Severe D, severe renal or moderate-severe hepatic impair **Disp:** Gelcaps 24 µg **SE:** N, HA, D, GI distention, abd pain **Labs:** Monitor LFTs and BUN/Cr; requires (–) PRG test before Tx **NIPE:** Utilize contraception; periodically reassess drug need; not for chronic use; suspend drug if D; ⊘ breast-feeding

Lutropin Alfa (Luveris) [Hormone] Uses: *Infertility* **Action:** Recombinant LH **Dose:** 75 units SC w/ 75–150 units FSH, 2 separate inj max 14 d **Caution:** [X, ?/M] **Contra:** Primary ovarian failure, uncontrolled thyroid/adrenal dysfunction, intracranial lesion, AUB, hormone-dependent GU tumor, ovarian cyst, PRG **Disp:** Inj 75 units **SE:** HA, N, ovarian hyperstimulation synd, breast pain, ovarian cysts; ↑ risk of multiple births **NIPE:** Rotate inj sites; do not exceed 14 d duration unless signs of imminent follicular development

Lymphocyte Immune Globulin [Antithymocyte Globulin, ATG] (Atgam) [Immunosuppressant]   WARNING: Should only be used by health care provider experienced in immunosuppressive Tx or management of solid organ and/or BM transplant patients. Adequate lab and supportive medical resources must be readily available in the facility for patient management Uses: *Allograft rejection in transplant pts; aplastic anemia if not candidates for BMT* **Action:** ↓ Circulating T lymphocytes **Dose:** *Adults. Prevent rejection:* 15 mg/kg/d IV ×14 d, then qod ×7; initial w/in 24 h before/after transplant. *Rx rejection:* Same except use 10–15 mg/kg/d; max 28 doses in 21 d. *Peds.* 5–25 mg/kg/d IV. **Caution:** [C, ?] **Contra:** h/o Rxn to other γ-globulin preparation, leukopenia, thrombocytopenia **Disp:** Inj 50 mg/mL **SE:** D/C w/ severe thrombocytopenia/leukopenia; rash, fever, chills, ↓ BP, HA, ↑ K⁺ **Notes:** Test dose: 0.1 mL

1:1000 dilution in NS **Interactions:** ↑ Immunosuppression *W/* azathioprine, corticosteroids, immunosuppressants **Labs:** ↑ LFTs **NIPE:** Risk of febrile Rxn

Magaldrate (Riopan, Lowsium) [OTC] [Antacid/Aluminum & Magnesium Salt] **Uses:** *Hyperacidity associated w/ peptic ulcer, gastritis, & hiatal hernia* **Action:** Low-Na antacid **Dose:** 5–10 mL PO between meals & hs **Caution:** [B, ?] **Contra:** Ulcerative colitis, diverticulitis, ileostomy/colostomy, renal insuff (Mg content) **Disp:** Susp (OTC) **SE:** GI upset **Notes:** <0.3 mg Na/tab or tsp **Interactions:** ↑ Effects *OF* levodopa, quinidine; ↓ effects *OF* allopurinol, anticoagulants, cefpodoxime, ciprofloxacin, clindamycin, digoxin, indomethacin, INH, ketoconazole, lincomycin, phenothiazine, quinolones, tetracyclines **NIPE:** ⊘ Other meds w/in 1–2 h

Magnesium Citrate (various) [OTC] [Laxative/Magnesium Salt] **Uses:** *Vigorous bowel preparation*; constipation **Action:** Cathartic laxative **Dose:** *Adults.* 120–300 mL PO PRN. *Peds.* 0.5 mL/kg/dose, to 200 mL PO max; w/ a beverage **Caution:** [B, +] **Contra:** Severe renal Dz, heart block, N/V, rectal bleeding **Disp:** Effervescent soln (OTC) **SE:** Abd cramps, gas **Interactions:** ↓ Effects *OF* anticoagulants, digoxin, fluoroquinolones, ketoconazole, nitrofurantoin, phenothiazine, tetracyclines **Labs:** ↑ Mg²⁺, ↓ protein, Ca²⁺, K⁺ **NIPE:** ⊘ Other meds w/in 1–2 h

Magnesium Hydroxide (Milk of Magnesia) [OTC] [Laxative/Magnesium Salt] **Uses:** *Constipation*, hyperacidity, Mg replacement **Action:** NS *Laxative* **Dose:** *Adults. Antacid:* 5–15 mL PO PRN qid, 2–4 tab PO PRN QID; *Laxative:* 30–60 mL PO daily or in ÷ doses *Peds.* <2 y: 0.5 mL/kg/dose PO PRN; (follow dose w/ 8 oz of H₂O **Caution:** [B, +] **Contra:** Renal insuff, intestinal obst, ileostomy/colostomy **Disp:** Chew tabs 311 mg; Liq 400, 800 mg/5 mL (OTC) **SE:** D, abd cramps **Interactions:** ↓ Effects *OF* chlordiazepoxide, dicumarol, digoxin, indomethacin, INH, quinolones, tetracyclines **Labs:** ↑ Mg²⁺, ↓ protein, Ca²⁺, K⁺ **NIPE:** ⊘ Other meds w/in 1–2 h

Magnesium Oxide (Mag-Ox 400, others) [OTC] [Antacid, Magnesium Supplement/Magnesium Salt] **Uses:** *Replace low Mg levels* **Action:** Mg supl **Dose:** 400–800 mg/d ÷ daily–qid w/ full glass of H₂O **Caution:** [B, +] **Contra:** Ulcerative colitis, diverticulitis, ileostomy/colostomy, heart block, renal insuff **Disp:** Caps 140 mg; tabs 400 mg (OTC) **SE:** D, N **Interactions:** ↓ Effects *OF* chlordiazepoxide, dicumarol, digoxin, indomethacin, INH, quinolones, tetracyclines **Labs:** ↑ Mg²⁺, ↓ protein, Ca²⁺, K⁺ **NIPE:** ⊘ Other meds w/in 1–2 h

Magnesium Sulfate (Various) [Magnesium Supplement/Magnesium Salt] **Uses:** *Replace low Mg²⁺*; preeclampsia & premature labor, cardiac arrest; AMI*; refractory ↓ K⁺ & ↓ Ca²⁺ **Action:** Mg²⁺ supl **Dose:** *Adults.* 3 g PO q6h × 4 PRN; *Supl:* 1–2 g IM or IV; repeat PRN. *Preeclampsia/premature labor:* 4 g load then 1–4 g/h IV inf; *Cardiac arrest:* 1–2 g IV push (2–4 mL 50% soln) in 10 mL D₅W *AMI:* Load 1–2 g in 50–100 mL D₅W, over 5–60 min IV; then 0.5–1.0 g/h IV up to 24 h (*ECC 2005*) *Peds.* 25–50 mg/kg/dose IM or IV q4–6h for 3–4 doses; repeat PRN; ↓ dose w/ low urine output or renal insuff

Caution: [B, +] **Contra:** Heart block, renal failure **Disp:** Inj 10, 20, 40, 80, 125, 500 mg/mL; bulk powder **SE:** CNS depression, D, flushing, heart block **Interactions:** ↑ CNS depression *W/* antidepressants, antipsychotics, anxiolytics, barbiturates, hypnotics, narcotics; EtOH; ↑ neuromuscular blockade *W/* aminoglycosides, atracurium, gallamine, pancuronium, tubocurarine, vecuronium **Labs:** ↑ Mg²⁺; ↓ protein, Ca²⁺, K⁺ **NIPE:** Check for absent patellar reflexes

Mannitol (Various) [Osmotic Diuretic] Uses: *Cerebral edema, ↑ intraocular pressure, renal impair, poisonings* **Action:** Osmotic diuretic **Dose:** *Test dose:* 0.2 g/kg/dose IV over 3–5 min; if no diuresis w/in 2 h, D/C. *Oliguria:* 50–100 g IV over 90 min; ↑ IOP: 0.5–2 g/kg IV over 30 min. *Cerebral edema:* 0.25–1.5 g/kg/dose IV >30 min. **Caution:** [C, ?] w/ CHF or volume overload **Contra:** Anuria, dehydration, HF, PE **Disp:** Inj 5, 10, 15, 20, 25% **SE:** May exacerbate CHF, N/V/D **Interactions:** ↑ Effects *OF* cardiac glycosides; ↓ effects *OF* barbiturates, imipramine, Li, salicylates **Labs:** ↑/↓ Electrolytes **NIPE:** Monitor for volume depletion

Measles, Mumps, Rubella, and Varicella Virus Vaccine Live [MMRV] (Proquad) [Vaccine/Live Attenuated] Uses: *Vaccination against measles, mumps, rubella, & varicella 12 mo–12 y or for 2nd dose of MMR* **Action:** Active immunization, live attenuated viruses **Dose:** 1 viral SQ inj **Caution:** [N/A] h/o cerebral injury or Szs (febrile Rxn) **Contra:** h/o anaphylaxis to neomycin, blood dyscrasia, lymphoma, leukemia, w/ immunosuppression, febrile illness, untreated TB **Disp:** Inj **SE:** Fever, inj site Rxn, rash **NIPE:** Allow 1 mo between inj & any other measles vaccine; limited avail; substitute MMR II or Varivax

Mecasermin (Increlex) [Human IGF-1] Uses: *Growth failure in IGF-1 deficiency or HGH antibodies* **Action:** Human IGF-1 **Dose:** *Peds.* 0.04–0.08 mg/kg SQ bid; may ↑ by 0.04 mg/kg to 0.12 mg/kg; take w/in 20 min of meal **Caution:** [C,+/–] **Disp:** Vial 40 mg **SE:** HA, inj site Rxn, V, hypoglycemia **Labs:** Rapid dose ↑ may cause hypoglycemia; ↑?LFTs **NIPE:** Limited distribution

Mechlorethamine (Mustargen) [Antineoplastic/Alkylating Agent] WARNING: Highly toxic, handle w/ care, limit use to experienced physicians **Uses:** *Hodgkin Dz & NHL, cutaneous T-cell lymphoma (mycosis fungoides), lung CA, CML, malignant pleural effusions*, & CLL **Action:** Alkylating agent, bifunctional **Dose:** Per protocol; 0.4 mg/kg single dose or 0.1 mg/kg/d for 4 d; 6 mg/m² 1–2 × mo **Caution:** [D, ?] **Contra:** Known infectious Dz **Disp:** Inj 10 mg **SE:** ↓ BM, thrombosis, thrombophlebitis at site; tissue damage w/ extrav (Na thiosulfate used topically to Rx); N/V, skin rash, amenorrhea, sterility (especially in men), secondary leukemia if treated for Hodgkin Dz **Interactions:** ↑ Risk of blood dyscrasias *W/* amphotericin B; ↑ risk of bleeding *W/* anticoagulants, NSAIDs, pit inhibitors, salicylates; ↑ myelosuppression *W/* antineoplastic drugs, radiation therapy; ↓ effects *OF* live virus vaccines **Labs:** ↑ Serum uric acid **NIPE:** Highly volatile; give w/in 30–60 min of prep; ↑ fluids to 2–3 L/d; ⊘ PRG, breast-feeding, vaccines, exposure to Infxn; ↑ risk of tinnitus

Meclizine (Antivert) [Antiemetic/Antivertigo/Anticholinergic]

Uses: *Motion sickness, vertigo* **Action:** Antiemetic, anticholinergic, & antihistaminic properties **Dose:** *Adults & Peds >12 y.* 12.5–100 mg PO tid–qid PRN **Caution:** [B, ?] **Disp:** Tabs 12.5, 25, 50 mg; chew tabs 25 mg; caps 25, 30 mg (OTC) **SE:** Drowsiness, xerostomia, & blurred vision **Interactions:** ↑ Sedation W/ antihistamines, CNS depressants, neuroleptics, EtOH; ↑ anticholinergic effects W/ anticholinergics, atropine, disopyramide, haloperidol, phenothiazine, quinidine **NIPE:** Use prophylactically

Medroxyprogesterone (Provera, Depo-Provera) [Antineoplastic/Progestin]

WARNING: May cause loss of bone density; associated w/ duration of use **Uses:** *Contraception; secondary amenorrhea, AUB caused by hormonal imbalance; endometrial CA* **Action:** Progestin supl **Dose:** *Contraception:* 150 mg IM q3mo depo or 104 mg SQ q3mo (depo SQ). *Secondary amenorrhea:* 5–10 mg/d PO for 5–10 d. *AUB:* 5–10 mg/d PO for 5–10 d beginning on the 16th or 21st d of menstrual cycle. *Endometrial CA:* 400–1000 mg/wk IM; ↓ in hepatic insuff **Caution:** [X, +] **Contra:** h/o thromboembolic disorders, hepatic Dz, PRG **Disp:** Tabs 2.5, 5, 10 mg; depo inj 150, 400 mg/mL; depo SQ inj 104 mg/0.65 mL **SE:** Breakthrough bleeding, spotting, altered menstrual flow, anorexia, edema, thromboembolic comps, depression, wt gain **Interactions:** ↓ Effects W/ aminoglutethimide, phenytoin, carbamazepine, phenobarbital, rifampin, rifabutin **NIPE:** Sunlight exposure may cause melasma; if GI upset take w/ food; perform breast exam & Pap smear before contraceptive therapy; obtain PRG test if last inj >3 mo

Megestrol Acetate (Megace) [Antineoplastic/Progestin]

Uses: *Breast/endometrial CAs; appetite stimulant in cachexia (CA & HIV)* **Action:** Hormone; progesterone analog **Dose:** *CA:* 40–320 mg/d PO in ÷ doses. *Appetite:* 800 mg/d PO ÷ dose **Caution:** [X, –] Thromboembolism **Contra:** PRG **Disp:** Tabs 20, 40 mg; soln 40 mg/mL; also available in 125 mg/mL (Megase ES) **SE:** DVT; edema, menstrual bleeding; photosens, insomnia, rash, ↓ BM **Interactions:** ↑ Effects OF warfarin **Labs:** ↑ LDH **NIPE:** ↑ Risk of photosensitivity—use sunscreen; do not D/C abruptly

Meloxicam (Mobic) [Analgesic/Anti-inflammatory/NSAIDs]

WARNING: May ↑ risk of cardiovascular events & GI bleeding **Uses:** *Osteoarthritis, RA, JRA* **Action:** NSAID w/ ↑ COX-2 activity **Dose:** *Adult.* 7.5–15 mg/d PO; *Peds (>2 y.)* 0.125 mg/kg/d, max 7.5 mg; ↓ in renal insuff; take w/ food **Caution:** [C, D (3rd tri) ?/–] Peptic ulcer, NSAID, or ASA sensitivity **Disp:** Tabs 7.5, 15 mg; susp. 7.5 mg/5 mL **SE:** HA, dizziness, GI upset, GI bleeding, edema **Interactions:** ↑ Effects OF ASA, anticoagulants, corticosteroids, Li, EtOH, tobacco; ↓ effects W/ cholestyramine; ↓ effects OF antihypertensives **Labs:** ↑ LFTs, BUN, Cr; ↓ HMG, WBCs, plat; **NIPE:** Take w/ food, may take several days for full effect

Melphalan [L-PAM] (Alkeran) [Antineoplastic/Alkylating Agent]

WARNING: Administered under the supervision of a qualified health care provider experienced in the use of chemotherapy; severe BM depression, leukemogenic, & mutagenic **Uses:** *Multiple myeloma, ovarian CAs*, breast & testicular CA, melanoma; allogenic & ABMT (high dose) **Action:** Bifunctional alkylating agent **Dose:** (Per protocol) 6 mg/d or 0.15–0.25 mg/kg/d for 4–7 d, repeat 4–6-wk intervals, or 1 mg/kg × 1 q4–6wk; 0.15 mg/kg/d for 5 d q6wk. *High-dose high-risk multiple myeloma:* Single dose 140 mg/m². *ABMT:* 140–240 mg/m² IV; ↓ in renal insuff **Caution:** [D, ?] **Contra:** Allergy or resistance **Disp:** Tabs 2 mg; inj 50 mg **SE:** ↓ BM, secondary leukemia, alopecia, dermatitis, stomatitis, & pulm fibrosis; rare allergic Rxns **Interactions:** ↑ Risk *OF* nephrotox *W/* cisplatin, cyclosporine; ↓ effects *W/* cimetidine, interferon alfa **Labs:** ↓ HMG, RBCs, WBCs, plt **NIPE:** ↑ Fluids, ⊘ PRG, breast-feeding; take PO on empty stomach.

Memantine (Namenda) [Anti-Alzheimer Agent/NMDA Receptor Antagonist]

Uses: *Moderate/severe Alzheimer Dz* **Action:** *N*-methyl-D-aspartate receptor antagonist **Dose:** Target 20 mg/d, start 5 mg/d, ↑ 5 mg/d to 20 mg/d, wait >1 wk before ↑ dose; use ÷ doses if >5mg/d **Caution:** [B, ?/–] Hepatic/mild–moderate renal impair **Disp:** Tabs 5, 10 mg, combo pack: 5 mg × 28 + 10 mg × 21; sol 2 mg/mL **SE:** Dizziness **Interactions:** ↑ Effects *W/* amantadine, carbonic anhydrase inhibitors, dextromethorphan, ketamine, Na bicarbonate; ↑ effects *W/* any drug, herb, food that alkalinizes urine **Labs:** Monitor BUN, SCr **NIPE:** Take w/o regard to food; EtOH ↑ adverse effects & ↓ effectiveness; renal clearance ↓ by alkaline urine (↓ 80% @ pH 8)

Meningococcal conjugate vaccine (Menactra) [Vaccine/Live]

Uses: *Immunize against N. meningitidis* (meningococcus)* **Action:** Active immunization; diphtheria toxoid conjugate of *N. meningitidis* A, C, Y, W-135 **Dose:** *Adults. 18–55 y:* 0.5 mL IM × 1 *Peds. 11–18 y:* 0.5 mL IM × 1 **Caution:** [C, ?/–] **Contra:** Allergy to class/compound/latex; w/ acute Infxn **Disp:** ↓ Inj **SE:** Local inj site Rxns, HA, fatigue, arthralgia, Guillain–Barré **Interactions:** ↓ Effects *W/* immunoglobulin if admin. w/in 1 mo **NIPE:** Pain & inflammation at inj site; keep epi (1:1000) available for anaphylactic/allergic Rxns; use polysaccharide >55 y

Meningococcal Polysaccharide Vaccine (Menomune A/C/Y/ W-135)

Uses: *Immunize against N. meningitidis* **Action:** Active immunization **Dose:** Adults & Peds >2 y: 0.5 mL SQ (not IM, intradermally, IV) may repeat 3–5 y if high risk **Caution:** [C, ?/–] **Contra:** Thimerosal/latex/sensitivity; w/ pertussis or typhoid vaccine, <2 y **Disp:** Inj **SE:** Local inj site Rxns, HA **NIPE:** Preferred in >55 y, conjugate vaccine (Menactra) in 11–55 y; active against serotypes A, C, Y, & W-135; not group B; keep epi (1:1000) available for Rxns

Meperidine (Demerol) [C–II] [Opioid Analgesic]

Uses: *Moderate–severe pain* **Action:** Narcotic analgesic **Dose:** *Adults.* 50–150 mg PO or IM/SQ q3–4h PRN. *Peds.* 1–1.5 mg/kg/dose PO or IM/SQ q3–4h PRN, up to 100 mg/dose; ↓ in elderly/renal impair **Caution:** [C/D (prolonged use or high dose at term), +] ↓ Sz threshold **Contra:** w/ MAOIs, renal failure **Disp:** Tabs 50, 100 mg; syrup 50 mg/5 mL; inj 10, 25, 50, 75, 100 mg/mL **SE:** Resp depression, Szs, sedation, constipation **Interactions:** ↑ Effects *W/* antihistamines, barbiturates, cimetidine,

MAOIs, neuroleptics, selegiline, TCAs, St. John's wort, EtOH; ↑ effects *OF* INH; ↓ effects *W/* phenytoin **Labs:** ↑ Serum amylase, lipase **NIPE:** Analgesic effects potentiated w/ hydroxyzine; 75 mg IM = 10 mg morphine IM

Meprobamate (Equinil, Miltown) [C-IV] [Antianxiety] Uses: *Short-term relief from anxiety* **Action:** Mild tranquilizer; antianxiety **Dose: Adults.** 400 mg PO tid–qid, max 2400 mg/d **Peds 6–12 y.** 100–200 mg bid–tid; ↓ in renal/liver impair **Caution:** [D, +/–] **Contra:** NAG, porphyria, PRG **Disp:** Tabs 200, 400 mg **SE:** Drowsiness, syncope, tachycardia, edema **Interactions:** ↑ Effects *W/* antihistamines, barbiturates, CNS depressants, narcotics, EtOH

Mercaptopurine [6-MP] (Purinethol) [Antineoplastic/Antimetabolite] Uses: *Acute leukemias*, 2nd-line Rx of CML & NHL, maint ALL in children, immunosuppressant w/ autoimmune Dzs (Crohn Dz) **Action:** Antimetabolite, mimics hypoxanthine **Dose: Adult.** 80–100 mg/m²/d or 2.5–5 mg/kg/d; maint 1.5–2.5 mg/kg/d; w/ allopurinol use 67–75% ↓ dose of 6-MP (interference w/ xanthine oxidase metabolism) **Peds.** Per protocol ↓ w/ renal/hepatic insuff; on empty stomach **Caution:** [D, ?] **Contra:** Severe hepatic Dz, BM suppression, PRG **Disp:** Tabs 50 mg **SE:** Mild hematotox, mucositis, stomatitis, D rash, fever, eosinophilia, jaundice, hepatitis **Interactions:** ↑ Effects *W/* allopurinol; ↑ risk of BM suppression *W/* trimethoprim-sulfamethoxazole; ↓ effects *OF* warfarin **Labs:** False ↑ serum glucose, uric acid; ↑ LFTs; ↓ HMG, RBCs, WBC, plt **NIPE:** ↑ Fluid intake to 2–3 L/d, may take 4+ wk for improvement; handle properly; limit use to experienced health care providers

Meropenem (Merrem) [Antibiotic/Carbapenem] Uses: *Intra-abd Infxns, bacterial meningitis* **Action:** Carbapenem; ↓ cell wall synth, a β-lactam. *Spectrum:* Excellent gram(+) (except MRSA & *E. faecium*); excellent gram(–) including extended-*Spectrum* β-lactamase producers; good anaerobic **Dose: Adults.** 1 to 2 g IV q8h. **Peds.** >3 mo, <50 kg 10–40 mg/kg IV q 8h; ↓ in renal insuff **Caution:** [B, ?] **Contra:** β-lactam sensitivity **Disp:** Inj 1 g, 500 mg **SE:** Less Sz potential than imipenem; D, thrombocytopenia **Interactions:** ↑ Effects *W/* probenecid **Labs:** ↑ LFTs, BUN, Cr, eosinophils ↓ HMG, Hct, WBCs, plt **NIPE:** Monitor for super Infxn; overuse ↑ bacterial resistance

Mesalamine (Asacol, Lialda, Pentasa, Rowasa) [Anti-inflammatory/Salicylate] Uses: *Mild–moderate distal ulcerative colitis, proctosigmoiditis, proctitis* **Action:** Unknown; may inhibit prostaglandins **Dose:** *Rectal:* 60 mL qhs, retain 8 h (enema), 500 mg bid–tid or 1000 mg qhs (supp) *PO:* Cap: 1 g PO qid, *Tab:* 1.6–2.4 g/d ÷ doses (tid–qid); delayed release 2.4–4.8 g PO daily 8 wk max, do not cut/crush/chew w/ food; ↓ initial dose in elderly **Caution:** [B, M] **Contra:** Salicylate sensitivity **Disp:** Tabs 400 mg; caps 250, 500 mg; delayed release tab (Lialda) 1.2 g; supp 500, 1000 mg; rectal susp 4 g/60 mL **SE:** HA, malaise, abd pain, flatulence, rash, pancreatitis, pericarditis **Interactions:** ↓ Effect *OF* digoxin **Labs:** ↑ LFTs, amylase, lipase; **NIPE:** May discolor urine yellow-brown

Mesna (Mesnex) [Uroprotectant/Antidote] Uses: *Prevent hemorrhagic cystitis due to ifosfamide or cyclophosphamide* Action: Antidote, reacts with acrolein and other metabolites to form stable compounds Dose: Per protocol; dose as % of ifosfamide or cyclophosphamide dose *IV bolus:* 20% (eg, 10–12 mg/kg) IV at 0, 4, 8 h, then 40% at 0, 1, 4, 7 h; *IV inf:* 20% prechemo, 50–100% w/ chemo, then 25–50% for 12 h following chemo; *Oral:* 20% IV dose at 0, 4, 8 h (mix with juice) Caution: [B; ?/–] Contra: Thiol sensitivity Disp: Inj 100 mg/mL; tabs 400 mg SE: ↓ BP, allergic Rxns, HA, GI upset, taste perversion Labs: ↑ LFTs NIPE: Hydration helps ↓ hemorrhagic cystitis; higher dose for BMT

Mesoridazine (Serentil) [Antipsychotic/Phenothiazine] WARNING: Can prolong QT interval in dose-related fashion; torsades de pointes reported Uses: *Schizophrenia*, acute & chronic alcoholism, chronic brain synd Action: Phenothiazine antipsychotic Dose: Initial, 25–50 mg PO or IV tid; ↑ to 300–400 mg/d max Caution: [C, ?/–] Contra: Phenothiazine sensitivity, coadministration w/ drugs that cause QTc prolongation, CNS depression Disp: Tabs 10, 25, 50, 100 mg; PO conc 25 mg/mL; inj 25 mg/mL SE: Low incidence of EPS; ↓ BP, xerostomia, constipation, skin discoloration, tachycardia, lowered Sz threshold, blood dyscrasias, pigmentary retinopathy at high doses Interactions: ↑ Effects *W/* antimalarials, BBs, chloroquine, TCAs, EtOH; ↑ effects *OF* antidepressants, nitrates, antihypertensives; ↑ QT interval *W/* amiodarone, azole antifungals, disopyramide, fluoxetine, macrolides, paroxetine, procainamide, quinidine, quinolones, TCAs, verapamil; ↓ effects *W/* attapulgite, barbiturates, caffeine, tobacco; ↓ effects of barbiturates, guanethidine, guanadrel, levodopa, Li, sympathomimetics Labs: False + PRG test; ↑ serum glucose, cholesterol; ↓ uric acid NIPE: Photosensitivity—use sunscreen

Metaproterenol (Alupent, Metaprel) [Bronchodilator/Beta-Adrenergic Agonist] Uses: *Asthma & reversible bronchospasm* Action: Sympathomimetic bronchodilator Dose: *Adults.* Inhal: 1–3 inhal q3–4h, 12 inhal max/24 h; wait 2 min between inhal. *PO:* 20 mg q6–8h. *Peds.* Inhal: 0.5 mg/kg/dose, 15 mg/dose max inhaled q4–6h by neb or 1–2 puffs q4–6h. *PO:* 0.3–0.5 mg/kg/dose q6–8h Caution: [C, ?/–] Contra: Tachycardia, other arrhythmias Disp: Aerosol 0.65 mg/inhal; soln for inhal 0.4%, 0.6%; tabs 10, 20 mg; syrup 10 mg/5 mL SE: Nervousness, tremor, tachycardia, HTN Interactions: ↑ Effects *W/* sympathomimetic drugs, xanthines; ↑ risk *OF* arrhythmias *W/* cardiac glycosides, halothane, levodopa, theophylline, thyroid hormones; ↑ HTN *W/* MAOIs; ↓ effects *W/* BBs NIPE: Separate additional aerosol use by 5 min; fewer β₁ effects than isoproterenol & longer acting

Metaxalone (Skelaxin) [Skeletal Muscle Relaxant] Uses: *Painful musculoskeletal conditions* Action: Centrally acting skeletal muscle relaxant Dose: 800 mg PO tid–qid Caution: [C, ?/–] Anemia Contra: Severe hepatic/renal impair Disp: Tabs 400, 800 mg SE: N/V, HA, drowsiness, hepatitis Interactions: ↑ Sedating effects *W/* CNS depressants, EtOH Labs: False + urine glucose using Benedict test

Metformin (Glucophage, Glucophage XR) [Hypoglycemic/ Biguanide] WARNING: Associated w/ lactic acidosis Uses: *Type 2 DM* Action: ↓ Hepatic glucose production & intestinal absorption of glucose; ↑ insulin sensitivity Dose: *Adults.* *Initial:* 500 mg PO bid; or 850 mg daily, may ↑ to 2550 mg/d max; take w/ AM & PM meals; can convert total daily dose to daily dose of XR *Peds 10–16 y.* 500 mg PO bid, ↑ 500 mg/wk to 2000 mg/d max in ÷ doses; do not use XR formulation in peds Caution: [B, +/–] avoid EtOH; hold dose before & 48 h after ionic contrast Contra: SCr >1.4 in females or >1.5 in males; hypoxemic conditions (eg acute CHF/sepsis) Disp: Tabs 500, 850, 1000 mg; XR tabs 500, 750, 1000 mg SE: Anorexia, N/V, rash, lactic acidosis (rare, but serious) Interactions: ↑ Effects W/ amiloride, cimetidine, digoxin, furosemide, MAOIs, morphine, procainamide, quinidine, quinine, ranitidine, triamterene, trimethoprim, vancomycin; ↓ effects W/ corticosteroids, CCBs, diuretics, estrogens, INH, OCPs, phenothiazine, phenytoin, sympathomimetics, thyroid drugs, tobacco Labs: Monitor LFTs, BUN/Cr, serum vitamin B_{12} NIPE: Take w/ food; ⊘ dehydration, EtOH, before surgery

Methadone (Dolophine) [C-II] [Opioid Analgesic] WARNING: Deaths, cardiac and respiratory have been reported during initiation and conversion of pain patients to methadone treatment from treatment with other opioids Uses: *Severe pain; detox w/ maint of narcotic addiction* Action: Narcotic analgesic Dose: *Adults.* 2.5–10 mg IM q3–8h or 5–15 mg PO q8h; titrate as needed *Peds.* 0.7 mg/kg/24 h PO or IM ÷ q8h; ↑ slowly to avoid resp depression; ↓ in renal impair Caution: [B/D (prolonged use/high doses at term), + (w/ doses =/> 20 mg/24 h)], severe liver Dz Disp: Tabs 5, 10, 40 mg; PO soln 5, 10 mg/5 mL; PO conc 10 mg/mL; inj 10 mg/mL SE: Resp depression, sedation, constipation, urinary retention, ↑ QT interval, arrhythmias Interactions: ↑ Effects W/ cimetidine, CNS depressants, protease inhibitors; EtOH; ↑ effects OF anticoagulants, EtOH, antihistamines, barbiturates, glutethimide, methocarbamol; ↓ effects W/ carbamazepine, nelfinavir, phenobarbital, phenytoin, primidone, rifampin, ritonavir Labs: ↑ Serum amylase, lipase, LFTs NIPE: Equianalgesic w/ parenteral morphine; longer 1/2-life

Methenamine (Hiprex, Urex, Others) [Urinary Anti-infective] Uses: *Suppress/eliminate bacteriuria associated w/ chronic/recurrent UTI* Action: Converted to formaldehyde & ammonia in acidic urine; nonspecific bactericidal action Dose: *Adults.* *Hippurate:* 0.5–1 g bid. *Mandelate:* 1 g qid PO pc & hs *Peds 6–12 y.* *Hippurate:* 25–50 mg/kg/d PO ÷ bid. *Mandelate:* 50–75 mg/kg/d PO ÷ qid (take w/ food, ascorbic acid w/ adequate hydration) Caution: [C, +] Contra: Renal insuff, severe hepatic Dz, & severe dehydration; sulfonamide allergy Disp: *Methenamine hippurate* (Hiprex, Urex): Tabs 1 g. *Methenamine mandelate:* 500 mg, 1g EC tabs SE: Rash, GI upset, dysuria, ↑ LFTs Interactions: ↓ Effects W/ acetazolamide, antacids Labs: ↑ LFTs NIPE: ↑ Fluids to 2–3 L/d; take w/ food

Methimazole (Tapazole) [Antithyroid Agent] Uses: *Hyperthyroidism, thyrotoxicosis*, prep for thyroid surgery or radiation **Action:** Blocks T_3 & T_4 formation **Dose:** *Adults.* Initial: 15–60 mg/d PO ÷ tid. Maint: 5–15 mg PO daily. *Peds.* Initial: 0.4–0.7 mg/kg/24 h PO ÷ tid. Maint: 1/3–2/3 of initial dose PO daily; w/ food **Caution:** [D, +/–] **Contra:** Breast-feeding **Disp:** Tabs 5, 10, 20 mg **SE:** GI upset, dizziness, blood dyscrasias **Interactions:** ↑ Effects OF digitalis glycosides, metoprolol, propranolol; ↓ effects OF anticoagulants, theophylline; ↓ effects W/ amiodarone **Labs:** ↑ LFTs, PT; follow clinically & w/ TFT **NIPE:** Take w/ food

Methocarbamol (Robaxin) [Skeletal Muscle Relaxant/Centrally Acting] Uses: *Relief of discomfort associated w/ painful musculoskeletal conditions* **Action:** Centrally acting skeletal muscle relaxant **Dose:** *Adults.* 1.5 g PO qid for 2–3 d, then 1-g PO qid maint therapy; IV form rarely indicated. *Peds.* 15 mg/kg/dose IV, may repeat PRN (OK for tetanus only), max 1.8 g/m²/d for 3 d **Caution:** [C, +] **Contra:** MyG, renal impair **Disp:** Tabs 500, 750 mg; inj 100 mg/mL **SE:** Can discolor urine; drowsiness; GI upset **Interactions:** ↑ Effects W/ CNS depressant, EtOH **Labs:** ↑ Urine 5-HIAA **NIPE:** Monitor for blurred vision, orthostatic hypotension

Methotrexate (Rheumatrex Dose Pack, Trexall) [Antineoplastic, Antirheumatic (DMARDs), Immunosuppressant/Antimetabolite] WARNING: Administration only by experienced health care provider; do not use in women of childbearing age unless absolutely necessary (teratogenic); impaired elimination w/ impaired renal Fxn, ascites, pleural effusion; severe myelosuppression if used with NSAIDs; hepatotox; can induce lung disease; D and ulcerative stomatitis require D/C; lymphoma risk; may cause tumor lysis synd; can cause severe skin Rxn, opportunistic infns; with RT can ↑ risk of tissue necrosis Uses: *ALL, AML, leukemic meningitis, trophoblastic tumors (choriocarcinoma, chorioadenoma, hydatidiform mole), breast, lung, head & neck CAs, Burkitt lymphoma, mycosis fungoides, osteosarcoma, Hodgkin Dz & NHL, psoriasis; RA* **Action:** ↓ Dihydrofolate reductase-mediated production of tetrahydrofolate **Dose:** *CA:* Per protocol. *RA:* 7.5 mg/wk PO 1/wk 1 or 2.5 mg q12h PO for 3 doses/wk; ↓ in renal/hepatic impair **Caution:** [D, –] **Contra:** Severe renal/hepatic impair, PRG/lactation **Disp:** Dose pack: 2.5 mg in 8, 12, 16, 20, or 24 doses; tabs 2.5 mg, 10 mg; inj 25 mg/mL **SE:** ↓ BM, N/V/D, anorexia, mucositis, hepatotox (transient & reversible; may progress to atrophy, necrosis, fibrosis, cirrhosis), rashes, dizziness, malaise, blurred vision, alopecia, photosens, renal failure, pneumonitis; rare pulm fibrosis; chemical arachnoiditis & HA w/ IT delivery **Notes:** Systemic levels *Therapeutic:* >0.01 μmole; *Toxic* >10 μmole over 24h **Interactions:** ↑ Effects W/ chloramphenicol, cyclosporine, etretinate, NSAIDs, phenylbutazone, phenytoin, penicillin, probenecid, salicylates, sulfonamides, sulfonylureas, EtOH; ↑ effects OF cyclosporine, tetracycline, theophylline; ↑ effects W/ antimalarials, aminoglycosides, binding resins, cholestyramine, folic acid;

↓ effects *OF* digoxin **Labs:** Monitor CBC, LFTs, Cr, MTX levels & CXR **NIPE:** "High dose" >500 mg/m^2 requires leucovorin rescue to ↓ tox; w/ intrathecal, use preservative-free/alcohol-free soln; ↑ risk *OF* photosensitivity—use sunscreen, ↑ fluids 2–3 L/d

Methyldopa (Aldomet) [Antihypertensive/Centrally Acting Antiadrenergic] Uses: *HTN* **Action:** Centrally acting antihypertensive **Dose:** *Adults.* 250–500 mg PO bid–tid (max 2–3 g/d) or 250 mg–1 g IV q6–8h. *Peds.* 10 mg/kg/24 h PO in 2–3 ÷ doses (max 40 mg/kg/24 h ÷ q6–12h) or 5–10 mg/kg/dose IV q6–8h to total dose of 20–40 mg/kg/24 h; ↓ in renal insuff/elderly **Caution:** [B (PO), C (IV), +] **Contra:** Liver Dz; MAOIs **Disp:** Tabs 125, 250, 500 mg; inj 50 mg/mL **SE:** Discolors urine; initial transient sedation/drowsiness frequent, edema, hemolytic anemia, hepatic disorders **Interactions:** ↑ Effects *W/* anesthetics, diuretics, levodopa, Li, methotrimeprazine, thioxanthenes, vasodilators, verapamil; ↑ effects *OF* haloperidol, Li, tolbutamide; ↓ effects *W/* amphetamines, Fe, phenothiazine, TCAs; ↓ effects *OF* ephedrine **Labs:** ↑ BUN, Cr; ↓ LFTs, HMG, RBC, WBC, plt **NIPE:** After 1–2 mo tolerance may develop

Methylergonovine (Methergine) [Oxytocic/Ergot Alkaloid] Uses: *Postpartum bleeding (uterine subinvolution)* **Action:** Ergotamine derivative **Dose:** 0.2 mg IM after placental delivery, may repeat 2–4-h intervals or 0.2–0.4 mg PO q6–12h for 2–7 d **Caution:** [C, ?] **Contra:** HTN, PRG **Disp:** Injectable 0.2 mg/mL; tabs 0.2 mg **SE:** HTN, N/V **Interactions:** ↑ Vasoconstriction *W/* ergot alkaloids, sympathomimetics, tobacco **NIPE:** ⊘ Smoking; give IV over >1 min w/ BP monitoring

Methylphenidate, Oral (Concerta, Ritalin, Ritalin SR, Others) [CII] [CNS Stimulant/Piperidine Derivative] WARNING: w/ h/o of drug or alcohol dependence; chronic use can lead to dependence or psychotic behavior; observe closely during withdrawal of drug Uses: *ADHD, narcolepsy* *depression* **Action:** CNS stimulant **Dose:** *Adults. Narcolepsy:* 10 mg PO 2–3 ×/d, 60 mg/d max. *Depression:* 2.5 mg qAM; ↑ slowly, 20 mg/d max; use regular release only *Peds.* Based on product; initial total daily dose of 15–20 mg; 90 mg/d max; administer once (ER/SR) or bid (regular) **Caution:** [C,+/–] h/o alcoholism or drug abuse; separate from MAOIs by 14 d **Disp:** Tabs 5, 10, 20 mg; Tabs SR (Ritalin SR) 20 mg; ER tabs (Concerta) 18, 27, 36, 54 mg **SE:** CV, CNS stimulation **Interactions:** ↑ Risk of hypertensive crisis *W/* MAOIs; ↑ effects *OF* anticonvulsants, anticoagulants, TCA, SSRIs; ↓ effects *OF* guanethidine, antihypertensives **Labs:** Monitor CBC, plts **NIPE:** Titrate dose; take 30–45 min before meals; do not chew or crush; concerta "ghost tablet" may appear in stool; see insert to convert to ER dose; see also transdermal methylphenidate; abuse and diversion concerns; D/C if Sz or agitation occurs

Methylphenidate, transdermal (Daytrana) [CII] [CNS Stimulant] WARNING: w/ h/o of drug or alcohol dependence; chronic use can lead to dependence or psychotic behavior; observe closely during withdrawal of drug

Uses: *ADHD in children 6–12 y* **Action:** CNS stimulant **Dose:** *Peds.* Apply to hip in AM (2 h before desired effect), remove 9 h later **Caution:** [C,+/–] sensitization may preclude subsequent use of oral forms; abuse and oral concerns **Disp:** Patches 10, 15, 20, 30 mg **SE:** Local Rxns, stimulation **Interactions:** ↑ Effects *OF* oral anticoagulants, phenobarbital, phenytoin, primidone, SSRIs, TCAs; ↑ risk *OF* hypertensive crisis *W/* MAOIs; caution *W/* pressor drugs **NIPE:** Titrate dose in weekly increments; effects last several hours following removal; rotate application sites; ⊘ expose patches to direct external sources of heat; eval BP, HR at baseline and periodically

Methylprednisolone (Solu-Medrol) [See Steroids and Table 3]

Metoclopramide (Reglan, Clopra, Octamide) [Antiemetic/ Dopamine Antagonist] **Uses:** *Diabetic gastroparesis, symptomatic GERD; chemo N/V, facilitate small-bowel intubation & UGI radiologic eval* stimulate gut in prolonged postop ileus **Action:** ↑ UGI motility; blocks dopamine in chemoreceptor trigger zone **Dose:** *Adults. Gastroparesis:* 10 mg PO 30 min ac & hs for 2–8 wk PRN, or same dose IV for 10 d, then PO. *Reflux:* 10–15 mg PO 30 min ac & hs. *Antiemetic:* 1–3 mg/kg/dose IV 30 min before chemo, then q2h × 2 doses, then q3h × 3 doses. *Peds. Reflux:* 0.1 mg/kg/dose PO qid. *Antiemetic:* 1–2 mg/kg/dose IV as adults **Caution:** [B, –] Drugs w/ extrapyramidal ADRs **Contra:** Sz disorders, GI obst **Disp:** Tabs 5, 10 mg; syrup 5 mg/5 mL; inj 5 mg/mL **SE:** Dystonic Rxns common w/ high doses, (Rx w/ IV diphenhydramine); restlessness, D, drowsiness **Interactions:** ↑ Risk *OF* serotonin synd *W/* sertraline, venlafaxine; ↑ effects *OF* acetaminophen, ASA, CNS depressants, cyclosporine, levodopa, Li, succinylcholine, tetracyclines, EtOH; ↓ effects *W/* anticholinergics, narcotics; ↓ effects *OF* cimetidine, digoxin **Labs:** ↑ Serum ALT, AST, amylase **NIPE:** Monitor for extrapyramidal effects

Metolazone (Mykrox, Zaroxolyn) [Antihypertensive/Thiazide Diuretic] **Uses:** *Mild–moderate essential HTN & edema of renal Dz or cardiac failure* **Action:** Thiazide-like diuretic; ↓ distal tubule Na reabsorption **Dose:** *Adult. HTN:* 2.5–5 mg/d PO (Zaroxolyn), 0.5–1 mg/d PO (Mykrox) *Edema:* 2.5–20 mg/d PO. *Peds.* 0.2–0.4 mg/kg/d PO ÷ q12h–daily **Caution:** [D, +] **Contra:** Thiazide/sulfonamide sensitivity, anuria **Disp:** Tabs: Mykrox (rapid acting) 0.5 mg, Zaroxolyn 2.5, 5, 10 mg **SE:** Monitor fluid/lytes; dizziness, ↓ BP, tachycardia, CP, photosens **Notes:** Mykrox & Zaroxolyn not bioequivalent **Interactions:** ↑ Effects *W/* antihypertensives, barbiturates, narcotics, nitrates, EtOH, food; ↑ effects *OF* digoxin, Li; ↑ hyperglycemia *W/* BBs, diazoxide; ↑ hypokalemia *W/* amphotericin B, corticosteroids, mezlocillin, piperacillin, ticarcillin; ↓ effects *W/* cholestyramine, colestipol, hypoglycemics, insulin, NSAIDs, salicylates; ↓ effects *OF* methenamine **Labs:** ↑ Serum and urine glucose, serum cholesterol, triglycerides, uric acid; ↓ K⁺, NA⁺, Mg⁺ **NIPE:** ↑ Risk of photosensitivity—use sunscreen; ↑ risk of gout; monitor electrolytes

Metoprolol (Lopressor, Toprol XL) [Antihypertensive/BB]

WARNING: Do not acutely stop therapy as marked worsening of angina can result **Uses:** *HTN, angina, AMI, CHF* **Action:** β-adrenergic receptor blocker **Dose:** *Adult. Angina:* 50–200 mg PO bid max 400 mg/d *HTN:* 50–200 mg PO bid max 450 mg/d. *AMI:* 5 mg IV q2min × 3 doses, then 50 mg PO q6h × 48 h, then 100 mg PO bid. *CHF:* 12–25 mg/d PO × 2 wk, ↑ at 2-wk intervals to 200 mg/max, use low dose in pts w/ greatest severity; 5 mg slow IV q5min, total 15 mg *(ECC 2005)*; ↓ in hepatic failure; take w/ meals **Caution:** [C, +] Uncompensated CHF, bradycardia, heart block **Contra:** Arrhythmia w/ tachycardia **Disp:** Tabs 25, 50, 100 mg; ER tabs 25, 50, 100, 200 mg; inj 1 mg/mL **SE:** Drowsiness, insomnia, ED, bradycardia, bronchospasm **Interactions:** ↑ Effects *W/* cimetidine, dihydropy- ridine, diltiazem, fluoxetine, hydralazine, methimazole, OCPs, propylthiouracil, quinidine, quinolones; ↑ effects *OF* hydralazine; ↑ bradycardia *W/* digoxin, dipyri- damole, verapamil; ↓ effects *W/* barbiturates, NSAIDs, rifampin; ↓ effects *OF* iso- proterenol, theophylline **Labs:** ↑ BUN, SCr, LFTs, uric acid **NIPE:** Take w/ food, ⊘ D/C abruptly—withdraw over 2 wk

Metronidazole (Flagyl, MetroGel) [Antibacterial, Antiproto- zoals]

WARNING: Carcinogenic in rats **Uses:** *Bone/joint, endocarditis, intra-abd, meningitis, & skin Infxns; amebiasis; trichomoniasis; bacterial vaginosis; PID; giardiasis; pseudomembranous colitis (C. difficile)* **Action:** Interferes w/ DNA synth. *Spectrum:* Excellent anaerobic *C. difficile,* also *H. pylori* in combo therapy **Dose:** *Adults. Anaerobic Infxns:* 500 mg IV q6–8h. *Amebic dysentery:* 750 mg/d PO for 5–10 d. *Trichomoniasis:* 250 mg PO tid for 7 d or 2 g PO × 1. *C. diffi- cile:* 500 mg PO or IV q8h for 7–10 d (PO preferred; IV only if pt NPO). *Vaginosis:* 1 applicatorful intravag bid or 500 mg PO bid for 7 d. *Acne rosacea/skin:* Apply bid. *Peds.* 30 mg/ kg PO/IV/d divided q6H, 4 g/d max÷. *Amebic dysentery:* 35–50 mg/kg/24 h PO in 3 ÷ doses for 5–10 d; Rx 7–10 d for *C. difficile;* ↓ in hepatic im- pair **Caution:** [B, M] Avoid EtOH **Contra:** 1st tri of PRG **Disp:** Tabs 250, 500 mg; XR tabs 750 mg; caps 375 mg; IV 500 mg/100mL; topical lotion & gel 0.75%; in- travag gel 0.75% (5 g/applicator 37.5 mg in 70-g tube), cream 1% **SE:** Disulfiram-like Rxn; dizziness, HA, GI upset, anorexia, urine discoloration **Interactions:** ↑ Effects *W/* cimetidine; ↑ effects *OF* carbamazepine, fluorouracil, Li, warfarin; ↓ effects *W/* barbiturates, cholestyramine, colestipol, phenytoin **Labs:** May cause ↓/zero values for LFTs, triglycerides, glucose **NIPE:** Take w/ food, possible metallic taste; for trichomoniasis, Rx pt's partner; no aerobic bacteria activity; use in combo w/ seri- ous mixed Infxns

Mexiletine (Mexitil) [Antiarrhythmic/Lidocaine Analogue]

WARNING: Mortality risks noted for flecainide and/or enceinte (type 1 antiar- rhythmias). Reserve for use in patients with life-threatening Ventricular Arrhythmias **Uses:** *Suppress symptomatic ventricular arrhythmias;* diabetic neuropathy **Ac- tion:** Class IB antiarrhythmic (Table 10) **Dose:** *Adults.* 200–300 mg PO q8h; 1200 mg/d max. *Peds.* 2.5–5 mg/kg PO q8h; w/ food or antacids **Caution:** [C, +] May worsen severe arrhythmias; interacts w/ hepatic inducers & suppressors (dosage changes) **Contra:** Cardiogenic shock or 2nd-/3rd-degree AV block w/o pacemaker **Disp:** Caps 150, 200, 250 mg **SE:** Lightheadedness, dizziness, anxiety, incoordination, GI upset, ataxia, hepatic damage, blood dyscrasias; **Interactions:** ↑ Effects **W/** fluvoxamine, quinidine, caffeine; ↑ effects **OF** theophylline; ↓ effects **W/** atropine, hydantoins, phenytoin, phenobarbital, rifampin, tobacco **Labs:** ↑ LFTs; ↓ plts; monitor LFTs & CBC **NIPE:** Take w/ food < GI upset

Miconazole (Monistat, others) [Antifungal] Uses: *Candidal Infxns, dermatomycoses (various tinea forms)* **Action:** Fungicide; alters fungal membrane permeability **Dose:** Apply to area bid for 2–4 wk. *Intravag:* 1 applicatorful or supp hs for 3 d (4% or 200 mg) or 7 d (2% or 100 mg) **Caution:** [C, ?] Azole sensitivity **Disp:** Topical cream 2%; lotion 2%; powder 2%; spray 2%; vag supp 100, 200 mg; vag cream 2%, 4% [OTC] **SE:** Vag burning **Interactions:** ↑ Effects **OF** anticoagulants, cisapride, loratadine, phenytoin, quinidine; ↓ effects **W/** amphotericin B; ↓ effects **OF** amphotericin B **Labs:** ↑ Protein **NIPE:** Antagonistic to amphotericin B in vivo

Miconazole/Zinc Oxide/Petrolatum (Vusion) [Antifungal] Uses: *Candidal diaper rash* **Action:** Combo antifungal **Dose:** *Peds > 4 wk.* Apply at each diaper change × 7d **Caution:** [C, ?] **Contra:** None **Disp:** Miconazole/zinc oxide/petrolatum oint 0.25%/81.35%/15% **SE:** None **NIPE:** Keep diaper dry

Midazolam (Hypnovel, Versed) [C-IV] [Sedative/Benzodiazepine] Uses: *Preop sedation, conscious sedation for short procedures & mechanically ventilated pts, induction of general anesthesia* **Action:** Short-acting benzodiazepine **Dose:** *Adults.* 1–5 mg IV or IM; titrate to effect. *Peds.* Preop: >6 mo 0.25–1 mg/kg PO, 20 mg max. *Conscious sedation:* 0.08 mg/kg × 1. >6 mo 0.1–0.15 mg/kg IM × 1 max 10 mg. *General anesthesia:* 0.025 –0.1 mg/kg IV q2min for 1–3 doses PRN to induce anesthesia (↓ in elderly, w/ narcotics or CNS depressants) **Caution:** [D, +/–] w/ CYP3A4 substrate (Table 11), multiple drug interactions **Contra:** NAG; w/ amprenavir, nelfinavir, ritonavir **Disp:** Inj 1, 5 mg/mL; syrup 2 mg/mL **SE:** Resp depression; ↓ BP w/ conscious sedation, N **Interactions:** ↑ Effects **W/** azole antifungals, antihistamines, cimetidine, CCBs, CNS depressants, erythromycin, INH, phenytoin, protease inhibitors, grapefruit juice, EtOH; ↓ effects **W/** rifampin, tobacco; ↓ effects **OF** levodopa **NIPE:** Monitor for resp depression; reversal w/ flumazenil

Mifepristone [RU 486] (Mifeprex) [Abortifacient/Synthetic Steroid] **WARNING:** Pt counseling & information required; associated w/ fatal Infxns & bleeding Uses: *Terminate intrauterine PRGs of <49 d* **Action:** Antiprogestin; ↑ prostaglandins, results in uterine contraction **Dose:** Administered w/ 3 office visits: day 1, three 200-mg tabs PO; day 3 if no abortion, two 200-mg tabs PO; on or about day 14, verify termination of PRG **Caution:** [X, –] **Contra**

Anticoagulation therapy, bleeding disorders **Disp:** Tabs 200 mg **SE:** Abd pain & 1–2 wk of uterine bleeding **Interactions:** ↑ Effects *W*/ azole antifungals, erythromycin, grapefruit juice; ↓ effects *W*/ carbamazepine, dexamethasone, phenytoin, phenobarbital, rifampin, St. John's wort **NIPE:** Give under supervision of health care provider only

Miglitol (Glyset) [Hypoglycemic/Alpha-Glucosidase Inhibitor] **Uses:** *Type 2 DM* **Action:** γ-Glucosidase inhibitor; delays digestion of carbohydrates **Dose:** Initial 25 mg PO tid; maint 50–100 mg tid (w/ 1st bite of each meal) **Caution:** [B, –] **Contra:** DKA, obst/inflammatory GI disorders; SCr >2 **Disp:** Tabs 25, 50, 100 mg **SE:** Flatulence, D, abd pain **Interactions:** ↑ Effects *W*/ celery, coriander, juniper berries, ginseng, garlic; ↓ effects w/ INH, niacin, intestinal absorbents, amylase, pancreatin ; ↓ effects *OF* digoxin, propranolol, ranitidine **Labs:** ⊘ Use w/ SCr >2 mg/dL **NIPE:** Use alone or w/ sulfonylureas

Milrinone (Primacor) [Vasodilator/Bipyridine Phosphodiesterase Inhibitor] **Uses:** *CHF*, Ca antagonist intoxication **Action:** Phosphodiesterase inhibitor, + inotrope & vasodilator; little chronotropic activity **Dose:** 50 µg/kg, then 0.375–0.75 µg/kg/min IV inf; ↓ in renal impair **Caution:** [C, ?] **Contra:** Allergy to drug; w/ amrinone **Disp:** Inj 200 µg/mL, 1 mg/mL **SE:** Arrhythmias, ↓ BP, HA **Interactions:** ↑ Hypotension *W*/ nesiritide **NIPE:** Monitor fluids, lytes, BP, HR

Mineral Oil [OTC] [Emollient Laxative] **Uses:** *Constipation* **Action:** Lubricant laxative **Dose:** *Adults.* 15–45 mL PO PRN. *Peds >6 y.* 5–25 mL PO qd **Caution:** [C, ?] N/V, difficulty swallowing, bedridden pts **Contra:** Colostomy/ileostomy, appendicitis, diverticulitis, UC **Disp:** Liq [OTC] **SE:** Lipid pneumonia **Interactions:** ↑ Effects *W*/ stool softeners; ↓ effects *OF* cardiac glycosides, OCPs, sulfonamides, vitamins, warfarin **NIPE:** Rectal incontinence

Minocycline (Solodyn) [Antibiotic/Tetracycline] **Uses:** *Acne* **Action:** Tetracycline, bacteriostatic **Dose:** *Adult and Peds >12 y* 1 mg/kg PO daily × 12wk; w/ food to ↓ irritation **Caution:** [C, ?] assoc w/ pseudomembranous colitis; w/ renal impair **Contra:** Allergy, women of childbearing potential **Disp:** Tabs ER 45, 90, 135 **SE:** D, HA, fever, rash, joint pain, fatigue, dizziness **Interactions:** ↑ Effects *W*/ digoxin, oral anticoagulants; ↑ risk of nephrotox *W*/ methoxyflurane; ↓ effects *W*/ antacids, cholestyramine, colestipol, laxatives, cimetidine, Fe products; ↓ effects *OF* hormonal contraceptives **Labs:** ↑ LFTs, BUN; ↓ HMG, plts, WBCs **NIPE:** Do not cut/crush/chew; keep away from children; risk of photosensitivity—use sunscreen; may take *W*/ food to < GI upset

Minoxidil (Loniten, Rogaine) [Antihypertensive/Vasodilator, Topical Hair Growth] **Uses:** *Severe HTN; male & female pattern baldness* **Action:** Peripheral vasodilator; stimulates vertex hair growth **Dose:** *Adults.* HTN: 2.5–80 mg PO ÷ daily–bid, max 100 mg/d. *Topical:* (Baldness)

Apply bid to area. **Peds.** 0.2–1 mg/kg/24 h ÷ PO q12–24h, max 50 mg/d; ↓ PO in elderly **Caution:** [C, +] **Contra:** Pheochromocytoma, component allergy **Disp:** Tabs 2.5, 5, 10 mg; topical soln (Rogaine) 2%, 5% **SE:** Pericardial effusion & volume overload w/ PO use; edema, ECG changes, wt gain **Interactions:** ↑ Hypotension **W/** guanethidine **Labs:** ↑ Alkaline phosphatase, BUN, Cr; ↓ HMG, Hct **NIPE:** Hypertrichosis w/ chronic use; take PO drug w/ food to < GI upset

Mirtazapine (Remeron, Remeron SolTab) [Tetracyclic Antidepressant] WARNING: Closely monitor for worsening depression or emergence of suicidality, particularly in ped pts **Uses:** *Depression* **Action:** α₂-antagonist antidepressant **Dose:** 15 mg PO hs, up to 45 mg/d hs **Caution:** [C, ?] w/ clonidine, CNS depressant use; CYP1A2, CYP3A4 inducers/inhibitors **Contra:** MAOIs w/in 14 d **Disp:** Tabs 15, 30, 45 mg; rapid dissolving tabs 15, 30, 45 mg **SE:** Somnolence, ↑ cholesterol, constipation, xerostomia, wt gain, agranulocytosis **Interactions:** ↑ Effects **W/** CNS depressants, fluvoxamine; ↑ risk **OF** HTN crisis **W/** MAOIs **Labs:** ↑ ALT, cholesterol, triglycerides **NIPE:** Handle rapid tabs with dry hands, do not cut or chew; Do not ↑ dose at intervals of less than 1–2 wk

Misoprostol (Cytotec) [Mucosal Protective Agent/Prostaglandin] WARNING: Use in PRG can cause abortion, premature birth, or birth defects; do not use to decrease ulcer risk in women of childbearing age **Uses:** *Prevent NSAID-induced gastric ulcers*; induce labor (cervical ripening); incomplete & therapeutic abortion **Action:** Prostaglandin (PGE-1), w/ antisecretory & mucosal protective properties; induces uterine contractions **Dose:** *Ulcer prevention:* 200 μg PO qid w/ meals; in females, start 2nd or 3rd day of next nl menstrual period; 25–50 μg for induction of labor (term); 400 μg on day 3 of mifepristone for PRG termination; take w/ food **Contra:** [X, –] **Contra:** PRG, component allergy **Disp:** Tabs 100, 200 μg **SE:** Can cause miscarriage w/ potentially dangerous bleeding; HA, GI common (D, abd pain, constipation) **Interactions:** ↑ HA & GI symptoms **W/** phenylbutazone

Mitomycin (Mutamycin) [Antineoplastic/Alkylating Agent] WARNING: Administer only by physician experienced in chemotherapy; myelosuppressive; can induce hemolytic uremic synd with irreversible renal failure **Uses:** *Stomach, pancreas*, breast, colon CA; squamous cell carcinoma of the anus; non-small-cell lung, head & neck, cervical; bladder CA (intravesically) **Action:** Alkylating agent; may generate oxygen-free radicals w/ DNA strand breaks **Dose:** Per protocol; 20 mg/m² q6–8wk or 10 mg/m² in combo w/ other myelosuppressive drugs; bladder CA 20–40 mg in 40 mL NS via a urethral catheter once/wk × 8 wk, followed by monthly × 12 mo for 1 y; ↓ in renal/hepatic impair **Caution:** [D, –] **Contra:** Thrombocytopenia, leukopenia, coagulation disorders, SCr >1.7 mg/dL **Disp:** Inj 5, 20, 40 mg **SE:** ↓ BM, (persists 3–8 wk after, may be cumulative; minimize w/ lifetime dose <50–60 mg/m²), N/V, anorexia, stomatitis, renal tox; microangiopathic hemolytic anemia w/ progressive renal failure (like hemolytic–uremic synd);

venoocclusive liver Dz, interstitial pneumonia, alopecia; extrav Rxns; contact dermatitis **Interactions:** ↑ Bronchospasm *W/* vinca alkaloids; ↑ BM suppression *W/* antineoplastics

Mitoxantrone (Novantrone) [Antineoplastic/Antibiotic]

WARNING: Administer only by health care provider experienced in chemotherapy; except for acute leukemia, do not use w/ ANC count of <1500 cells/mm³; severe neutropenia can result in Infxn, follow CBC; cardiotoxic (CHF), secondary AML reported **Uses:** *AML (w/ cytarabine), ALL, CML, PCA, MS, Lung CA* breast CA, & NHL **Action:** DNA-intercalating agent; ↓ DNA synth by interacting with topoisomerase II **Dose:** Per protocol; ↓ w/ hepatic impair, leukopenia, thrombocytopenia **Caution:** [D, –] Reports of secondary AML (monitor CBC) **Contra:** PRG, significant ↓ in LVEF **Disp:** Inj 2 mg/mL **SE:** ↓ BM, N/V, stomatitis, alopecia (infrequent), cardiotox, urine discoloration **Interactions:** ↑ BM suppression *W/* antineoplastics; ↓ effects *OF* live virus vaccines **Labs:** ↑ AST, ALT, uric acid **NIPE:** ↑ Fluids to 2–3 L/d, maintain hydration ⊘ vaccines, Infxn; cardiac monitoring prior to each dose

Modafinil (Provigil) [Analeptic/CNS Stimulant] Uses: * Improve wakefulness in pts w/ narcolepsy & excess daytime sleepiness* **Action:** Alters dopamine & norepinephrine release, ↓ GABA-mediated neurotransmission **Dose:** 200 mg PO q AM; ↓ dose 50% w/elderly/hepatic impair **Caution:** [C,?/–] CV Dz; **Contra:** Component allergy **Disp:** Tabs 100, 200 mg **SE:** HA, N, D, paresthesias, rhinitis, agitation **Interactions:** ↑ Effects *OF* CNS stimulants, diazepam, phenytoin, propranolol, TCAs, warfarin; ↓ effect *OF* cyclosporine, OCPs, theophylline **Labs:** ↑ Glucose, AST, GTT **NIPE:** Take w/o regard to food; monitor BP; use barrier contraception

Moexipril (Univasc) [Antihypertensive/ACEI] Uses: *HTN, postMI,* DN **Action:** ACE inhibitor **Dose:** 7.5–30 mg in 1–2 ÷ doses 1 h ac ↓ in renal impair **Caution:** [C (1st tri, D 2nd & 3rd tri), ?] **Contra:** ACE inhibitor sensitivity **Disp:** Tabs 7.5, 15 mg **SE:** ↓ BP, edema, angioedema, HA, dizziness, cough **Interactions:** ↑ Effects *W/* diuretics, antihypertensives, EtOH, probenecid, garlic; ↑ effects *OF* insulin, Li; ↑ risk *OF* hyperkalemia with K supl, K-sparing diuretics; ↓ effects *W/* antacids, ASA, NSAIDS, ephedra, yohimbe, ginseng **Labs:** ↑ BUN, Cr, K⁺, ↓ Na⁺ **NIPE:** May alter sense of taste, may cause cough, ⊘ salt substitutes, ⊘ PRG, use barrier contraception

Molindone (Moban) [Antipsychotic] Uses: *Psychotic disorders* **Action:** Piperazine phenothiazine **Dose:** *Adults.* 50–75 mg/d PO, ↑ to max of 225 mg/d in 3–4 d intervals if necessary. *Peds. 3–5 y:* 1–2.5 mg/d PO in 4 ÷ doses. *5–12 y:* 0.5–1.0 mg/kg/d in 4 ÷ doses **Caution:** [C, ?] NAG **Contra:** Drug/EtOH CNS depression **Disp:** Tabs 5, 10, 25, 50 mg **SE:** ↓ BP, tachycardia, arrhythmias, EPS, Szs, constipation, xerostomia, blurred vision **Interactions:** ↑ Effects *W/* antihypertensives; ↑ hyperkalemia *W/* K-sparing diuretics, K supls, salt substitutes, trimethoprim; ↑ effects *OF* insulin, Li; ↓ effects *W/* ASA, NSAIDs **Labs:** ↑ Serum

K^+, BUN, Cr; monitor lipid profile, fasting glucose, HgB A1-c **NIPE:** Take w/o food; monitor for persistent cough

Montelukast (Singulair) [Bronchodilator/Leukotriene Receptor Antagonist]
Uses: *Prophylaxis & Rx of chronic asthma, seasonal allergic rhinitis* **Action:** Leukotriene receptor antagonist **Dose:** *Asthma: Adults & Peds >15 y.* 10 mg/d PO taken in PM. *Peds.* 2–5 y: 4 mg/d PO taken in PM. 6–14 y: 5 mg/d PO in PM. **Caution:** [B, M] **Contra:** Component allergy **Disp:** Tabs 10 mg; chew tabs 4, 5 mg; granules 4 mg/packet **SE:** HA, dizziness, fatigue, rash, GI upset, Churg–Strauss synd **Interactions:** ↑ ↓ Effects W/ phenobarbital, rifampin **Labs:** ↑ AST, ALT **NIPE:** Not for acute asthma

Morphine (Avinza XR, Duramorph, Infumorph, MS Contin, Kadian SR, Oramorph SR, Infumorph, Roxanol) [C-II] [Analgesic/Opioid Agonist]
Uses: *Relief of severe pain* **AMI Action:** Narcotic analgesic **Dose:** *Adults.* **PO:** 5–30 mg q4h PRN; SR tabs 15–60 mg q8–12h (do not chew/crush). **IV/IM:** 2.5–15 mg q2–6h; supp 10–30 mg q4h. **IT:** *(Duramorph, Infumorph).* Per protocol **Peds.** >6 mo 0.1–0.2 mg/kg/dose IM/IV q2–4h PRN to 15 mg/dose max; 0.2–0.5 mg/kg PO q4–6h PRN; 0.3–0.6 mg/kg SR tabs PO q12h; 2–4 mg IV (over 1–5 min) every 5–30 min *(ECC 2005)* **Caution:** [B (D w/ prolonged use/high doses at term), +/–] **Contra:** Severe asthma, resp depression, GI obst **Disp:** Immediate-release tabs 10, 15, 30 mg; MS Contin CR tabs 15, 30, 60, 100, 200 mg; Oramorph SR CR tabs 15, 30, 60, 100 mg; Kadian SR caps 20, 30, 50, 60, 80, 100 mg; Avinza XR caps 30, 60, 90, 120 mg; soln 10, 20, 100 mg/5 mL; supp 5, 10, 20, 30 mg; inj 2, 4, 5, 8, 10, 15, 25, 50 mg/mL; Duramorph/Astramorph inj 0.5, 1 mg/mL; Infumorph 10, 25 mg/mL, supp 5, 10, 20, 30 mg **SE:** Narcotic SE (resp depression, sedation, constipation, N/V, pruritus); granulomas w/ IT **Interactions:** ↑ Effects W/ cimetidine, CNS depressants, dextroamphetamine, TCAs, EtOH, kava kava, valerian, St. John's wort; ↑ effects OF warfarin; ↑ risk OF HTN crisis W/ MAOIs; ↓ effects W/ opioids, phenothiazines **Labs:** ↑ Serum amylase, lipase **NIPE:** May require scheduled dosing to relieve severe chronic pain; do not crush/chew SR/CR forms

Morphine liposomal (DepoDur) [Analgesic/Opioid Agonist]
Uses: *Long-lasting epidural analgesia* **Action:** ER morphine analgesia **Dose:** 10–20 mg lumbar epidural inj (C-section 10 mg after cord clamped) **Caution:** [C,+/–] elderly, biliary Dz (sphincter of Oddi spasm) **Contra:** Ileus, resp depression, asthma, obst airway, suspected/known head injury ↑ ICP, allergy to morphine. **Disp:** Inj 10 mg/mL **SE:** Hypoxia, resp depression, ↓ BP, retention, N/V, constipation, flatulence, pruritus, pyrexia, anemia, HA, dizziness, tachycardia, insomnia, ileus **NIPE:** Effect =48 h; not for IT/IV/IM

Moxifloxacin (Avelox, Vigamox ophthalmic) [Antibiotic/Fluoroquinolone]
Uses: *Acute sinusitis & bronchitis, skin/soft tissue Infxns, conjunctivitis, & community-acquired pneumonia* **Action:** 4th-gen quinolone; ↓ DNA gyrase. *Spectrum:* Excellent gram(+) except MRSA & E. faecium; good gram(–) except P. aeruginosa, S. maltophilia, & Acinetobacter sp; good anaerobic

coverage **Dose:** 400 mg/d PO/IV; avoid cation products, antacids. *Ophth:* 1 gtt tid ×7d; take PO 4 h before or 8 h after antacids **Caution:** [C, ?/–] Quinolone sensitivity; interactions w/ Mg-, Ca-, Al-, Fe-containing products & class IA & III antiarrhythmic agents **Contra:** Quinolone/component sensitivity **Disp:** Tabs 400 mg, inj, ophth 0.5% **SE:** Dizziness, N, QT prolongation, Szs, photosens, tendon rupture **Interactions:** ↑ Effects *W/* probenecid; ↑ effects *OF* diazepam, theophylline, caffeine, metoprolol, propranolol, phenytoin, warfarin; ↓ effects *W/* antacids, didanosine, Fe salts, Mg, sucralfate, NaHCO₃, Zn **Labs:** ↑ LFTs, BUN, SCr, amylase, PT, triglycerides, cholesterol; ↓ HMG, Hct **NIPE:** ⊘ Give to children <18 y; ↑ fluids to 2–3 L/d

Multivitamins, Oral [OTC]   (Table 13)

Mupirocin (Bactroban) [Topical Anti-infective]   **Uses:** *Impetigo; eradicate MRSA in nasal carriers* **Action:** ↓ Bacterial protein synth **Dose:** *Topical:* Apply small amount to area 3 ×/d × 5–14 d. *Nasal:* Apply bid in nostrils × 5d **Caution:** [B, ?] **Contra:** Do not use w/ other nasal products **Disp:** Oint 2%; cream 2% **SE:** Local irritation, rash. **Interactions:** ↓ Bacterial action *W/* chloramphenicol **NIPE:** Instruct patient to contact health care provider if no improvement in 3–5 d

Muromonab-CD3 (Orthoclone OKT3) [Immunosuppressant/ Monoclonal Antibody]   WARNING: Can cause anaphylaxis; monitor fluid status   **Uses:** *Acute rejection following organ transplantation* **Action:** Murine Ab, blocks T-cell Fxn **Dose:** Per protocol **Adults.** 5 mg/d IV for 10–14 d. **Peds.** 0.1 mg/kg/d IV for 10–14 d **Caution:** [C, ?/–] w/ h/o Szs, PRG, uncontrolled HTN, **Contra:** Murine sensitivity, fluid overload **Disp:** Inj 5 mg/5 mL **SE:** Anaphylaxis, pulm edema, fever/chills w/ 1st dose (premedicate w/ steroid/ APAP/antihistamine) **Interactions:** ↑ Effects *W/* immunosuppressives; ↑ effects *OF* live virus vaccines; ↑ risk *OF* CNS effects & encephalopathy *W/* indomethacin **Labs:** ↑ BUN, Cr **NIPE:** ⊘ Immunizations, exposure to Infxn; monitor during inf; use 0.22-µg filter

Mycophenolic Acid (Myfortic) [Immunosuppressant/My-cophenolic Acid Derivative]   WARNING: ↑ Risk of Infxns, possible development of lymphoproliferative disorders   **Uses:** *Prevent rejection after renal transplant* **Action:** Cytostatic to lymphocytes **Dose:** **Adults.** 720 mg PO bid. **Peds.** BSA 400 mg/m² max 720 mg bid; ↓ in renal insuff/neutropenia; take on empty stomach **Caution:** [C, ?/–] **Contra:** Component allergy **Disp:** DR tabs 180, 360 mg **SE:** N/V/D, pain, fever, HA, Infxn, PRG, anemia, leukopenia, edema **Interactions:** ↓ *OF* phenytoin, theophylline; ↓ effects *W/* antacids, cholestyramine, Fe **Labs:** ↑ Cholesterol; monitor CBC **NIPE:** If GI distress-take w/ food; avoid crowds & people w/ Infxns

Mycophenolate Mofetil (CellCept) [Immunosuppressant/ Mycophenolic Acid Derivative]   WARNING: ↑ Risk of Infxns, possible development of lymphoma   **Uses:** *Prevent organ rejection after transplant* **Action:** ↓ Immunologically mediated inflammatory responses **Dose:** **Adults.** 1 g PO bid; **Peds.** BSA 1.2–1.5 m²: 750 mg PO bid; BSA >1.5 m²: 1 g PO bid; may taper up to 600 mg/m² PO bid; used w/ steroids & cyclosporine; ↓ in renal insuff or neutropenia. *IV:* Inf over >2 h. *PO:* Take on empty stomach, do not open capsules **Caution:** [C, ?/–] **Contra:** Component allergy; IV use in polysorbate 80 allergy

Disp: Caps 250, 500 mg; susp 200 mg/mL, inj 500 mg **SE:** N/V/D, pain, fever, HA, Infxn, HTN, anemia, leukopenia, edema **Interactions:** ↑ Effects W/ acyclovir, ganciclovir, probenecid; ↑ effects OF acyclovir, ganciclovir; ↓ effects W/ antacids, cholestyramine, cyclosporine, Fe, food; ↓ effects OF OCPs, phenytoin, theophylline **Labs:** ↑ Cholesterol; monitor CBC **NIPE:** Use barrier contraception during and 6 wk after drug therapy; ⊘ exposure to Infxn; take w/o food

Nabilone (Cesamet) [CII] [Synthetic Cannabinoid] WARNING: Psychotomimetic Rxns, may persist for 72 h following D/C; caregivers should be present during initial use or dosage modification; patients should not operate heavy machinery; avoid alcohol, sedatives, hypnotics, other psychoactive substances **Uses:** *Refractory chemo-induced emesis* **Action:** Synthetic cannabinoid **Dose:** *Adults.* 1–2 mg PO bid 1–3 h before chemo, 6 mg/d max; may continue for 48 h beyond final chemo dose **Caution:** [C,?/–] Elderly, HTN, HF, underlying psychiatric illness, substance abuse; high protein binding w/ 1st-pass metabolism may lead to drug interactions **Disp:** Caps 1 mg **SE:** Drowsiness, vertigo, xerostomia, euphoria, ataxia, HA, difficulty concentrating, tachycardia, ↓ BP **Interactions:** ↑ CNS depression W/ benzodiazepines, barbiturates, CNS depressants, EtOH; ↑ effects W/ opioids; ↑ effects OF opioids; cross-tolerance W/ opioids **NIPE:** May require initial dose evening before chemo; Rx only quantity for single cycle

Nabumetone (Relafen) [Analgesic, Anti-inflammatory, Antipyretic/NSAID] WARNING: May ↑risk of cardiovascular events & GI bleeding **Uses:** *Arthritis & pain* **Action:** NSAID; ↓ prostaglandins **Dose:** 1000–2000 mg/d ÷ daily–bid w/ food **Caution:** [C (D 3rd tri), +] severe hepatic Dz **Contra:** Peptic ulcer, NSAID sensitivity, after CABG surgery **Disp:** Tabs 500, 750 mg **SE:** Dizziness, rash, GI upset, edema, peptic ulcer **Interactions:** ↑ Effects W/ aminoglycosides; ↑ effects OF anticoagulants, hypoglycemics, Li, MTX, thrombolytics; ↑ GI effects W/ ASA, corticosteroids, K supls, NSAIDs, EtOH; ↓ effects OF antihypertensives, diuretics **NIPE:** Photosensitivity—use sunscreen

Nadolol (Corgard) [Antihypertensive, Antianginal/BB] **Uses:** *HTN & angina* migraine prophylaxis **Action:** Competitively blocks β-adrenergic receptors (β₁, β₂) **Dose:** 40–80 mg/d; ↑ to 240 mg/d (angina) or 320 mg/d (HTN) at 3–7 d intervals; ↓ in renal insuff & elderly **Caution:** [C (1st tri; D if 2nd or 3rd tri), +] **Contra:** Uncompensated CHF, shock, heart block, asthma **Disp:** Tabs 20, 40, 80, 120, 160 mg **SE:** Nightmares, paresthesias, ↓ BP, bradycardia, fatigue **Interactions:** ↑ Effects W/ antihypertensives, diuretics, nitrates, EtOH; ↑ effects OF aminophylline, lidocaine; ↑ risk of HTN W/ clonidine, ephedrine, epinephrine, MAOIs, phenylephrine, pseudoephedrine; ↑ bradycardia W/ digitalis glycosides, ephedrine, epinephrine, phenylephrine, pseudoephrine ↓ effects W/ ampicillin, antacids, clonidine, NSAIDs, thyroid meds; ↓ effects OF glucagon, theophylline **NIPE:** May ↑ cold sensitivity; ⊘ D/C abruptly

Nafcillin (Nallpen) [Antibiotic/Penicillinase-Resistant Penicillin] **Uses:** *Infxns due to susceptible strains of Staphylococcus sp &*

Streptococcus sp * **Action:** Bactericidal β-lactamase-resistant penicillin; ↓ cell wall synth. *Spectrum:* Good gram(+) except MRSA and *Enterococcus* sp, no gram (–), poor anaerobe **Dose:** *Adults.* 1–2 g IV q4–6h. *Peds.* 50–200 mg/kg/d ÷ q4–6h **Caution:** [B, ?] PCN allergy **Disp:** Inj powder l, 2 g **SE:** Interstitial nephritis, D, fever, N **Interactions:** ↑ Effects *OF* MTX; ↓ effects *W/* chloramphenicol, macrolides, tetracyclines; ↓ effects *OF* cyclosporine, OCPs, tacrolimus, warfarin **Labs:** ↑ Serum protein; no adjustments for renal Fxn **NIPE:** Aminoglycosides not compatible, risk of drug inactivation w/ fruit juice/carbonated drinks; monitor for super Infxn

Naftifine (Naftin) [Antifungal/Antibiotic] **Uses:** *Tinea pedis, cruris, & corporis* **Action:** Allylamine antifungal, ↓ cell membrane ergosterol synth **Dose:** Apply daily (cream) or bid (gel) **Caution:** [B, ?] **Contra:** Component sensitivity **Disp:** 1% cream; gel **SE:** Local irritation

Nalbuphine (Nubain) [Analgesic/Narcotic Agonist-Antagonist] **Uses:** *Moderate–severe pain; preop & obstetric analgesia* **Action:** Narcotic agonist–antagonist; ↓ ascending pain pathways **Dose:** *Adults.* 10–20 mg IM or IV q3–6h PRN; max of 160 mg/d; 20 mg max 1 × dose *Peds.* 0.2 mg/kg IV or IM, 20 mg max; ↓ in hepatic insuff **Caution:** [B (D w/ prolonged/high doses at term), ?] **Contra:** Sulfite sensitivity **Disp:** Inj 10, 20 mg/mL **SE:** CNS depression, drowsiness; caution w/ opiate use, ↓ BP **Interactions:** ↑ CNS depression *W/* cimetidine, CNS depressants; EtOH ↑ effects *OF* digitoxin, phenytoin, rifampin **Labs:** ↑ Serum amylase, lipase **NIPE:** Monitor for resp depression

Naloxone (Narcan) [Antidote/Opioid Antagonist] **Uses:** *Opioid addiction (diagnosis) & OD* **Action:** Competitive narcotic antagonist **Dose:** *Adults.* 0.4–2 mg IV, IM, or SQ q2–3 min; total dose 10 mg max *Peds.* 0.01–0.1 mg/kg/dose IV, IM, or SQ; repeat IV q3min × 3 doses PRN **Caution:** [B, ?] May precipitate acute withdrawal in addicts **Disp:** Inj 0.4, 1 mg/mL; neonatal inj 0.02 mg/mL **SE:** ↓ BP, tachycardia, irritability, GI upset, pulm edema **Interactions:** ↓ Effects *OF* opiates **NIPE:** If no response after 10 mg, suspect nonnarcotic cause

Naltrexone (Depade, ReVia, Vivitrol) [Opioid Antagonist] **WARNING:** Can cause hepatic injury, contraindicated w/ active liver Dz **Uses:** *EtOH & narcotic addiction* **Action:** Antagonizes opioid receptors **Dose:** *EtOH and narcotic addiction:* 50 mg/d PO; do not give until opioid-free for 7–10 d; *EtOH dependence:* 380 mg IM q4wks (Vivitrol) **Caution:** [C, M] **Contra:** Acute hepatitis, liver failure, opioid use **Disp:** Tabs 50 mg; inj 380 mg (Vivitrol) **SE:** May cause hepatotox; insomnia, GI upset, joint pain, HA, fatigue **Interactions:** ↑ Lethargy & somnolence *W/* thioridazine; ↓ effects *OF* opioids **Labs:** ↑ LFTs **NIPE:** Give IM in gluteal muscle & rotate

Naphazoline (Albalon, AK-Con, Naphcon, others), Naphazoline & Pheniramine Acetate (Naphcon A) [Ophthalmic Antihistamine] **Uses:** *Relieve ocular redness & itching caused by allergy* **Action:** Sympathomimetic (α-adrenergic vasoconstrictor) & antihistamine (pheniramine) **Dose:** 1–2 gtt up to qid, 3-d max **Caution:** [C, +] **Contra:**

NAG, in children, w/ contact lenses **SE:** CV stimulation, dizziness, local irritation **Disp:** Ophthalmic 0.012, 0.025, 0.1%/15 mL; naphazoline & pheniramine 0.025%/0.3% soln; **Interactions:** ↑ Risk of HTN crisis W/ MAOIs, TCAs

Naproxen (Aleve [OTC], Naprosyn, Anaprox) [Analgesic, Anti-inflammatory, Antipyretic/NSAID] **WARNING:** May ↑ risk of cardiovascular events & GI bleeding **Uses:** *Arthritis & pain* **Action:** NSAID; ↓ prostaglandins **Dose:** *Adults & Peds >12 y.* 200–500 mg bid–tid to 1500 mg/d max; ↓ in hepatic impair **Caution:** [B (D 3rd tri), +] **Contra:** NSAID or ASA triad sensitivity, peptic ulcer, post CABG for pain, 3rd tri PRG **Disp:** Tabs. 220, 250, 375, 500 mg; *Delayed release:* 375 mg, 500 mg; *Controlled release:* 375 mg, 550 mg; susp 125 mL/5 mL. **SE:** Dizziness, pruritus, GI upset, peptic ulcer, edema **Interactions:** ↑ Effects W/ aminoglycosides; ↑ effects OF anticoagulants, hypoglycemics, Li, MTX, thrombolytics; ↑ GI effects W/ ASA, corticosteroids, K supls, NSAIDs, EtOH; ↓ effects OF antihypertensives, diuretics **Labs:** ↑ BUN, Cr, LFTs, PT **NIPE:** Take W/ food to < GI upset

Naratriptan (Amerge) [Migraine Suppressant/5-HT Agonist] **Uses:** *Acute migraine* **Action:** Serotonin 5-HT$_1$ receptor antagonist **Dose:** 1–2.5 mg PO once; repeat PRN in 4 h; 5 mg/24 h max; ↓ in mild renal/hepatic insuff, take w/ fluids **Caution:** [C, M] **Contra:** Severe renal/hepatic impair, avoid w/ angina, ischemic heart Dz, uncontrolled HTN, cerebrovascular synds, & ergot use **Disp:** Tabs 1, 2.5 mg **SE:** Dizziness, sedation, GI upset, paresthesias, ECG changes, coronary vasospasm, arrhythmias **Interactions:** ↑ Effects W/ MAOIs, SSRIs; ↑ effects OF ergot drugs; ↓ effects W/ nicotine

Natalizumab (Tysabri) [Immunomodulator/Monoclonal Antibody] **WARNING:** Cases of progressive multifocal leukoencephalopathy (PML) reported **Uses:** *Relapsing MS to delay disability and ↓ recurrences* **Action:** Adhesion molecule inhibitor **Dose:** *Adults.* 300 mg IV q4wk; 2nd-line Tx only **Contra:** PML; immune compromise or w/ immunosuppressant **Caution:** [C,?/–] Baseline MRI to rule out PML **Disp:** Vial 300 mg **SE:** Infxn, immunosuppression; inf Rxn precluding subsequent use; HA, fatigue, arthralgia **Interactions:** ↑ Risk of Infxn W/ corticosteroids, immunosuppressants **Labs:** ↑ LFTs **NIPE:** Give slowly to ↓ Rxns; D/C immediately w/ signs of PML (weakness, paralysis, vision loss, impaired speech, cognitive ↓); eval at 3 and 6 mo, then q6mo thereafter; limited distribution [TOUCH risk mgmt program (800) 456-2255]

Nateglinide (Starlix) [Hypoglycemic/Amino Acid Derivative] **Uses:** *Type 2 DM* **Action:** ↑ Pancreatic insulin release **Dose:** 120 mg PO tid 1–30 min ac; ↓ to 60 mg tid if near target HbA$_{1c}$ **Caution:** [C, –] w/ CYP2C9/3A4 metabolized drug (Table 11) **Contra:** DKA, type 1 DM **Disp:** Tabs 60, 120 mg **SE:** Hypoglycemia, URI **Interactions:** ↑ Effects of hypoglycemia W/ nonselective BBs, MAOIs, NSAIDs, salicylates, ↓ effects W/ corticosteroids, niacin, sympathomimetics, thiazide diuretics, thyroid meds **Labs:** ↓ Glucose **NIPE:** ⊘ Take med if meal skipped

Nedocromil (Tilade) [Anti-inflammatory/Respiratory Inhalant]

Uses: *Mild–moderate asthma* **Action:** Anti-inflammatory agent **Dose:** *Inhal:* 2 inhal qid **Caution:** [B, ?/–] **Contra:** Component allergy **Disp:** Met-dose inhal 1.75 mg/spray **SE:** Chest pain, dizziness, dysphonia, rash, GI upset, Infxn **NIPE:** May take 2–4 wk for full therapeutic effect; not for acute asthma

Nefazodone [Antidepressant/Serotonin Modulator] WARN-

ING: Fatal hepatitis & liver failure possible, D/C if LFT >3× ULN, do not retreat; closely monitor for worsening depression or emergence of suicidality, particularly in ped pts **Uses:** *Depression* **Action:** ↓ Neuronal uptake of serotonin & norepinephrine **Dose:** Initial 100 mg PO bid; usual 300–600 mg/d in 2 ÷ doses **Caution:** [C, ?] **Contra:** w/ MAOIs, pimozide, carbamazepine, alprazolam; active liver Dz **Disp:** Tabs 50, 100, 150, 200, 250, 500 mg **SE:** Postural ↓ BP & allergic Rxns; HA, drowsiness, xerostomia, constipation, GI upset, liver failure **Interactions:** ↑ Risk of hypotension W/ antihypertensives, nitrates; ↑ effects OF alprazolam, CCB, digoxin, HMG-CoA reductase inhibitors, triazolam; ↑ risk of QT prolongation W/ astemizole, cisapride, pimozide; ↑ risk of serious and/or fatal Rxn W/ MAOIs; ↓ effects OF propranolol **Labs:** ↑ LFTs, cholesterol; ↓ Hct **NIPE:** Take w/o food; may take 2–4 wk for full therapeutic effects; monitor HR, BP

Nelarabine (Arranon) [Antineoplastic/Antimetabolite]

WARNING: Fatal neurotox possible **Uses:** *T-cell ALL or T-cell LBL unresponsive >2 other regimens* **Action:** Nucleoside analog **Dose:** *Adults.* 1500 mg/m^2 IV over 2 h days 1, 3, 5 of 21-d cycle *Peds.* 650 mg/m^2 IV over 1 h on days 1–5 of 21-d cycle **Caution:** [D,?/–] **Disp:** Vial 250 mg **SE:** Neuropathy, ataxia, Sz, coma, hematologic tox, GI upset, HA, blurred vision **Labs:** Monitor CBC **NIPE:** Prehydration, urinary alkalinization, allopurinol before dose

Nelfinavir (Viracept) [Antiretroviral/Protease Inhibitor]

Uses: *HIV Infxn* **Action:** Protease inhibitor causes immature, noninfectious virion production **Dose:** *Adults.* 750 mg PO tid or 1250 mg PO bid. *Peds.* 25–35 mg/kg PO tid; take w/ food **Caution:** [B, ?] Many drug interactions **Contra:** Phenylketonuria, triazolam/midazolam use or drug dependent on CYP3A4 (Table 11) **Disp:** Tabs 250, 625 mg; powder 50 mg/g; **SE:** Food ↓ absorption; interacts w/ St. John's wort; dyslipidemia, lipodystrophy, D, rash **Interactions:** ↑ Effects W/ erythromycin, ketoconazole, indinavir, ritonavir; ↑ effects OF barbiturates, carbamazepine, cisapride, ergot alkaloids, erythromycin, lovastatin, midazolam, phenytoin, saquinavir, simvastatin, triazolam; ↓ effects W/ barbiturates, carbamazepine, phenytoin, rifabutin, rifampin, St. John's Wort; ↓ effects OF OCP **Labs:** ↑ LFTs **NIPE:** Take W/ food; use barrier contraception

Neomycin, Bacitracin, & Polymyxin B (Neosporin Ointment) (See Bacitracin, Neomycin, & Polymyxin B Topical)

Neomycin, Colistin, & Hydrocortisone (Cortisporin-TC Otic Drops); Neomycin, Colistin, Hydrocortisone, & Thonzonium (Cortisporin-TC Otic Susp) [Antibiotic/Aminoglycoside] Uses: *External

otitis,* Infxns of mastoid/fenestration cavities **Action:** Antibiotic w/ anti-inflammatory **Dose:** *Adults.* 4–5 gtt in ear(s) tid–qid. *Peds.* 3–4 gtt in ear(s) tid–qid **Contra:** Component allergy; HSV, vaccinia, varicella **Caution:** [C, ?] **Disp:** Otic gtt & susp **SE:** Local irritation

Neomycin & Dexamethasone (AK-Neo-Dex Ophthalmic, NeoDecadron Ophthalmic) [Antibiotic/Corticosteroid] Uses:
Steroid-responsive inflammatory conditions of the cornea, conjunctiva, lid, & anterior segment **Action:** Antibiotic w/ anti-inflammatory corticosteroid **Dose:** 1–2 gtt in eye(s) q3–4h or thin coat tid–qid until response, then ↓ to daily **Caution:** [C, ?] **Disp:** Cream neomycin 0.5%/dexamethasone 0.1%; oint neomycin 0.35%/dexamethasone 0.05%; soln neomycin 0.35%/dexamethasone 0.1% **SE:** Local irritation **NIPE:** Use under ophthalmologist's supervision

Neomycin & Polymyxin B (Neosporin Cream) [OTC] [Antibiotic] Uses:
Infxn in minor cuts, scrapes, & burns **Action:** Bactericidal **Dose:** Apply bid–qid **Caution:** [C, ?] **Contra:** Component allergy **Disp:** Cream neomycin 3.5 mg/polymyxin B 10,000 units/g **SE:** Local irritation **NIPE:** Different from Neosporin oint

Neomycin, Polymyxin B, & Dexamethasone (Maxitrol) [Antibiotic/Corticosteroid] Uses:
Steroid-responsive ocular conditions w/ bacterial Infxn **Action:** Antibiotic w/ anti-inflammatory corticosteroid **Dose:** 1–2 gtt in eye(s) q3–4h; apply oint in eye(s) tid–qid **Contra:** Component allergy; viral fungal, TB eye Dz **Caution:** [C, ?] **Disp:** Oint neomycin sulfate 3.5 mg/polymyxin B sulfate 10,000 units/dexamethasone 0.1%/g; susp identical/5 mL **SE:** Local irritation **NIPE:** Use under supervision of ophthalmologist

Neomycin-Polymyxin Bladder Irrigant [Neosporin GU Irrigant] [Antibiotic] Uses:
Continuous irrigant prevent bacteriuria & gram(−) bacteremia associated w/ indwelling catheter **Action:** Bactericidal; not for *Serratia* sp or streptococci **Dose:** 1 mL irrigant in 1 L of 0.9% NaCl; cont bladder irrigation w/ 1 L of soln/24 h **Caution:** [D] **Contra:** Component allergy **Disp:** Soln neomycin sulfate 40 mg & polymyxin B 200,000 units/mL; amp 1, 20 mL **SE:** Neomycin ototox or nephrotox (rare) **NIPE:** Potential for bacterial/fungal super Infxn; not for inj

Neomycin, Polymyxin, & Hydrocortisone (Cortisporin Ophthalmic & Otic) [Antibiotic/Anti-inflammatory] Uses:
Ocular & otic bacterial Infxns **Action:** Antibiotic & anti-inflammatory **Dose:** *Otic:* 3–4 gtt in the ear(s) tid–qid. *Ophth:* Apply a thin layer to the eye(s) or 1 gtt daily–qid **Caution:** [C, ?] **Disp:** Otic susp; ophth soln; ophth oint **SE:** Local irritation

Neomycin, Polymyxin B, & Prednisolone (Poly-Pred Ophthalmic) [Antibiotic/Corticosteroid] Uses:
Steroid-responsive ocular conditions w/ bacterial Infxn **Action:** Antibiotic & anti-inflammatory **Dose:** 1–2 gtt in eye(s) q4–6h; apply oint in eye(s) tid–qid **Caution:** [C, ?] **Disp:** Susp neomycin 0.35%/polymyxin B 10,000 units/prednisolone 0.5%/mL **SE:** Irritation **NIPE:** Use under supervision of ophthalmologist

Neomycin Sulfate (Neo-Fradin, generic) [Antibiotic] WARN-ING: Systemic absorption of oral route may cause neuro/oto/nephrotox may result; respiratory paralysis possible with any route of admin **Uses:** *Hepatic coma, bowel prep* **Action:** Aminoglycoside, poorly absorbed PO; ↓ GI bacterial flora **Dose:** *Adults.* 3–12 g/24 h PO in 3–4 ÷ doses. *Peds.* 50–100 mg/kg/24 h PO in 3–4 ÷ doses **Caution:** [C, ?/–] Renal failure, neuromuscular disorders, hearing impair **Contra:** Intestinal obst **Disp:** Tabs 500 mg; PO soln 125 mg/5 mL **SE:** Hearing loss w/ long-term use; rash, N/V **NIPE:** Do not use parenterally (↑ tox); part of the Condon bowel prep; also topical form

Neomycin Sulfate, Topical (Myciguent [OTC]) [Antibiotic] **Uses:** *Prevent skin Infxn* **Action:** Topical aminoglycoside **Dose:** Apply to skin and rub in **Caution:** [C, ?/–] **Contra:** Component allergy **Disp:** Cream 0.5% **SE:** Itching, rash, redness

Nepafenac (Nevanac) [Analgesic, Anti-inflammatory, Antipyretic/NSAID] **Uses:** *Inflammation post-cataract surgery* **Action:** NSAID **Dose:** 1 gtt in eye(s) tid 1 d before, and continue 14 d after surgery **Contra:** NSAID/ASA sensitivity **Caution:** [C,?/–] May ↑ bleeding time, delay healing, cause keratitis **Disp:** Susp 3 mL **SE:** Capsular opacity, visual changes, foreign body sensation, inc. IOP **Interactions:** ↑ Effects *OF* oral anticoagulants **NIPE:** Prolonged use ↑ corneal risk; remove contact lenses during use; shake well before use, separate from other drops by >5 min

Nesiritide (Natrecor) [Vasodilator/Human B-Type Natriuretic Peptide] **Uses:** *Acutely decompensated CHF* **Action:** Human B-type natriuretic peptide **Dose:** 2 µg/kg IV bolus, then 0.01 µg/kg/min IV **Caution:** [C, ?/–] When vasodilators are not appropriate **Contra:** SBP <90, cardiogenic shock **Disp:** Vials 1.5 mg **SE:** ↓ BP, HA, GI upset, arrhythmias **Interactions:** ↑ Hypotension *W/* ACEIs, nitrates **Labs:** ↑ Cr **NIPE:** Requires continuous BP monitoring; some studies indicate ↑ in mortality

Nevirapine (Viramune) [Antiretroviral/NNRTI] WARNING: Reports of fatal hepatotox even after short-term use; severe life-threatening skin Rxns (Stevens–Johnson, tox epidermal necrolysis, & allergic Rxns); monitor closely during 1st 8 wk of Rx **Uses:** *HIV Infxn* **Action:** Nonnucleoside RT inhibitor **Dose:** *Adults.* Initial 200 mg/d PO × 14 d, then 200 mg bid. *Peds.* <8 y: 4 mg/kg/d × 14 d, then 7 mg/kg bid. > 8 y: 4 mg/kg/d × 14 d, then 4 mg/kg bid max 200 mg/dose for peds (w/o regard to food) **Caution:** [B, +/–] OCP **Disp:** Tabs 200 mg; susp 50 mg/5 mL **SE:** Life-threatening rash; HA, fever, D, neutropenia, hepatitis **Interactions:** ↑ Effects *W/* clarithromycin, erythromycin; ↓ effects *W/* rifabutin, rifampin, St. John's wort; ↓ effects *OF* clarithromycin, indinavir, ketoconazole, methadone, OCPs, protease inhibitors, warfarin **NIPE:** Use barrier contraception; HIV resistance when given as monotherapy; always use in combo w/ atleast 1 additional antiretroviral agent; ⊘ women if CD4 >250 or men >400 unless benefit > risk of hepatotox

Niacin (Niaspan, Slo-Niacin) [Antilipemic/Vitamin B Complex]

Uses: *Adjunct in significant hyperlipidemia* **Action:** Nicotinic acid, vitamin B_3; ↓ lipolysis; ↓ esterification of triglycerides; ↑ lipoprotein lipase **Dose:** 1–6 g ÷ doses PO tid; 9 g/d max (w/ food) **Caution:** [A (C if doses >RDA), +] **Contra:** Liver Dz, peptic ulcer, arterial hemorrhage **Disp:** SR caps 125, 250, 400, 500 mg; tabs 50, 100, 250, 500 mg; SR tabs 150, 250, 500, 750, 1000 mg; elixir 50 mg/5 mL **SE:** Upper body/facial flushing & warmth; GI upset, flatulence, exacerbate peptic ulcer; HA, paresthesias, liver damage, gout, or altered glucose control in DM **Interactions:** ↑ Effects **OF** antihypertensives, anticoagulants; ↓ effects **OF** hypoglycemics, probenecid, sulfinpyrazone **Labs:** ↑ LFTs, glucose, uric acid **NIPE:** EtOH & hot beverages ↑ flushing; flushing ↓ by taking ASA or NSAID 30–60 min prior to dose

Nicardipine (Cardene) [Antianginal/Antihypertensive/CCB]

Uses: *Chronic stable angina & HTN*; prophylaxis of migraine **Action:** CCB **Dose:** *Adults.* *PO:* 20–40 mg PO tid. *SR:* 30–60 mg PO bid. *IV:* 5 mg/h IV cont inf; ↑ by 2.5 mg/h q15min to max 15 mg/h. *Peds.* *PO:* 20–30 mg PO q8h. *IV:* 0.5–5 μg/kg/min; ↓ in renal/hepatic impair **Caution:** [C, ?/–] Heart block, CAD **Contra:** Cardiogenic shock **Disp:** Caps 20, 30 mg; SR caps 30, 45, 60 mg; inj 2.5 mg/mL **SE:** Flushing, tachycardia, ↓ BP, edema, HA **Notes:** PO-to-IV conversion: 20 mg tid = 0.5 mg/h, 30 mg tid = 1.2 mg/h, 40 mg tid = 2.2 mg/h **Interactions:** ↑ Effects **W/** cimetidine, grapefruit juice; ↑ effects **OF** cyclosporine; ↑ hypotension **W/** antihypertensives, fentanyl, nitrates, quinidine, EtOH; ↑ dysrhythmias **W/** digoxin, disopyramide, phenytoin; ↓ effects **W/** NSAIDs, rifampin; high-fat food **Labs:** ↑ LFTs **NIPE:** ↑ Risk of photosensitivity—use sunscreen; take w/ food (not high fat)

Nicotine Gum (Nicorette, Others) [OTC] [Smoking Deterrent/ Cholinergic]

Uses: *Aid to smoking cessation, relieve nicotine withdrawal* **Action:** Systemic delivery of nicotine **Dose:** Chew 9–12 pieces/d PRN; max 24 pieces/d **Caution:** [C, ?] **Contra:** Life-threatening arrhythmias, unstable angina **Disp:** 2 mg, 4 mg/piece; mint, orange, original flavors **SE:** Tachycardia, HA, GI upset, hiccups **Interactions:** ↑ Effects **W/** cimetidine; ↑ effects **OF** catecholamines, cortisol; ↑ hemodynamic & A-V blocking effects **OF** adenosine; ↓ effects **W/** coffee, cola **NIPE:** Chew 30 min for full dose of nicotine; ↓ absorption **W/** coffee, soda, juices, wine w/in 15 min; must stop smoking & perform behavior modification for max effect

Nicotine Nasal Spray (Nicotrol NS) [Smoking Deterrent/ Cholinergic]

Uses: *Aid to smoking cessation, relieve nicotine withdrawal* **Action:** Systemic delivery of nicotine **Dose:** 0.5 mg/actuation; 1–2 sprays/h, 10 sprays/h; max **Caution:** [D, M] **Contra:** Life-threatening arrhythmias, unstable angina **Disp:** Nasal inhaler 10 mg/mL **SE:** Local irritation, tachycardia, HA, taste perversion **Interactions:** ↑ Effects **W/** cimetidine, blue cohash; ↑ effects **OF** catecholamines, cortisol; ↑ hemodynamic & A-V blocking effects **OF** adenosine **NIPE:** ⊘ in pts **W/** chronic nasal disorders or severe reactive airway Dz; ↑ incidence of cough; must stop smoking & perform behavior modification for max effect

Nicotine Transdermal (Habitrol, Nicoderm CQ [OTC], Nicotrol [OTC], Others) [Smoking Deterrent/Cholinergic] Uses: *Aid to smoking cessation; relief of nicotine withdrawal* **Action:** Systemic delivery of nicotine **Dose:** Individualized; 1 patch (14–21 mg/d), & taper over 6 wk **Caution:** [D, M] **Contra:** Life-threatening arrhythmias, unstable angina **Disp:** *Habitrol & Nicoderm CQ:* 7, 14, 21 mg of nicotine/24 h; *Nicotrol:* 5, 10, 15 mg/24 h **SE:** Insomnia, pruritus, erythema, local site Rxn, tachycardia **Interactions:** ↑ Effects *OF* cimetidine, blue cohash; ↑ effects *OF* catecholamines, cortisol; ↑ hemodynamic & A-V blocking effects *OF* adenosine; ↑ HTN *W/* bupropion **NIPE:** Change application site daily; Nicotrol worn for 16 h to mimic smoking patterns; others worn for 24 h; must stop smoking & perform behavior modification for max effect

Nifedipine (Procardia, Procardia XL, Adalat, Adalat CC) [Antihypertensive, Antianginal/CCB] Uses: *Vasospastic or chronic stable angina & HTN*; tocolytic **Action:** CCB **Dose:** *Adults.* SR tabs 30–90 mg/d. *Tocolysis:* 10–20 mg PO q4–6h. *Peds.* 0.6–0.9 mg/kg/24 h ÷ tid–qid **Caution:** [C, +] Heart block, aortic stenosis **Contra:** Immediate-release preparation for urgent or emergent HTN; acute MI **Disp:** Caps 10, 20 mg; SR tabs 30, 60, 90 mg **SE:** HA common on initial Rx; reflex tachycardia may occur w/ regular release dosage forms; peripheral edema, ↓ BP, flushing, dizziness **Interactions:** ↑ Effects *W/* antihypertensives, azole antifungals, cimetidine, cisapride, CCBs, diltiazem, famotidine, nitrates, quinidine, ranitidine, EtOH, grapefruit juice; ↑ effects *OF* digitalis glycosides, phenytoin, vincristine; ↓ effects *W/* barbiturates, nafcillin, NSAIDs, phenobarbital, rifampin, St. John's wort, tobacco; ↓ effects *OF* of quinidine **Labs:** ↑ LFTs **NIPE:** Adalat CC & Procardia XR not interchangeable; SL administration not OK; take w/o regard to food; ↑ risk of photosensitivity—use sunscreen

Nilutamide (Nilandron) [Antineoplastic/Antiandrogen] **WARNING:** Interstitial pneumonitis possible; most cases in 1st 3 mo; follow CXR before Rx Uses: *Combo w/ surgical castration for met CAP* **Action:** Nonsteroidal antiandrogen **Dose:** 300 mg/d PO in ÷ doses × 30 d, then 150 mg/d **Caution:** Not used in females **Contra:** Severe hepatic impair, resp insuff **Disp:** Tabs 150 mg **SE:** Interstitial pneumonitis, hot flashes, ↓ libido, impotence, N/V/D, gynecomastia, hepatic dysfunction **Interactions:** ↑ Effects *OF* phenytoin, theophylline, warfarin **Labs:** ↑ LFTs (monitor) **NIPE:** Take w/o regard to food; visual adaptation may be delayed; may cause Rxn when taken w/ EtOH

Nimodipine (Nimotop) [Cerebral Vasodilator/CCB] Uses: *Prevent vasospasm following subarachnoid hemorrhage* **Action:** CCB **Dose:** 60 mg PO q4h for 21 d; ↓ in hepatic failure **Caution:** [C, ?] **Contra:** Component allergy **Disp:** Caps 30 mg **SE:** ↓ BP, HA, constipation **Interactions:** ↑ Effects *W/* other CCB; grapefruit juice, EtOH; ↓ effects *W/* ephedra, St. John's wort, any food **Labs:** ↑ LFTs **NIPE:** Give via NG tube if caps cannot be swallowed whole, PO administration only; ↑ risk of photosensitivity—use sunscreen

Nisoldipine (Sular) [Antihypertensive/CCB] Uses: *HTN* Action: CCB Dose: 10–60 mg/d PO; ↓ start doses w/ elderly or hepatic impair Caution: [C, ?] Disp: ER tabs 10, 20, 30, 40 mg SE: Edema, HA, flushing Interactions: ↑ Effects W/ antihypertensives, cimetidine, nitrates, EtOH, high-fat foods; ↓ effects W/ phenytoin, St. John's wort NIPE: Do not take w/ grapefruit juice or high-fat meal

Nitazoxanide (Alinia) [Antiinfective/Antiprotozoal] Uses: *Cryptosporidium* sp or *Giardia* sp-induced D in pts 1–11 y* Action: Antiprotozoal interferes w/ pyruvate ferredoxin oxidoreductase Spectrum: Cryptosporidium sp, Giardia sp Dose: *Peds. 12–47 mo:* 5 mL (100 mg) PO q12h × 3 d. *4–11 y:* 10 mL (200 mg) PO q12h × 3 d; *= 12 y:* 500 mg q12h for 3 d take w/ food Caution: [B, ?] Disp: 100 mg/5 mL PO susp, 500 tab SE: Abd pain Interactions: ↑ Effects W/ warfarin NIPE: Susp contains sucrose, interacts w/ highly protein-bound drugs

Nitrofurantoin (Macrodantin, Furadantin, Macrobid) [Urinary Anti-infective] WARNING: Pulm Rxns possible Uses: *Prevention & Rx UTI* Action: Bacteriostatic; interferes w/ carbohydrate metabolism. Spectrum: Some gram(+) & (–) bacteria; *Pseudomonas* sp, *Serratia* sp, & most *Proteus* sp-resistant Dose: *Adults. Suppression:* 50–100 mg/d PO. *Rx:* 50–100 mg PO qid. *Peds. Suppression:* 1–2 mg/kg/d in 1–2 ÷ doses, max 100 mg/d. *Rx:* 5–7 mg/kg/24 h in 4 ÷ doses (w/ food/milk/antacid) Caution: [B, +] Avoid w/ CrCl <60 mL/min, PRG at term Contra: Renal failure, infants <1 mo Disp: Caps 25, 50, 100 mg; susp 25 mg/5 mL SE: GI effects, dyspnea, various acute/chronic pulm Rxns, peripheral neuropathy Interactions: ↑ Effects W/ probenecid, sulfinpyrazone; ↓ effects W/ antacids, quinolones Labs: ↑ Serum bilirubin, alk phos NIPE: Take W/ food; may discolor urine; Macrocrystals (Macrodantin) cause < N than other forms

Nitroglycerin (Nitrostat, Nitrolingual, Nitro-Bid Ointment, Nitro-Bid IV, Nitrodisc, Transderm-Nitro, Others) [Antianginal, Vasodilator/Nitrate] Uses: *Angina pectoris, acute & prophylactic therapy, CHF, BP control* Action: Relaxes vascular smooth muscle, dilates coronary arteries Dose: *Adults. SL:* 1 tab q5min SL PRN for 3 doses. *Translingual:* 1–2 met-doses sprayed onto PO mucosa q3–5min, max 3 doses. *PO:* 2.5–9 mg tid. *IV:* 5–20 μg/min, titrated to effect. *Topical:* Apply 1/2 in. of oint to chest wall tid, wipe off at night. *TD:* 0.2–0.4 mg/h/patch daily; *IV bolus:* 12.5–25 μg; inf at 10–20 μg/min. *SL:* 0.3–0.4 mg, repeat q5min. *Aerosol spray:* Spray 0.5–1.0 s at 5-min intervals *(ECC 2005)* Peds. 0.25–0.5 μg/kg/min IV, titrate. Caution: [B, ?] Restrictive cardiomyopathy Contra: *IV:* Pericardial tamponade, constrictive pericarditis. *PO:* w/ sildenafil, tadalafil, vardenafil, head trauma, NAG Disp: SL tabs 0.3, 0.4, 0.6 mg; translingual spray 0.4 mg/dose; SR caps 2.5, 6.5, 9; SR tabs 2.6, 6.5, 9.0 mg; inj 0.1, 0.2, 0.4 mg/mL (premixed); 5 mg/mL injection soln; oint 2%; TD patches 0.1, 0.2, 0.4, 0.6 mg/h; buccal CR 2, 3 mg SE: HA, ↓ BP, lightheadedness, GI upset Interactions: ↑ Hypotensive effects W/ antihypertensives, phenothiazines, sildenafil, tadalafil, vardenafil, EtOH; ↓ effects W/ ergot alkaloids; ↓ effects OF

SL tabs & spray **W/** antihistamines, phenothiazine, TCAs **Labs:** False ↑ cholesterol, triglycerides **NIPE:** Replace SL tabs q6mo & keep in original container; nitrate tolerance w/ chronic use after 1–2 wk; minimize by providing nitrate-free period daily, using shorter-acting nitrates tid, & removing LA patches & oint before sleep to ↓ tolerance

Nitroprusside (Nipride, Nitropress) [Antihypertensive/Vasodilator] Uses: *Hypertensive crisis, CHF, controlled ↓ BP periop (↓ bleeding)*, aortic dissection, pulm edema **Action:** ↓ Systemic vascular resistance **Dose:** *Adult & Peds.* 0.5–10 μg/kg/min IV inf, titrate; usual dose 3 μg/kg/min **Caution:** [C, ?] ↓ Cerebral perfusion **Contra:** High output failure, compensatory HTN **Disp:** Inj 25 mg/mL **SE:** Excessive hypotensive effects, palpitations, HA **Interactions:** ↑ Effects **W/** antihypertensives, anesthetics, sildenafil, tadalafil, vardenafil; ↑ risk of arrhythmias **W/** TCA **Labs** **NIPE:** Discard colored soln other than light brown; thiocyanate (metabolite w/ renal excretion) w/ tox at 5–10 mg/dL, more likely if used for >2–3 d; w/ aortic dissection use w/ β-blocker

Nizatidine (Axid, Axid AR [OTC]) [Gastric Antisecretory/H₂ Receptor Antagonist] Uses: *Duodenal ulcers, GERD, heartburn* **Action:** H₂-Receptor antagonist **Dose:** *Adults. Active ulcer:* 150 mg PO bid or 300 mg PO hs; maint 150 mg PO hs. *GERD:* 150 mg PO bid. *Heartburn:* 75 mg PO bid. *Peds. GERD:* 10 mg/kg PO bid in ÷ doses, 150 mg bid max; ↓ in renal impair **Caution:** [B, +] **Contra:** H₂-Receptor antagonist sensitivity **Disp:** Caps 75 [OTC], 150, 300 mg; sol 15 mg/mL **SE:** Dizziness, HA, constipation, D **Interactions:** ↑ Effects *OF* salicylates, EtOH; ↓ effects **W/** antacids, tomato/mixed veg juice **Labs:** ↑ LFTs, uric acid **NIPE:** Smoking ↑ gastric acid secretion

Norepinephrine (Levophed) [Adrenergic Agonist/Vasopressor/Sympathomimetic] Uses: *Acute ↓ BP, cardiac arrest (adjunct)* **Action:** Peripheral vasoconstrictor of arterial/venous beds **Dose:** *Adults.* 8–30 μg/min IV, titrate. *Peds.* 0.05–0.1 μg/kg/min IV, titrate **Caution:** [C, ?] **Contra:** ↓ BP due to hypovolemia **Disp:** Inj 1 mg/mL **SE:** Bradycardia, arrhythmia **Notes:** Correct volume depletion as much as possible before vasopressors; interaction w/ TCAs leads to severe HTN; use large vein to avoid extrav; phentolamine 5–10 mg/10 mL NS injected locally for extrav **Interactions:** ↑ HTN **W/** antihistamines, BBs, ergot alkaloids, guanethidine, MAOIs, methyldopa, oxytocic meds, TCAs; ↑ risk of arrhythmias **W/** cyclopropane, halothane **Labs:** ↑ Glucose **NIPE:** Correct volume depletion as much as possible before vasopressors; use large vein to avoid extrav; phentolamine 5–10 mg/10 mL NS injected locally for extrav

Norethindrone Acetate/Ethinyl Estradiol Tablets (Femhrt) (See Estradiol/ Norethindrone Acetate) [Progestin & Estrogen]

Norfloxacin (Noroxin, Chibroxin Ophthal) [Antibiotic/Fluoroquinolone] Uses: *Complicated & uncomplicated UTI due to gram(−) bacteria, prostatitis, gonorrhea*, infectious D, conjunctivitis **Action:** Quinolone, ↓ DNA gyrase, bactericidal *Spectrum:* Broad gram(+) & (−) E. faecalis, E. coli,

K. pneumoniae, P. mirabilis, P. aeruginosa, S. epidermidis, S. saprophyticus **Dose:** 400 mg PO bid; *Gonorrhea:* 800 mg single dose; *Prostatitis:* 400 mg PO bid; *Gastroenteritis, travelers D:* 400 mg PO × 3–5 d ↓ w/ renal impair *Adults & Peds. >1 y:* *Ophth:* 1 gtt each eye qid for 7 d **Caution:** [C, –] Tendinitis/tendon rupture, quinolone sensitivity **Contra:** h/o allergy or tendonitis w/ fluoroquinolones **Disp:** Tabs 400 mg; ophth 3 mg/mL **SE:** Photosens, HA, GI; ocular burning w/ ophth **Interactions:** ↑ Effects **W/** probenecid; ↑ effects of diazepam, theophylline, caffeine, metoprolol, propranolol, phenytoin, warfarin; ↓ effects **W/** antacids, didanosine, Fe salts, Mg, sucralfate, NaHCO$_3$, Zn; ↓ effects **W/** food **Labs:** ↑ LFTs, BUN, SCr **NIPE:** ⊘ Give to children <18 y except for opth sol; ↑ fluids to 2–3 L/d; may cause photosensitivity—use sunscreen; good conc in the kidney & urine, poor blood levels; not for urosepsis

Norgestrel (Ovrette) [Progestin] Uses: *PO contraceptive* Action: Prevent follicular maturation & ovulation **Dose:** 1 tab/d; begin day 1 of menses **Caution:** [X, ?] **Contra:** Thromboembolic disorders, breast CA, PRG, severe hepatic Dz **Disp:** Tabs 0.075 mg **SE:** Edema, breakthrough bleeding, thromboembolism **Interactions:** ↓ Effects **W/** barbiturates, carbamazepine, hydantoins, griseofulvin, penicillins, rifampin, tetracyclines, St. John's wort **NIPE:** Photosensitivity—use sunscreen; D/C drug if suspect PRG—use barrier contraception until confirmed progestin-only products have ↑ risk of failure in prevention of PRG

Nortriptyline (Aventyl, Pamelor) [Antidepressant/TCA] Uses: *Endogenous depression* Action: TCA; ↑ synaptic CNS levels of serotonin &/or norepinephrine **Dose:** *Adults.* 25 mg PO tid–qid; >150 mg PO not OK. *Elderly.* 10–25 mg hs. *Peds. 6–7 y:* 10 mg/d. *8–11 y:* 10–20 mg/d. *>11 y:* 25–35 mg/d, ↓ w/ hepatic insuff **Caution:** [D, +/–] NAG, CV Dz **Contra:** TCA allergy, use w/ MAOI **Disp:** Caps 10, 25, 50, 75 mg; soln 10 mg/5 mL **SE:** ↑ Anticholinergic (blurred vision, retention, xerostomia) **Interactions:** ↑ Effects **W/** antihistamines, CNS depressants, cimetidine, fluoxetine, OCP, phenothiazine, quinidine, EtOH; ↑ effects **OF** anticoagulants; ↑ risk of HTN **W/** clonidine, levodopa, sympathomimetics; ↓ effects **W/** barbiturates, carbamazepine, rifampin **Labs:** ↑ Serum bilirubin, alkaline phosphatase **NIPE:** Concurrent use **W/** MAOIs have resulted in HTN, Szs, death; ↑ risk of photosensitivity—use sunscreen; max effect after 2 wk

Nystatin (Mycostatin) [Anti-infective/Antifungal] Uses: *Mucocutaneous Candida Infxns (oral, skin, vag)* Action: Alters membrane permeability. *Spectrum:* Susceptible *Candida* sp **Dose:** *Adults & children.* PO: 400,000–600,000 units PO "swish & swallow" qid. *Vag:* 1 tab vag hs × 2 wk. *Topical:* Apply bid–tid to area. *Peds.* Infants: 200,000 units PO q6h. **Caution:** [B (C PO), +] **Disp:** PO susp 100,000 units/mL; PO tabs 500,000 units; troches 200,000 units; vag tabs 100,000 units; topical cream/oint 100,000 units/g, powder 100,000 units/g **SE:** GI upset, Stevens–Johnson synd **NIPE:** Store susp up to 10 d in refrigerator; not absorbed PO; not for systemic Infxns

Octreotide (Sandostatin, Sandostatin LAR) [Antidiarrheal/ Hormone] Uses: *↓ Severe D associated w/ carcinoid & neuroendocrine GI tumors (eg, VIPoma, ZE synd)*; bleeding esophageal varices Action: LA peptide; mimics natural hormone somatostatin Dose: *Adults.* 100–600 μg/d SQ/IV in 2–4 ÷ doses; start 50 μg daily–bid. *Sandostatin LAR (depot):* 10–30 mg IM q4wk *Peds.* 1–10 μg/kg/24 h SQ in 2–4 ÷ doses. Caution: [B, +] Hepatic/renal impair Disp: Inj 0.05, 0.1, 0.2, 0.5, 1 mg/mL; 10, 20, 30 mg/5 mL LAR depot SE: N/V, abd discomfort, flushing, edema, fatigue, cholelithiasis, hyper/hypoglycemia, hepatitis Interactions: ↓ Effects *OF* cyclosporine, vitamin B_{12} Labs: Small ↑ LFTs, ↓ serum thyroxine, vitamin B_{12} NIPE: May alter effects of hypoglycemics

Ofloxacin (Floxin, Ocuflox Ophthalmic) [Antibiotic/Fluoroquinolone] Uses: *Lower resp tract, skin & skin structure, & UTI, prostatitis, uncomplicated gonorrhea, & *Chlamydia* Infxns; topical (bacterial conjunctivitis; otitis externa; if perforated ear drum >12 y)* Action: Bactericidal; ↓ DNA gyrase. *Broad spectrum gram(+) & (–): S. pneumonias, S. aureus, S. pyogenes, H. influenzae, P. mirabilis, N. gonorrhoeae, C. trachomatis, E. coli* Dose: *Adults.* 200–400 mg PO bid or IV q12h. *Adults & Peds >1 y. Ophth:* 1–2 gtt in eye(s) q2–4h for 2 d, then qid × 5 more d. *Adults & Peds >12 y. Otic:* 10 gtt in ear(s) bid for 10 d. *Peds 1–12 y. Otic:* 5 gtt in ear(s) for 10 d. ↓ in renal impair, take on empty stomach Caution: [C, –] ↓ Absorption w/ antacids, sucralfate, Al-, Ca-, Mg-, Fe-, Zn-containing drugs Contra: Quinolone allergy Disp: Tabs 200, 300, 400 mg; inj 20, 40 mg/mL; ophth & otic 0.3% SE: N/V/D, photosens, insomnia, HA, local irritation Notes: Ophth form OK in ears Interactions: ↑ Effects *W/* cimetidine, probenecid; ↑ effects *OF* procainamide, theophylline, warfarin; ↑ risk of tendon rupture *W/* corticosteroids; ↓ effects *W/* antacids, antineoplastics, Ca, didanosine, Fe, NaHCO₃, sucralfate, Zn NIPE: Take w/o food; use sunscreen; ↑ fluids to 2–3 L/d

Olanzapine (Zyprexa, Zyprexa, Zydis) [Antipsychotic/ Thienobenzodiazepine] WARNING: Mortality in elderly w/ dementia-related psychosis Uses: *Bipolar mania, schizophrenia*, psychotic disorders, acute agitation in schizophrenia Action: Dopamine & serotonin antagonist; Dose: *Bipolar/schizophrenia:* 5–10 mg/d, ↑ weekly PRN, 20 mg/d max; *Agitation:* 5–10 mg IM q2–4h PRN, 30 mg d/max Caution: [C, –] Disp: Tabs 2.5, 5, 7.5, 10, 15, 20 mg; PO disint tabs 5, 10, 15, 20 mg; Inj 10 mg SE: HA, somnolence, orthostatic ↓ BP, tachycardia, dystonia, xerostomia, constipation Interactions: ↑ Effects *W/* fluvoxamine; ↑ sedation *W/* CNS depressants, EtOH; ↑ Szs *W/* anticholinergics, CNS depressants; ↑ hypotension *W/* antihypertensives, diazepam; ↓ effects *W/* activated charcoal, carbamazepine, omeprazole, rifampin, St. John's wort, tobacco; ↓ effects *OF* dopamine agonists, levodopa Labs: ↑ LFTs NIPE: ↑ Risk *OF* tardive dyskinesia, photosensitivity—use sunscreen, body temp impairment; takes weeks to titrate dose; smoking ↓ levels; may be confused w/ Zyrtec

Olopatadine (Patanol) [Ophthalmic Antihistamine] Uses: *Allergic conjunctivitis* Action: H_1-receptor antagonist Dose: 1–2 gtt in eye(s)

bid –allow 6–8 h between doses **Caution:** [C, ?] **Disp:** Soln 0.1% 5 mL **SE:** Local irritation, HA, rhinitis **NIPE:** ⊘ In children <3 y; may reinsert contacts 10 min later if eye not red

Olsalazine (Dipentum) [Anti-inflammatory/Aminosalicylic Acid Derivative]   Uses: *Maint remission in UC* **Action:** Topical anti-inflammatory **Dose:** 500 mg PO bid (w/ food) **Caution:** [C, M] Salicylate sensitivity **Disp:** Caps 250 mg **SE:** D, HA, blood dyscrasias, hepatitis **Interaction:** ↑ Effects *OF* anticoagulants **Labs:** ↑ LFTs **NIPE:** Food < GI upset

Omalizumab (Xolair) [Antiasthmatic/Monoclonal Antibody]   **WARNING:** Reports of anaphylaxis 2–24 h after administration, even in previously treated patients   **Uses:** *Moderate–severe asthma in >/=12 y w/ reactivity to an allergen & when Sxs inadequately controlled w/ inhaled steroids* **Action:** Anti-IgE Ab **Dose:** 150–375 mg SQ q2–4wk (dose/frequency based on serum IgE level & BW, see package insert) **Caution:** [B,?/–] **Contra:** Component allergy, acute bronchospasm **Disp:** 150 mg single-use 5-mL vial **SE:** Site Rxn, sinusitis, HA, anaphylaxis reported in 3 pts **Interactions:** No drug interaction studies done **NIPE:** ⊘ D/C abruptly; not for acute bronchospasm; admin w/in 8 h of reconstitution and store in refrigerator; continue other asthma medications as indicated

Omega-3 fatty acid [fish oil] (Louaza) [Lipid Regulator/ Ethyl Ester]   Uses: *Rx hypertriglyceridemia* **Action:** Omega-3-acid ethyl esters, ↓ thrombus inflammation & triglycerides **Dose:** *Hypertriglyceridemia:* 4 g/d divided in 1–2 doses **Caution:** PRG risk factor [C,-] w/ anticoagulant use, w/ bleed risk **Contra:** Hypersensitivity to components **Disp:** 1000-mg gelcap **SE:** Dyspepsia, N, GI pain, rash, flulike Sxs **Interactions:** ↑ Effects *OF* anticoagulants **Labs:** Monitor triglycerides, LDL, ALT **NIPE:** Only FDA approved fish oil supplement; not for exogenous hypertriglyceridemia (type 1 hyperchylomicronemia); many OTC products; D/C after 2 mo if TG levels do not ↓; previously called "Omacor"

Omeprazole (Prilosec, Zegerid) [Anti-Ulcer Agent/Proton Pump Inhibitor]   Uses: *Duodenal/gastric ulcers, ZE synd, GERD*, *H. pylori* Infxns **Action:** Proton-pump inhibitor **Dose:** 20–40 mg PO daily–bid; Zegerid powder/mix; in small cup w/ 2 Tbsp H₂O (not food or other Liq) refill and drink **Caution:** [C, –] **Disp:** DR tabs 20 mg; DR caps 10, 20, 40 mg; Zegerid powder for oral susp: 20, 40 mg. Zegerid caps 20, 40 mg **SE:** HA, D **Interactions:** ↑ Effects *OF* clarithromycin,digoxin, phenytoin, warfarin; ↓ effects *W/* sucralfate; ↓ effects *OF* ampicillin, cyanocobalamin, ketoconazole **Labs:** ↑ LFTs; **NIPE:** Combo (ie, antibiotic) Rx for *H. pylori,* take Zegerid 1 h before meals preferably in AM

Ondansetron (Zofran, Zofran ODT) [Antiemetic/5-HT Antagonist]   Uses: *Prevent chemo-associated & postop N/V* **Action:** Serotonin receptor antagonist **Dose:** *Chemo: Adults & Peds.* 0.15 mg/kg/dose IV prior to chemo, then 4 & 8 h after 1st dose or 4–8 mg PO tid; 1st dose 30 min prior to chemo & give on a schedule, not PRN. *Postop: Adults.* 4 mg IV immed preanesthesia or postop. **Peds.** <40 kg: 0.1 mg/kg. >40 kg: 4 mg IV; ↓ dose w/ hepatic impair **Caution:** [B, +/–] **Disp:** Tabs 4, 8, 24 mg, soln 4 mg/5 mL, inj 2 mg/mL, 32 mg/50 mL; Zofran ODT tab, 4, 8 mg **SE:** D, HA, constipation, dizziness **Interactions:** ↓ Effects W/ cimetidine, phenobarbital, rifampin **Labs:** ↑ LFTs **NIPE:** Food ↑ absorption

Oprelvekin (Neumega) [Thrombopoietic Growth Factor]
WARNING: Allergic Rxn w/ anaphylaxis reported; D/C w/ any allergic Rxn **Uses:** *Prevent ↓ plt w/ chemo* **Action:** ↑ Proliferation & maturation of megakaryocytes (interleukin-11) **Dose:** *Adults.* 50 μg/kg/d SQ for 10–21 d. **Peds.** >12 y: 75–100 μg/kg/d SQ for 10–21 d. <12 y: Use only in clinical trials. **Caution:** [C, ?/–] **Disp:** 5 mg powder for inj **SE:** Tachycardia, palpitations, arrhythmias, edema, HA, dizziness, insomnia, fatigue, fever, N, anemia, dyspnea, allergic Rxns including anaphylaxis **Interactions:** None noted **Labs:** ↓ HMG, albumin **NIPE:** Monitor for peripheral edema; use med w/in 3 h of reconstitution

Oral Contraceptives, Biphasic, Monophasic, Triphasic, Progestin Only (Table 6) [Progestin/Hormone] **WARNING:** Cigarette smoking ↑ risk of serious CV side effects; ↑ risk w/ >15 cig/d, >35 y; strongly advise women on OCPs not to smoke **Uses:** *Birth control; regulation of anovulatory bleeding; dysmenorrhea; endometriosis; polycystic ovaries; acne* (Note: FDA approvals vary widely, see insert) **Action:** *Birth control:* Suppresses LH surge, prevents ovulation; progestins thicken cervical mucus; ↓ fallopian tubule cilia, ↓ endometrial thickness to ↓ chances of fertilization. *Anovulatory bleeding:* Cyclic hormones mimic body's natural cycle & regulate endometrial lining, results in regular bleeding q28d; may ↓ uterine bleeding & dysmenorrhea **Dose:** Start day 1 menstrual cycle or 1st Sunday after onset of menses; 28-d cycle pills take daily; 21-d cycle pills take daily, no pills during last 7 d of cycle (during menses); some available as transdermal patch **Caution:** [X, +] Migraine, HTN, DM, sickle cell Dz, gallbladder Dz; monitor for breast Dz, ✓ K+ if taking drugs with ↑ K+ risk **Contra:** AUB, PRG, estrogen-dependent malignancy, ↑ hypercoagulation/liver Dz, hemiplegic migraine, smokers >35 y **Disp:** 28-d cycle pills (21 active pills + 7 placebo or Fe supplement); 21-d cycle pills (21 active pills) **SE:** Intramenstrual bleeding, oligomenorrhea, amenorrhea, ↑ appetite/wt gain, ↓ libido, fatigue, depression, mood swings, mastalgia, HA, melasma, ↑ vaginal discharge, acne/greasy skin, corneal edema, N **NIPE:** Taken correctly, 99.9% effective for contraception; no STDs prevention, use additional barrier contraceptive; long-term, can ↓ risk of ectopic PRG, benign breast Dz, ovarian & uterine CA. *Rx for menstrual cycle control:* Start w/monophasic × 3 mo before switching to another brand; w/ continued bleed, change to pill w/↑estrogen; *Rx for birth control:* Choose pill w/ lowest SE profile for particular pt; SEs numerous; due to estrogenic excess or progesterone deficiency; each pill's SE profile can be unique (see insert); newer extended cycle combo have shorter/fewer hormone free intervals ? ↓ PRG risk; OCP troubleshooting SE w/ suggested OCP:

- *Absent menstrual flow:* ↑ Estrogen, ↓ progestin: Brevicon, Necon 1/35, Norinyl 1/35, Modicon, Necon 1/50, Norinyl 1/50, Ortho-Cyclen, Ortho-Novum 1/50, Ortho-Novum 1/35, Ovcon 35
- *Acne:* Use ↑ estrogen, ↓ androgenic: Brevicon, Cyclen, Demulen 1/50, Othro-Tri Cyclen, Mircette, Modicon, Necon, Ortho Evra, Yasmin
- *Break through bleed:* ↑ Estrogen, ↑ progestin, ↓ androgenic: Demulen 1/50, Desogen, Estrostep, Loestrin 1/20, Ortho-Cept, Ovcon 50, Yasmin, Zovia 1/50E
- *Breast tenderness or ↑ wt:* ↓ Estrogen, ↓ progestin: use ↓ estrogen pill than current; Alesse, Levlite, Loestrin 1/20 Fe, Ortho Evra Yasmin
- *Depression:* ↓ Progestin: Alesse, Brevicon, Levlite, Modicon, Necon, Ortho Evra, Ovcon 35, Othro-Cyclen, Ortho-TriCyclen Tri-Levlen, Triphasil, Trivora
- *Endometriosis:* ↓ Estrogen, ↑ progestin: Demulen 1/35, Loestrin 1.5/30, Loestrin 1/20 Fe, LoOvral, Levlen, Levora, Nordette, Zovia 1/35; continuous w/0 placebo pills or w/ 4 d of placebo pills
- *HA:* ↓ Estrogen, ↓ progestin: Alesse, Levlite, Ortho Evra
- *Moodiness or irritability:* ↓ Progestin: Alesse, Brevicon, Levlite, Modicon, Necon 1/35, Ortho Evra, Ortho-Cyclen, Ortho Tri-Cyclen, Ovcon 35, Tri-Levlen, Triphasil, Trivora
- *Severe menstrual cramping:* ↑ Progestin: Demulen 1/50, Desogen, Loestrin 1.5/30, Mircette, Ortho-Cept ,Yasmin, Zovia 1/50E, Zovia 1/35E

Orlistat (Xenical, Alli [OTC]). [Obesity Management/GI Lipase Inhibitor]
Uses: *Manage obesity w/ BMI ≥30 kg/m^2 or ≥27 kg/m^2 w/ other risk factors; type 2 DM, dyslipidemia* **Action:** Reversible inhibitor of gastric & pancreatic lipases. **Dose:** 120 mg PO tid w/ a fat-containing meal; Alli (OTC) 60 mg po tid w/ fat-containing meals **Caution:** [B, ?] May ↓ cyclosporine & warfarin dose requirements **Contra:** Cholestasis, malabsorption **Disp:** Capsules 120 mg **SE:** Abd pain/discomfort, fatty stools, fecal urgency **Interactions:** ↑ Effects *OF* pravastatin; ↓ effects *OF* cyclosporine, fat-soluble vitamins **Labs:** Monitor INR if taking warfarin, ↓ serum glucose, total cholesterol, LDL **NIPE:** Do not use if meal contains no fat; GI effects ↑ w/ higher-fat meals; supplement w/ fat-soluble vitamins

Orphenadrine (Norflex) [Skeletal Muscle Relaxant]
Uses: *Muscle spasms* **Action:** Central atropine-like effects cause indirect skeletal muscle relaxation, euphoria, analgesia **Dose:** 100 mg PO bid, 60 mg IM/IV q12h **Caution:** [C, +] **Contra:** NAG, GI obst, cardiospasm, MyG **Disp:** Tabs 100 mg; SR tabs 100 mg; inj 30 mg/mL **SE:** Drowsiness, dizziness, blurred vision, flushing, tachycardia, constipation **Interactions:** ↑ CNS depression *W/* anxiolytics, butorphanol, hypnotics, MAOIs, nalbuphine, opioids, pentazocine, phenothiazine, tramadol, TCAs, kava kava, valerian, EtOH; ↑ effects *W/* anticholinergics **NIPE:** Impaired body temp regulation

Oseltamivir (Tamiflu) [Antiviral/Neuraminidase Inhibitor]
Uses: *Prevention & Rx influenza A & B* **Action:** ↓ Viral neuraminidase **Dose:**

Adults. Treatment 75 mg PO bid × 5 d *Prophylaxis:* 75 mg PO daily × 10 d *Peds. PO bid dosing:* <15 kg: 30 mg. *15–23 kg:* 45 mg. *24–40 kg:* 60 mg. >40 kg adult dose. ↓ w/ renal impair **Caution:** [C, ?/–] **Contra:** Component allergy **Disp:** Caps 75 mg, powder 12 mg/mL **SE:** N/V, insomnia, reports of neuropsychiatric events in children (self-injury, confusion, delirium) **Interaction:** ↑ Effects *W/* probenecid **NIPE:** Take w/ regard to food; initiate w/in 48 h of Sx onset or exposure

Oxacillin (Prostaphlin) [Antibiotic/Penicillin] Uses: *Infxns due to susceptible *S. aureus* & *Streptococcus* sp* **Action:** Bactericidal; ↓ Cell wall synth. *Spectrum:* Excellent gram(+), poor gram(–) **Dose:** *Adults.* 250–500 mg (2g severe) IM/IV q4–6h. *Peds.* 150–200 mg/kg/d IV ÷ q4–6h; ↓ w/ sig renal Dz Caution: [B, M] **Contra:** PCN sensitivity **Disp:** Powder for inj 500 mg, 1, 2, 10 g, soln 250 mg/5 mL **SE:** GI upset, interstitial nephritis, blood dyscrasias **Interactions:** ↑ Effects *W/* disulfiram, probenecid; ↑ effects *OF* anticoagulants, MTX; ↓ effects *W/* chloramphenicol, tetracyclines, carbonated drinks, fruit juice, food; ↓ effects *OF* OCPs **NIPE:** Take w/o food

Oxaliplatin (Eloxatin) [Antineoplastic/Alkylating Agent]
WARNING: Administer w/ supervision of health care provider experienced in chemo. Appropriate management is possible only w/ adequate diagnostic & Rx facilities. Anaphylactic-like Rxns reported Uses: *Adjuvant Rx stage-III colon CA (primary resected) & met colon CA w/ 5-FU* **Action:** Metabolized to platinum derivatives, crosslink DNA **Dose:** Per protocol; see insert. *Premedicate:* Antiemetic w/ or w/o d examethasone **Caution:** [D, –] see Warning **Contra:** Allergy to components or platinum **Disp:** Inj 50, 100 mg **SE:** Anaphylaxis, granulocytopenia, paresthesia, N/V/D, stomatitis, fatigue, neuropathy, hepatotox **Interactions:** ↑ Effects *OF* nephrotoxic drugs **Labs:** ↑ Bilirubin, Cr, LFTs; ↓ HMG, K⁺, neutrophils, plts, WBC **NIPE:** Monitor CBC, plts, LFTs, BUN & Cr before each chemotherapy cycle; ↑ acute neurologic symptoms *W/* cold exposure / cold Liq 5-FU & Leucovorin are given in combo; epi, corticosteroids, & antihistamines alleviate severe Rxns

Oxaprozin (Daypro, Daypro ALTA) [Analgesic, Anti-inflammatory, Antipyretic/NSAID] WARNING: May ↑ risk of cardiovascular events & GI bleeding Uses: *Arthritis & pain* **Action:** NSAID; ↓ prostaglandins synth **Dose:** 600–1200 mg/d (÷ dose may help GI tolerance); ↓ in renal/hepatic impair **Caution:** [C (D in 3rd tri or near term), ?], peptic ulcer, bleeding disorders **Contra:** ASA/NSAID sensitivity perioperative pain w/ CABG **Disp:** Daypro ALTA tab 600 mg; caplets 600 mg **SE:** CNS inhibition, sleep disturbance, rash, GI upset, peptic ulcer, edema, renal failure, anaphylactoid Rxn with ASA triad (asthmatic w/ rhinitis, nasal polyps and bronchospasm w/ NSAID use) **Interactions:** ↑ Effects *OF* aminoglycosides, anticoagulants, ASA, Li, MTX, ↓ effects *OF* antihypertensives, diuretics **NIPE:** ↑ Risk of photosensitivity—use sunscreen; take w/ food

Oxazepam [C-IV] [Anxiolytic/Benzodiazepines] Uses: *Anxiety, acute EtOH withdrawal*, anxiety w/ depressive Sxs **Action:** Benzodiazepine;

metabolite of diazepam **Dose:** *Adults.* 10–15 mg PO tid–qid; severe anxiety & EtOH withdrawal may require up to 30 mg qid. *Peds.* 1 mg/kg/d ÷ doses **Caution:** [D, ?] **Contra:** Component allergy, NAG **Disp:** Caps 10, 15, 30 mg; tabs 15 mg **SE:** Sedation, ataxia, dizziness, rash, blood dyscrasias, dependence **Interactions:** ↑ CNS effects **W/** anticonvulsants, antidepressants, antihistamines, barbiturates, MAOIs, opioids, phenothiazine, kava kava, lemon balm, sassafras, valerian, EtOH; ↑ effects **W/** cimetidine; ↓ effects **W/** OCPs, phenytoin, theophylline, tobacco; ↓ effects **OF** levodopa **Labs:** False ↑ serum glucose **NIPE:** ⊘ D/C abruptly

Oxcarbazepine (Trileptal) [Anticonvulsant/Carbamazepine]
Uses: *Partial Szs*, bipolar disorders **Action:** Blocks voltage-sensitive Na⁺ channels, stabilization of hyperexcited neural membranes **Dose:** *Adults.* 300 mg PO bid, ↑ weekly to target maint 1200–2400 mg/d. *Peds.* 8–10 mg/kg bid, 600 mg/d max, ↑ weekly to target maint dose; ↓ w/ renal insuff **Caution:** [C, –] Carbamazepine sensitivity; **Contra:** Components sensitivity **Disp:** Tabs 150, 300, 600 mg; Susp 300 mg/5 mL **SE:** ↓ Na⁺, HA, dizziness, fatigue, somnolence, GI upset, diplopia, concentration difficulties, fatal skin/multiorgan hypersensitivity Rxns **Interactions:** ↑ Effects **W/** benzodiazepines, EtOH; ↑ effects **OF** phenobarbital, phenytoin; ↓ effects **W/** barbiturates, carbamazepine, phenobarbital, valproic acid, verapamil; ↓ effects **OF** CCBs, OCPs **Labs:** ↓ Thyroid levels, serum Na; ✓ Na⁺ if fatigued **NIPE:** Take w/o regard to food; use barrier contraception; do not abruptly D/C,; advise about Stevens–Johnson synd and topic epidermal necrolysis

Oxiconazole (Oxistat) [Antifungal] **Uses:** *Tinea cruris, corporis, pedis, versicolor* **Action:** ? ↓ Ergosterols in fungal cell membrane **Spectrum:** Most *E.floccosum, T. mentagrophytes, T. rubrum, M. furfur* **Dose:** Apply thin layer daily–bid **Caution:** [B, M] **Contra:** Component allergy **Disp:** Cream, lotion 1% **SE:** Local irritation

Oxybutynin (Ditropan, Ditropan XL) [GU Antispasmodic/Anticholinergic] **Uses:** *Symptomatic relief of urgency, nocturia, incontinence w/ neurogenic or reflex neurogenic bladder* **Action:** Anicholinergic, relaxes bladder smooth muscle, ↑ bladder capacity **Dose:** *Adults & Peds.* >5 y: 5 mg PO tid–qid; XR 5 mg PO daily; ↑ to 30 mg/d PO (5 & 10 mg/tab). *Peds. 1–5 y:* 0.2 mg/kg/dose bid–qid (syrup 5 mg/5 mL); ↓ in elderly; periodic drug holidays OK **Caution:** [B, ?] **Contra:** NAG, MyG, GI/GU obst, ulcerative colitis, megacolon **Disp:** Tabs 5 mg; XR tabs 5, 10, 15 mg; syrup 5 mg/5 mL **SE:** Anticholinergic (drowsiness, xerostomia, constipation, tachycardia) **Interactions:** ↑ Effects **W/** CNS depressants, EtOH; ↑ effects **OF** atenolol, digoxin, nitrofurantoin; ↑ anticholinergic effects **W/** antihistamines, anticholinergics; ↓ effects **OF** haloperidol, levodopa **NIPE:** ↓ Temp regulation; ↑ photosensitivity—use sunscreen; ER form shell expelled in stool

Oxybutynin Transdermal System (Oxytrol) [GU Antispasmodic/Anticholinergic] **Uses:** *Rx OAB* **Action:** Anicholinergic, relaxes bladder smooth muscle, ↑ bladder capacity ↑ **Dose:** One 3.9 mg/d system apply 2×/wk (every 3–4 d) to abdomen, hip, or buttock **Caution:** [B, ?/–] **Contra:** GI/GU obst, NAG **Disp:** 3.9 mg/d transdermal patch **SE:** Anticholinergic, itching/redness at site **Interactions:** ↑ Effects **W/** anticholinergics **NIPE:** Metabolized by the cytochrome P450 CYP3A4 enzyme system; do not apply to same site w/in 7 d

Oxycodone [Dihydrohydroxycodeinone] (OxyContin, OxyIR, Roxicodone) [C-II] [Opioid Analgesic]   WARNING: High abuse potential; CR only for extended chronic pain, not for PRN use; 80 mg ER tabs only for opioid tolerant patients   **Uses:** *Moderate/severe pain, usually in combo w/ nonnarcotic analgesics* **Action:** Narcotic analgesic **Dose:** *Adults.* 5 mg PO q6h PRN (immed release); *Mod-severe chronic pain* 10–160 mg PO q12h (XR) *Peds.* *6–12 y:* 1.25 mg PO q6h PRN. *>12 y:* 2.5 mg q6h PRN; ↓ w/ severe liver/renal Dz, elderly; w/ food **Caution:** [B (D if prolonged use/near term), M] **Contra:** Allergy, resp depression, acute asthma, ileus w/ microsomal morphine **Disp:** Immed-release caps (OxyIR) 5 mg; tabs (Percolone) 5 mg; CR Roxicodone tabs 5, 15, 30 mg; XR (OxyContin) 10, 20, 40, 80 mg; Liq 5 mg/5 mL; soln conc 20 mg/mL **SE:** ↓ BP, sedation, dizziness, GI upset, constipation, risk of abuse **Interactions:** ↑ CNS & resp. depression **W/** amitriptylline, barbiturates, cimetidine, clomipramine, MAOIs, nortriptyline, protease inhibitors, TCAs **Labs:** ↑ Serum amylase, lipase **NIPE:** Take w/ food; OxyContin for chronic CA pain; do not crush/chew/cut ER prod; sought after as drug of abuse

Oxycodone & Acetaminophen (Percocet, Tylox) [C-II] [Narcotic Analgesic]   **Uses:** *Moderate–severe pain* **Action:** Narcotic analgesic **Dose:** *Adults.* 1–2 tabs/caps PO q4–6h PRN (acetaminophen max dose 4 g/d). *Peds.* Oxycodone 0.05–0.15 mg/kg/dose q4–6h PRN, 5 mg/dose max **Caution:** [C (D prolonged use or near term), M] **Contra:** Allergy, resp depression **Disp:** Percocet tabs, mg oxycodone/mg APAP: 2.5/325, 5/325, 7.5/325, 10/325, 7.5/500, 10/650; Tylox caps 5 mg oxycodone, 500 mg APAP; soln 5 mg oxycodone & 325 mg APAP/5 mL **SE:** ↓ BP, sedation, dizziness, GI upset, constipation **Interactions:** ↑ CNS & resp depression **W/** amitriptylline, barbiturates, cimetidine, clomipramine, MAOIs, nortriptylline, protease inhibitors, TCAs **Labs:** False ↑ serum amylase, lipase **NIPE:** Take w/ food

Oxycodone & Aspirin (Percodan, Percodan-Demi) [C-II] [Narcotic Analgesic/Nonsteroidal Analgesic]   **Uses:** *Moderate–moderately severe pain* **Action:** Narcotic analgesic w/ NSAID **Dose:** *Adults.* 1–2 tabs/ caps PO q4–6h PRN. *Peds.* Oxycodone 0.05–0.15 mg/kg/dose q4–6h PRN, up to 5 mg/dose; ↓ in severe hepatic failure **Caution:** [D (prolonged use or near term), M] Peptic ulcer **Contra:** Component allergy, children (<16 y) with viral Infxn, resp depression, ileus **Disp:** *Percodan* 4.5 mg oxycodone hydrochloride, 0.38 mg oxycodone terephthalate, 325 mg ASA; *Percodan-Demi* 2.25 mg oxycodone hydrochloride, 0.19 mg oxycodone terephthalate, 325 mg ASA **SE:** Sedation, dizziness, GI upset, constipation **Interactions:** ↑ CNS & resp depression **W/**

amitriptyline, barbiturates, cimetidine, clomipramine, MAOIs, nortriptylline, protease inhibitors, TCAs; ↑ effects *OF* anticoagulants **Labs:** ↑ Serum amylase, lipase **NIPE:** Take w/ food

Oxycodone/Ibuprofen (Combunox) [C-II] [Narcotic Analgesic/NSAID]
WARNING: May ↑ risk of serious CV events; contra in periop CABG pain; ↑ risk of GI events such as bleeding   **Uses:** *Short-term (not >7 d) management of acute moderate–severe pain* **Action:** Narcotic w/ NSAID **Dose:** 1 tab q6h PRN 4 tab max/24 h; 7 d max. **Caution:** [C, –] w/ impaired renal/hepatic Fxn; COPD, CNS depression **Contra:** Paralytic ileus, 3rd tri PRG, allergy to ASA or NSAIDs, where opioids are contraindicated **Disp:** Tabs 5 mg oxycodone/400 mg ibuprofen **SE:** N/V, somnolence, dizziness, sweating, flatulence **Interactions:** ↑ CNS & resp. depression *W/* amitriptyline, barbiturates, cimetidine, clomipramine, MAOIs, nortriptyline , protease inhibitors, TCAs; ↑ effects *W/* ASA, corticosteroids, probenecid, EtOH; ↑ effects *OF* aminoglycosides, anticoagulants, digoxin, hypoglycemics, Li, MTX; ↑ risks of bleeding *W/* abciximab, cefotetan, valproic acid, thrombolytic drugs, warfarin, ticlopidine, garlic, ginger, ginkgo biloba; ↓ effects *W/* feverfew; ↑ effects *OF* antihypertensives **Labs:** ↑ Serum amylase, lipase, LFTs, BUN, Cr **NIPE:** Take w/ food; monitor renal Fxn; abuse potential w/ oxycodone

Oxymorphone (Opana, Opana ER) [C-II] [Opioid Analgesic]
WARNING: (Opana ER) Abuse potential, CR only for chronic pain; do not consume EtOH-containing beverages, may cause fatal OD   **Uses:** *Moderate/severe pain, sedative* **Action:** Narcotic analgesic **Dose:** 10–20 mg PO q4–6h PRN if opioid-naïve or 1–1.5 mg SC/IM q4–6h PRN or 0.5 mg IV q4–6h PRN; start 20 mg/dose max PO; Chronic pain: XR 5 mg PO q12h; if opioid-naïve ↑ PRN 5–10 mg PO q12h q3–7d; take 1h qc or 2h ac; ↓ dose w/ elderly, renal/hepatic impair **Caution:** [B, ?] **Contra:** ↑ ICP, severe resp depression, w/ EtOH or liposomal morphine, severe hepatic impair **Disp:** Tab 5, 10 mg; ER 5, 10, 20, 40 **SE:** ↓ BP, sedation, GI upset, constipation, histamine release **Interactions:** ↑ Effects *W/* CNS depressants, cimetidine, neuroleptics, EtOH; ↓ effects *W/* phenothiazines **Labs:** ↑ Amylase, lipase **NIPE:** Related to hydromorphone

Oxytocin (Pitocin) [Oxytocic/Hormone]
Uses: *Induce labor, control postpartum hemorrhage*; promote milk letdown in lactating women **Action:** Stimulate muscular contractions of the uterus & milk flow during nursing **Dose:** 0.0005–0.001 units/min IV inf; titrate 0.001–0.002 units/min q30–60min. *Breastfeeding:* 1 spray in both nostrils 2–3 min before feeding **Caution:** [Uncategorized, no anomalies expected, +/–] **Contra:** Where vaginal delivery not favorable, fetal distress **Disp:** Inj 10 units/mL; nasal soln 40 units/mL **SE:** Uterine rupture, fetal death; arrhythmias, anaphylaxis, H_2O intox **Interactions:** ↑ Pressor effects *W/* sympathomimetics **NIPE:** Monitor vital signs; nasal form for breast-feeding only

Paclitaxel (Taxol, Abraxane) [Antineoplastic/Antimitotic]
WARNING: Administration only by health care provider experienced in chemotherapy; fatal anaphylaxis and hypersensitivity possible; severe myelosuppression

possible **Uses:** *Ovarian & breast CA, PCa*, Kaposi sarcoma, NSCLC **Action:** Mitotic spindle poison; promotes microtubule assembly & stabilization against de-polymerization **Dose:** per protocols; use glass or polyolefin containers (eg, nitroglycerin tubing set); PVC sets leach plasticizer; ↓in hepatic failure **Caution:** [D, –] **Contra:** Neutropenia <1500 WBC/mm³; solidtumors, component allergy **Disp:** Inj 6 mg/mL, 5 mg/mL albumin bound (Abraxane) **SE:** ↓ BM, peripheral neuropathy, transient ileus, myalgia, bradycardia, ↓ BP, mucositis, N/V/D, fever, rash, HA, phlebitis; hematologic tox schedule-dependent; leukopenia dose-limiting by 24-h inf; neurotox limited w/ short (1–3 h) inf; allergic Rxns (dyspnea, ↓ BP, urticaria, rash) **Interactions:** ↑ Effects W/ cyclosporine, dexamethasone, diazepam,ketoconazole, midazolam, quinidine, teniposide, verapamil, vincristine; ↑ risk of bleeding W/ anticoagulants, plt inhibitors, thrombolytics; ↑ myelosuppression when cisplatin is admin before paclitaxel; ↓ effects W/ carbamazepine, phenobarbital; ↓ effects of live-virus vaccines **Labs:** ↑ AST, alkaline phosphatase, triglycerides **NIPE:** ⊘ PRG, breast-feeding, live-virus vaccines; use barrier contraception; maintain hydration; allergic Rxn usually w/in 10 min of inf; minimize w/ corticosteroid, antihistamine pretreatment

Palivizumab (Synagis) [Antiviral/Monoclonal Antibody]
Uses: *Prevent RSV Infxn* **Action:** MoAb **Dose:** *Peds.* 15 mg/kg IM monthly, typically Nov–Apr **Caution:** [C, ?] Renal/hepatic dysfunction **Contra:** Component allergy **Disp:** Vials 50, 100 mg **SE:** URI, rhinitis, cough, local irritation **Labs:**↑ LFT **NIPE:** Use drug w/in 6 h after reconstitution; ⊘ inj in gluteal site; for prophylaxis

Palifermin (Kepivance) [Growth Factor/Keratinocyte Growth Factor]
Uses: *Oral mucositis w/ BMT* **Action:** Synthetic keratinocyte GF **Dose:** *Phase 1:* 60 µg/kg IV daily × 3, 3rd dose 24–48 h before chemo *Phase 2:* 60 µg/kg IV daily × 3, immediately after stem cell inf **Caution:** [C, ?/–] **Contra:** N/A **Disp:** Inj 6.25 mg/vial **SE:** Unusual mouth sensations, tongue thickening, rash **LABS:** ↑ Amylase, lipase **NIPE:** Eval for rash & taste alterations; *E coli*-derived; separate phases by 4 d; safety unknown w/ nonhematologic malignancies

Palonosetron (Aloxi) [Antiemetic/5-HT3 Antagonist]
WARNING: May ↑ QTc interval **Uses:** *Prevention acute & delayed N/V w/ emetogenic chemo* **Action:** 5-HT3 receptor antagonist **Dose:** 0.25 mg IV 30 min prior to chemo; do not repeat w/in 7 d **Caution:** [B, ?] **Contra:** Component allergy **Disp:** 0.25 mg/5 mL vial **SE:** HA, constipation, dizziness, abd pain, anxiety **Interactions:** Potential for drug interactions low

Paliperidone (Invega) [Benzisoxazole]
WARNING: Not for dementia-related psychosis **Uses:** *Schizophrenia* **Action:** Risperidone metabolite, antagonizes dopamine receptors **Dose:** 6 mg PO qAM, 12 mg/d max; CrCl 50–79; 6 mg/d max; CrCl 10–49 3 mg/d max **Caution:** [C; ?/–] w/ bradycardia, ↓ K⁺/Mg²⁺, renal/hepatic impair **Contra:** Risperidone hypersensitivity, w/ phenothiazine, ranolazine, ziprasidone, prolonged QT, h/o arrhythmia **Disp:** ER Tabs 3, 6, 9 mg

SE: Impaired temp regulation, ↑ QT and HR, HA, anxiety, dizziness, N, dry mouth, fatigue, EPS **Interactions:** ↑ Risk of prolongation of QT W/ Class 1A & III antiarrhythmics, chlorpromazine, chlorpromazine, thioridazine, gatifloxacin, moxifloxacin, EtOH **Labs:** Monitor LFTs **NIPE:** Do not chew/cut/crush pill; monitor for orthostatic effects

Pamidronate (Aredia) [Antihypercalcemic/Bisphosphonate]
Uses: *↑ Ca²⁺ of malignancy, Paget Dz, palliate symptomatic bone metastases* **Action:** ↓ NI & abnormal bone resorption **Dose:** ↑ Ca²⁺: 60 mg IV over 4 h or 90 mg IV over 24 h. *Paget Dz:* 30 mg/d IV slow inf for 3 d **Caution:** [D, ?/–] Avoid invasive dental procedures w/ use **Contra:** PRG **Disp:** Inj 30, 60, 90 mg **SE:** Fever, inj site Rxn, uveitis, fluid overload, HTN, abd pain, N/V, constipation, UTI, bone pain, hypophosphatemia; jaw osteonecrosis, perform dental exam pretherapy **Interactions:** ↓ Serum Ca levels W/ foscarnet; ↓ effects W/ Ca, vitamin D **Labs:** ↓ K⁺, Ca²⁺, Mg²⁺ **NIPE:** ⊘ Ingest food W/ Ca or vitamins W/ minerals before or 2–3 h after admin of drug

Pancrelipase (Pancrease, Cotazym, Creon, Ultrase) [Pancreatic Enzyme] **Uses:** *Exocrine pancreatic secretion deficiency (eg, CF, chronic pancreatitis, pancreatic insuff), steatorrhea of malabsorption* **Action:** Pancreatic enzyme supl **Dose:** 1–3 caps (tabs) w/ meals & snacks; ↑ to 8 caps (tabs); do not crush or chew EC products; dose-dependent on digestive requirements of pt; avoid antacids **Caution:** [C, ?/–] **Contra:** Pork product allergy, acute pancreatitis **Disp:** Caps, tabs **SE:** N/V, abd cramps **Notes:** Individualize therapy **Interactions:** ↓ Effects W/ antacids w/ Ca or Mg; ↓ effects OF Fe **Labs:** ↑ Serum and urine uric acid **NIPE:** Take w/ food; stress adherence to diet (usually low-fat, high-protein, high-calorie)

Pancuronium (Pavulon) [Skeletal Muscle Relaxant/Nondepolarizing Neuromuscular Blocking Agent] **Uses:** *Paralysis w/ mechanical ventilation* **Action:** Nondepolarizing neuromuscular blocker **Dose:** *Adults.* 2–4 mg IV q2–4h PRN. *Peds.* 0.02–0.1 mg/kg/dose q2–4h PRN; ↓ in renal/hepatic impair; intubate pt & keep on controlled ventilation; use adequate sedation or analgesia **Caution:** [C, ?/–] **Contra:** Component or bromide sensitivity **Disp:** Inj 1, 2 mg/mL **SE:** Tachycardia, HTN, pruritus, other histamine Rxns **Interactions:** ↑ Effects W/ amikacin, clindamycin, Li, quinidine, succinylcholine, gentamicin, streptomycin, verapamil; ↓ effects W/ carbamazepine, phenytoin, theophylline **NIPE:** Neuromuscular blocker does not alter pain, use analgesics for pain

Panitumumab (Vectibix) [Human Epidermal Growth Factor Receptor (EGFR) Inhibitor] **WARNING:** Derm tox common (89%) and severe in 12%; can be associated w/ Infxn (sepsis, abscesses requiring I&D); w/ severe derm tox, hold or D/C and monitor for Infxns; severe inf Rxns (anaphylactic Rxn, bronchospasm, fever, chills, hypotension) in 1%; w/ severe Rxns, immediately D/C inf & possibly permanent discontinuation **Uses:** *Rx EGFR-expressing metastatic colon CA* **Action:** Anti-EGFR MoAB **Dose:** 6 mg/kg IV inf over 60 min q14d; doses >1000 mg over 90 min. ↓ inf rate by 50% w/ grade 1–2 inf Rxn, D/C permanently w/ grade 3–4 Rxn. For derm tox, hold until <grade 2 tox. If improves <1 mo, restart 50% original dose. If tox recurs or resoln >1 mo permanently D/C. If ↓ dose tolerated, ↑ dose by 25% **Caution:** [C; -] D/C nursing during, 2 mo after **Disp:** Vial 20 mg/mL **SE:** Rash, acneiform dermatitis, pruritus, paronychia, ↓ Mg²⁺, abd pain, N/V/D, constipation, fatigue, dehydration, photosens, conjunctivitis, ocular hyperemia, ↑ lacrimation, stomatitis, mucositis, pulm fibrosis, severe derm tox, inf Rxns **Labs:** ✓ Lytes; **NIPE:** May impair female fertility; wear sunscreen/hats, limit sun exposure

Pantoprazole (Protonix) [Gastric Acid Suppressant/Proton Pump Inhibitor] **Uses:** *GERD, erosive gastritis*, ZE synd, PUD **Action:** Proton-pump inhibitor **Dose:** 40 mg/d PO; do not crush/chew tabs; 40 mg IV/d (not >3 mg/min, use Protonix filter) **Caution:** [B, ?/–] **Disp:** Tabs, delayed release 20, 40 mg; powder for inj 40 mg **SE:** Chest pain, anxiety, GI upset **Interactions:** ↑ Effects *OF* warfarin; ↑ effects of photosensitivity *W/* St. John's wort; ↓ effects *OF* ketoconazole **Labs:**↑ Serum glucose, lipids, LFTs; monitor PT, INR **NIPE:** ⊘ Sun exposure—use sunscreen; take w/o regard to food; antacids will not effect drug absorption

Paregoric [Camphorated Tincture of Opium] [C-III] [Narcotic Antidiarrheal] **Uses:** *D*, Pain & neonatal opiate withdrawal synd **Action:** Narcotic **Dose:** *Adults.* 5–10 mL PO daily-qid PRN. *Peds.* 0.25–0.5 mL/kg daily–qid. *Neonatal withdrawal:* 3–6 gtt PO q3–6 h PRN to relieve Sxs × 3–5 d, then taper over 2–4 wk **Caution:** [B (D w/ prolonged use/high dose near term, +] **Contra:** Toxic diarrhea; convulsive disorder **Disp:** Liq 2 mg morphine = 20 mg opium/5 mL **SE:** ↓ BP, sedation, constipation **Interactions:** ↓ Effects *OF* ampicillin esters, azole antifungals, Fe salts **Labs:** ↑ LFTs, SCr **NIPE:** Take w/o regard to food; contains anhydrous morphine from opium; short-term use only

Paroxetine (Paxil, Paxil CR) [Antidepressant/SSRI] **WARNING:** Closely monitor for worsening depression or emergence of suicidality, particularly in ped pts **Uses:** *Depression, OCD, panic disorder, social anxiety disorder*, PMDD **Action:** SSRI **Dose:** 10–60 mg PO single daily dose in AM; CR 25 mg/d PO; ↑ 12.5 mg/wk (max range 26–62.5 mg/d) **Caution:** [D, ?/] **Contra:** MAOI **Disp:** Tabs 10, 20, 30, 40 mg; susp 10 mg/5 mL; CR 12.5, 25, 37.5 mg **SE:** Sexual dysfunction, HA, somnolence, dizziness, GI upset, D, xerostomia, tachycardia **Interactions:** ↑ Effects *W/* cimetidine; ↑ effects *OF* BBs, dexfenfluramine, dextromethorphan, fenfluramine, haloperidol, MAOIs, theophylline, thioridazine, TCAs, warfarin, St. John's wort, EtOH; ↓ effects *W/* cyproheptadine, phenobarbital, phenytoin; ↓ effects *OF* digoxin, phenytoin **Labs:** ↑ Alk phosp, bilirubin, glucose **NIPE:** Take w/o regard to food, may take up to 4 wk for full effect

Pegfilgrastim (Neulasta) [Colony Stimulating Factor] **Uses:** *↓ Frequency of Infxn in pts w/ nonmyeloid malignancies receiving myelosuppressive anti-CA drugs that cause febrile neutropenia* **Action:** Granulocyte and macrophage stimulating factor **Dose:** *Adults.* 6 mg SQ × 1/chemo cycle. *Peds.* 100 μg/kg SQ × 1/chemo cycle **Caution:** [C, M] In sickle cell **Contra:** Allergy to *E. coli*-derived proteins or filgrastim **Disp:** *Syringes:* 6 mg/0.6 mL **SE:** Splenic rupture, HA, fever, weakness, fatigue, dizziness, insomnia, edema, N/V/D, stomatitis, anorexia, constipation, taste perversion, dyspepsia, abd pain, granulocytopenia, neutropenic fever, ↑ LFT & uric acid, arthralgia, myalgia, bone pain, ARDS, alopecia, worsen sickle cell Dz **Interactions:** ↑ Effects *W*/ Li **Labs:** ↑ LFTs, uric acid, alkaline phosphatase, LDH **NIPE:** ⊘ Exposure to Infxn; never give between 14 d before & 24 h after dose of cytotoxic chemo

Peg Interferon Alfa-2a (Pegasys) [Antiviral/Immunomodulator] **WARNING:** Can cause or aggravate fatal or life-threatening neuropsychiatric, autoimmune, ischemic, and infectious disorders. Monitor patients closely

Uses: *Chronic Hep C w/ compensated liver Dz* **Action:** Biologic response modifier **Dose:** 180 μg (1 mL) SQ qwk × 48 wk; ↓ in renal impair **Caution:** [C, X if used *W*/ ribavirin; ?/–] **Contra:** Autoimmune hepatitis, decompensated liver Dz **Disp:** 180 μg/mL inj **SE:** Depression, insomnia, suicidal behavior, GI upset, neutro & thrombocytopenia, alopecia, pruritus **Interactions:** ↑ Effects *OF* theophylline; ↑ risk of anemia *W*/ ribavirin **Labs:** Monitor CBC; ↑ ALT, triglycerides; ↓ HMG, Hct, plts, WBC **NIPE:** ⊘ Exposure to Infxn; use barrier contraception; may aggravate neuropsychiatric, autoimmune, ischemic, & infectious disorders

Peg Interferon Alfa-2b (PEG-Intron) [Antiviral/Immunomodulator] **WARNING:** Can cause or aggravate fatal or life-threatening neuropsychiatric, autoimmune, ischemic, and infectious disorders. Monitor patients closely

Uses: *Rx Hep C* **Action:** Immune modulation **Dose:** 1 μg/kg/wk SQ; 1.5 μg/kg/wk combined w/ ribavirin **Caution:** [C, X if used *W*/ ribavirin; ?/–] w/ h/o psychiatric **Contra:** Autoimmune hepatitis, decompensated liver Dz, hemoglobinopathy **Disp:** Vials 50, 80, 120, 150 μg/0.5 mL; Redipen 50, 80,120,150 μg/5 mL; reconstitute w/ 0.7 mL w/ sterile water **SE:** Depression, insomnia, suicidal behavior, GI upset, neutropenia, thrombocytopenia, alopecia, pruritus **Interactions:** ↑ Myelosuppression *W*/ antineoplastics; ↑ effects *OF* doxorubicin, theophylline; ↑ neurotox *W*/ vinblastine **Labs:** ↑ ALT, ↓ neutrophils, plts; monitor CBC/plts **NIPE:** Maintain hydration; use barrier contraception; give hs or w/ APAP to ↓ flulike Sxs; use immediately or store in refrigerator × 24 h; do not freeze

Pemetrexed (Alimta) [Antineoplastic/Folate Antagonist]

Uses: *w/ cisplatin in nonresectable mesothelioma* NSCLC **Action:** Antifolate antineoplastic **Dose:** 500 mg/m² IV over 10 min every 3 wk; hold if CrCl <45 mL/min; give w/ vitamin B₁₂ (1000 μg IM every 9 wk) & folic acid (350–1000 μg PO daily); start 1 wk before; dexamethasone 4 mg PO bid × 3 start 1 d before each Rx **Caution:** [D, –] w/ renal/hepatic/ BM impair **Contra:** Component sensitivity **Disp:** 500-mg vial **SE:** Neutropenia, thrombocytopenia, N/V/D, anorexia, stomatitis, renal failure, neuropathy, fever, fatigue, mood changes, dyspnea, anaphylactic

Rxns **Interactions:** ↑ Effects W/ NSAIDs, probenecid due to decreased pemetrexed clearance **Labs:** ↑ Cr, LFTs; ↓ HMG, Hct; monitor CBC/ plts **NIPE:** ⊘ PRG & lactation; ⊘ use NSAIDs 5 d before, during, or 5 d after treatment

Pemirolast (Alamast) [Mast Cell Stabilizer] **Uses:** *Allergic conjunctivitis* **Action:** Mast cell stabilizer **Dose:** 1–2 gtt in each eye qid **Caution:** [C, ?/–] **Disp:** 0.1% (1 mg/mL) in 10-mL bottles **SE:** HA, rhinitis, cold/flu Sxs, local irritation **NIPE:** Wait 10 min before inserting contacts

Penbutolol (Levatol) [Antihypertensive/BB] **Uses:** *HTN* **Action:** β-adrenergic receptor blocker, β₁, β₂ **Dose:** 20–40 mg/d; ↓ in hepatic insuff **Caution:** [C 1st tri; D if 2nd/3rd tri, M] **Contra:** Asthma, cardiogenic shock, cardiac failure, heart block, bradycardia, COPD, pulm edema **Disp:** Tabs 20 mg **SE:** Flushing, ↓ BP, fatigue, hyperglycemia, GI upset, sexual dysfunction, bronchospasm **Interactions:** ↑ Effects W/ CCBs, fluoroquinolones; ↑ bradycardia W/ adenosine, amiodarone, digitalis, dipyridamole, epinephrine, neuroleptics, phenylephrine, physostigmine, tacrine; ↑ effects OF lidocaine, verapamil; ↓ effects W/ antacids, NSAIDs; ↓ effects OF insulin, hypoglycemics, theophylline **Labs:** ↑ Serum glucose, BUN, K⁺, lipoprotein, triglycerides, uric acid **NIPE:** ↑ Cold sensitivity

Penciclovir (Denavir) [Antiviral] **Uses:** *Herpes simplex (herpes labialis/cold sores)* **Action:** Competitive inhibitor of DNA polymerase **Dose:** Apply at 1st sign of lesions, then q2h while awake × 4 d **Caution:** [B, ?/–] **Contra:** Allergy, previous Rxn to famciclovir **Disp:** Cream 1% [OTC] **SE:** Erythema, HA **NIPE:** ⊘ Recommended in lactation or in children; ⊘ apply to mucous membranes or near eyes

Penicillin G, Aqueous (Potassium or Sodium) (Pfizerpen, Pentids) [Antibiotic/Penicillin] **Uses:** *Bacteremia, endocarditis, pericarditis, resp tract Infxns, meningitis, neurosyphilis, skin/skin structure Infxns* **Action:** Bactericidal; ↓ cell wall synth. *Spectrum:* Most gram(+) (not staphylococci), streptococci, N. *meningitidis*, syphilis, clostridia, & anaerobes (not *Bacteroides*) **Dose:** *Adults.* 400,000–800,000 units PO qid; IV doses vary depending on indications; range 0.6–24 million units/d in ÷ doses q4h. *Peds. Newborns <1 wk:* 25,000–50,000 units/kg/dose IV q12h. *Infants 1 wk–<1 mo:* 25,000–50,000 units/kg/dose IV q8h. *Children:* 100,000–300,000 units/kg/24h IV ÷ q4h; ↓ in renal impair **Caution:** [B, M] **Contra:** Allergy **Disp:** Tabs 200,000, 250,000, 400,000, 800,000 units; susp 200,000, 400,000 units/5 mL; powder for inj **SE:** Allergic Rxns; interstitial nephritis, D, Szs **Notes:** Contains 1.7 mEq of K⁺/million units **Interactions:** ↑ Effects W/ probenecid; ↑ effects OF MTX; ↑ risk of bleeding W/ anticoagulants; ↓ effects W/ chloramphenicol, macrolides, tetracyclines; ↓ effects OF OCPs **Labs:** ↑ K⁺, eosinophils; ↓ serum albumin **NIPE:** Monitor for super Infxn; use barrier contraception

Penicillin G Benzathine (Bicillin) [Antibiotic/Penicillin] **Uses:** *Single-dose regimen for streptococcal pharyngitis, rheumatic fever, glomerulonephritis prophylaxis, & syphilis* **Action:** Bactericidal; ↓ cell wall synth.

Spectrum: See Penicillin G **Dose:** *Adults.* 1.2–2.4 million units deep IM inj q2–4wk. *Peds.* 50,000 units/kg/dose, 2.4 million units/dose max; deep IM inj q2–4 wk **Caution:** [B, M] **Contra:** Allergy **Disp:** IM 300,000, 600,000 units/mL; Bicillin L-A benzathine salt only; Bicillin C-R combo of benzathine & procaine (300,000 units procaine w/ 300,000 units benzathine/mL or 900,000 units benzathine w/ 300,000 units procaine/2 mL) **SE:** Inj site pain, acute interstitial nephritis, anaphylaxis **Interactions:** ↑ Effects *W/* probenecid; ↑ penicillin 1/2 life *W/* ASA, furosemide, indomethacin, sulfonamides, thiazide diuretics; ↑ risk of bleeding *W/* anticoagulants; ↓ effects *W/* chloramphenicol, macrolides, tetracyclines; ↓ effects *OF* OCPs **Labs:** ↑ Eosinophils; ↓ serum albumin **NIPE:** Monitor for super Infxn; sustained action, detectable levels up to 4 wk; drug of choice for noncongenital syphilis

Penicillin G Procaine (Wycillin, Others) [Antibiotic/Penicillin] **Uses:** *Infxns of respir tract, skin/soft tissue, scarlet fever, syphilis* **Action:** Bactericidal; ↓ cell wall synth. *Spectrum:* PCN G-sensitive organisms that respond to low, persistent serum levels **Dose:** *Adults.* 0.6–4.8 million units/d in ÷ doses q12–24h; give probenecid at least 30 min prior to PCN to prolong action. *Peds.* 25,000–50,000 units/kg/d IM ÷ daily–bid **Caution:** [B, M] **Contra:** Allergy **Disp:** Inj 300,000, 500,000, 600,000 units/mL **SE:** Pain at inj site, interstitial nephritis, anaphylaxis **Interactions:** ↑ Effects *W/* probenecid; ↑ penicillin 1/2 life *W/* ASA, furosemide, indomethacin, sulfonamides, thiazide diuretics; ↑ risk of bleeding *W/* anticoagulants; ↓ effects *W/* chloramphenicol, macrolides, tetracyclines; ↓ effects *OF* OCPs **Labs:** ↑ Eosinophils; ↓ serum albumin **NIPE:** Monitor for super Infxn; use barrier contraception; LA parenteral PCN; levels up to 15 h

Penicillin V (Pen-Vee K, Veetids, Others) [Antibiotic/Penicillin] **Uses:** Susceptible streptococci Infxns, otitis media, URIs, skin/soft tissue Infxns (PCN-sensitive staph) **Action:** Bactericidal; ↓ cell wall synth. *Spectrum:* Most gram(+), including strep **Dose:** *Adults.* 250–500 mg PO q6h, q8h, q12h. *Peds.* 25–50 mg/kg/25h PO in 4 doses; ↓ in renal impair; on empty stomach **Caution:** [B, M] **Contra:** Allergy **Disp:** Tabs 125, 250, 500 mg; susp 125, 250 mg/5 mL **SE:** GI upset, interstitial nephritis, anaphylaxis, convulsions **Interactions:** ↑ Effects *W/* ASA, probenecid; ↑ effects *OF* MTX; ↑ risk of anaphylaxes *W/* BB; ↓ effects *W/* chloramphenicol, macrolides, tetracyclines; ↓ effects *OF* OCPs **Labs:** ↑ Eosinophils; ↓ serum albumin, WBC **NIPE:** Monitor for super Infxn; use barrier contraception; well-tolerated PO PCN; 250 mg = 400,000 units of PCN G

Pentamidine (Pentam 300, NebuPent) [Antiprotozoal] **Uses:** *Rx & prevention of PCP* **Action:** ↓ DNA, RNA, phospholipid, & protein synth **Dose:** *Rx: Adults & Peds.* 4 mg/kg/24 h IV daily for 14–21 d. *Prevention. Adults & Peds >5 y.* 300 mg once q4wk, give via Respirgard II neb; ↓ w/ IV in renal impair **Caution:** [C, ?] **Contra:** Component allergy, use w/ didanosine **Disp:** Inj 300 mg/vial; aerosol 300 mg **SE:** Pancreatic cell necrosis w/ hyperglycemia; pancreatitis, CP, fatigue, dizziness, rash, GI upset, renal impair, blood dyscrasias (leukopenia & thrombocytopenia) **Interactions:** ↑ Nephrotoxic effects W/ amino-glycosides, amphotericin B, capreomycin, cidofovir, cisplatin, cyclosporine, colistin, ganciclovir, methoxyflurane, polymyxin B, vancomycin; ↑ BM suppression W/ antineoplastics, radiation therapy **Labs:** ↑ LFTs, serum K+, ↓ HMG, Hct, plts, WBCs; ↑ or ↓ glucose; monitor glucose and CBC **NIPE:** Reconstitute W/ sterile H₂O only, inhalation may cause metallic taste; ↑ fluids to 2–3 L/d; monitor pancreatic Fxn monthly for 1st 3 mo; monitor for ↓ BP following IV dose

Pentazocine (Talwin, Talwin Compound, Talwin NX) [C-IV] [Narcotic Analgesic]
Uses: *Moderate–severe pain* **Action:** Partial narcotic agonist–antagonist **Dose:** *Adults.* 30 mg IM or IV; 50–100 mg PO q3–4h PRN. *Peds. 5–8 y:* 15 mg IM q4h PRN. *8–14 y:* 30 mg IM q4h PRN; ↓ in renal/hepatic impair **Caution:** [C (1st tri, D w/ prolonged use/high dose near term), +/–] **Contra:** Allergy, ↑ ICP (unless ventilated) **Disp:** Talwin compound tab 12.5 mg + 325 mg ASA; Talwin NX 50 mg + 0.5 mg naloxone; inj 30 mg/mL **SE:** Considerable dysphoria; drowsiness, GI upset, xerostomia, Szs **Notes:** 30–60 mg IM = 10 mg of morphine IM **Interactions:** ↑ CNS depression W/ antihistamines, barbiturates, hypnotics, phenothiazine, EtOH; ↑ effects W/ cimetidine; ↑ effects OF digitoxin, phenytoin, rifampin; ↓ effects OF opioids **Labs:** ↑ Serum amylase, lipase **NIPE:** May cause withdrawal in pts using opioids; Talwin NX has naloxone to curb abuse by non-oral route.

Pentobarbital (Nembutal, others) [C-II] [Anticonvulsant, Sedative/Hypnotic/Barbiturate]
Uses: *Insomnia, convulsions*, induce coma following severe head injury **Action:** Barbiturate **Dose:** *Adults. Sedative:* 20–40 mg PO or PR q6–12h. *Hypnotic:* 100–200 mg PO or PR hs PRN. *Induced coma:* Load 5–10 mg/kg IV, then maint 1–3 mg/kg/h IV inf to maint burst suppression on EEG. *Peds. Hypnotic:* 2–6 mg/kg/dose PO hs PRN. *Induced coma:* As adult **Caution:** [D, +/–] Severe hepatic impair **Contra:** Allergy **Disp:** Caps 50, 100 mg; elixir 18.2 mg/5 mL (= 20 mg pentobarbital); supp 30, 60, 120, 200 mg; inj 50 mg/mL **SE:** Resp depression, ↓ BP w/ aggressive IV use for cerebral edema; bradycardia, ↓ BP, sedation, lethargy, resp ↓, hangover, rash, Stevens–Johnson synd, blood dyscrasias **Interactions:** ↑ Effects W/ MAOIs, narcotic analgesics, EtOH; ↓ effects OF anticoagulants, BBs, corticosteroids, cyclosporine, digoxin, doxycycline, griseofulvin, neuroleptics, OCPs, quinidine, theophylline, verapamil **NIPE:** Tolerance to sedative–hypnotic effect w/in 1–2 wk

Pentosan Polysulfate Sodium (Elmiron) [Urinary Analgesic]
Uses: *Relieve pain/discomfort w/ interstitial cystitis* **Action:** Bladder wall buffer **Dose:** 100 mg PO tid; on empty stomach w/ H₂O 1 h ac or 2 h pc **Caution:** [B, ?/–] **Contra:** Allergy **Disp:** Caps 100 mg **SE:** Alopecia, N/D, HA, thrombocytopenia **Interactions:** Risk of ↑ anticoagulation W/ anticoagulants, ASA, thrombolytics **Labs:** ↑ LFTs **NIPE:** Reassess after 3 mo

Pentoxifylline (Trental) [Hemorheologic/Xanthine Derivative]
Uses: *Rx symptoms of peripheral vascular Dz* **Action:** ↓ Blood cell viscosity,

restores RBC flexibility **Dose:** *Adults.* 400 mg PO tid pc; Rx min 8 wk for effect; ↓ to bid w/ GI/CNS SEs **Caution:** [C, +/–] **Contra:** Cerebral/retinal hemorrhage **Disp:** Tabs CR 400 mg; Tabs XR 400 mg **SE:** Dizziness, HA, GI upset **Interactions:** ↑ Risk of bleeding *W/* anticoagulants, NSAIDs; ↑ effects *OF* antihypertensives, theophylline **NIPE:** Take *W/* food to < GI upset

Perindopril Erbumine (Aceon) [Antihypertensive/ACEI] Uses: *HTN*, CHF, DN, post-MI **Action:** ACE inhibitor **Dose:** 4–8 mg/d;16 mg/day max; avoid w/ food; ↓ in elderly/renal impair **Caution:** [C (1st tri, D 2nd & 3rd tri), ?/–] ACE-inhibitor-induced angioedema **Contra:** Bilateral RAS, primary hyperaldosteronism **Disp:** Tabs 2, 4, 8 mg **SE:** HA, ↓ BP, dizziness, GI upset, cough **Interactions:** ↑ Effects *W/* antihypertensives, diuretics; ↑ effects *OF* cyclosporine, insulin, Li, sulfonylureas, tacrolimus; ↓ effects *W/* NSAIDs **Labs:** ↑ Serum K⁺, LFTs, uric acid, cholesterol, Cr **NIPE:** ↓ Effects if taken *W/* food; risk of persistent cough; OK *W/* diuretics

Permethrin (Nix, Elimite) [OTC] [Scabicides/Pediculicides] Uses: *Rx lice/scabies* **Action:** Pediculicide **Dose:** *Adults & Peds.* Lice: Saturate hair & scalp; allow 10 min before rinsing; *Scabies:* Apply cream head to toe; leave for 8–14 hours, wash w/ H₂O **Caution:** [B, ?/–] **Contra:** Allergy **Disp:** Topical lotion 1%; cream 5% **SE:** Local irritation **NIPE:** Drug remains on hair up to 2 wk, reapply in 1 wk if live lice; disinfect clothing, bedding, combs, & brushes, lotion not OK in peds <2 y, may repeat after 7 d

Perphenazine (Trilafon) [Antipsychotic, Antiemetic/Phenothiazine] Uses: *Psychotic disorders, severe N*, intractable hiccups **Action:** Phenothiazine, blocks brain dopaminergic receptors **Dose:** *Adults: Antipsychotic:* 4–16 mg PO tid; max 64 mg/d. *Hiccups:* 5 mg IM q6h PRN or 1 mg IV at intervals not <1–2 mg/min; 5 mg max. *Peds. 1–6 y:* 4–6 mg/d PO in ÷ doses. *6–12 y:* 6 mg/d PO in ÷ doses. *>12 y:* 4–16 mg PO bid–qid; ↓ in hepatic insuff **Caution:** [C, ?/–] NAG, severe ↑/↓ BP **Contra:** Phenothiazine sensitivity, BM depression, severe liver or cardiac Dz **Disp:** Tabs 2, 4, 8, 16 mg; PO conc 16 mg/ 5 mL; inj 5 mg/mL **SE:** ↓ BP, tachycardia, bradycardia, EPS, drowsiness, Szs, photosens, skin discoloration, blood dyscrasias, constipation **Interactions:** ↑ Effects *W/* antidepressants; ↑ effects *OF* anticholinergics, antidepressants, propranolol, phenytoin; ↑ CNS effects *W/* CNS depressants, EtOH; ↓ effects *W/* antacids, Li, phenobarbital, caffeine, tobacco; ↓ effects *OF* levodopa, Li **Labs:** ↑ Serum cholesterol, glucose, LFTs; ↓ HMG, plts, WBCs **NIPE:** Take oral dose *W/* food; risk of photosensitivity—use sunscreen

Phenazopyridine (Pyridium, Others) [Urinary Analgesic] Uses: *Lower urinary tract irritation* **Action:** Local anesthetic on urinary tract mucosa **Dose:** *Adults.* 100–200 mg PO tid. *Peds 6–12 y.* 12 mg/kg/24 h PO in 3 ÷ doses; ↓ in renal insuff **Caution:** [B, ?] Hepatic Dz **Contra:** Renal failure **Disp:** Tabs 95, 97.2, 100, 200 mg **SE:** GI disturbances; red-orange urine color (can stain clothing); HA, dizziness, acute renal failure, methemoglobinemia **Labs:** Interferes

W/ urinary tests for glucose, ketones, bilirubin, protein, steroids **NIPE:** Urine may turn red-orange in color and can stain clothing; take pc

Phenelzine (Nardil) [Antidepressant/MAOI] **WARNING:** Antidepressants increase the risk of suicidal thinking and behavior in children and adolescents w/ major depressive disorder and other psychiatric disorders **Uses:** *Depression* **Action:** MAOI **Dose:** 15 mg PO tid. *Elderly:* 15–60 mg/d ÷ doses **Caution:** [C, –] Interacts w/ SSRI, ergots, triptans **Contra:** CHF, h/o liver Dz, pheochromocytoma **Disp:** Tabs 15 mg **SE:** Postural ↓ BP; edema, dizziness, sedation, rash, sexual dysfunction, xerostomia, constipation, urinary retention **Interactions:** ↑ HTN Rxn *W/* amphetamines, fluoxetine, levodopa, metaraminol, phenylephrine, phenylpropanolamine, pseudoephedrine, reserpine, sertraline, tyramine, EtOH, foods *W/* tyramine, caffeine, tryptophan; ↑ effects *OF* barbiturates, narcotics, sedatives, sumatriptan, TCAs, ephedra, ginseng **Labs:** ↓ Glucose, false + ↑ in bilirubin & uric acid **NIPE:** May take 2–4 wk for effect; avoid tyramine-containing foods (eg, cheeses)

Phenobarbital [C-IV] [Anticonvulsant, Sedative/ Hypnotic/Barbiturate] **Uses:** *Sz disorders*, insomnia, anxiety **Action:** Barbiturate **Dose:** *Adults. Sedative–hypnotic:* 30–120 mg/d PO or IM PRN. *Anticonvulsant:* Load 10–12 mg/kg in 3 ÷ doses, then 1–3 mg/kg/24 h PO, IM, or IV. *Peds. Sedative–hypnotic:* 2–3 mg/kg/24 h PO or IM hs PRN. *Anticonvulsant:* Load 15–20 mg/kg ÷ in 2 equal doses 4 h apart, then 3–5 mg/kg/24h PO ÷ in 2–3 doses; ↓ w/ CrCl <10 **Caution:** [D, M] **Contra:** Porphyria, hepatic impair, dyspnea, airway obst **Disp:** Tabs 15, 16, 30, 32, 60, 65, 100 mg; elixir 15, 20 mg/5 mL; inj 30, 60, 65, 130 mg/mL **SE:** Bradycardia, ↓ BP, hangover, Stevens–Johnson synd, blood dyscrasias, resp depression **Notes:** *Levels: Trough:* Just before next dose; *Therapeutic: Peak:* 15–40 μg/mL; *Toxic: Trough:* >40 μg/mL; *1/2 life:* 40–120h **Interactions:** ↑ CNS depression *W/* CNS depressants, anesthetics, antianxiety meds, antihistamines, narcotic analgesics, EtOH, Indian snakeroot, kava kava; ↑ effects *W/* chloramphenicol, MAOIs, procarbazine, valproic acid; ↓ effects *W/* rifampin; ↓ effects *OF* anticoagulants, BBs, carbamazepine, clozapine, corticosteroids, doxorubicin, doxycycline, estrogens, felodipine, griseofulvin, haloperidol, methadone, metronidazole, OCPs, phenothiazine, quinidine, TCAs, theophylline, verapamil **Labs:** ↓ Bilirubin **NIPE:** May take 2–3 wk for full effects; ⊘ D/C abruptly; tolerance develops to sedation; paradoxic hyperactivity seen in ped pts; long 1/2-life allows single daily dosing

Phenylephrine, nasal (Neo-Synephrine Nasal) (OTC) [Vasopressor/Decongestant] **Uses:** *Nasal congestion* **Action:** α-Adrenergic agonist **Dose:** *Adults.* 1–2 sprays/nostril q4h (usual 0.25%) PRN. *Peds. 6 mo–2 y:* 0.125% 1–2 drops/nostril q3–4h, *2–6 y:* 0.125% 2–3 drops/nostril q3–4h, *6–12 y:* 1–2 sprays/nostril q4h 0.25% 2–3 drops **Caution:** [C, +/–] HTN, acute pancreatitis, hepatitis, coronary Dz, NAG, hyperthyroidism **Contra:** Bradycardia, arrhythmias **Disp:** Nasal soln 0.125, 0.25, 0.5, 1%; Liq 7.5 mg/5 mL; drops 2.5 mg/mL

SE: Arrhythmias, HTN, nasal irritation, dryness, sneezing, rebound congestion w/ prolonged use, HA **NIPE:** Do not use >3 d

Phenylephrine, Ophthalmic (Neo-Synephrine Ophthalmic, AK-Dilate, Zincfrin [OTC]) [Vasopressor/Decongestant]
Uses: * Mydriasis, ocular redness [OTC], periop mydriasis, posterior synechiae, uveitis w/ posterior synechiae* **Action:** α-Adrenergic agonist **Dose: Adults.** *Redness:* 1 gtt 0.12% q3–4h PRN; *Eye mydriasis:* 1 gtt 2.5% (15 min–1 h for effect); *Preop:* 1 gtt 2.5–10% 30–60 min preop; *Ocular disorders:* 1 gtt 2.5–10% daily–tid **Peds.** As adult, only use 2.5% for exam, preop, and ocular conditions **Caution:** [C (may cause late-term fetal anoxia/bradycardia), +/–] HTN, w/ elderly w/ CAD, **Contra:** NAG **Disp:** Ophth soln 0.12% (Zincfrin OTC), 2.5, 10%; **SE:** Tearing, HA, irritation, eye pain, photophobia, arrhythmia, tremor

Phenylephrine, Oral (Sudafed PE, SudoGest PE, Nasop, Lusonal, AH-chew D, Sudafed PE dissolve) (OTC) [Vasopressor/Decongestant]   **WARNING:** Prescribers should be aware of full prescribing info before use   **Uses:** *Nasal congestion* **Action:** α-Adrenergic agonist **Dose: Adults.** 10–20 mg PO q4h PRN, max 60 mg/d **Peds.** 5 mg PO q4h PRN, max 60 mg/d **Caution:** [C, +/–] HTN, acute pancreatitis, hepatitis, coronary Dz, NAG, hyperthyroidism **Contra:** MAOI w/in 14 d, NAG, severe ↑ BP or CAD, urinary retention **Disp:** Liq 7.5 mg/5 mL; drops 2.5 mg/mL; tabs 5, 10 mg; chew tabs 10 mg; tabs OD 10 mg; strips 10 mg. **SE:** Arrhythmias, HTN, HA, agitation, anxiety, tremor, palpitations **Interactions:** ↑ Risk of HTN crisis W/ MAOIs; ↑ risk of pressor effects W/ BB; ↑ risk of arrhythmias W/epinephrine, isoproterenol; ↓ effects OF guanethidine, methyldopa, reserpine

Phenylephrine, Systemic (Neo-Synephrine) [Vasopressor/Adrenergic]   **WARNING:** Prescribers should be aware of full prescribing info before use   **Uses:** *Vascular failure in shock, allergy, or drug-induced ↓ BP* **Action:** α-Adrenergic agonist **Dose: Adults.** *Mild–moderate ↓ BP:* 2–5 mg IM or SQ ↑ BP for 2 h; 0.1–0.5 mg IV ↑ BP for 15 min. *Severe ↓ BP/shock:* Cont inf at 100–180 µg/min; after BP stable, maint 40–60 µg/min **Peds.** ↓ BP: 5–20 µg/kg/dose IV q10–15 min or 0.1–0.5 µg/kg/min IV inf, titrate to effect. **Caution:** [C, +/–] HTN, acute pancreatitis, hepatitis, coronary Dz, NAG, hyperthyroidism **Contra:** Bradycardia, arrhythmias **Disp:** Inj 10 mg/mL **SE:** Arrhythmias, HTN, peripheral vasoconstriction ↑ w/ oxytocin, MAOIs, & TCAs; HA, weakness, necrosis, ↓ renal perfusion **Interactions:** ↑ HTN W/ BBs, MAOIs; ↑ pressor response W/ guanethidine, methyldopa, reserpine, TCAs; **NIPE:** Restore blood volume if loss has occurred; use large veins to avoid extrav; phentolamine 10 mg in 10–15 mL of NS for local inj to Rx extrav

Phenytoin (Dilantin) [Anticonvulsant/Hydantoin]   **Uses:** *Sz disorders* **Action:** ↓ Sz spread in the motor cortex **Dose:** *Load:* **Adults & Peds.** 15–20 mg/kg IV, 25 mg/min max or PO in 400-mg doses at 4-h intervals. *Maint:* **Adults.** Initial, 200 mg PO or IV bid or 300 mg hs; then follow levels. **Peds.**

4–7 mg/kg/24h PO or IV ÷ daily–bid; avoid PO susp (erratic absorption) **Caution:** [D, +] **Contra:** Heart block, sinus bradycardia **Disp:** Dilantin Infatab chew 50 mg; Dilantin/Phenytek caps 100 mg; caps, XR 30, 100, 200, 300 mg; susp 125 mg/5 mL; inj 50 mg/mL **SE:** Nystagmus/ataxia early signs of tox; gum hyperplasia w/ long-term use. *IV:* ↓ BP, bradycardia, arrhythmias, phlebitis; peripheral neuropathy, rash, blood dyscrasias, Stevens–Johnson synd **Notes:** *Levels: Trough:* Just before next dose; *Therapeutic: Peak:* 10–20 μg/mL; *Toxic:* >20 μg/mL; Phenytoin albumin bound, levels = bound & free phenytoin; w/ ↓ albumin & azotemia, low levels may be therapeutic (nl free levels) **Interactions:** ↑ Effects W/ amiodarone, allopurinol, chloramphenicol, disulfiram, INH, omeprazole, sulfonamides, quinolones, trimethoprim; ↑ effects OF Li; ↓ effects W/ cimetidine, cisplatin, diazoxide, folate, pyridoxine, rifampin; ↓ effects OF azole antifungals, benzodiazepines, carbamazepine, corticosteroids, cyclosporine, digitalis glycosides, doxycycline, furosemide, levodopa, OCPs, quinidine, tacrolimus, theophylline, thyroid meds, valproic acid **Labs:** ↑ Serum cholesterol, glucose, alkaline phosphatase **NIPE:** Take w/ food; may alter urine color; use barrier contraception; ⊘ D/C abruptly; do not change dosage at intervals <7–10 d, hold tube feeds 1 h before and after dose if using oral susp

Physostigmine (Antilirium) [Antimuscarinic Antidote/Reversible Cholinesterase Inhibitor] Uses: *Antidote for TCA, atropine, & scopolamine OD; glaucoma* **Action:** Reversible cholinesterase inhibitor **Dose:** *Adults.* 0.5–2 mg IV or IM q20min. *Peds.* 0.01–0.03 mg/kg/dose IV q15–30min up to 2 mg total if needed **Caution:** [C, ?] **Contra:** GI/GU obst, CV Dz **Disp:** Inj 1 mg/mL **SE:** Rapid IV admin associated w/ Szs; cholinergic SE: sweating, salivation, lacrimation, GI upset, asystole, changes in HR **Interactions:** ↑ Resp depression W/ succinylcholine, ↑ effects W/ cholinergics, jaborandi tree, pill-bearing spurge **Labs:** ↑ ALT, AST, serum amylase; excessive readministration can result in cholinergic crisis; crisis reversed W/ atropine

Phytonadione [Vitamin K] (AquaMEPHYTON, Others) [Blood Modifier/Vitamin K] Uses: *Coagulation disorders due to faulty formation of factors II, VII, IX, X*; hyperalimentation **Action:** Cofactor for production of factors II, VII, IX, & X **Dose:** *Adults & Children. Anticoagulant-induced prothrombin deficiency:* 1–10 mg PO or IV slowly. *Hyperalimentation:* 10 mg IM or IV qwk. *Infants.* 0.5–1 mg/dose IM, SQ, or PO **Caution:** [C, +] **Contra:** Allergy **Disp:** Tabs 5 mg; inj 2, 10 mg/mL **SE:** Anaphylaxis from IV dosage; give IV slowly; GI upset (PO), inj site Rxns **Interactions:** ↓ Effects W/ antibiotics, cholestyramine, colestipol, salicylates, sucralfate; ↓ effects OF oral anticoagulants **Labs:** Falsely ↑ urine steroids **NIPE:** W/ parenteral Rx, 1st change in pt usually seen in 12–24 h; use makes recoumadinization more difficult

Pimecrolimus (Elidel) [Topical Immunomodulator] WARNING: Associated with rare skin malignancies and lymphoma, limit to area, not for age <2 y Uses: *Atopic dermatitis* refractory, severe perianal itching **Action:**

Inhibits T-lymphocytes **Dose:** *Adult and Peds >2 y:* Apply bid; use at least 1 wk following resoln **Caution:** [C, ?/–] w/ local Infxn, lymphadenopathy; immunocompromise; avoid <2 y of age **Contra:** Allergy component, <2 y **Disp:** Cream 1% **SE:** Phototox, local irritation/burning, flulike Sxs, may ↑ malignancy **NIPE:** Apply to dry skin only; wash hands after use; theoretical CA risk; 2nd line/short-term use only

Pindolol (Visken) [Antihypertensive/BB] Uses: *HTN* Action:
β-Adrenergic receptor blocker, β$_1$, β$_2$, ISA **Dose:** 5–10 mg bid, 60 mg/d max; ↓ in hepatic/renal failure **Caution:** [B (1st tri; D if 2nd or 3rd tri), +/–] **Contra:** Uncompensated CHF, cardiogenic shock, bradycardia, heart block, asthma, COPD **Disp:** Tabs 5, 10 mg **SE:** Insomnia, dizziness, fatigue, edema, GI upset, dyspnea; fluid retention may exacerbate CHF **Interactions:** ↑ HTN & bradycardia *W/* amphetamines, ephedrine, phenylephrine; ↑ Effects *W/* antihypertensives, diuretics; ↓ effects *W/* NSAIDs; ↓ effect *OF* hypoglycemics **Labs:** ↑ LFTs, uric acid **NIPE:** ⊘ D/C abruptly; ↑ cold sensitivity

Pioglitazone HCL/Glimepiride (Duetact) [Hypoglycemic/Thiazolidinedione & Sulfonylurea] Uses: Type 2 DM as adjunct to diet
and exercise **Action:** Combined ↑ insulin resistance, ↑ pancreatic insulin secretion, ↓ hepatic glucose output and production **Dose:** Initially 1 tab PO OD with the 1st main meal **Caution:** [C, –] **Contra:** Hepatic impair, DKA **Disp:** Tabs pioglitazone HCL/glimepiride: 30 mg/2mg, 30 mg/4 mg **SE:** ↑ Risk of CV mortality, hypoglycemia, wt gain, HA, edema, N, URI **Interactions:** ↑ Effects *W/* ASA, BB, chloramphenicol, ketoconazole, MAOIs, NSAIDs, probenecid, salicylates, sulfonamides, ↓ effects *W/* corticosteroids, diuretics, estrogens, isoniazid, phenothiazine, phenytoin, sympathomimetics, thyroid drugs ↓ effects *OF* OCPs **Labs:** ↑ LFTs, ↓ HMG, Hct **NIPE:** Take w/ 1st main meal of the day; use barrier contraception; ⊘ use in type 1 DM

Pioglitazone/Metformin (ActoPlus Met) [Hypoglycemic/Thiazolidinedione & Biguanide] WARNING: Can cause lactic acidosis,
which is fatal in 50% of cases **Uses:** *Type 2 DM as adjunct to diet and exercise* **Action:** Combined ↑ insulin sensitivity w/ ↓ hepatic glucose release **Dose:** Initial 1 tab PO daily or bid, titrate; max daily pioglitazone 45 mg & metformin 2550 mg **Caution:** [C, –] Stop w/ radiologic contrast agents **Contra:** Renal impair, acidosis **Disp:** Tabs pioglitazone mg/metformin mg: 15/500, 15/850 **SE:** Lactic acidosis, hypoglycemia, edema, wt gain, URI, HA, GI upset, liver damage **Interactions:** ↑ Effects *W/* amiloride, cimetidine, digoxin, furosemide, ketoconazole, MAOIs, morphine, procainamide, quinidine, quinine, ranitidine, triamterene, trimethoprim, vancomycin; ↓ effects *OF* OCPs; ↓ effects *W/* corticosteroids, CCBs, diuretics, estrogens, INH, OCPs, phenothiazine, phenytoin, sympathomimetics, thyroid drugs, tobacco **Labs:** ↑ LFTs, ↓ HMG, Hct; monitor serum glucose **NIPE:** Take w/o regard to food; use barrier contraception; ⊘ dehydration, EtOH; ↑ fracture risk in women receiving pioglitazone

Pioglitazone (Actos) [Hypoglycemic/Thiazolidinedione] Uses: *Type 2 DM* **Action:** ↑ Insulin sensitivity **Dose:** 15–45 mg/d PO **Caution:** [C, –] **Contra:** Hepatic impair **Disp:** Tabs 15, 30, 45 mg **SE:** Wt gain, URI, HA, hypoglycemia, edema **Interactions:** ↑ Effects W/ ketoconazole; ↓ effects OF OCPs **Labs:** ↑ LFTs, ↓ HMG, Hct **NIPE:** Take w/o regard to food; use barrier contraception; ↑ fracture risk in women

Piperacillin (Pipracil) [Antibiotic/Penicillin-4th Generation] Uses: *Infxns of skin, bone, resp &, urinary tract, abdomen, sepsis* **Action:** 4th-gen PCN; bactericidal; ↓ cell wall synth. *Spectrum:* Primarily gram(+), better *Enterococcus* sp, *H. influenza,* not *Staphylococcus* sp; gram(–) *E. coli, Proteus* sp, *Shigella* sp, *Pseudomonas* sp, not β-lactamase-producing **Dose:** *Adults.* 2–4 g IV q4–6h. *Peds.* 200–300 mg/kg/d IV ÷ q4–6h; ↓ in renal failure **Caution:** [B, M] **Contra:** PCN sensitivity **Disp:** Powder for inj: 2, 3, 4, 40 g **SE:** ↓ Plt aggregation, interstitial nephritis, renal failure, anaphylaxis, hemolytic anemia **Interactions:** ↑ Effects W/ probenecid; ↑ effects OF anticoagulants, MTX; ↓ effects W/ macrolides, tetracyclines; ↓ effects OF OCPs **Labs:** ↑ LFTs, BUN, Cr, + direct Coombs test, ↓ K⁺ **NIPE:** Inactivation of aminoglycosides if drugs given together—admin at least 1 h apart; often used w/ aminoglycoside

Piperacillin–Tazobactam (Zosyn) [Antibiotic/Extended Spectrum Penicillin, Beta-Lactamase Inhibitor] Uses: *Infxns of skin, bone, resp & urinary tract, abdomen, sepsis* **Action:** PCN plus β-lactamase inhibitor; bactericidal; ↓ cell wall synth. *Spectrum:* Good gram(+), excellent gram(–);anaerobes & β-lactamase producers **Dose:** *Adults.* 3.375–4.5 g IV q6h; ↓ in renal insuff **Caution:** [B, M] **Contra:** PCN or β-lactam sensitivity **Disp:** Powder for inj: frozen, premix inj 3.25, 3.375, 4.5 g **SE:** D, HA, insomnia, GI upset, serum sickness-like Rxn, pseudomembranous colitis **Interactions:** ↑ Effects W/ probenecid; ↑ effects OF anticoagulants, MTX; ↓ effects W/ macrolides, tetracyclines; ↓ effects OF OCPs **Labs:** ↑ LFTs, BUN, Cr, + direct Coombs test, ↓ K⁺ **NIPE:** Inactivation of aminoglycosides if drugs given together—admin at least 1 h apart; often used w/ aminoglycoside

Pirbuterol (Maxair) [Bronchodilator/Sympathomimetic] Uses: *Prevention & Rx reversible bronchospasm* **Action:** β₂-Adrenergic agonist **Dose:** 2 inhal q4–6h; max 12 inhal/d **Caution:** [C, ?/–] **Disp:** Aerosol 0.2 mg/actuation **SE:** Nervousness, restlessness, trembling, HA, taste changes, tachycardia **Interactions:** ↑ Effects W/ epinephrine, sympathomimetics; ↑ vascular effects W/ MAOIs, TCAs; ↓ effects W/ BBs **NIPE:** Rinse mouth after use; shake well before use; teach patient proper inhaler technique

Piroxicam (Feldene) [Bronchodilator/Beta-Adrenergic Agonist] **WARNING:** May ↑ risk of cardiovascular events & GI bleeding Uses: *Arthritis & pain* **Action:** NSAID; ↓ prostaglandins **Dose:** 10–20 mg/d **Caution:** [B (1st tri; D if 3rd tri or near term), +] GI bleeding **Contra:** ASA/NSAID sensitivity **Disp:** Caps 10, 20 mg **SE:** Dizziness, rash, GI upset, edema, acute renal failure, peptic ulcer **Interactions:** ↑ Effects W/ probenecid; ↑ effects OF aminoglycosides, anticoagulants, hypoglycemics, Li, MTX; ↑ risk of bleeding **W/** ASA, corticos teroids, NSAIDs, feverfew, garlic, ginger, ginkgo biloba, EtOH; ↓ effect **W/** ASA antacids, cholestyramine; ↓ effect **OF** IBs, diuretics **Labs:** ↑ BUN, Cr, LFTs **NIPE** Take w/food, full effect after 2 wk admin, ↑ risk of photosensitivity—use sunscreen

Plasma Protein Fraction (Plasmanate, Others) [Plasma Volume Expander]
Uses: *Shock & ↓ BP* **Action:** Plasma volume expander **Dose** Initial, 250–500 mL IV (not >10 mL/min); subsequent inf based on response. **Peds** 10–15 mL/kg/dose IV; subsequent inf based on response **Caution:** [C, +] **Contra** Renal insuff, CHF **Disp:** Inj 5% **SE:** ↓ BP w/ rapid inf; hypocoagulability, meta bolic acidosis, PE **NIPE:** 130–160 mEq NaL; not substitute for RBC

Pneumococcal 7-Valent Conjugate Vaccine (Prevnar) [Vaccine
Uses: *Immunization against pneumococcal Infxns in infants & children* **Action** Active immunization **Dose:** 0.5 mL IM/dose; series of 3 doses; 1st dose age 2 mo then doses q2mo, 4th dose at age 12–15 mo **Caution:** [C, +] Thrombocytopenia **Contra:** Diphtheria toxoid sensitivity, febrile illness **Disp:** Inj **SE:** Local Rxns arthralgia, fever, myalgia

Pneumococcal Vaccine, Polyvalent (Pneumovax-23) [Vaccine/ Inactive Bacteria]
Uses: *Immunization against pneumococcal Infxns i pts at high risk (eg, all = 65 y of age)* **Action:** Active immunization **Dose:** 0.5 ml IM. **Caution:** [C, ?] **Contra:** *Do not* vaccinate during immunosuppressive therapy **Disp:** Inj 0.5 mL **SE:** Fever, inj site Rxn, hemolytic anemia, thrombocytopenia anaphylaxis **Interactions:** ↓ Effects **W/** corticosteroids, immunosuppressants

Podophyllin (Podocon-25, Condylox Gel 0.5%, Condylox [Antimitotic Effect]
Uses: *Topical therapy of benign growths (genital & perianal warts [condylomata acuminata]*, papillomas, fibromas) **Action:** Direc antimitotic effect; exact mechanism unknown **Dose:** *Condylox gel & Condylox* Apply bid for 3 consecutive d/wk for 4 wk; 0.5 mL/d max; *Podocon-25:* Use spar ingly on the lesion, leave on for 1–4 h, thoroughly wash off **Caution:** [X, ?] Immuno suppression **Contra:** DM, bleeding lesions **Disp:** Podocon-25 (w/ benzoin) 15-ml bottles; Condylox gel 0.5% 35 g clear gel; Condylox soln 0.5% 35 g clear **SE** Local Rxns, significant absorption; anemias, tachycardia, paresthesias, GI upse renal/hepatic damage **NIPE:** Podocon-25 applied by the clinician; do not dispense directly to patient; ⊘ use on warts on mucous membranes; ⊘ use near eyes

Polyethylene Glycol [PEG]-Electrolyte Soln (GoLYTELY, CoLyte [Laxative]
Uses: *Bowel prep prior to examination or surgery* **Action:** Os motic cathartic **Dose:** *Adults.* Following 3–4-h fast, drink 240 mL of soln q10mi until 4 L consumed or until BMs are clear. *Peds.* 25–40 mL/kg/h for 4–10 h **Cau tion:** [C, ?] **Contra:** GI obst, bowel perforation, megacolon, ulcerative coliti **Disp:** Powder for recons to 4 L **SE:** Cramping or N, bloating **Interactions:** Drug taken within 1 h of polyethylene glycol administration may not be absorbed **NIPE** Instruct pt to drink solution rapidly q10min until finished; 1st BM should occur i approximately 1 h; chilled soln more palatable

Polyethylene Glycol [PEG] 3350 (MiraLax) [Laxative] Uses: *Occasional constipation* Action: Osmotic laxative Dose: 17 g powder (1 heaping Tbsp) in 8 oz (1 cup) of H_2O & drink; max 14 d Caution: [C, ?] R/O bowel obst before use Contra: GI obst, allergy to PEG Disp: Powder for recons; bottle cap holds 17 g SE: Upset stomach, bloating, cramping, gas, severe D, hives NIPE: May take 2–4 d for BM; can add to H_2O, juice, soda, coffee, or tea

Polymyxin B & Hydrocortisone (Otobiotic Otic) [Antibiotic-otic/Anti-inflammatory] Uses: *Superficial bacterial Infxns of external ear canal* Action: Antibiotic/anti-inflammatory combo Dose: 4 gtt in ear(s) tid–qid Caution: [B, ?] Disp: Soln polymyxin B 10,000 units/hydrocortisone 0.5%/mL SE: Local irritation NIPE: Clean ear before instillation of gtts; ⊘ use w/ perforated eardrum; useful in neomycin allergy

Posaconazole (Noxafil) [Anti-infective/Antifungal] Uses: *Prevent Aspergillus & Candida Infxns in severely immunocompromised* Action: ↓ Cell membrane ergosterol synth Dose: *Adult. Invasive fungal prophylaxis:* 200 mg PO tid; *Oropharyngeal candidiasis:* 100 mg PO daily × 13 d, if refractory 40 mg PO bid; *Peds. >13 y:* 200 mg PO tid; w/ meal Caution: [C; ?] Multiple drug interactions; ↑ QT, cardiac diseases, severe renal/liver impair Contra: Component hypersensitivity; w/ many drugs including alfuzosin, astemizole, alprazolam, phenothiazine, terfenadine, triazolam, others Disp: Sol 40 mg/mL SE: ↑ QT, ↑ LFTs, hepatic failure, fever, N/V/D, HA, abd pain, anemia, ↓ plt, ↓ K⁺ rash, dyspnea, cough, anorexia, fatigue Interactions: ↑ Effects *OF* CCB, cyclosporine, midazolam, sirolimus, statins, tacrolimus, vinca alkaloids; ↓ effects *W/* cimetidine, phenytoin, rifabutin Labs:? ↑ LFTs; ↓ K+ , plts; monitor LFTs, electrolytes, CBC NIPE: Monitor for breakthrough fungal Infxns; ⊘ for children <13 y

Potassium Citrate (Urocit-K) Uses: *Alkalinize urine, prevention of urinary stones (uric acid, Ca stones if hypocitraturia)* Action: Urinary alkalinizer Dose: 1 packet dissolved in H_2O or 15–30 mL after meals and hs 10–20 mEq PO tid w/ meals, max 100 mEq/d Caution: [A, +] Contra: Severe renal impair, dehydration, ↑ K⁺, peptic ulcer; w/ K⁺-sparing diuretics, salt substitutes Disp: 540, 1080 mg tabs SE: GI upset, metabolic alkalosis Interactions: ↑ Risk of hyperkalemia *W/* ACEIs, K⁺-sparing diuretics Labs: ↑ K⁺, ↓ Ca²⁺ NIPE: Take w/in 30 min of meals or hs snack; tabs 540 mg = 5 mEq, 1080 mg = 10 mEq

Potassium Citrate & Citric Acid (Polycitra-K) [Urinary Alkalinizer] Uses: *Alkalinize urine, prevent urinary stones (uric acid, Ca stones if hypocitraturia)* Action: Urinary alkalinizer Dose: 10–20 mEq PO tid w/ meals, max 100 mEq/d Caution: [A, +] Contra: Severe renal impair, dehydration, ↑ K⁺, peptic ulcer; w/ use of K⁺-sparing diuretics or salt substitutes Disp: Soln 10 mEq/ 5 mL; powder 30 mEq/packet SE: GI upset, metabolic alkalosis Interactions: ↑ Risk of hyperkalemia *W/* ACEIs, K⁺-sparing diuretics Labs: ↑ K⁺, ↓ Ca²⁺

Potassium Iodide [Lugol Soln] (SSKI, Thyro-Block) [Iodine Supplement] Uses: *Thyroid storm*, ↓ vascularity before thyroid surgery, block thyroid uptake of radioactive iodine, thin bronchial secretions **Action:** Iodine supl **Dose:** *Adults & Peds >2 y. Preop thyroidectomy:* 50–250 mg PO tid (2–6 gtt strong iodine soln); give 10 d preop. *Peds 1 y. Thyroid crisis:* 300 mg (6 gtt SSKI q8h). *Peds <1 y.* 1/2 adult dose **Caution:** [D, +] ↑ K^+, TB, PE, bronchitis, renal impair **Contra:** Iodine sensitivity **Disp:** Tabs 130 mg; soln (SSKI) 1 g/mL; Lugol soln, strong iodine 100 mg/mL; syrup 325 mg/5 mL **SE:** Fever, HA, urticaria, angioedema, goiter, GI upset, eosinophilia **Interactions:** ↑ Risk of hypothyroidism W/ antithyroid drugs and Li; ↑ risk of hyperkalemia W/ ACEIs, K^+-sparing diuretics, K supls **Labs:** May alter TFTs **NIPE:** Take pc w/ food or milk

Potassium Supplements (Kaon, Kaochlor, K-Lor, Slow-K, Micro-K, Klorvess, others) [K+ Supplement/Electrolyte]
Uses: *Prevention or Rx of ↓ K^+* (eg, diuretic use) **Action:** K^+ supl **Dose:** *Adults* 20–100 mEq/d PO ÷ daily–bid; IV 10–20 mEq/h, max 40 mEq/h & 150 mEq/ (monitor K^+ levels frequently w/ high-dose IV). *Peds.* Calculate K^+ deficit; 1–3 mEq/kg/d PO ÷ daily–qid; IV max dose 0.5–1 mEq/kg/h **Caution:** [A, +] Renal insuff, use w/ NSAIDs & ACE inhibitors **Contra:** ↑ K^+ **Disp:** PO forms (Table 7), inj **SE:** GI irritation; bradycardia; ↑ K^+, heart block **Interactions:** ↑ Effects W/ ACEI, K^+-sparing diuretics, salt substitutes **Labs:** Follow K^+; Cl^- salt OK w/ alkalosis **NIPE:** Take w/ food; mix powder & Liq w/ beverage (unsalted tomato juice etc); w/ acidosis use acetate, bicarbonate, citrate, or gluconate salt

Pramipexole (Mirapex) [Antiparkinson Agent/Dopamine Agonist] **Uses:** *Parkinson Dz* **Action:** Dopamine agonist **Dose:** 1.5–4.5 mg/ PO, initial 0.375 mg/d in 3 ÷ doses; titrate slowly **Caution:** [C, ?/–] ↓ renal impai **Contra:** Component allergy **Disp:** Tabs 0.125, 0.25, 0.5, 1, 1.5 mg **SE:** Postural ↓ BP, asthenia, somnolence, abnormal dreams, GI upset, EPS **Interactions:** ↑ Effects W/ cimetidine, diltiazem, quinidine, quinine, ranitidine, triamterene, verapamil; ↑ effects OF levodopa; ↑ CNS depression W/ CNS depressants, EtOH ↓ effects W/ antipsychotics, butyrophenones, metoclopramide, phenothiazines, thioxanthenes **NIPE:** May take w/ food; ⊘ D/C abruptly

Pramoxine (Anusol Ointment, ProctoFoam-NS, Others) [Topical Anesthetic] **Uses:** *Relief of pain & itching from hemorrhoids, anorectal surgery*; topical for burns & dermatosis **Action:** Topical anesthetic **Dose:** Apply freely to anal area q3h **Caution:** [C, ?] **Disp:** [OTC] All 1%; foam (Proctofoam), cream, oint, lotion, gel, pads, spray **SE:** Contact dermatitis, mucosal thinning w/ chronic use **NIPE:** ⊘ Use on large areas

Pramoxine + Hydrocortisone (Enzone, Proctofoam-HC) [Topical Anesthetic/Anti-inflammatory] **Uses:** *Relief of pain & itching from hemorrhoids* **Action:** Topical anesthetic, anti-inflammatory **Dose:** Apply freely to anal area tid–qid **Caution:** [C, ?/–] **Disp:** *Cream* pramoxine 1% acetate 0.5/1%; *foam* pramoxine 1% hydrocortisone 1%; *lotion* pramoxine 1% hydrocortisone 0.25/1/2.5%, pramoxine 2.5% & hydrocortisone 1% **SE:** Contact dermatitis, mucosal thinning w/ chronic use **NIPE:** ⊘ Use on large areas

Pravastatin (Pravachol) [Antilipemic/HMG-CoA Reductase Inhibitor] Uses: * ↓ Cholesterol* Action: HMG-CoA reductase inhibitor Dose: 10–80 mg PO hs; ↓ in significant renal/hepatic impair Caution: [X –] w/ gemfibrozil Contra: Liver Dz or persistent LFT ↑ Disp: Tabs 10, 20, 40, 80 mg SE: Use caution w/ concurrent gemfibrozil; HA, GI upset, hepatitis, myopathy, renal failure Interactions: ↑ Risk of myopathy & rhabdomyolysis W/ clarithromycin, clofibrate, cyclosporine, danazol, erythromycin, fluoxetine, gemfibrozil, niacin, nefazodone, troleandomycin; ↑ effects W/ azole antifungals, cimetidine, grapefruit juice; ↓ effects W/ cholestyramine, isradipine Labs: ↑ LFTs NIPE: ⊘ PRG, breast-feeding; take w/o regard to food; full effect may take up to 4 wk; ↑ risk of photosensitivity—use sunscreen

Prazosin (Minipress) [Antihypertensive/Alpha Blocker] Uses: * HTN* Action: Peripherally acting α-adrenergic blocker Dose: Adults. 1 mg PO tid; can ↑ to 20 mg/d max PRN. Peds. 0.05–0.1 mg/kg/d in 3 div doses; max 0.5 mg. kg/d Caution: [C, ?] Contra: Component allergy, concurrent use of PDE-5 inhibitors Disp: Caps 1, 2, 5 mg; tabs XR 2.5, 5 mg XR SE: Dizziness, edema, palpitations, fatigue, GI upset Interactions: ↑ Hypotension W/ antihypertensives, diuretics, nitrates, EtOH; ↓ effects W/ NSAIDs, butcher's broom Labs: ↑ Serum Na levels, vanillylmandelic acid level; alters test for pheochromocytoma NIPE: ⊘ D/C abruptly; can cause orthostatic ↓ BP, take the 1st dose hs; tolerance develops to this effect; tachyphylaxis may result

Prednisolone [Corticosteroid] [See Steroids and Table 3] Interactions: ↑ Effects W/ clarithromycin, erythromycin, estrogen, ketoconazole, OCPs, troleandomycin; ↓ effects W/ antacids, aminoglutethimide, barbiturates, cholestyramine, colestipol, phenytoin, rifampin; ↓ effects OF anticoagulants, hypoglycemics, INH, salicylates, vaccine toxoids Labs: False—skin allergy tests; false ↑ cortisol, digoxin, theophylline NIPE: ⊘ Use live-virus vaccines, ⊘ D/C abruptly; take w/ food

Prednisone [Corticosteroid] [See Steroids and Table 3] Interactions: ↑ Effects W/ clarithromycin, cyclosporine, erythromycin, estrogen, ketoconazole, OCPs, troleandomycin; ↓ effects W/ antacids, aminoglutethimide, barbiturates, carbamazepine, cholestyramine, colestipol, phenytoin, rifampin; ↓ effects OF anticoagulants, hypoglycemics, INH, salicylates, vaccine toxoids Labs: False skin allergy tests, false ↑ cortisol, digoxin, theophylline NIPE: Take w/ food; ⊘ use live-virus vaccine, ⊘ D/C abruptly, Infxn may be masked

Pregabalin (Lyrica) [Antinociceptive/Antiseizure] Uses: *DM peripheral neuropathy pain; postherpetic neuralgia; fibromyalgia; adjunct w/ adult partial onset Sz* Action: Nerve transmission modulator, antinociceptive, antiseizure effect; mechanism; related to gabapentin Dose: Neuropathic pain: 50 mg PO tid; ↑ to 300 mg/d w/in 1 wk based on response, 300 mg/d max; Postherpetic neuralgia: 75–150 mg bid, or 50–100 mg tid; start 75 mg bid or 50 mg tid; ↑ to 300 mg/d w/in 1 wk PRN; if pain persists after 2–4 wk, ↑ to 600 mg/d; Epilepsy:

Start 150 mg/d (75 mg bid or 50 mg ~~tid~~) ~~may~~ ↑ to max 600 mg/d; ↓ w/ renal insuff; w/ or w/o food **Caution:** [X, –] w/ significant renal impair (see insert), w/ elderly & severe CHF avoid abrupt D/C **Contra:** PRG **Disp:** Caps 25, 50, 75, 100, 150, 200, 225, 300 mg **SE:** Dizziness, drowsiness, xerostomia, edema, blurred vision, wt gain, difficulty concentrating **NIPE:** Avoid abrupt D/C; w/ D/C, taper over at least 1 wk

Probenecid (Benemid, others) [Uricosuric/Analgesic] Uses: *Prevent gout & hyperuricemia; prolongs levels of PCNs & cephalosporins* **Action:** Uricosuric, renal tubular blocker of organic anions **Dose:** *Adults. Gout:* 250 mg bid × 1 wk, then 0.5 g PO bid; can ↑ by 500 mg/mo up to 2–3 g/d. *Antibiotic effect:* 1–2 g PO 30 min before dose *Peds >2 y.* 25 mg/kg, then 40 mg/kg PO ÷ qid **Caution:** [B, ?] **Contra:** High-dose ASA, moderate–severe renal impair, age <2 y **Disp:** Tabs 500 mg **SE:** HA, GI upset, rash, pruritus, dizziness, blood dyscrasias **Interactions:** ↑ Effects *OF* acyclovir, allopurinol; ↑ effects *OF* benzodiazepines, cephalosporins, ciprofloxacin, clofibrate, dapsone, dyphylline, MTX, NSAIDs, olanzapine, rifampin, sulfonamides, sulfonylureas zidovudine; ↓ effects *W/* niacin, EtOH; ↑ effects *OF* penicillamine **Labs:** False + urine glucose; false ↑ level of theophylline **NIPE:** Take w/ food, ↑ fluids to 2–3 L/d; ⊘ ASA, NSAIDs, salicylates; do not use during acute gout attack

Procainamide (Pronestyl, Pronestyl SR, Procanbid) [Antiarrhythmic] **WARNING:** Positive ANA titer or SLE w/ prolonged use; only use in life-treating arrhythmias; hematologic tox can be severe, follow CBC **Uses:** *Supraventricular/ventricular arrhythmias* **Action:** Class 1A antiarrhythmic (Table 10) **Dose:** *Adults. Recurrent VF/VT:* 20 mg/min IV (total 17 mg/kg max). *Maint:* 1–4 mg/min. *Stable wide-complex tachycardia of unknown origin, AF w/ rapid rate in WPW:* 20 mg/min IV until arrhythmia suppression, ↓ BP, or QRS widens >50%, then 1–4 mg/min. *Chronic dosing:* 50 mg/kg/d PO in ÷ doses q4–6h; *Recurrent VF/VT:* 20–50 mg/min IV; max total 17 mg/kg. *Others:* 20 mg/min IV until one these: arrhythmia stopped, hypotension, QRS widens >50%, total 17 mg/kg; then 1–4 mg/min *(ECC 2005) Peds. Chronic maint:* 15–50 mg/kg/24 h PO ÷ q3–6h; ↓ in renal/hepatic impair **Caution:** [C, +] **Contra:** Complete heart block, 2nd- or 3rd-degree heart block w/o pacemaker, torsades de pointes, SLE **Disp:** Tabs & caps 250, 500 mg; SR tabs 500, 750, 1000 mg; inj 100, 500 mg/mL **SE:** ↓ BP, lupus-like synd, GI upset, taste perversion, arrhythmias, tachycardia, heart block, angioneurotic edema, blood dyscrasias **Notes:** *Levels: Trough:* Just before next dose: *Therapeutic:* 4–10 μg/mL; NAPA+ procaine 5–30 μg/mL *Toxic:* >10 μg/mL; NAPA+ procaine >30 μg/mL; *1/2-life:* procaine 3–5 h, NAPA 6–10 h **Interactions:** ↑ Effects *W/* acetazolamide, amiodarone, cimetidine, ranitidine, trimethoprim; ↑ effects *OF* anticholinergics, antihypertensives; ↓ effects *W/* procaine, EtOH **Labs:** ↑ LFTs **NIPE:** Take w/ food if GI upset; ⊘ crush SR tab

Procarbazine (Matulane) [Antineoplastic/Alkylating Agent] **WARNING:** Highly toxic; handle w/ care **Uses:** *Hodgkin Dz*, NHL, brain & lung tumors **Action:** Alkylating agent; ↓ DNA & RNA ~~synth~~ **Dose:** Per protoco

Caution: [D, ?] w/ EtOH ingestion **Contra:** Inadequate BM reserve **Disp:** Caps 50 mg **SE:** ↓ BM, hemolytic Rxns (w/ G6PD deficiency), N/V/D; disulfiram-like Rxn; cutaneous & constitutional Sxs, myalgia, arthralgia, CNS suppression, azoospermia, cessation of menses **Interactions:** ↑ CNS depression *W/* antihistamines, barbiturates, MAOIs, CNS depressants, narcotics, phenothiazine; ↑ risk of HTN *W/* guanethidine, levodopa, MAOIs, methyldopa, sympathomimetics, TCAs, tyramine-containing foods; ↓ effects *OF* digoxin **NIPE:** Disulfiram-like Rxn w/ EtOH; ↑ fluids to 2–3 L/d; ↑ risk of photosensitivity—use sunscreen; ⊘ exposure to Infxn

Prochlorperazine (Compazine) [Antiemetic, Antipsychotic/ Phenothiazine] Uses: *N/V, agitation, & psychotic disorders* Action: Phenothiazine; blocks postsynaptic dopaminergic CNS receptors **Dose:** *Adults.* Antiemetic: 5–10 mg PO tid–qid or 25 mg PR bid or 5–10 mg deep IM q4–6h. *Antipsychotic:* 10–20 mg IM acutely or 5–10 mg PO tid–qid for maint; ↑ doses may be required for antipsychotic effect. **Peds.** 0.1–0.15 mg/kg/dose IM q4–6h or 0.4 mg/kg/24 h PO ÷ tid–qid **Caution:** [C, +/–] NAG, severe liver/cardiac Dz **Contra:** Phenothiazine sensitivity, BM suppression; age <2 y old or wt <9 kg **Disp:** Tabs 5, 10, 25 mg; SR caps 10, 15 mg; syrup 5 mg/5 mL; supp 2.5, 5, 25 mg; inj 5 mg/mL **SE:** EPS common; Rx w/ diphenhydramine or benztropine **Interactions:** ↑ Effects *W/* chloroquine, indomethacin, narcotics, procarbazine, SSRIs, pyrimethamine; ↑ effects *OF* antidepressants, BBs, EtOH; ↓ effects *W/* antacids, anticholinergics, barbiturates, tobacco; ↓ effects *OF* guanethidine, levodopa, Li **Labs:** False + urine bilirubin, amylase, phenylketonuria, ↑ serum prolactin **NIPE:** ⊘ D/C abruptly; ↑ risk of photosensitivity—use sunscreen; urine may turn pink/red

Promethazine (Phenergan) [Antihistamine, Antiemetic, Sedative/Phenothiazine] Uses: *N/V, motion sickness* Action: Phenothiazine; blocks CNS postsynaptic mesolimbic dopaminergic receptors **Dose:** *Adults.* 12.5–50 mg PO, PR, or IM bid–qid PRN. **Peds.** 0.1–0.5 mg/kg/dose PO or IM q2–6h PRN **Caution:** [C, +/–] Use w/ agents w/ respiratory depressant effects **Contra:** Component allergy, NAG, age <2 y **Disp:** Tabs 12.5, 25, 50 mg; syrup 6.25 mg/5 mL, 25 mg/5 mL; supp 12.5, 25, 50 mg; inj 25, 50 mg/mL **SE:** Drowsiness, tardive dyskinesia, EPS, lowered Sz threshold, ↓ BP, GI upset, blood dyscrasias, photosens, respiratory depression in children **Interactions:** ↑ Effects *W/* CNS depressants, MAOIs, EtOH; ↑ effects *OF* antihypertensives; ↓ effects *W/* anticholinergics, barbiturates, tobacco; ↓ effect *OF* levodopa **NIPE:** Effects skin allergy tests; use sunscreen for photosensitivity

Propafenone (Rythmol) [Antiarrhythmic] WARNING: Excess mortality or nonfatal cardiac arrest rate possible; avoid use in asymptomatic and symptomatic non-life-threatening ventricular arrhythmias **Uses:** *Life-threatening ventricular arrhythmias, AF* **Action:** Class IC antiarrhythmic (Table 10) **Dose:** *Adults.* 150–300 mg PO q8h. **Peds.** 8–10 mg/kg/d ÷ in 3–4 doses; may ↑ 2 mg/kg/d, 20 mg/kg/d max **Caution:** [C, ?] w/ amprenavir, ritonavir, MI w/in 2 y, w/liver/renal impair **Contra:** Uncontrolled CHF, bronchospasm, cardiogenic shock, AV block

w/o pacer, **Disp:** Tabs 150, 225, 300 mg; XR caps 225, 425 mg **SE:** Dizziness, unusual taste, 1st-degree heart block, arrhythmias, prolongs QRS & QT intervals; fatigue, GI upset, blood dyscrasias **Interactions:** ↑ Effects *W/* cimetidine, quinidine; ↑ effects *OF* anticoagulants, BBs, digitalis glycosides, theophylline; ↓ effects *W/* rifampin, phenobarbital, rifabutin **Labs:** ↑ ANA titers **NIPE:** Take w/o regard to food

Propantheline (Pro-Banthine) [Antimuscarinic] Uses: *PUD*, symptomatic Rx of small intestine hypermotility, spastic colon, ureteral spasm, bladder spasm, pylorospasm **Action:** Antimuscarinic **Dose:** *Adults.* 15 mg PO ac & 30 mg PO hs; ↓ in elderly. *Peds.* 2–3 mg/kg/24h PO ÷ tid–qid **Caution:** [C, ?] **Contra:** NAG, ulcerative colitis, toxic megacolon, GI/GU obst **Disp:** Tabs 7.5, 15 mg **SE:** Anticholinergic (eg, xerostomia, blurred vision) **Interactions:** ↑ Anticholinergic effects *W/* antihistamines, antidepressants, atropine, haloperidol, phenothiazines, quinidine, TCAs; ↑ effects *OF* atenolol, digoxin; ↓ effects *W/* antacids **NIPE:** May cause heat intolerance, ↑ risk of photosensitivity—use sunscreen

Propofol (Diprivan) [Anesthetic] Uses: *Induction & maint of anesthesia; sedation in intubated pts* **Action:** Sedative–hypnotic; mechanism unknown; acts in 40 sec **Dose:** *Adults. Anesthesia:* 2–2.5 mg/kg (also *ECC 2005*), then 0.1–0.2 mg/kg/ min inf; *ICU sedation:* 5 µg/kg/min IV × 5 min, ↑ PRN 5–10 µg/kg/min q5–10 min 5–50 µg/kg/min cont inf; *Peds. Anesthesia:* 2.5–3.5 mg/kg induction; then 125–300 µg/kg/min; ↓ in elderly, debilitated, ASA II/IV pts **Caution:** [B, +] **Contra:** If general anesthesia contraindicated, sensitivity to egg, egg products, soybeans, soybean products **Disp:** Inj 10 mg/mL **SE:** ↓ BP, pain at site, apnea, anaphylaxis **Notes:** 1 mL has 0.1 g fat **Interactions:** ↑ Effects *W/* antihistamines, opioids, hypnotics, EtOH **Labs:** ↑ Serum cortisol levels; may ↑ triglycerides w/ extended dosing

Propoxyphene (Darvon); Propoxyphene & Acetaminophen (Darvocet); & Propoxyphene & Aspirin (Darvon Compound-65, Darvon-N + Aspirin) [C-IV] [Narcotic Analgesic] WARNING: Excessive doses alone or in combo w/ other CNS depressants can be cause of death; use w/ caution in depressed or suicidal patients Uses: *Mild-moderate pain* **Action:** Narcotic analgesic **Dose:** 1–2 PO q4h PRN; ↓ in hepatic impair, elderly **Caution:** [C (D if prolonged use), M] Hepatic impair (APAP), peptic ulcer (ASA); severe renal impair, h/o EtOH abuse **Contra:** Allergy, suicide risk, h/o drug abuse **Disp:** *Darvon:* Propoxyphene HCl caps 65 mg. *Darvon-N:* Propoxyphene napsylate 100-mg tabs. *Darvocet-N:* Propoxyphene napsylate 50 mg/ APAP 325 mg. *Darvocet-N 100:* Propoxyphene napsylate 100 mg/APAP 650 mg. *Darvon Compound-65:* Propoxyphene HCl caps 65-mg/ASA 389 mg/caffeine 32 mg. *Darvon-N w/ ASA:* Propoxyphene napsylate 100 mg/ASA 325 mg **SE:** OD can be lethal; ↓ BP, dizziness, sedation, GI upset **Interactions:** ↑ CNS depression *W/* antidepressants, antihistamines, barbiturates, glutethimide, methocarbamol, protease inhibitors, EtOH, St. John's wort; ↑ effects *OF* BBs, carbamazepine

MAOIs, phenobarbital, TCAs, warfarin; ↓ effects **W/** tobacco **Labs:** ↑ LFTs, serum amylase, lipase **NIPE:** Take w/ food if GI upset

Propranolol (Inderal) [Antihypertensive, Antianginal, Antiarrhythmic/BB]

Uses: *HTN, angina, MI, hyperthyroidism, essential tremor, hypertrophic subaortic stenosis, pheochromocytoma; prevents migraines & atrial arrhythmias* **Action:** β-Adrenergic receptor blocker, β_1, β_2; only β-blocker to block conversion of T_4 to T_3 **Dose:** *Adults. Angina:* 80–320 mg/d PO ÷ bid–qid or 80–160 mg/d SR. *Arrhythmia:* 10–80 mg PO tid–qid or 1 mg IV slowly, repeat q5 min, 5 mg max. *HTN:* 40 mg PO bid or 60–80 mg/d SR, ↑ weekly to max 640 mg/d. *Hypertrophic subaortic stenosis:* 20–40 mg PO tid–qid. *MI:* 180–240 mg PO ÷ tid–qid. *Migraine prophylaxis:* 80 mg/d ÷ qid–tid, ↑ weekly 160–240 mg/d ÷ tid–qid max; wean if no response in 6 wk. *Pheochromocytoma:* 30–60 mg/d ÷ tid–qid. *Thyrotoxicosis:* 1–3 mg IV × 1; 10–40 mg PO q6h. *Tremor:* 40 mg PO bid, ↑ PRN 320 mg/d max; 0.1 mg/kg slow IV push, divided 3 equal doses q2–3min, max 1 mg/min; repeat in 2 min PRN *(ECC 2005)* *Peds. Arrhythmia:* 0.5–1.0 mg/kg/d ÷ tid–qid, ↑ PRN q3–7d to 60 mg/d max; 0.01–0.1 mg/kg IV over 10 min, 1 mg max. *HTN:* 0.5–1.0 mg/kg ÷ bid–qid, ↑ PRN q3–7d to 2 mg/kg/d max; ↓ in renal impair **Caution:** [C (1st tri, D if 2nd or 3rd tri). +] **Contra:** Uncompensated CHF, cardiogenic shock, bradycardia, heart block, PE, severe resp Dz **Disp:** Tabs 10, 20, 40, 80 mg; SR caps 60, 80, 120, 160 mg; oral soln 4, 8 mg/mL; inj 1 mg/mL **SE:** Bradycardia, ↓ BP, fatigue, GI upset, ED **Interactions:** ↑ Effects **W/** antihypertensives, cimetidine, hydralazine, neuroleptics, nitrates, propylthiouracil, theophylline, EtOH; ↑ effects *OF* digitalis, glycosides, hypoglycemics, hydralazine, lidocaine, neuroleptics; ↓ effects **W/** NSAIDs, phenobarbital, phenytoin, rifampin, tobacco **Labs:** ↑ LFTs, BUN; ↑ or ↓ serum glucose; ↓ plts, thyroxine; **NIPE:** ⊘ D/C abruptly; ↑ cold sensitivity

Propylthiouracil [PTU] [Antithyroid Agent/Thyroid Hormone Antagonist]

Uses: *Hyperthyroidism* **Action:** ↓ Production of T_3 & T_4 & conversion of T_4 to T_3 **Dose:** *Adults.* Initial: 100 mg PO q8h (may need up to 1200 mg/d); after pt euthyroid (6–8 wk), taper dose by 1/2 q4–6wk to maint, 50–150 mg/24 h; can usually D/C in 2–3 y; ↓ in elderly *Peds.* Initial: 5–7 mg/kg/24 h PO ÷ q8h. *Maint:* 1/3–2/3 of initial dose **Caution:** [D, –] **Contra:** Allergy **Disp:** Tabs 50 mg **SE:** Fever, rash, leukopenia, dizziness, GI upset, taste perversion, SLE-like synd **Interactions:** ↑ Effects **W/** iodinated glycerol, Li, KI, NaI **Labs:** ↑ LFTs, PT; ↑ effects of anticoagulants; monitor TFT **NIPE:** Take w/ food for GI upset; omit dietary sources of I; full effects take 6–12 wk; monitor pt clinically;

Protamine (Generic) [Heparin Antagonist]

Uses: *Reverse heparin effect* **Action:** Neutralize heparin by forming a stable complex **Dose:** Based on degree of heparin reversal; give IV slowly; 1 mg reverses approx 100 units of heparin given in the preceding 3–4 h, 50 mg max **Caution:** [C, ?] **Contra:** Allergy **Disp:** Inj 10 mg/mL **SE:** Follow coags; anticoag effect if given w/o heparin; ↓ BP, bradycardia, dyspnea, hemorrhage **Interactions:** Incompatible **W/** many penicillins & cephalosporins—⊘ mix

Pseudoephedrine (Sudafed, Novafed, Afrinol, Others) [OTC] [Decongestant/Sympathomimetic] Uses: *Decongestant* Action: Stimulates α-adrenergic receptors w/ vasoconstriction Dose: *Adults.* 30–60 mg PO q6–8h *Peds.* 4 mg/kg/24 h PO ÷ qid; ↓ in renal insuff Caution: [C, +] Contra: Poorly controlled HTN or CAD, w/ MAOIs Disp: Tabs 30, 60 mg; caps 60 mg; SR tabs 120, 240 mg; Liq 7.5 mg/0.8 mL, 15, 30 mg/5 mL SE: HTN, insomnia, tachycardia, arrhythmias, nervousness, tremor Interactions: ↑ Risk of HTN crisis W/ MAOIs; ↑ effects W/ BBs, sympathomimetics; ↓ effects W/ TCAs; ↓ effect OF methyldopa, reserpine NIPE: Found in many OTC cough/cold preparations; OTC restricted distribution

Psyllium (Metamucil, Serutan, Effer-Syllium) [Laxative] Uses: *Constipation & colonic diverticular Dz * Action: Bulk laxative Dose: 1 tsp (7 g) in glass of H_2O PO daily–tid Caution: [B, ?] Effer-Syllium (effervescent psyllium) usually contains K^+ caution w/ renal failure; phenylketonuria (in products w/ aspartame) Contra: Suspected bowel obst Disp: Granules 4, 25 g/tsp; powder 3.5 g/packet, caps 0.52g (3 g/6 caps), wafers 3.4 g/dose SE: D, abd cramps, bowel obst, constipation, bronchospasm Interactions: ↓ Effects OF digitalis glycosides, K-sparing diuretics, nitrofurantoin, salicylates, tetracyclines, warfarin NIPE: Psyllium dust inhalation may cause wheezing, runny nose, watery eyes

Pyrazinamide (Generic) [Antitubercular] Uses: *Active TB in combo w/ other agents* Action: Bacteriostatic; unknown mechanism Dose: *Adults.* 15–30 mg/kg/24 h PO ÷ tid–qid; max 2 g/d; dosing based on lean body wt; ↓ dose in renal/hepatic impairment *Peds.* 15–30 mg/kg/d PO ÷ daily–bid; ↓ w/ renal/hepatic impair Caution: [C, +/–] Contra: Severe hepatic damage, acute gout Disp: Tabs 500 mg SE: Hepatotox, malaise, GI upset, arthralgia, myalgia, gout, photosens Interactions: ↓ Effects OF probenecid Labs: ↑ Uric acid NIPE: ↑ Risk of photosensitivity—use sunscreen; ↑ fluids to 2 L/d; Use in combo w/ other anti-TB drugs; consult *MMWR* for latest TB recommendations; dosage regimen differs for "directly observed" therapy

Pyridoxine [Vitamin B_6] [Vitamin B_6 Supplement] Uses: *Rx & prevention of vitamin B_6 deficiency* Action: Vitamin B_6 supl Dose: *Adults. Deficiency:* 10–20 mg/d PO. *Drug-induced neuritis:* 100–200 mg/d; 25–100 mg/d prophylaxis. *Peds.* 5–25 mg/d × 3 wk Caution: [A (C if doses exceed RDA), +] Contra: Component sensitivity Disp: Tabs 25, 50, 100 mg; inj 100 mg/mL SE: Allergic Rxns, HA, N Interactions: ↓ Effects OF levodopa, phenobarbital, phenytoin Labs: ↑ AST; ↓ folic acid NIPE: Antidote for isoniazid poisoning

Quadrivalent Human Papillomavirus (HPV Types 6, 11, 16, 18) Recombinant Vaccine (Gardasil) [Vaccine] Uses: Prevent cervical CA, genital warts, cervical adenocarcinoma in situ, cervical intraepithelial neoplasia grades 2 & 3, vulvar intraepithelial neoplasia grades 2 & 3, vaginal intraepithelial neoplasia grades 2 & 3, cervical intraepithelial neoplasia grade 1 caused by HPV types 6, 11, 16, 18 Dose: 0.5 mL IM inj in deltoid or upper thigh *Peds.* <9 y:

Not recommended; *Females.* 9–26 y: Give 1st, 2nd dose 2 mo >1st, 3rd dose 6 mo >1st dose **Caution:** [B, –]; **Disp:** 0.5 mL for IM inj **SE:** Inj site reaction, fever **Interactions:** ↓ Response W/ immunosuppressants **NIPE:** May not protect all recipients; not a substitute for routine cervical screening

Quazepam (Doral) [C-IV] [Sedative/Hypnotic/Benzodiazepine] **Uses:** *Insomnia* **Action:** Benzodiazepine **Dose:** 7.5–15 mg PO hs PRN; ↓ in elderly & hepatic failure **Caution:** [X, ?/–] NA glaucoma **Contra:** PRG, sleep apnea **Disp:** Tabs 7.5, 15 mg **SE:** Sedation, hangover, somnolence, resp depression **Interactions:** ↑ Effects W/ azole antifungals, cimetidine, digoxin, disulfiram, INH, levodopa, macrolides, neuroleptics, phenytoin, quinolones, SSRIs, verapamil, grapefruit juice, EtOH; ↓ effects W/ carbamazepine, rifampin, rifabutin, tobacco **NIPE:** ⊘ Breastfeed, PRG; ⊘ D/C abruptly; use barrier contraception

Quetiapine (Seroquel, Seroquil XR) [Antipsychotic] **WARNING:** Closely monitor pts for worsening depression or emergence of suicidality, particularly in ped pts; ↑ mortality in elderly with dementia-related psychosis **Uses:** *Acute exacerbations of schizophrenia* **Action:** Serotonin & dopamine antagonism **Dose:** 150–750 mg/d; initiate at 25–100 mg bid–tid; slowly ↑ dose; XR: 400–800 mg PO qPM, start 300 mg/d, ↑ 300 mg/d, 800 mg/d max ↓ dose w/ hepatic & geriatric pts **Caution:** [C, –] **Contra:** Component allergy **Disp:** Tabs 25, 50, 100, 200, 300, 400 mg; Tabs XR 150, 200, 300, 400 XR **SE:** Confusion w/ nefazodone; HA, somnolence, HA, ↓ wt, ↓ BP, dizziness, cataracts, neuroleptic malignant synd, tardive dyskinesia, ↑ QT internal **Interactions:** ↑ Effects W/ azole antifungals, cimetidine, macrolides, EtOH; ↑ effects OF antihypertensives, lorazepam; ↓ effects W/ barbiturates, carbamazepine, glucocorticoids, phenytoin, rifampin, thioridazine; ↓ effects OF dopamine antagonists, levodopa **Labs:** ↑ LFTs, cholesterol, triglycerides **NIPE:** ↑ risk OF cataract formation, tardive dyskinesia; take w/o regard to food; ↓ body temp regulation

Quinapril (Accupril) [Antihypertensive/ACEI] **WARNING:** ACE inhibitors used during PRG can cause fetal injury & death **Uses:** *HTN, CHF, DN, post-MI* **Action:** ACE inhibitor **Dose:** 10–80 mg PO daily; ↓ in renal impair **Caution:** [D, +] w/ RAS, volume depletion **Contra:** ACE inhibitor sensitivity, angioedema, PRG **Disp:** Tabs 5, 10, 20, 40 mg **SE:** Dizziness, HA, ↓ BP, impaired renal Fxn, angioedema, taste perversion, cough **Interactions:** ↑ Effects W/ diuretics, antihypertensives; ↑ effects OF insulin, Li; ↓ effects W/ ASA, NSAIDs; ↓ effects OF quinolones, tetracyclines **Labs:** ↑ K+, ↓ LFTs **NIPE:** ↓ Absorption W/ high-fat foods; ↑ risk of cough

Quinidine (Quinidex, Quinaglute) [Antiarrhythmic/Antimalarial] **Uses:** *Prevention of tachydysrhythmias, malaria* **Action:** Class 1A antiarrhythmic **Dose:** *Adults.* *AF/flutter conversion:* After digitalization, 200 mg q2–3h × 8 doses; ↑ daily to 3–4 g max or nl rhythm. *Peds.* 15–60 mg/kg/24 h PO in 4–5 ÷ doses; ↓ in renal impair **Caution:** [C, +] w/ ritonavir **Contra:** Digitalis tox & AV block; conduction disorders **Disp:** *Sulfate:* Tabs 200, 300 mg; SR tabs 300 mg.

Gluconate: SR tabs 324 mg; inj 80 mg/mL **SE:** Extreme ↓ BP w/ IV use; syncope, QT prolongation, GI upset, arrhythmias, fatigue, cinchonism (tinnitus, hearing loss, delirium, visual changes), fever, hemolytic anemia, thrombocytopenia, rash **Notes:** *Levels: Trough:* Just before next dose; *Therapeutic:* 2–5 μg/mL; *Toxic:* >10 μg/mL; *1/2 life:* 6–8h; sulfate salt 83% quinidine; gluconate salt 62% quinidine **Interactions:** ↑ Effects *W/* acetazolamide, antacids, amiodarone, azole antifungals, cimetidine, K, macrolides, NaHCO₃, thiazide diuretics, lily-of-the-valley, pheasant's eye herb, scopolia root, squill; ↑ effects *OF* anticoagulants, dextromethorphan, digitalis glycosides, disopyramide, haloperidol, metoprolol, nifedipine, procainamide, propafenone, propranolol, TCAs, verapamil; ↓ effects *W/* barbiturates, disopyramide, nifedipine, phenobarbital, phenytoin, rifampin, sucralfate **NIPE:** Take w/ food, ↑ risk of photosensitivity—use sunscreen; use w/ drug that slows AV conduction (eg, digoxin, diltiazem, β-blocker)

Quinupristin–Dalfopristin (Synercid) [Antibiotic/Streptogramin]
Uses: *Vancomycin-resistant Infxns due to *E. faecium* & other gram(+)* **Action:** ↓ Ribosomal protein synth. **Spectrum:** Vanco-resistant *E. faecium,* methicillin-susceptible *S. aureus, S. pyogenes;* not against *E. faecalis* **Dose:** *Adults & Peds.* 7.5 mg/kg IV q8–12h (central line preferred); incompatible w/ NS or heparin; flush IV w/ dextrose; ↓ w/ hepatic failure **Caution:** [B, M] Multiple drug interactions (eg, cyclosporine) **Contra:** Component allergy **Disp:** Inj 500 mg (150 mg quinupristin/350 mg dalfopristin) 600 mg (180 quinupristin/420 mg dalfopristin) **SE:** Hyperbilirubinemia, arthralgia, myalgia **Interactions:** ↑ Effects *OF* CCBs, carbamazepine, cyclosporine, diazepam, disopyramide, docetaxel, lovastatin, methylprednisolone, midazolam, paclitaxel, protease inhibitors, quinidine, tacrolimus, vinblastine **Labs:** ↑ ALT, AST, bilirubin; **NIPE:** Inf site Rxns & pain

Rabeprazole (AcipHex) [Antiulcer Agent/Proton Pump Inhibitor]
Uses: *PUD, GERD, ZE* **H. pylori Action:** Proton-pump inhibitor **Dose:** 20 mg/d; may ↑ to 60 mg/d; *H. pylori* 20 mg PO bid × 7 d (w/ amoxicillin and clarithromycin); do not crush/chew tabs **Caution:** [B, ?/–] **Disp:** Tabs 20 mg ER **SE:** HA, fatigue, GI upset **Interactions:** ↑ Effects *OF* cyclosporine, digoxin; ↓ effects *OF* ketoconazole **Labs:** ↑ LFTs, TSH **NIPE:** Take w/o regard to food; ↑ risk of photosensitivity—use sunscreen

Raloxifene (Evista) [Selective Estrogen Receptor Modulator]
Uses: *Prevent osteoporosis* **Action:** Partial antagonist of estrogen, behaves like estrogen **Dose:** 60 mg/d **Caution:** [X, –] **Contra:** Thromboembolism, PRG **Disp:** Tabs 60 mg **SE:** Chest pain, insomnia, rash, hot flashes, GI upset, hepatic dysfunction **Interactions:** ↓ Effects *W/* ampicillin, cholestyramine **NIPE:** ⊘ PRG, breast-feeding; take w/o regard to food; ↑ risk of venous thromboembolic effects

Ramelteon (Rozerem) [Hypnotic]
Uses: *Short-term RX of insomnia esp w/ difficulty of sleep onset* **Action:** Hypnotic agent **Dose:** 8 mg tabs PO w/in 30 min of bedtime **Caution:** [C, –] **Contra:** Severe hepatic impair; concurrent use of fluvoxamine **Disp:** 8 mg tabs **SE:** HA, N, somnolence, fatigue, dizziness, URI,

depression, D, myalgia, arthralgia **Interactions:** ↑ Effects W/ CYP1A2 inhibitors (fluvoxamine), CYP3A4 inhibitors (ketoconazole), and CYP2C9 inhibitors (fluconazole); ↓ effects W/ CYP450 inducers (rifampin) **Labs:** ↓ Testosterone levels & ↑ prolactin levels noted **NIPE:** High-fat foods delay effect; ⊘ use in pts W/ severe sleep apnea & severe COPD

Ramipril (Altace) [Antihypertensive/ACEI] **WARNING:** ACE inhibitors used during PRG can cause fetal injury & death **Uses:** *HTN, CHF, DN, post-MI* **Action:** ACE inhibitor **Dose:** 2.5–20 mg/d PO ÷ daily–bid; ↓ in renal failure **Caution:** [D, +] **Contra:** ACE-inhibitor-induced angioedema **Disp:** Caps 1.25, 2.5, 5, 10 mg **SE:** Cough, HA, dizziness, ↓ BP, renal impair, angioedema **Interactions:** ↑ Effects W/ α-adrenergic blockers, loop diuretics; ↑ effects OF insulin, Li; ↑ risk of hyperkalemia W/ K⁺, K-sparing diuretics, K salt substitutes, trimethoprim, ↓ effects W/ ASA, NSAIDs, food **Labs:** ↑ BUN, Cr, K⁺, ↓ HMG, Hct, cholesterol **NIPE:** ↑ Risk of photosensitivity—use sunscreen; ↑ risk of cough esp w/ capsaicin; take w/o food; OK in combo w/ diuretics

Ranibizumab (Lucentis) [Vascular Endothelial GF Inhibitor] **Uses:** *Neovascular "wet" macular degeneration* **Action:** Vascular endothelial growth factor inhibitor **Dose:** 0.5 mg intravitreal inj qmo **Caution:** [C; ?] h/o thromboembolism **Contra:** periocular Infxn **Disp:** Inj **SE:** Endophthalmitis, retinal detachment/hemorrhage, cataract, intraocular inflammation, conjunctival hemorrhage, eye pain, floaters

Ranitidine Hydrochloride (Zantac) [Antiulcer Agent/H₂-Receptor Antagonist] **Uses:** *Duodenal ulcer, active benign ulcers, hypersecretory conditions, & GERD* **Action:** H₂-receptor antagonist **Dose:** *Adults.* *Ulcer:* 150 mg PO bid, 300 mg PO hs, or 50 mg IV q6–8h; or 400 mg IV/d cont inf, then maint of 150 mg PO hs. *Hypersecretion:* 150 mg PO bid, up to 600 mg/d. *GERD:* 300 mg PO bid; maint 300 mg PO hs. *Dyspepsia:* 75 mg PO daily–bid *Peds.* 0.75–1.5 mg/kg/dose IV q6–8h or 1.25–2.5 mg/kg/dose PO q12h; ↓ in renal insuff/failure **Caution:** [B, +] **Contra:** Component allergy **Disp:** Tabs 75 [OTC], 150, 300 mg; Caps 150, 300 mg; effervescent tabs 150 mg; syrup 15 mg/mL; inj 25 mg/mL **SE:** Dizziness, sedation, rash, GI upset **Interactions:** ↑ Effects OF glipizide, glyburide, procainamide, warfarin; ↓ effects W/ antacids, tobacco; ↓ effects OF diazepam **Labs:** ↑ SCr, ALT **NIPE:** ASA, NSAIDs, EtOH, caffeine ↑ stomach acid production; PO & parenteral doses differ

Ranolazine (Ranexa) [Antianginal] **Uses:** *Chronic angina* **Action:** ↓ ischemia-related Na⁺ entry into myocardium **Dose:** *Adults.* 500 mg PO bid to 1000 mg PO bid **Contra:** w/ hepatic impair, CYP3A inhibitors (Table 11); w/ agents that ↑ QT interval **Caution:** [C, ?/–] HTN may develop w/ renal impairment **Disp:** SR tabs 500 mg **SE:** Dizziness, HA, constipation, arrhythmias **Labs:** ↓ K⁺ **NIPE:** Not 1st line; use w/ amlodipine, nitrates, β-blockers

Rasagiline Mesylate (Azilect) [Anti-Parkinson Agent/MAO B Inhibitor] **Uses:** *Early Parkinson disease monotherapy; levodopa adjunct w/ advanced Dz* **Action:** MAO B inhibitor **Dose:** *Adults. Early Dz:* 1 mg PO daily, start 0.5 mg PO daily w/ levodopa; ↓ w/ CYP1A2 inhibitors or hepatic impair **Contra:** MAOIs, sympathomimetic amines, meperidine, methadone, tramadol, propoxyphene, dextromethorphan, mirtazapine, cyclobenzaprine, St. John's wort, sympathomimetic vasoconstrictors, general anesthetics, SSRIs **Caution:** [C, ?] Avoid tyramine-containing foods; moderate/severe hepatic impairment **Disp:** Tabs 0.5, 1 mg **SE:** Arthralgia, indigestion, dyskinesia, hallucinations, ↓ wt, postural ↓ BP, N, V, constipation, xerostomia, rash, sedation, CV conduction disturbances **Interactions:**↑ Risk of HTN crisis *W/* tyramine-containing foods; ↑ effects *W/* ciprofloxacin; ↑ CNS tox/death *W/* TCA, SSRIs, MAOIs **Labs:** Monitor LFTs **NIPE:** Rare melanoma reported; do periodic dermatologic exams; D/C 14 d prior to elective surgery; D/C fluoxetine 5 wk before starting rasagiline; initial ↓ levodopa dose recommended

Rasburicase (Elitek) [Antigout Agent/Antimetabolite]
Uses: *Reduce ↑ uric acid due to tumor lysis (peds)* **Action:** Catalyzes uric acid **Dose:** *Peds.* 0.15 or 0.20 mg/kg IV over 30 min, daily × 5 **Caution:** [C, ?/–] Falsely ↓ uric acid values **Contra:** Anaphylaxis, screen for G6PD deficiency to avoid hemolysis, methemoglobinemia **Disp:** 1.5 mg inj **SE:** Fever, neutropenia, GI upset, HA, rash **Labs:** ↓ Neutrophils **NIPE:** Place blood test tube for uric acid level on ice to stop enzymatic Rxn; removed by dialysis

Repaglinide (Prandin) [Hypoglycemic/Meglitinide]
Uses: *Type 2 DM* **Action:** ↑ pancreatic insulin release **Dose:** 0.5–4 mg ac, PO start 1–2 mg, ↑ to 16 mg/d max; take be **Caution:** [C, ?/–] **Contra:** DKA, type 1 DM **Disp:** Tabs 0.5, 1, 2 mg **SE:** HA, hyper-/hypoglycemia, GI upset **Interactions:** ↑ Effects *W/* ASA, BBs, chloramphenicol, erythromycin, ketoconazole, miconazole, MAOIs, NSAIDs, probenecid, sulfa drugs, warfarin, celery, coriander, dandelion root, fenugreek, garlic, ginseng, juniper berries; ↓ effects *W/* barbiturates, carbamazepine, CCBs, corticosteroids, diuretics, estrogens, INH, OCPs, phenytoin, phenothiazines, rifampin, sympathomimetics, thiazide diuretics, thyroid drugs **NIPE:** Take 15 min before meal; skip drug if meal skipped

Retapamulin (Altabax) [Pleuromutilin Antibiotic]
Uses: *Topical Rx impetigo in patients >9 mo* **Action:** Pleuromutilin antibiotic; *Spectrum: S. aureus (MRSA), S. pyogenes* **Dose:** Apply bid × 5 d **Caution:** [B; ?] **Disp:** 10 mg/1 g **SE:** Local irritation **NIPE:** Prolonged use may result in super Infxn

Reteplase (Retavase) [Tissue Plasminogen Activator]
Uses: *Post-AMI* **Action:** Thrombolytic **Dose:** 10 units IV over 2 min, 2nd dose in 30 min, 10 units IV over 2 min; 10 units IV bolus over 2 min; 30 min later, 10 units IV bolus over 2 min NS flush before and after each dose (*ECC 2005*) **Caution:** [C, ?/–] **Contra:** Internal bleeding, spinal surgery/trauma, h/o CNS AVM, uncontrolled ↓ BP, sensitivity to thrombolytics **Disp:** Inj 10.8 units/2 mL **SE:** Bleeding, allergic Rxns **Interactions:** ↑ Risk of bleeding *W/* ASA, abciximab, dipyridamole, heparin, NSAIDs, oral anticoagulants, vitamin K antagonists **Labs:**

↓ Fibrinogen, plasminogen **NIPE:** Monitor ECG during Rx for ↑ risk of reperfusion arrhythmias

Ribavirin (Virazole, Copegus) [Antiviral/Nucleoside Analogue]

WARNING: Monotherapy for chronic Hep C ineffective; hemolytic anemia possible, teratogenic and embryocidal **Uses:** *RSV Infxn in infants [Virazole]; Hep C (in combo w/ interferon alfa-2b [Copegus])* **Action:** **Dose:** *RSV:* 6 g in 300 mL sterile H_2O, inhale over 12–18 h. *Hep C:* 600 mg PO bid in combo w/ interferon alfa-2b (see Rebetron) **Caution:** [X, ?] May accumulate on soft contact lenses **Contra:** PRG, autoimmune hepatitis, CrCl <50 mL/min **Disp:** Powder for aerosol 6 g; tabs 200, 400, 600 mg, caps 200 mg, soln 40 mg/mL, **SE:** Fatigue, HA, GI upset, anemia, myalgia, alopecia, bronchospasm **Interactions:** ↓ Effects *W/* Al, Mg, simethicone; ↓ effect *OF* zidovudine **Labs:** ↑ LFTs; ↓ HMG, Hct, plts, WBC; monitor labs **NIPE:** ⊘ PRG, breast-feeding; PRG test monthly; ↑ risk of photosensitivity—use sunscreen; take w/o regard to food; Virazole aerosolized by a SPAG

Rifabutin (Mycobutin) [Antibiotic/Antitubercular]

Uses: *Prevent M. avium complex Infxn in AIDS pts w/ CD4 count <100* **Action:** ↓ DNA-dependent RNA polymerase activity **Dose:** *Adults.* 150–300 mg/d PO. *Peds. 1 y:* 15–25 mg/kg/d PO. *2–10 y:* 4.4–18.8 mg/kg/d PO. *14–16 y:* 2.8–5.4 mg/kg/d PO **Caution:** [B; ?/–] WBC <1000/mm³ or plts <50,000/mm³; ritonavir **Contra:** Allergy **Disp:** Caps 150 mg **SE:** Discolored urine, rash, neutropenia, leukopenia, myalgia **Interactions:** ↑ Effects *W/* ritonavir; ↓ effects *OF* anticoagulants, anticonvulsants, barbiturates, benzodiazepines, BBs, corticosteroids, methadone, morphine, OCPs, quinidine, theophylline, TCAs **Labs:** ↑ LFTs **NIPE:** Urine and body fluids may turn reddish brown in color, discoloration of soft contact lenses, use barrier contraception, take w/o food; SE/interactions similar to Rifampin

Rifampin (Rifadin) [Antibiotic/Antitubercular]

Uses: *TB & Rx & prophylaxis of N. meningitidis, H. influenzae, or S. aureus carriers*; adjunct w/ severe *S. aureus* **Action:** ↓ DNA-dependent RNA polymerase **Dose:** *Adults.* N. meningitidis & H. influenzae carrier: 600 mg/d PO for 4 d; *TB:* 600 mg PO or IV daily or 2 ×/wk w/ combo regimen. *Peds.* 10–20 mg/kg/dose PO or IV daily–bid; ↓ in hepatic failure **Caution:** [C, +] Amprenavir, multiple drug interactions **Contra:** Allergy, active N. meningitidis Infxn, w/ saquinavir/ritonavir **Disp:** Caps 150, 300 mg; inj 600 mg **SE:** Red-orange colored bodily fluids, ↑ LFTs, flushing, HA **Interactions:** ↓ Effects *W/* aminosalicylic acid; ↓ effects *OF* acetaminophen, aminophylline, amiodarone, anticoagulants, barbiturates, BBs, CCBs, chloramphenicol, clofibrate, delavirdine, digoxin, disopyramide, doxycycline, enalapril, estrogens, haloperidol, hypoglycemics, hydantoins, methadone, morphine, nifedipine, ondansetron, OCPs, phenytoin, protease inhibitors, quinidine, repaglinide, sertraline, sulfapyridine, sulfones, tacrolimus, theophylline, thyroid drugs, tocainide, TCAs, theophylline, verapamil, zidovudine, zolpidem **Labs:** ↑ LFTs, uric acid **NIPE:** Use barrier contraception; take w/o food, reddish brown color in urine and body fluids; stains soft contact lenses; Never use as single agent w/ active TB

Rifapentine (Priftin) [Antibiotic/Antitubercular]

Uses: *Pulm TB* Action: ↓ DNA-dependent RNA polymerase. Spectrum: M. tuberculosis Dose: Intensive phase: 600 mg PO 2 ×/wk for 2 mo; separate doses by >3 d. Continuation phase: 600 mg/wk for 4 mo; part of 3–4 drug regimen Caution: [C, red-orange breast milk] ↓ protease inhibitor efficacy, antiepileptics, β-blockers, CCBs Contra: Rifamycins allergy Disp: 150-mg tabs SE: Neutropenia, hyperuricemia, HTN, HA, dizziness, rash, GI upset, blood dyscrasias, ↑ LFTs, hematuria, discolored secretions Interactions: ↓ Effects OF anticoagulants, BBs, CCBs, corticosteroids, cyclosporine, digoxin, fluoroquinolones, methadone, metoprolol, OCPs, phenytoin, propranolol, protease inhibitors, rifampin, sulfonylureas, TCAs, theophylline, verapamil, warfarin Labs: ↑ LFTs-monitor; plts, uric acid; ↓ HMG, neutrophil, WBCs NIPE: May take with food; body fluids, teeth, tongue, feces may become orange-red; may permanently discolor soft contact lenses; use barrier contraception

Rifaximin (Xifaxan) [Antibiotic/Rifamycin Antibacterial]

Uses: *Travelers' diarrhea (noninvasive strains of E. coli) in patients >12 y* Action: Not absorbed, derivative of rifamycin. Spectrum: E. coli Dose: 1 tab PO daily × 3 d Caution: [C, ?/–] h/o allergy; pseudomembranous colitis Contra: Allergy to rifamycins Disp: Tabs 200 mg SE: Flatulence, HA, abd pain, GI distress, fever Interactions: None significant Labs: None noted NIPE: May be taken w/o regard to food; ⊘ crush/chew tabs-swallow whole; D/C if Sxs worsen or persist >24–48 h, or w/ fever or blood in stool

Rimantadine (Flumadine) [Antiviral]

Uses: *Prophylaxis & Rx of influenza A viral Infxns* Action: Antiviral Prophylaxis: Adults & Peds >9 y. 100 mg PO bid. Peds 1–9 y. 5 mg/kg/d PO, 150 mg/d max; daily w/ severe renal/hepatic impair & elderly; initiate w/in 48 h of Sx onset Caution: [C, –] w/ cimetidine; avoid w/ PRG, breast-feeding Contra: Component & amantadine allergy Disp: Tabs 100 mg; syrup 50 mg/5 mL SE: Orthostatic ↓ BP, edema, dizziness, GI upset, ↓ Sz threshold Interactions: ↑ Effects W/ cimetidine; ↓ effects W/ acetaminophen, ASA NIPE: See CDC (MMWR) for current influenza A guidelines

Rimexolone (Vexol Ophthalmic) [Steroid]

Uses: *Postop inflammation & uveitis* Action: Steroid Dose: Adults & Peds >2 y. Uveitis: 1–2 gtt/h AM & q2h PM, taper to 1 gtt q4h; Postop: 1–2 gtt qid =2 wk Caution: [C, ?/–] Ocular Infxns Disp: Susp 1% SE: Blurred vision, local irritation NIPE: Shake well, ⊘ touch eye w/ dropper; taper dose

Risedronate (Actonel w/calcium) [Biphosphonate/Hormone]

Uses: *Paget Dz; Rx/ prevent glucocorticoid-induced/postmenopausal osteoporosis* Action: Bisphosphonate; ↓ osteoclast-mediated bone resorption Dose: Paget Dz: 30 mg/d PO for 2 mo. Osteoporosis Rx/prevention: 5 mg daily or 35 mg qwk; 30 min before 1st food/drink of the day; stay upright for at least 30 min after **Caution:** [C, ?/–] Ca supls & antacids ↓ absorption **Contra:** Component allergy, ↓ Ca²⁺, esophageal abnormalities, unable to stand/sit for 30 min, CrCl <30 mL/min **Disp:** Tabs 5, 30, 35, 75 mg; Risedronate 35 mg (4 tabs)/Ca carbonate 1250 mg (24 tabs) **SE:** HA, D, abd pain, arthralgia; flulike Sxs, rash, esophagitis, bone pain **Interactions:** ↓ Effects W/ antacids, ASA, Ca²⁺, food **Labs:** Interference W/ bone-imaging agents **Labs:** Monitor LFT, Ca²⁺, PO³⁻, K⁺ **NIPE:** EtOH intake and cigarette smoking promote osteoporosis

Risperidone, oral (Risperdal, Risperdal M-Tab) [Antipsychotic] WARNING: ↑ mortality in elderly with dementia-related psychosis **Uses:** *Psychotic disorders (schizophrenia)*, dementia of the elderly, bipolar disorder, mania, Tourette disorder, autism **Action:** Benzisoxazole antipsychotic **Dose:** *Adults.* 0.5–6 mg PO bid; M-Tab 1–6 mg/d start 1–2 mg/d, titrate q3–7d *Peds/Adolescents.* 0.25 mg PO bid, ↑ q5–7d; ↓ start dose w/ elderly, renal/hepatic impair **Caution:** [C, –], ↑ BP w/ antihypertensives, clozapine **Contra:** Component allergy **Disp:** Tabs 0.25, 0.5, 1, 2, 3, 4 mg; soln 1 mg/mL, M-Tab (orally disintegrating) tabs 0.5, 1, 2, 3, 4 mg **SE:** Orthostatic ↑ BP, EPS w/ high dose, tachycardia, arrhythmias, sedation, dystonias, neuroleptic malignant synd, sexual dysfunction, constipation, xerostomia, blood dyscrasias, cholestatic jaundice, wt **Interactions:** ↑ Effects W/ clozapine, CNS depressants, EtOH; ↑ effects OF antihypertensives; ↑ effects w/ carbamazepine; ↓ effects OF levodopa **Labs:** ↑ LFTs, serum prolactin **NIPE:** ↑ Risk photosensitivity—use sunscreen, extrapyramidal effects; may alter body temp regulation; several wks to see effect; several wks for effect

Risperidone, parenteral (Risperdal Consta) [Antipsychotic] WARNING: Not approved for dementia-related psychosis; ↑ mortality risk in elderly dementia pts on atypical antipsychotics; most deaths due to CV or infectious events **Uses:** *Schizophrenia* **Dose:** Benzisoxazole antipsychotic **Dose:** 25 mg q2wk IM may ↑ to max 50 mg q2wk; w/ renal/hepatic impair start PO Risperdal 0.5 mg PO bid × 1 wk titrate weekly **Caution:** [C, –], ↑ BP w/ antihypertensives, clozapine **Contra:** Component allergy **Disp:** Inj 25, 37.5, 50 mg/vial **SE:** See risperidone **Interactions:** ↑ Effects W/ clozapine, CNS depressants, EtOH; ↑ effects OF antihypertensives; ↓ effects w/ carbamazepine; ↑ effects OF levodopa **Labs:** ↑ LFTs, serum prolactin **NIPE:** ↑ Risk photosensitivity—use sunscreen, extrapyramidal effects; may alter body temp regulation; several wks to see effect; long-acting injection

Ritonavir (Norvir) [Antiretroviral/Protease Inhibitor] WARNING: Life-threatening adverse events when used with certain nonsedating antihistamines, sedative hypnotics, antiarrhythmics, or ergot alkaloids due to inhibited drug metabolism **Uses:** *HIV* **Actions:** Protease inhibitor; ↓ maturation of immature noninfectious virions to mature infectious virus **Dose:** *Adults.* Initial 300 mg PO bid, titrate over 1 wk to 600 mg PO bid (titration will ↓ GI SE). *Peds >1 mo.* 250 mg/m² titrate to 400 mg bid (adjust w/ amprenavir, indinavir, nelfinavir, & saquinavir); w/ food **Caution:** [B, +] w/ ergotamine, amiodarone, bepridil, flecainide, propafenone, quinidine, pimozide, midazolam, triazolam **Contra:** Component

Allergy Disp: Caps 100 mg; soln 80 mg/mL **SE:** ↑ triglycerides, ↑ LFTs, N/V/D/C, abd pain, taste perversion, anemia, weakness, HA, fever, malaise, rash, paresthesias **Interactions:** ↑ Effects W/ erythromycin, interleukins, grapefruit juice, food; ↑ effects OF amiodarone, astemizole, atorvastatin, barbiturates, bepridil, bupropion, cerivastatin, cisapride, clorazepate, clozapine, clarithromycin, desipramine, diazepam, encainide, ergot alkaloids, estazolam, flecainide, flurazepam, indinavir, ketoconazole, lovastatin, meperidine, midazolam, nelfinavir, phenytoin, pimozide, piroxicam, propafenone, propoxyphene, quinidine, rifabutin, saquinavir, sildenafil, simvastatin, SSRIs, TCAs, terfenadine, triazolam, troleandomycin, zolpidem; ↓ effects W/ barbiturates, carbamazepine, phenytoin, rifabutin, rifampin, St. John's wort, tobacco; ↓ effects OF didanosine, hypnotics, methadone, OCPs, sedatives, theophylline, warfarin **Labs:** ↑ Serum glucose, LFTs, triglycerides, uric acid **NIPE:** Food ↑ absorption; use barrier contraception; disulfiramlike Rxn w/ disulfiram, metronidazole; refrigerate

Rivastigmine (Exelon) [Cholinesterase Inhibitor/Anti-Alzheimer Agent]
Uses: *Mild–moderate dementia in Alzheimer Dz* **Action:** Enhances cholinergic activity **Dose:** 1.5 mg bid; ↑ to 6 mg bid, w/ ↑ at 2-wk intervals (w/ food) **Caution:** [B, ?] w/ β-Blockers, CCBs, smoking, neuromuscular blockade, digoxin **Contra:** Rivastigmine or carbamate allergy **Disp:** Caps 1.5, 3, 4.5, 6 mg; soln 2 mg/mL **SE:** Dose-related GI effects, N/V/D, dizziness, insomnia, fatigue, tremor, diaphoresis, HA, wt loss (in 18–26%) **Interactions:** ↑ Risk OF GI bleed W/ NSAIDs; ↓ effects W/ nicotine; ↓ effects OF anticholinergics **NIPE:** Take w/ food; swallow caps whole, do not break/chew/crush; avoid EtOH

Rivastigmine transdermal (Exelon) [Cholinesterase Inhibitor/Anti-Alzheimer Agent]
Uses: *Mild/moderate Alzheimer and Parkinson disease dementia* **Action:** Acetylcholinesterase inhibitor **Dose:** Initial 4.6-mg patch/d applied to back, chest, upper arm, ↑ 9.5 mg after 4 wk if tolerated **Caution:** [?; ?] Sick sinus synd, conduction defects, asthma, COPD, urinary obst, Sz **Contra:** Hypersensitivity to rivastigmine, other carbamates **Disp:** Transdermal patch 5 cm^2 (4.6 mg/24 h), 10 cm^2 (9.5 mg/24 h) **SE:** N/V/D

Rizatriptan (Maxalt, Maxalt MLT) [Antimigraine Agent/5-HT$_1$ Agonist]
Uses: *Rx acute migraine* **Action:** Vascular serotonin receptor agonist **Dose:** 5–10 mg PO, repeat in 2 h, PRN, 30 mg/d max **Caution:** [C, M] **Contra:** Angina, ischemic heart Dz, ischemic bowel Dz, hemiplegic/basilar migraine, uncontrolled HTN, ergot or serotonin 5-HT$_1$ agonist use w/in 24 h, MAOI use w/in 14 d **Disp:** Tab 5, 10 mg; MLT: OD tabs 5, 10 mg. **SE:** Chest pain, palpitations, N, V, asthenia, dizziness, somnolence, fatigue **Interactions:** ↑ Vasospastic effects W/ ergots, 5-HT agonists; ↓ effects W/ MAOIs, propranolol **NIPE:** Treatment for migraines—not for prophylaxis

Rocuronium (Zemuron) [Skeletal Muscle Relaxant]
Uses: *Skeletal muscle relaxation during rapid-sequence intubation, surgery, or mechanical ventilation* **Action:** Nondepolarizing neuromuscular blocker **Dose:** *Rapid sequence*

intubation: 0.6–1.2 mg/kg IV. *Continuous inf:* 5–12.5 µg/kg/min IV; adjust/titrate based on monitoring; ↓ in hepatic impair **Caution:** [C, ?] Aminoglycosides, vancomycin, tetracycline, polymyxin enhance blockade **Contra:** Component or pancuronium allergy **Disp:** Inj preservative free 10 mg/mL **SE:** BP changes, tachycardia **Interactions:** ↑ Effects W/ MAOIs, propranolol; ↑ vasospastic Rxn W/ ergot-containing drugs; ↑ risk of hyperreflexia, incoordination, weakness W/ SSRIs **NIPE:** Food delays drug action; ○ take >30 mg/24 h

Ropinirole (Requip) [Dopamine Agonist/Anti-Parkinson Agent] **Uses:** *Rx of Parkinson Dz, restless leg synd* **Action:** Dopamine agonist **Dose:** Initial 0.25 mg PO tid, weekly ↑ 0.25 mg/dose, to 3 mg max, max 4 mg for RLS **Caution:** [C, ?/–] Severe CV, renal, or hepatic impair **Contra:** Component allergy **Disp:** Tabs 0.25, 0.5, 1, 2, 3, 4, 5 mg **SE:** Syncope, postural ↓ BP, N/V, HA, somnolence, dose-related hallucinations, dyskinesias, dizziness **Interactions:** ↑ Risk of bleeding W/ ASA, NSAIDs, feverfew, garlic, ginger, horse chestnut, red clover, EtOH, tobacco; ↑ effects OF amitriptyline, Li, MTX, theophylline, warfarin; ↑ risk of photosensitivity W/ dong quai—use sunscreen, St. John's wort; ↓ effects W/ antacids, rifampin; ↓ effects OF ACEIs, diuretics **Labs:** ↑ ALT, AST **NIPE:** Take W/ food; D/C w/ 7-d taper

Rosiglitazone (Avandia) [Hypoglycemic/Thiazolidinedione] **Uses:** *Type 2 DM* **Action:** Thiazolidinedione; ↑ insulin sensitivity **Dose:** 4–8 mg/d PO or in 2 ÷ doses (w/o regard to meals) **Caution:** [C, –] w/ ESRD, CHF, edema, **Contra:** DKA, severe CHF, ALT >2.5 ULN **Disp:** Tabs 2, 4, 8 mg **SE:** May ↑ CV & CA risk; wt gain, hyperlipidemia, HA, edema, fluid retention, worsen CHF, hyper-/hypoglycemia, hepatic damage w/ ↑ LFTs **Interactions:** ↑ Risk of hypoglycemia W/ insulin, ketoconazole, oral hypoglycemics, fenugreek, garlic, ginseng, glucomannan; ↓ effects OF OCPs **Labs:** ↑ ALT, total cholesterol, LDL, HDL, ↓ HMG, Hct **NIPE:** Use barrier contraception; not recommended in class III, IV heart Dz

Rosiglitazone/Metformin (Avandamet) [Hypoglycemic/Thiazolidinedione & Biguanide] **WARNING:** Associated w/ lactic acidosis **Uses:** Type 2 DM **Action:** ↓ Hepatic glucose production & intestinal absorption of glucose; ↑ insulin sensitivity **Dose:** *Adults.* Initial: 2 mg/500 mg PO OD or bid with AM and PM meal; increase by 2 mg/500 mg/d after 4 wk; max 8 mg/2000 mg/d. *Peds.* Not recommended. **Caution:** [C, –] Hold dose before & 48 h after ionic contrast; not for DKA; w/ ESRD (renal elimination) **Contra:** SCr >1.4 in females or >1.5 in males; hypoxemic conditions (eg, acute CHF/sepsis); active liver Dz; metabolic acidosis **Disp:** Tabs Rosiglitazone/Metformin: (mg/mg) 2/500, 4/500, 2/1000, 4/1000 **SE:** Wt gain, hyperlipidemia, HA, edema, fluid retention, exacerbated CHF, hyper-/hypoglycemia, hepatic damage, anorexia, N/V, rash, lactic acidosis (rare, but serious) **Interactions:** ↑ Risk of hypoglycemia W/ insulin, ketoconazole, fenugreek, garlic, ginseng, glucomannan; ↑ effects W/ amiloride, cimetidine, digoxin, furosemide, MAOIs, morphine, procainamide, quinidine, quinine, ranitidine, triamterene, trimethoprim, vancomycin; ↓ effects *W/* corticosteroids, CCBs, diuretics, estrogens, INH, OCPs, phenothiazine, phenytoin, sympathomimetics, thyroid drugs, tobacco; ↓ effects *OF* OCPs **Labs:** ↑ LFTs, lipids, SCr ↓ HMG, Hct; monitor LFTs, SCr baseline & periodically **NIPE:** Use barrier contraception; take w/ food; ⊘ dehydration, EtOH, before surgery

Rosuvastatin (Crestor) [Antilipemic/HMG-CoA Reductase Inhibitor] Uses: *Rx primary hypercholesterolemia & mixed dyslipidemia* **Action:** HMG-CoA reductase inhibitor **Dose:** 5–40 mg PO daily; max 5 mg/d w/cyclosporine, 10 mg/d w/gemfibrozil or CrCl <30 mL/min (avoid Al-/Mg-based antacids for 2 h after) **Caution:** [X, ?/–] **Contra:** Active liver Dz, unexplained ↑ LFT **Disp:** Tabs 5, 10, 20, 40 mg **SE:** Myalgia, constipation, asthenia, abd pain, N, myopathy, rarely rhabdomyolysis **Interactions:** ↑ Effects *OF* warfarin; ↑ risk of myopathy *W/* cyclosporine, fibrates, niacin, statins **Labs:** ↑ Warfarin; ↑ LFTs; monitor LFTs at baseline, 12 wk, then q6mo; ↑ urine protein, HMG **NIPE:** ⊘ PRG or breast-feeding; ↓ dose in Asian patients

Rotavirus vaccine, live, oral, pentavalent (RotaTeq) [Vaccine] Uses: *Prevent rotavirus gastroenteritis* **Action:** Active immunization **Dose:** *Peds.* Single dose PO at 2, 4, 6 mo **Caution:** [?, ?] **Disp:** Oral susp 2-mL single-use tubes **SE:** D, V **Interactions:** ↓ Effects *W/* immunosuppressants such as irradiation, chemotherapy or high dose steroids **NIPE:** Begin series by 12 wk and conclude by 32 wk of age; ⊘ take with oral polio vaccine

Salmeterol (Serevent Diskus) [Bronchodilator/Sympathomimetic] **WARNING:** Long-acting β₂-agonists, such as salmeterol, may ↑ the risk of asthma-related death. Should not be used alone, only as additional therapy for patients not controlled on other asthma medications **Uses:** *Asthma, exercise-induced asthma, COPD* **Action:** Sympathomimetic bronchodilator, β₂-agonist **Dose:** *Adults & Peds = 12 y.* 1 diskus-dose inhaled bid **Caution:** [C, ?/–] **Contra:** Acute asthma; w/in 14 d of MAOI **Disp:** 50 µg/dose, dry powder discus, metered dose inhaler, 21 µg/activation **SE:** HA, pharyngitis, tachycardia, arrhythmias, nervousness, GI upset, tremors **Interactions:** ↑ CV Effects *W/* MAOIs, TCAs; ↓ effects *W/* BBs **Labs:** ↑ Glucose; ↓ serum K⁺ **NIPE:** Shake canister before use, inhale q12h, not for acute exacerbations; also prescribe short-acting β-agonist

Saquinavir (Fortovase, Invirase) [Antiretroviral/Protease Inhibitor] **WARNING:** Invirase and Fortovase not bioequivalent/interchangeable; must use Invirase in combo w/ ritonavir, which provides saquinavir plasma levels = to those w/ Fortovase **Uses:** *HIV Infxn* **Action:** HIV protease inhibitor **Dose:** 1200 mg PO tid w/in 2 h pc (dose adjust w/ ritonavir, delavirdine, lopinavir, & nelfinavir) **Caution:** [B, +] w/ ketoconazole, statins, sildenafil **Contra:** w/ rifampin, severe hepatic impair, allergy, sun exposure w/o sunscreen/clothing, triazolam, midazolam, ergots, **Disp:** Caps 200, tabs 500 mg **SE:** Dyslipidemia, lipodystrophy, rash, hyperglycemia, GI upset, weakness **Interactions:** ↑ Risk of life-threatening arrhythmias *W/* amiodarone, astemizole, bepridil, cisapride, flecainide, propafenone, pimozide, quinidine, terfenadine; ↑ risk of myopathy *W/* HMG-CoA reductase inhibitors; ↑ risk of peripheral vasospasm & ischemia *W/* ergot derivatives; ↑ effects *W/* delavirdine, indinavir, ketoconazole, macrolide antibiotics, nelfinavir, ritonavir, grapefruit juice, garlic, St. John's wort, food; ↑ effects *OF* amitriptyline, benzodiazepines, CCB, lovastatin, macrolide antibiotics, phenytoin, sildenafil, simvastatin, terfenadine, TCAs, verapamil; ↓ effects *W/* barbiturates, carbamazepine, dexamethasone, efavirenz, phenytoin, rifabutin, rifampin, St. John's wort; ↓ effects *OF* OCPs **Labs:** ↑ LFTs, ↓ neutrophils **NIPE:** Take 2 h after meal; use barrier contraception; ↑ risk of photosensitivity; use sunscreen

Sargramostim [GM-CSF] (Leukine) [Hematopoietic Drug/Colony-Stimulating Factor] Uses: *Myeloid recovery following BMT or chemo* Action: Recombinant GF, activates mature granulocytes & macrophages Dose: *Adults & Peds.* 250 μg/m²/d IV for 21 d (BMT) Caution: [C, ?/–] Lithium, corticosteroids Contra: >10% blasts, allergy to yeast, concurrent chemo/RT Disp: Inj 250, 500 μg SE: Bone pain, fever, ↓ BP, tachycardia, flushing, GI upset, myalgia Interactions: ↑ Effects *W/* corticosteroids, Li Labs: ↑ BUN, LFTs NIPE: ⊘ Exposure to Infxn; rotate inj sites; use APAP PRN for pain

Scopolamine, Scopolamine Transdermal and Ophthalmic (Scopace, Transderm-Scop) [Antiemetic/Antivertigo/Anticholinergic] Uses: *Prevent N/V associated w/ motion sickness, anesthesia, opiates; mydriatic*, cycloplegic, Rx uveitis & iridocyclitis Action: Anticholinergic, inhibits iris and ciliary bodies, antiemetic Dose: 1 mg/ 72 h, 1 patch behind ear q3d; apply >4 h before exposure; cycloplegic 1–2 gtt 1 h pre, uveitis 1–2 gtt up to qid max; ↓ in elderly Caution: [C, +] w/ APAP, levodopa, ketoconazole, digitalis, KCl Contra: NAG, GI, or GU obst, thyrotoxicosis, paralytic ileus Disp: Patch 1.5 mg, (releases 1 mg over 72 h), ophth 0.25% SE: Xerostomia, drowsiness, blurred vision, tachycardia, constipation Interactions: ↑ Effects *W/* antihistamines, antidepressants, disopyramide, opioids, phenothiazine, quinidine, TCAs, EtOH NIPE: Do not blink excessively after eye gt, wait 5 min before dosing other eye; antiemetic activity w/ patch requires several hours; ⊘ D/C abruptly; wash hands after applying patch; may cause heat intolerance

Secobarbital (Seconal) [C-II] [Anticonvulsant, Sedative/Hypnotic/Barbiturate] Uses: *Insomnia, short-term use*, preanesthetic agent Action: Rapid-acting barbiturate Dose: *Adults.* 100–200 mg hs, 100–300 mg preop. *Peds.* 2–6 mg/kg/dose, 100 mg/max, ↓ in elderly Caution: [D, +] CYP2C9, 3A3/4, 3A5/7 inducer (Table 11); ↑ tox w/ other CNS depressants Contra: Porphyria, PRG w/ voriconazole, PRG Disp: Caps 50, 100 mg SE: Tolerance in 1–2 wk; resp depression, CNS depression, porphyria, photosens Interactions: ↑ Effects *W/* MAOIs, valproic acid, EtOH, kava kava, valerian; ↑ effects *OF* meperidine; ↓ effects *OF* anticoagulants, BBs, CCBs, CNS depressants, chloramphenicol, corticosteroids, cyclosporine, digitoxin, disopyramide, doxycycline, estrogen, griseofulvin, methadone, neuroleptics, OCPs, propafenone, quinidine, tacrolimus, theophylline

NIPE: Tolerance in 1–2 wk; ~~photosensitivity~~; ⊘ PRG, ~~breast-feeding~~; use barrier contraception

Selegiline, Oral (Eldepryl, Zelapar) [Anti-Parkinson Agent/ MAOB Inhibitor] Uses: * Parkinson Dz* Action: MAOI Dose: 5 mg PO bid; 1.25–2.5 OD tabs PO qAM (before breakfast w/o Liq) 2.5 mg/d max; ↓ in elderly Caution: [C, ?] w/ drugs that induce CYP3A4 (Table 11) (eg, phenytoin, carbamazepine, nafcillin, phenobarbital, and rifampin); avoid w/ antidepressants Contra: w/ meperidine, MAOI, dextromethorphan, general anesthesia w/in 10 d, pheochromocytoma Disp: Tabs/caps 5 mg; OD Tabs 1.25 mg SE: N, dizziness, orthostatic ↓ BP, arrhythmias, tachycardia, edema, confusion, xerostomia Interactions: ↑ Risk of serotonin syndrome W/ dextroamphetamine, dextromethorphan, fenfluramine, meperidine, methylphenidate, sibutramine, venlafaxine; ↑ risk of hypertension W/ dextroamphetamine, levodopa, methylphenidate, SSRIs, tyramine-containing foods, EtOH, ephedra, ginseng, ma-huang, St. John's wort Labs: + for amphetamine on urine drug screen NIPE: ↓ Carbidopa/levodopa if used in combo; see transdermal form

Selegiline, Transdermal (Emsam) [Anti-Parkinson Agent/ MAO B Inhibitor] WARNING: May ↑ risk of suicidal thinking and behavior in children and adolescents with major depression disorder Uses: *Depression* Action: MAOI Dose: Adults. Apply patch daily to upper torso, upper thigh, or outer upper arm Contra: Tyramine-containing foods w/ 9- or 12-mg doses; serotonin-sparing agents Caution: [C, –] ↑ Carbamazepine and oxcarbazepine levels Disp: XR Patches 6, 9, 12 mg SE: Local Rxns requiring topical steroids; HA, insomnia, orthostatic, ↓ BP, serotonin synd, suicide risk Interactions: ↑ Risk of serotonin synd W/ dextroamphetamine, dextromethorphan, fenfluramine, meperidine, methylphenidate, sibutramine, venlafaxine; ↑ risk of hypertension W/ dextroamphetamine, levodopa, methylphenidate, SSRIs, tyramine-containing foods, EtOH, ephedra, ginseng, ma-huang, St. John's wort; NIPE: ⊘ EtOH & tyramine-containing foods; rotate site; see oral form

Selenium Sulfide (Exsel Shampoo, Selsun Blue Shampoo, Selsun Shampoo) [Antiseborrheic] Uses: *Scalp seborrheic dermatitis*, scalp itching & flaking due to *dandruff*; tinea versicolor Action: Antiseborrheic Dose: Dandruff, seborrhea: Massage 5–10 mL into wet scalp, leave on 2–3 min rinse, repeat; use 2 × wk, then once q1–4wk PRN. Tinea versicolor: Apply 2.5% daily × on area & lather w/ small amounts of water; leave on 10 min, then rinse Caution: [C, ?] Contra: Open wounds Disp: Shampoo [OTC]; 2.5% lotion SE: Dry or oily scalp, lethargy, hair discoloration, local irritation NIPE: ⊘ Use on excoriated skin; may cause reversible hair loss; rinse thoroughly after use; DO NOT use more than 2 ×/wk

Sertaconazole (Ertaczo) [Antifungal] Uses: *Topical Rx interdigital tinea pedis* Action: Imidazole antifungal. Spectrum: T. rubrum, T. mentagrophytes, E. floccosum Dose: Adults & Peds > 12. Apply between toes & immediate surrounding healthy skin bid × 4 wk **Caution:** [C, ?] **Contra:** Component allergy **Disp:** 2% cream **SE:** Contact dermatitis, dry/burning skin, tenderness **NIPE:** Use in immunocompetent pts; not for oral, intravag, ophthalmic use; avoid occlusive dressings; avoid contact with mucous membranes

Sertraline (Zoloft) [Antidepressant/SSRI] WARNING: Closely monitor pts for worsening depression or emergence of suicidality, particularly in ped pts **Uses:** *Depression, panic disorders, obsessive–compulsive disorder (OCD), posttrauma tress disorders (PTSD)*, social anxiety disorder, eating disorders, premenstrual disorders **Action:** ↓ Neuronal uptake of serotonin **Dose:** *Adults. Depression:* 50–200 mg/d PO. *PTSD:* 25 mg PO daily × 1 wk, then 50 mg PO daily, 200 mg/d max *Peds. 6–12 y:* 25 mg PO daily; *13–17 y:* 50 mg PO daily **Caution:** [C, ?/–] w/ haloperidol (serotonin synd), sumatriptan, linezolid, hepatic impair **Contra:** MAOI use w/in 14 d; concomitant pimozide **Disp:** Tabs 25, 50, 100, 150, 200 mg; 20 mg/mL oral **SE:** Activate manic/hypomanic state, ↓ wt, insomnia, somnolence, fatigue, tremor, xerostomia, N/D, dyspepsia, ejaculatory dysfunction, ↓ libido, hepatotox **Interactions:** ↑ Effects *W/* cimetidine, tryptophan, St. John's wort; ↑ effects *OF* benzodiazepines, phenytoin, TCAs, warfarin, EtOH; ↑ risk of serotonin synd *W/* MAOIs **Labs:** ↑ LFTs, triglycerides, ↓ uric acid **NIPE:** ⊘ D/C abruptly; take w/o regard to food

Sevelamer (Renagel) [Phosphate Binder] Uses: *↓ Serum phosphorus in ESRD* **Action:** Binds intestinal PO^{3+} **Dose:** 2–4 caps PO tid w/ meals; adjust based on PO^{3+}, max 4 g/dose **Caution:** [C, ?] **Contra:** Hypophosphatemia, Bowel obst **Disp:** Caps 403 mg, tabs 400, 800 mg **SE:** BP changes, N/V/D, dyspepsia, thrombosis **Notes:** 800 mg sevelamer = 667 mg Ca acetate **Interactions:** ↓ Effects *OF* antiarrhythmics, anticonvulsants, ciprofloxacin when given *W/* sevelamer **Labs:** ↑ alk phosp **NIPE:** Must be admin w/ meals; take daily multivitamin, may ↓ fat-soluble vitamin absorption; take 1 h before or 3 h after other meds; do not open or chew capsules

Sibutramine (Meridia) [C-IV] [Anorexic/CNS Stimulant] Uses: *Obesity* **Action:** Blocks uptake of norepinephrine, serotonin, dopamine **Dose:** 10 mg/d PO, may ↓ to 5 mg after 4 wk **Caution:** [C, –] w/ SSRIs, lithium, dextromethorphan, opioids **Contra:** MAOI w/in 14 d, uncontrolled HTN, arrhythmias **Disp:** Caps 5, 10, 15 mg **SE:** HA, insomnia, xerostomia, constipation, rhinitis, tachycardia, HTN **Interactions:** ↑ Risk of serotonin synd *W/* dextromethorphan, ergots, fentanyl, Li, meperidine, MAOIs, naratriptan, pentazocine, rizatriptan, sumatriptan, SSRIs, tromethorphan, tryptophan, zolmitriptan, St. John's wort; ↓ effects *W/* cimetidine, erythromycin, ketoconazole; ↑ CNS depression *W/* EtOH **Labs:** ↑ LFTs **NIPE:** ⊘ EtOH; take early in the day to avoid insomnia; use w/ low-calorie diet, monitor BP & HR

Sildenafil (Viagra, Revatio) [Vasodilator/PDE 5 Inhibitor] Uses: *Viagra:* *Erectile dysfunction*, *Revatio:* *Pulm artery HTN* **Action:** ↓ Phosphodiesterase type 5 (responsible for cGMP breakdown); ↑ cGMP activity to relax smooth muscles & ↑ flow to corpus cavernosum and pulm vasculature; ? antiproliferative on pulm artery smooth muscle **Dose:** *ED:* 25–100 mg PO 1 h before sexual activity, max 1 × d; ↓ if >65 y; avoid fatty foods w/ dose; *Revatio Pulm HTN:* 20 mg PO tid **Caution:** [B, ?] CYP3A4 inhibitors (Table 11) **Contra:** w/ nitrates or if sex activity not advised; retinitis pigmentosa; hepatic/severe renal impair **Disp:** Tabs (Viagra) 25, 50, 100 mg, tabs (Revatio) 20 mg **SE:** HA; flushing; dizziness; blue haze visual change, hearing loss **Interactions:** ↑ Effects w/ amlodipine, cimetidine, erythromycin, indinavir, itraconazole, ketoconazole, nelfinavir, protease inhibitors, ritonavir, saquinavir, grapefruit juice; ↑ risk of hypotension w/ amlodipine, antihypertensives, nitrates; ↓ effects w/ rifampin **NIPE:** High-fat food delays absorption; ↑ risk of cardiac arrest if used w/ nitrates; cardiac events in absence of nitrates debatable

Silver Nitrate (Dey-Drop, others) [Antiseptic/Astringent]

Uses: *Removal of granulation tissue & warts; prophylaxis in burns* **Action:** Caustic antiseptic & astringent **Dose:** *Adults & Peds.* Apply to moist surface 2–3 × wk for several wk or until effect **Caution:** [C, ?] **Contra:** Do not use on broken skin **Disp:** Topical impregnated applicator sticks, soln 0.5, 10, 25, 50%; ophth 1% amp; topical ointment 10% **SE:** May stain tissue black, usually resolves; local irritation, methemoglobinemia **NIPE:** D/C if redness or irritation develop; no longer used in US for newborn prevention of GC conjunctivitis

Silver Sulfadiazine (Silvadene, Others) [Antibiotic]

Uses: *Prevention & Rx of Infxn in 2nd- & 3rd-degree burns* **Action:** Bactericidal **Dose:** *Adults & Peds.* Aseptically cover the area w/ 1/16-in. coating bid **Caution:** [B unless near term, ?/–] **Contra:** Infants <2 mo, PRG near term **Disp:** Cream 1% **SE:** Itching, rash, skin discoloration, blood dyscrasias, hepatitis, allergy **Interactions:** May inactivate topical proteolytic enzymes; **Labs:** ↓ WBCs; monitor LFTs, BUN, Cr **NIPE:** Photosensitivity—use sunscreen; systemic absorption w/ extensive application

Simethicone (Mylicon, Others) [OTC] [Antiflatulent]

Uses: Flatulence **Action:** Defoaming, alters gas bubble surface tension action **Dose:** *Adults & Peds.* >2 y: 40–125 mg PO pc & hs PRN; 500 mg/D max; <2 y: 20 mg PO qid PRN, 2–12 y: 40 mg PO qid PRN, >12 y–adult **Caution:** [C, ?] **Contra:** GI Intestinal perforation or obst **Disp:** [OTC] Tabs 80, 125 mg; caps 125 mg; Softgels 125, 166, 180 mg, susp 40 mg/0.6 mL, Chew tabs 80, 125 mg **SE:** N/D **Interactions:** ↑ Effects of topical proteolytic enzymes **NIPE:** Available in combo products OTC

Simvastatin (Zocor) [Antilipemic/HMG-CoA Reductase Inhibitor]

Uses: ↓ Cholesterol **Action:** HMG-CoA reductase inhibitor **Dose:** *Adult.* 5–80 mg PO; w/ meals; ↓ in renal insuff **Peds.** 10–17 y: 10 mg, 40 mg/daily max. **Caution:** [X, –] Avoid concurrent use of gemfibrozil **Contra:** PRG, liver Dz **Disp:** Tabs 5, 10, 20, 40, 80 mg **SE:** HA, GI upset, myalgia, myopathy (muscle pain, tenderness or weakness with creatine kinase 10 × ULN), hepatitis **Interactions:**

↑ Effects *OF* digoxin, warfarin; ↑ risk of myopathy/rhabdomyolysis *W/* amiodarone, cyclosporine, CYP3A4 inhibitors, fibrates, HIV protease inhibitors, macrolides, niacin, verapamil, grapefruit juice; ↓ effects *W/* cholestyramine, colestipol, fluvastatin, isradipine, propranolol **Labs:** ↑ LFTs, monitor **NIPE:** Take w/ food and in the evening; ⊘ PRG, breast-feeding; combo with ezetimibe/simvastatin

Sirolimus [Rapamycin] (Rapamune) [Immunosuppressant]
WARNING: Use only by health care provider experienced in immunosuppression; immunosuppression w/ lymphoma ↑ Infxns risk; do not use in lung transplant (fatal bronchial anastomotic dehiscence) **Uses:** *Prophylaxis of organ rejection in new Tx pts* **Action:** ↓ T-lymphocyte activation **Dose:** *Adults >40 kg.* 6 mg PO on day 1, then 2 mg/d PO. *Adults <40 kg & Peds = 13 y.* 3 mg/m² load, then 1 mg/m²/d in (H₂O/OJ; no grapefruit juice w/ sirolimus); take 4 h after cyclosporine; ↓ in hepatic impair **Caution:** [C, ?/–] Grapefruit juice, ketoconazole **Contra:** Component allergy **Disp:** Soln 1 mg/mL, tab 1, 2 mg **SE:** HTN, edema, CP, fever, HA, insomnia, acne, rash, ↑ cholesterol, GI upset, ↑↓ K⁺, Infxns, blood dyscrasias, arthralgia, tachycardia, renal impair, hepatic artery thrombosis, graft loss & death in de novo liver transplant (↑ hepatic artery thrombosis), delayed wound healing **Notes:** Levels not needed except in liver failure (trough 9–17 ng/mL) **Interactions:** ↑ Effects *W/* azole antifungals, cimetidine, cyclosporine, diltiazem, macrolides, nicardipine, protease inhibitors, verapamil, grapefruit juice; ↓ effects *W/* carbamazepine, phenobarbital, phenytoin, rifabutin, rifapentine, rifampin; ↓ effects *OF* live virus vaccines **Labs:** ↑ LFTs, BUN, Cr, cholesterol, triglycerides **NIPE:** Take w/o regard to food; ⊘ PRG while taking drug and for 12 wk after drug D/C

Sitagliptin (Januvia) [Hypoglycemic/DPP-4 Inhibitor] **Uses:**
Type 2 DM **Action:** Dipeptidyl peptidase-4 (DDP-4) inhibitor, ↑ insulin synth/release **Dose:** 100 mg PO daily; ↓ w/ renal impair **Caution:** [B; ?] **Contra:** DKA, type 1 DM **Disp:** Tabs 25, 50, 100 **SE:** URI, HA, D, abd pain, arthralgia **Interactions:** Monitor digoxin levels **Labs:** Monitor LFTs, BUN/Cr **NIPE:** ⊘ Children <18 y; monitor renal function; start drug at low dose and periodically increase

Sitagliptin/Metformin (Janumet) [Hypoglycemic/DPP-4 Inhibitor/Biguanide] **WARNING:** Associated w/ lactic acidosis **Uses:** *Adjunct to diet and exercise in type 2 DM* **Action:** See individual agents **Dose:** 1 tab PO bid, titrate; 100 mg sitagliptin & 2000 mg metformin/d max; w/ meals **Caution:** [B, ?/–] **Contra:** Type 1 DM, DKA **Disp:** Tabs 50/500, 50/1000 (mg/mg) **SE:** Nasopharyngitis, N/V/D, flatulence, abd discomfort, dyspepsia, asthenia, HA **Interactions:** ↑ Effects *W/* amiloride, cimetidine, digoxin, furosemide, MAOIs, morphine, procainamide, quinidine, quinine, ranitidine, triamterene, trimethoprim, vancomycin; ↓ effects *W/* corticosteroids, CCBs, diuretics, estrogens, INH, OCPs, phenothiazine, phenytoin, sympathomimetics, thyroid drugs, tobacco; monitor digoxin levels **Labs:** Monitor LFTs, BUN/Cr **NIPE:** ⊘ Children <18 y; monitor renal function; start drug at low dose & periodically increase; hold w/ contrast study

Smallpox Vaccine (Dryvax) [Vaccine] WARNING: Acute myocarditis and other infectious complications possible; contra in immunocompromised, eczema or exfoliative skin conditions, infants <1 y Uses: Immunization against smallpox(Variola virus) Action: Active immunization (live attenuated cowpox virus) Dose: *Adults (routine nonemergency) or all ages (emergency).* 2–3 punctures w/ bifurcated needle dipped in vaccine into deltoid, posterior triceps muscle; ✓ site for Rxn in 6–8 d; if major Rxn, site scabs, & heals, leaving scar; if mild/equivocal Rxn, repeat w/ 15 punctures Caution: [X, N/A] Contra: *Nonemergency use:* Febrile illness, immunosuppression, h/o eczema & their household contacts. *Emergency:* No absolute contraindications Disp: Vial for recons: 100 million pock-forming units/mL SE: Malaise, fever, regional lymphadenopathy, encephalopathy, rashes, spread of inoculation to other sites administered; Stevens–Johnson synd, eczema vaccinatum w/ severe disability NIPE: Virus transmission possible until scab separates from skin (14–21 d); avoid infant contact for 14 d; intradermal use only

Sodium Bicarbonate [NaHCO₃] [Antacid/Alkalinizing Agent]
Uses: *Alkalinization of urine*, RTA, *metabolic acidosis*, ↑ K⁺, TCA OD* Action: Alkalinizing agent Dose: *Adults. Cardiac arrest:* Initiate ventilation, 1 mEq/kg IV bolus; repeat 1/2 dose q10 min PRN *(ECC 2005); Metabolic acidosis:* 2–5 mEq/kg IV over 8 h & PRN based on acid–base status. *Alkalinize urine:* 4 g (48 mEq) PO, then 1–2 g q4h; adjust based on urine pH; 2 amp/1 L D₅W at 100–250 mL/h IV, monitor urine pH & serum bicarbonate. *Chronic renal failure:* 1–3 mEq/kg/d. *Distal RTA:* 1 mEq/kg/d PO. *Peds > 1 y.* Cardiac arrest: See Adult dosage. *Peds < 1 y.* ECC: Initiate ventilation, 1:1 dilution 1 mEq/mL dosed 1 mEq/kg IV; can repeat w/ 0.5 mEq/kg in 10 min × 1 or based on acid–base status. *Chronic renal failure:* See adult dosage. *Distal RTA:* 2–3 mEq/kg/d PO. *Proximal RTA:* 5–10 mEq/kg/d PO; titrate based on serum bicarbonate. *Urine alkalinization:* 84–840 mg/kg/d (1–10 mEq/kg/d) in ÷ doses; adjust based on urine pH Caution: [C, ?] Contra: Alkalosis, ↑ Na⁺, severe pulm edema, ↓ Ca²⁺ Disp: Powder, tabs; 300 mg = 3.6 mEq; 325 mg = 3.8 mEq; 520 mg = 6.3 mEq; 600 mg = 7.3 mEq; 650 mg = 7.6 mEq; inj 1 mEq/1 mL, 4.2% (0.5 mEq/10 mL), 7.5% (8.92 mEq/10 mL), 8.4% (10 mEq/10 mL) vial or amp SE: Belching, edema, flatulence, ↑ Na⁺, metabolic alkalosis Notes: 1 g neutralizes 12 mEq of acid; 50 mEq bicarb = 50 mEq Na; can make 3 amps in 1 L D₅W to = D₅NS w/ 150 mEq bicarb Interactions: ↑ Effects *OF* anorexiants, amphetamines, ephedrine, flecainide, mecamylamine, pseudoephedrine, quinidine, sympathomimetics; ↓ effects *OF* Li, MTX, salicylates, tetracyclines Labs: ↑ K⁺, lactate NIPE: ⊘ Take w/in 2 h of other drugs; ↑ risk of milk-alkali syndrome w/ long-term use or when taken w/ milk

Sodium Citrate/Citric Acid (Bicitra) [Alkalinizing Agent]
Uses: *Chronic metabolic acidosis, alkalinize urine; dissolve uric acid & cysteine stones* Action: Urinary alkalinizer Dose: *Adults.* 2–6 tsp (10–30 mL) diluted in 1–3 oz H₂O pc & hs. *Peds.* 1–3 tsp (5–15 mL) diluted in 1–3 oz H₂O pc & hs; best

after meals **Caution:** [C, +] **Contra:** Al-based antacids; severe renal impair or Na-restricted diets **Disp:** 15- or 30-mL unit dose: 16 (473 mL) or 4 (118 mL) fl oz **SE:** Tetany, metabolic alkalosis, ↑ K⁺, GI upset; avoid use of multiple 50-mL amps; can cause ↑ Na⁺/hyperosmolality **Notes:** 1 mL = 1 mEq Na & 1 mEq bicarb **Interactions:** ↑ Effects *OF* amphetamines, ephedrine, flecainide, pseudoephedrine, quinidine; ↓ effects *OF* barbiturates, chlorpropamide, Li, salicylates **NIPE:** Dilute W/ water;

Sodium Oxybate (Xyrem) [C-III] [Inhibitory Neurotransmitter] **WARNING:** Known drug of abuse even at recommended doses; confusion, depression, resp. depression may occur **Uses:** *Narcolepsy-associated cataplexy* **Action:** Inhibitory neurotransmitter **Dose:** *Adults & Peds = 16 y.* 2.25 g PO qhs, 2nd dose 2.5–4 h later; may ↑ 9 g/d max **Caution:** [B, ?/–] **Contra:** Succinic semialdehyde dehydrogenase deficiency; potentiates EtOH **Disp:** 500 mg/mL 180-mL PO soln **SE:** Confusion, depression, ↓ diminished level of consciousness, incontinence, significant V, resp depression, psychiatric Sxs **Interactions:** ↑ Risk of CNS depression W/ sedatives, hypnotics, EtOH **NIPE:** Dilute w/ 2 oz water, ⊘ eat w/in 2 h of taking this drug; may lead to dependence; synonym for γ-hydroxybutyrate (GHB), abused as a "date rape drug"; controlled distribution (prescriber & pt registration); must be administered when pt in bed

Sodium Phosphate (Visicol) [Laxative] **Uses:** *Bowel prep prior to colonoscopy* **Action:** Hyperosmotic laxative **Dose:** 3 tabs PO w/ at least 8 oz clear Liq every 15 min (20 tabs total night before procedure; 3–5 h before colonoscopy, repeat) **Caution:** [C, ?] Renal impair, electrolyte disturbances **Contra:** Megacolon, bowel obst, CHF, ascites, unstable angina, gastric retention, bowel perforation, colitis, hypomotility. **Disp:** Tablets 0.398, 1.102 g **SE:** ↑ QT, ↑ PO³⁻,↓ K⁺, Na, D, flatulence, cramps, abd bloating/pain **Interactions:** May bind with Al- & Mg-containing antacids and sucralfate; ↑ risk *OF* hypoglycemia W/ bisphosphonates; ↓ absorption *OF* other meds **Labs:** Monitor electrolytes **NIPE:** Drink clear Liq 12 h before start of this med; ⊘ take w/ drugs that prolong QT interval, ⊘ take other laxatives

Sodium Polystyrene Sulfonate (Kayexalate) [Potassium Removing Resin] **Uses:** *Rx of ↑ K⁺* **Action:** Na⁺/K⁺ ion-exchange resin **Dose:** *Adults.* 15–60 g PO or 30–60 g PR q6h based on serum K⁺. *Peds.* 1 g/kg/dose PO or PR q6h based on serum K⁺ (given w/ agar, eg, sorbitol, to promote movement through the bowel) **Caution:** [C, M] **Contra:** ↑ Na⁺ **Disp:** Powder; susp 15 g/ 60 mL sorbitol **SE:** ↑ Na⁺, ↓ K⁺, Na retention, GI upset, fecal impaction **Interactions:** ↑ Risk of systemic alkalosis W/ Ca- or Mg-containing antacids **NIPE:** Mix W/ chilled fluid other than OJ; enema acts more quickly than PO; PO most effective

Solifenacin (VESIcare) [Antispasmodic/Muscarinic Receptor Antagonist] **Uses:** *OAB* **Action:** Antimuscarinic, ↓ detrusor contractions **Dose:** 5 mg PO daily, 10 mg/d max; ↓ w/ renal/hepatic impair **Caution:** [C, ?/–] Bladder outflow or GI obst, ulcerative colitis, MyG, renal/hepatic impair, QT prolongation risk **Contra:** NAG, urinary/gastric retention **Disp:** Tabs 5, 10 mg **SE:** Constipation, xerostomia, dyspepsia, blurred vision **Interactions:** ↑ Effects *OF* azole antifungals & other CYP3A4 inhibitors; ↑ risk *OF* prolonged QT interval *W/* amiodarone, amitriptyline, bepridil, disopyramide, erythromycin, gatifloxacin, haloperidol, imipramine, moxifloxacin, quinidine, pimozide, procainamide, sparfloxacin, thioridazine; other drugs that prolong QT **Labs:** Monitor BUN, CR, LFTs **NIPE:** Take w/ or w/o food, swallow whole W/ H₂O; do not ↑ dose w/ severe renal/moderate hepatic impair

Sorafenib (Nexavar) [Antineoplastic/Kinase Inhibitor]
Uses: *Advanced RCC* met liver CA **Action:** Kinase inhibitor **Dose:** *Adults.* 400 mg PO bid on empty stomach **Caution:** [D, –] w/ irinotecan, doxorubicin, warfarin; avoid conception (male/female) **Disp:** Tabs 200 mg **SE:** Hand–foot synd; treatment-emergent hypertension; bleeding, ↑ INR, cardiac infarction/ischemia; ↑ pancreatic enzymes, hypophosphatemia, lymphopenia, anemia, fatigue, alopecia, pruritus, D, GI upset, HA, neuropathy **NIPE:** Monitor BP 1st 6 wk; may require ↓ dose (daily or every other day); impaired metabolism w/ Asian descent; unknown effect on wound healing, D/C before major surgery

Sorbitol (generic) [Laxative]
Uses: *Constipation* **Action:** Laxative **Dose:** 30–60 mL PO of a 20–70% soln PRN **Caution:** [B, +] **Contra:** Anuria **Disp:** Liq 70% **SE:** Edema, electrolyte losses, lactic acidosis, GI upset, xerostomia **NIPE:** ⊘ Use unless soln clear; may be vehicle for many Liq formulations (eg, zinc, Kayexalate)

Sotalol (Betapace) [Antiarrhythmic, Antihypertensive/BB]
WARNING: Monitor pts for 1st 3 d of Rx to ↓ risks of arrhythmia **Uses:** *Ventricular arrhythmias, AF* **Action:** β-adrenergic-blocking agent **Dose:** *Adults.* 80 mg PO bid; may be ↑ to 240–320 mg/d *Peds. Neonates:* 9 mg/m² tid. *1–19 mo:* 20.4 mg/m² tid. *20–23 mo:* 29.1 mg/m² tid; = >2 y: 30 mg/m² tid; to max dose of 90 mg/m² tid ↓ w/ renal impair **Caution:** [B (1st tri) (D if 2nd or 3rd tri), +] **Contra:** Asthma, COPD, bradycardia, ↑ prolonged QT interval, 2nd- or 3rd-degree heart block w/o pacemaker, cardiogenic shock, uncontrolled CHF, CrCl <40 mL/min **Disp:** Tabs 80, 120, 160, 240 mg **SE:** Bradycardia, CP, palpitations, fatigue, dizziness, weakness, dyspnea **Interactions:** ↑ Effects *W/* ASA, antihypertensives, nitrates, OCPs, fluoxetine, prazosin, sulfinpyrazone, verapamil, EtOH; ↑ risk of prolonged QT interval *W/* amiodarone, amitriptyline, bepridil, disopyramide, erythromycin, gatifloxacin, haloperidol, imipramine, moxifloxacin, quinidine, pimozide, procainamide, sparfloxacin, thioridazine; ↑ effects *OF* lidocaine; ↓ effects *W/* antacids, clonidine, NSAIDs, thyroid drugs; ↓ effects *OF* hypoglycemics, terbutaline, theophylline **Labs:** ↑ BUN, serum glucose, triglycerides, K⁺, uric acid **NIPE:** May ↑ sensitivity to cold; D/C MAOIs 14 d before drug; take w/o food; Betapace should not be substituted for Betapace AF because of differences in labeling

Sotalol (Betapace AF) [Antiarrhythmic, Antihypertensive/BB]
WARNING: To minimize risk of induced arrhythmia, pts initiated/reinitiated on Betapace AF should be placed for a minimum of 3 d (on their maint dose) in a

facility that can provide cardiac resuscitation, continuous ECG monitoring, & calculations of CrCl; Betapace should not be substituted for Betapace AF because of labeling differences **Uses:** *Maintain sinus rhythm for symptomatic A fib/flutter* **Action:** β-Adrenergic-blocking agent **Dose:** *Adults.* Initial CrCl >60 mL/min: 80 mg PO q12h. CrCl 40–60 mL/min: 80 mg PO q24h; ↑ to 120 mg during hospitalization; monitor QT interval 2–4 h after each dose, w/ dose reduction or D/C if QT interval >500 ms. *Peds. Neonates:* 9 mg/m² tid. *1–19 mo:* 20 mg/m² tid. *20–23 mo:* 29.1 mg/m² tid. =*2 y:* 30 mg/m² tid; can double all doses as max daily dose; allow ≈ 36 h between dosage titrations **Caution:** [B (1st tri; D if 2nd or 3rd tri), +] if converting from previous antiarrhythmic therapy **Contra:** Asthma, bradycardia, prolonged QT interval, 2nd- or 3rd-degree heart block w/o pacemaker, cardiogenic shock, uncontrolled CHF, CrCl <40 mL/min **Disp:** Tabs 80, 120, 160 mg **SE:** Bradycardia, CP, palpitations, fatigue, dizziness, weakness, dyspnea **Interactions:** ↑ Risk of prolonged QT interval *W/* amiodarone, amitriptyline, bepridil, disopyramide, erythromycin, gatifloxacin, haloperidol, imipramine, moxifloxacin, quinidine, pimozide, procainamide, sparfloxacin, TCAs, thioridazine; ↑ effects *W/* general anesthesia, phenytoin administered IV, verapamil ↑ effects *OF* insulin, oral hypoglycemics; ↑ risk of hypotension *W/* antihypertensives, ASA, bismuth sub-salicylate, Mg salicylate, sulfinpyrazone, nitrates, OCPs, EtOH; ↑ CV reactions CCB, digoxin; ↑ risk *OF* severe HTN if used w/in 14 d of MAOIs; ↓ effects *W/* antacids; ↑ effects *OF* β-adrenergic bronchodilators, dopamine, dobutamine, theophylline **Labs:** ↑ ANA titers, BUN, K⁺, serum glucose, LFTs, triglycerides, uric acid; monitor QT interval **NIPE:** ⊘ D/C abruptly after long-term use; take w/o food; administer antacids 2hr < or > sotalol; Betapace should not be substituted for Betapace AF because of differences in labeling

Spironolactone (Aldactone) [Potassium Sparing Diuretic]

Uses: *Hyperaldosteronism, ascites from CHF or cirrhosis* **Action:** Aldosterone antagonist; K⁺-sparing diuretic **Dose:** *Adults.* 25–100 mg PO qid; CHF (NYHA class III–IV) 25–50 mg/d. *Peds.* 1–3.3 mg/kg/24 h PO ÷ bid–qid. *Neonates:* 0.5–1 mg/kg/dose q8h; w/ food **Caution:** [D, +] **Contra:** ↑ K⁺, renal failure, anuria **Disp:** Tabs 25, 50, 100 mg **SE:** ↑ K⁺ & gynecomastia, arrhythmia, sexual dysfunction, confusion, dizziness, D/N/V, abnormal menstruation **Interactions:** ↑ Risk of hyperkalemia *W/* ACEIs, K supls, K⁺-sparing diuretics, ↑ K diet; ↑ effects *OF* Li; ↓ effects *W/* salicylates; ↓ effects *OF* anticoagulants **Labs:** ↑ K⁺ BUN **NIPE:** Take w/ food; ↑ risk of gynecomastia; maximum effects of drug may take 2–3 wk

Stavudine (Zerit) [Antiretroviral/Reverse Transcriptase Inhibitor]

WARNING: Lactic acidosis & severe hepatomegaly w/ steatosis & pancreatitis reported **Uses:** *Advanced HIV* **Action:** Reverse transcriptase inhibitor **Dose:** *Adults.* >60 kg: 40 mg bid. <60 kg: 30 mg bid. *Peds. Birth–13 d:* 0.5 mg/kg q12h. >*14 d & <30 kg:* 1 mg/kg q12h. =*30 kg:* Adult dose; ↓ in renal insuff failure **Caution:** [C, +/-] **Contra:** Allergy **Disp:** Caps 15, 20, 30, 40 mg; soln 1 mg/mL **SE:** Peripheral neuropathy, HA, chills, fever, malaise, rash, GI upset, anemias, lactic acidosis, pancreatitis **Interactions:** ↑ Risk of pancreatitis *W/* didanosine;

↑ effects W/ probenecid; ↓ effects W/ zidovudine **Labs:** ↑ LFTs **NIPE:** Take *W/O* regard to food; take *W/* plenty of H_2O

Steroids, Systemic [Glucocorticoid] (See Also Table 3) The following relates only to the commonly used systemic glucocorticoids

Uses: *Endocrine disorders* (adrenal insuff), *rheumatoid disorders*, collagen–vascular Dzs, derm Dzs, allergic states, cerebral edema*, nephritis, nephrotic synd, immunosuppression for transplantation, ↑ Ca^{2+}, malignancies (breast, lymphomas), preop (in any pt who has been on steroids in the previous year, known hypoadrenalism, preop for adrenalectomy); inj into joints/tissue **Action:** Glucocorticoid **Dose:** Varies w/ use & institutional protocols

- *Adrenal insuff, acute: Adults.* Hydrocortisone: 100 mg IV; then 300 mg/d ÷ q6h; convert to 50 mg PO q8h × 6 doses, taper to 30–50 mg/d ÷ bid. *Peds.* Hydrocortisone: 1–2 mg/kg IV, then 150–250 mg/d ÷ tid.
- *Adrenal insuff, chronic (physiologic replacement):* May need mineralocorticoid supl such as Florinef. *Adults.* Hydrocortisone 20 mg PO qAM, 10 mg PO qPM; cortisone 0.5–0.75 mg/kg/d ÷ bid; cortisone 0.25–0.35 mg/kg/d IM; dexamethasone 0.03–0.15 mg/kg/d or 0.6–0.75 mg/m²/d ÷ q6–12h PO, IM, IV. *Peds.* Hydrocortisone: 0.5–0.75 mg/kg/d PO tid; hydrocortisone succinate 0.25–0.35 mg/kg/d IM.
- *Asthma, acute: Adults.* Methylprednisolone: 60 mg PO/IV q6h or dexamethasone 12 mg IV q6h. *Peds.* Prednisolone: 1–2 mg/kg/d or prednisone 1–2 mg/kg/d ÷ daily–bid for up to 5 d; Methylprednisolone: 2–4 mg/kg/d IV ÷ tid; Dexamethasone: 0.1–0.3 mg/kg/d ÷ q6h.
- *Congenital adrenal hyperplasia: Peds.* Initial hydrocortisone 30–36 mg/m²/d PO ÷ 1/3 dose qAM, 2/3 dose qPM; maint 20–25 mg/m²/d ÷ bid.
- *Extubation/airway edema: Adults.* Dexamethasone: 0.5–1 mg/kg/d IM/IV ÷ q6h (start 24 h prior to extubation; continue × 4 more doses). *Peds.* Dexamethasone: 0.1–0.3 mg/kg/d ÷ q6h × 3 3–5 d (start 48–72 h before extubation).
- *Immunosuppressive/anti-inflammatory: Adults & Older Peds.* Hydrocortisone: 15–240 mg PO, IM, IV q12h; Methylprednisolone: 4–48 mg/d PO, taper to lowest effective dose; Methylprednisolone Na succinate: 10–80 mg/d IM. *Adults.* Prednisone or prednisolone: 5–60 mg/d PO ÷ daily–qid. *Infants & Younger Children.* Hydrocortisone: 2.5–10 mg/kg/d PO ÷ q6–8h; 1–5 mg/kg/d IM/IV ÷ bid.
- *Nephrotic synd: Peds.* Prednisolone or prednisone: 2 mg/kg/d PO tid–qid until urine is protein-free for 5 d, use up to 28 d; for persistent proteinuria, 4 mg/kg/dose PO qod max 120 mg/d for an additional 28 d; maint 2 mg/kg/dose qod for 28 d; taper over 4–6 wk (max 80 mg/d).
- *Septic shock (controversial): Adults.* Hydrocortisone: 500 mg–1 g IM/IV q2–6h. *Peds.* Hydrocortisone: 50 mg/kg IM/IV, repeat q4–24 h PRN.
- *Status asthmaticus: Adults & Peds.* Hydrocortisone: 1–2 mg/kg/dose IV q6h; then ↓ by 0.5–1 mg/kg q6h.

- *Rheumatic Dz:* **Adults.** *Intra-articular:* Hydrocortisone acetate: 25–37.5 mg large joint, 10–25 mg small joint; methylprednisolone acetate 20–80 mg large joint, 4–10 mg small joint. *Intrabursal:* Hydrocortisone acetate: 25–37.5 mg. *Intraganglial:* Hydrocortisone acetate: 25–37.5 mg. *Tendon sheath:* Hydrocortisone acetate: 5–12.5 mg.
- *Periop steroid coverage:* Hydrocortisone 100 mg IV night before surgery, 1 h preop, intraop, & 4, 8, 12 h postop; postop day 1 100 mg IV q6h; postop day 2 100 mg IV q8h; postop day 3 100 mg IV q12h; postop day 4 50 mg IV q12h; postop day 5 25 mg IV q12h; resume prior PO dosing if chronic use or D/C if only periop coverage required.
- *Cerebral edema:* Dexamethasone: 10 mg IV; then 4 mg IV q4–6h.

Caution: [C, ?/–] **Contra:** Active varicella Infxn, serious Infxn except TB, fungal Infxns **Disp:** Table 3 **SE:** ↑ appetite, hyperglycemia, ↓ K⁺, osteoporosis, nervousness, insomnia, "steroid psychosis," adrenal suppression **NIPE:** Never abruptly D/C steroids, especially in chronic Rx; taper dose; hydrocortisone succinate for systemic, acetate for intra-articular

Streptokinase (Streptase, Kabikinase) [Plasminogen Activator/Thrombolytic Enzyme]

Uses: *Coronary artery thrombosis, acute massive PE, DVT, & some occluded vascular grafts* **Action:** Activates plasminogen to plasmin that degrades fibrin **Dose:** *Adults.* **PE:** Load 250,000 units peripheral IV over 30 min, then 100,000 units/h IV for 24–72 h. *Coronary artery thrombosis:* 1.5 million units IV over 60 min. *DVT or arterial embolism:* Load as w/ PE, then 100,000 units/h for 72 h; 1.5 million IU in a 1 h inf *(ECC 2005)* **Peds.** 3500–4000 units/kg over 30 min, then 1000–1500 units/kg/h. *Occluded catheter (controversial):* 10,000–25,000 in NS to final volume of catheter (leave in for 1 h, aspirate & flush w/ NS) **Caution:** [C, +] **Contra:** Streptococcal Infxn or streptokinase in last 6 mo, active bleeding, CVA, TIA, spinal surgery/trauma in last month, vascular anomalies, severe hepatic/renal Dz, endocarditis, pericarditis, severe uncontrolled HTN **Disp:** Powder for inj 250,000, 750,000, 1,500,000 units **SE:** Bleeding, ↓ BP, fever, bruising, rash, GI upset, hemorrhage, anaphylaxis **Interactions:** ↑ Risk of bleeding *W/* anticoagulants, ASA, heparin, indomethacin, NSAIDs, dong quai, feverfew, garlic, ginger, horse chestnut, red clover **Labs:** ↑ PT, PTT **NIPE:** If inf inadequate to keep clotting time 2–5× control, see package for adjustments; antibodies remain 3–6 mo following dose

Streptomycin [Antibiotic/Aminoglycoside]

WARNING: Neuro/oto/renal tox possible; neuromuscular blockage w/resp paralysis possible **Uses:** *TB*, streptococcal or enterococcal endocarditis **Action:** Aminoglycoside, ↓ protein synth **Dose:** *Adults.* *Endocarditis:* 1 g q12h 1–2 wk, then 500 mg q12h 1–4 wk; *TB:* 15 mg/kg/d (up to 1 g), directly observed therapy (DOT) 2 × wk 20–30 mg/kg/dose (max 1.5 g); DOT 3 × wk 25–30 mg/kg/dose (max 1 g). *Peds.* 15 mg/kg/d; DOT 2 × wk 20–40 mg/kg/dose (max 1 g); DOT 3 × wk 25–30 mg/kg/dose (max 1 g); ↓ w/in renal failure insuff, either IM or IV over 30–60 min

Caution: [D, +] **Contra:** PRG **Disp:** Inj 400 mg/mL (1-g vial) **SE:** ↑ Incidence of vestibular & auditory tox, ↑ neurotox risk in pts w/ impaired renal function **Notes:** Monitor levels: *Peak* 20–30 μg/mL, *Trough* <5 μg/mL; *Toxic peak* > 50, *Trough* > 10; IV over 30–60 min **Interactions:** ↑ Risk of nephrotox *W/* amphotericin B, cephalosporins, cisplatin, methoxyflurane, polymyxin B, vancomycin; ↑ risk of ototox *W/* carboplatin, furosemide, mannitol, urea; ↑ effects *OF* anticoagulants **Labs:** False + urine glucose, false ↑ urine protein **NIPE:** ↑ Fluid intake

Streptozocin (Zanosar) [Alkylating Agent/Nitrosourea]
Uses: *Pancreatic islet cell tumors* & carcinoid tumors **Action:** DNA–DNA (interstrand) cross-linking; DNA, RNA, & protein synth inhibitor **Dose:** Per protocol; ↓ in renal failure **Caution:** w/ renal failure [D, ?/–] **Contra:** w/ rotavirus vaccine, PRG **Disp:** Inj 1 g **SE:** N/V/D, duodenal ulcers, depression, ↓ BM rare (20%) & mild; nephrotox (proteinuria & azotemia dose related), hypophosphatemia dose limiting; hypo-/hyperglycemia; inj site Rxns **Interactions:** ↑ Risk of nephrotox *W/* aminoglycosides, amphotericin B, cisplatin, vancomycin; ↑ effects *OF* doxorubicin; ↓ effects *W/* phenytoin **Labs:** Monitor Cr **NIPE:** ⊘ PRG, breast-feeding; ↑ fluid intake to 2–3 L/d

Succimer (Chemet) [Chelating Agent]
Uses: *Lead poisoning (levels >45 μg/mL)* **Action:** Heavy-metal chelating agent **Dose:** *Adults & Peds.* 10 mg/kg/dose q8h × 5 d, then 10 mg/kg/dose q12h for 14 d; ↓ in renal impair **Caution:** [C, ?] **Contra:** Allergy **Disp:** Caps 100 mg **SE:** Rash, fever, GI upset, hemorrhoids, metallic taste, drowsiness, ↑ LFTs **Labs:** ↑ LFTs; monitor lead levels **NIPE:** ⊘ Take *W/* other chelating agents; ↑ fluid intake to 2–3 L/d may open capsules

Succinylcholine (Anectine, Quelicin, Sucostrin, others) [Skeletal Muscle Relaxant]
WARNING: Risk of cardiac arrest from hyperkalemic rhabdomyolysis **Uses:** *Adjunct to general anesthesia, facilitates ET intubation; induce skeletal muscle relaxation during surgery or mechanical ventilation* **Action:** Depolarizing neuromuscular blocker; rapid onset, short duration (3–5 min) **Dose:** *Adults.* Rapid sequence intubation 1–2 mg/kg IV over 10–30 s or 2–4 mg/kg IM *(ECC 2005)* *Peds.* 1–2 mg/kg/dose IV, then by 0.3–0.6 mg/kg/dose q5min use of CI not OK; ↓ w/ severe renal/hepatic impair **Caution:** See Warning [C, M] **Contra:** w/ malignant hyperthermia risk, myopathy, recent major burn, multiple trauma, extensive skeletal muscle denervation, NAG, pseudocholinesterase deficiency **Disp:** Inj 20, 50, 100 mg/mL **SE:** Fasciculations, ↑ intraocular, intragastric, intracranial pressure, salivation, myoglobinuria, malignant hyperthermia, resp depression, or prolonged apnea; multiple drugs potentiate; CV effects (arrhythmias, ↓ BP, brady/tachycardia) **Interactions:** ↑ Effects *W/* amikacin, gentamicin, neomycin, streptomycin, Li, MAOIs, opiates; ↓ effect *W/* diazepam **Labs:** ↑ Serum K⁺ **NIPE:** May be given IVP/inf/IM deltoid; hyperkalemic rhabdomyolysis in children with undiagnosed myopathy such as Duchenne muscular dystrophy

Sucralfate (Carafate) [Antiulcer Agent/Pepsin Inhibitor]

Uses: *Duodenal ulcers*, gastric ulcers, stomatitis, GERD, preventing stress ulcers, esophagitis **Action:** Forms ulcer-adherent complex that protects against acid, pepsin, & bile acid **Dose:** *Adults.* 1 g PO qid, 1 h prior to meals & hs. *Peds.* 40–80 mg/kg/d ÷ q6h; continue 4–8 wk until healing demonstrated by x-ray or endoscopy; separate from other drugs by 2 h; on empty stomach ac **Caution:** [B, +] **Contra:** Component allergy **Disp:** Tabs 1 g; susp g/10 mL **SE:** Constipation; D, dizziness, xerostomia **Interactions:** ↓ Effects *OF* cimetidine, digoxin, levothyroxine, phenytoin, quinolones, quinidine, ranitidine, tetracyclines, theophylline, warfarin **NIPE:** Take w/o food; Al may accumulate in renal failure

Sulfacetamide (Bleph-10, Cetamide, Sodium Sulamyd) [Antibiotic/Sulfonamide]

Uses: *Conjunctival Infxns* **Action:** Sulfonamide antibiotic **Dose:** 10% oint apply qid & hs; soln for keratitis apply q2–3h based on severity **Caution:** [C, M] **Contra:** Sulfonamide sensitivity; age <2 mo **Disp:** susp: sulfacetamide 10%/ prednisolone 0.25%, sulfacetamide 10%/ prednisolone 0.5%, sulfacetamide 10%/ prednisolone 0.2% **SE:** Irritation, burning; blurred vision, brow ache, Stevens–Johnson synd, photosens **Interactions:** ↓ Effects *W/* tetracyclines **NIPE:** Not compatible *W/* Ag-containing preps; purulent exudate inactivates drug; ↑ risk of photosensitivity—use sunscreen

Sulfacetamide & Prednisolone (Blephamide, Others) [Antibiotic, Anti-inflammatory]

Uses: *Steroid-responsive inflammatory ocular conditions w/ Infxn or a risk of Infxn* **Action:** Antibiotic & anti-inflammatory **Dose:** *Adults & Peds >2 y.* Apply oint lower conjunctival sac daily–qid; soln 1–3 gtt 2–3 h while awake **Caution:** [C, ?/–] Sulfonamide sensitivity; age <2 mo **Disp:** Oint: sulfacetamide/prednisolone (%/%) 10/0.5, 10/0.2, 10/0.25; Susp: sulfacetamide/prednisolone (%/%) 10/0.25, 10/0.5, 10/0.2 **SE:** Irritation, burning, blurred vision, brow ache, Stevens–Johnson synd, photosens **Interactions:** ↑ Effects *W/* tetracyclines **NIPE:** Not compatible *W/* Ag-containing preps; purulent exudate inactivates drug; ↑ risk of sensitivity to light; ⊘ D/C abruptly; OK ophth susp use as otic agent

Sulfasalazine (Azulfidine, Azulfidine EN) [Anti-inflammatory, Antirheumatic (DMARD)/Sulfonamide]

Uses: *Ulcerative colitis, RA, juvenile RA*, active Crohn Dz, ankylosing spondylitis, psoriasis **Action:** Sulfonamide; actions unclear **Dose:** *Adults.* Initial, 1 g PO tid–qid; ↑ to max of 8 g/d in 3–4 ÷ doses; maint 500 mg PO qid. *Peds.* Initial, 40–60 mg/kg/24 h PO ÷ q4–6h; maint, 20–30 mg/kg/24 h PO ÷ q6h. *RA >6 y:* 30–50 mg/kg/d in 2 doses, start w/ 1/4–1/3 maint dose, ↑ weekly until dose reached at 1 mo, 2 g/d max; ↓ in renal failure **Caution:** [B (D if near term), M] **Contra:** Sulfonamide or salicylate sensitivity, porphyria, GI/GU obst; avoid in hepatic impair **Disp:** Tabs 500 mg; EC delayed-release tabs 500 mg **SE:** GI upset; discolors urine; dizziness, HA, photosens, oligospermia, anemias, Stevens–Johnson synd **Interactions:** ↑ Effects *OF* oral anticoagulants, oral hypoglycemics, MTX, phenytoin, zidovudine; ↓ effects

W/ antibiotics; ↓ effects *OF* digoxin, folic acid, Fe, procaine, proparacaine, sulfonylureas, tetracaine **Labs:** ↑ LFTs, BUN, Cr; ↓ plts, WBCs **NIPE:** Take pc; ↑ fluids to 2–3 L/d; ↑ risk of photosensitivity—use sunscreen; skin & urine may become yellow-orange; may stain contact lenses

Sulfinpyrazone [Uricosuric/Antigout Agent] Uses: *Acute & chronic gout* **Action:** ↓ renal tubular absorption of uric acid **Dose:** 100–200 mg PO bid for 1 wk, ↑ PRN to maint of 200–400 mg bid; max 800 mg/d; take w/ food or antacids, & plenty of fluids; avoid salicylates **Caution:** [C (D if near term), ?/–] **Contra:** Renal impair, avoid salicylates; peptic ulcer; blood dyscrasias, near term PRG, allergy **Disp:** Tabs 100 mg; caps 200 mg **SE:** N/V, stomach pain, urolithiasis, leukopenia **Interactions:** ↑ Effects *OF* oral anticoagulants, oral hypoglycemics, MTX; ↓ effects *W/* ASA, cholestyramine, niacin, salicylates, EtOH; ↓ effects *OF* acetaminophen, theophylline, verapamil **Labs:** ↑ BUN, Cr; ↓ plts, WBCs **NIPE:** Take w/ food, ↑ fluids to 2–3 L/d

Sulindac (Clinoril) [Analgesic, Anti-inflammatory, Antipyretic/ NSAID] WARNING: May ↑ risk of cardiovascular events & GI bleeding Uses: *Arthritis & pain* **Action:** NSAID; ↓ prostaglandins **Dose:** 150–200 mg bid, 400 mg/d max; w/ food **Caution:** [B (D if 3rd tri or near term), ?] **Contra:** NSAID or ASA sensitivity, w/ ketorolac, ulcer, GI bleeding, postop pain in CABG **Disp:** Tabs 150, 200 mg **SE:** Dizziness, rash, GI upset, pruritus, edema, ↓ renal blood flow, renal failure (? fewer renal effects than other NSAIDs), peptic ulcer, GI bleeding **Interactions:** ↑ Effects *W/* NSAIDs, probenecid; ↑ effects *OF* aminoglycosides, anticoagulants, cyclosporine, digoxin, Li, MTX, K-sparing diuretics ↑ risk of bleeding *W/* ASA, anticoagulants, NSAIDs, thrombolytics, EtOH, dong quai, feverfew, garlic, ginger, horse chestnut, red clover; ↓ effects *W/* antacids, ASA; ↓ effects *OF* antihypertensives, diuretics, hydralazine **Labs:** ↑ LFTs, BUN Cr, K+ **NIPE:** Take w/ food; ↑ risk of photosensitivity—use sunscreen; may take several weeks for full drug effect

Sumatriptan (Imitrex) [Antimigraine Agent/Selective 5-HT₁ Receptor Agonist] Uses: *Rx acute migraine* **Action:** Vascular serotonin receptor agonist **Dose:** *Adults. SQ:* 6 mg SQ as a single dose PRN; repeat PRN in 1 h to a max of 12 mg/24 h. *PO:* 25 mg, repeat in 2 h, PRN, 100 mg/d max PO dose; max 300 mg/d. *Nasal spray:* 1 spray into 1 nostril, repeat in 2 h to 40 mg/24 h max. *Peds. Nasal spray:* 6–9 y: 5–20 mg/d. 12–17 y: 5–20 mg, up to 40 mg/d **Caution:** [C, M] **Contra:** Angina, ischemic heart Dz, uncontrolled HTN, severe hepatic impair, ergot use, MAOI use w/in 14 d **Disp:** Orally disintegrating tabs 25 50, 100 mg; Inj 6, 8, 12 mg/mL; orally disintegrating tabs 25, 50, 100 mg, orally disintegrating tabs 25, 50, 100 mg; nasal spray 5, 10, 20 mg/spray **SE:** Pain & bruising at site; dizziness, hot flashes, paresthesias, CP, weakness, numbness, coronary vasospasm, HTN **Interactions:** ↑ Effects of weakness, incoordination and hyper reflexia *W/* ergots, MAOIs, and SSRIs, horehound, St. John's Wort **Labs:** ↑ LFT **NIPE:** Admin drug as soon as possible after onset of migraine

Sunitinib (Sutent) [Kinase Inhibitor] Uses: *Advanced GI stromal tumor refractory/intolerant of imatinib; advanced RCC* Action: Kinase inhibitor Dose: *Adults.* 50 mg PO daily × 4 wk, followed by 2 wk holiday = 1 cycle; ↓ to 37.5 mg w/ CYP3A4 inhibitors (Table 11), to ↑ 87.5 mg w/ CYP3A4 inducers Contra: w/ atazanavir Caution: [D, –] Multiple interactions require dose modification (eg, St. John's Wort) Disp: Caps 12.5, 25, 50 mg SE: ↓ WBC & plt, bleeding, ↑ BP, ↓ ejection fraction, ↑ QT interval, pancreatitis, DVT, Sz, adrenal insuff, N/V/D, skin discoloration, oral ulcers, taste perversion, hypothyroidism LABS: Monitor CBC, plts, chemistries at cycle onset; baseline cardiac Fxn recommended NIPE: ↓ Dose in 12.5-mg increments if not tolerated

Tacrine (Cognex) [Anti-Alzheimer Agent/Centrally Acting Reversible Cholinesterase Inhibitor] Uses: *Mild–moderate Alzheimer dementia* Action: Cholinesterase inhibitor Dose: 10–40 mg PO qid to 160 mg/d; separate doses from food Caution: [C, ?] Contra: Previous tacrine-induced jaundice Disp: Caps 10, 20, 30, 40 mg SE: ↑ LFT, HA, dizziness, GI upset, flushing, confusion, ataxia, myalgia, bradycardia Interactions: ↑ Effects *W*/ cimetidine, quinolones; ↑ effects *OF* cholinesterase inhibitors, succinylcholine, theophylline; ↓ effects w/ tobacco, food; ↓ effects *OF* anticholinergics Labs: ↑ LFTs NIPE: If taken w/ food ↓ drug plasma levels by 30%; may take up to 6 wk for ALT elevations—monitor LFTs; serum conc >20 mg/mL have more SE

Tacrolimus [FK 506] (Prograf, Protopic) [Immunosuppressant/Macrolide] WARNING: ↑ Risk of Infxn and lymphoma Uses: *Prevent organ rejection*, eczema Action: Macrolide immunosuppressant Dose: *Adults. IV:* 0.05–0.1 mg/kg/d cont inf. *PO:* 0.15–0.3 mg/kg/d ÷ 2 doses. *Peds. IV:* 0.03–0.05 mg/kg/d as cont inf. *PO:* 0.15–0.2 mg/kg/d PO ÷ q 12 h. *Adults & Peds. Eczema:* Apply bid, continue 1 wk after clearing; ↓ in hepatic/renal impair Caution: [C, –] w/ cyclosporine; avoid topical if <2 y of age Contra: Component allergy, castor oil allergy w/ IV form Disp: Caps 0.5, 1, 5 mg; inj 5 mg/mL; oint 0.03, 0.1% SE: Neuro & nephrotox, HTN, edema, HA, insomnia, fever, pruritus, ↓/↑ K+, hyperglycemia, GI upset, anemia, leukocytosis, tremors, paresthesias, pleural effusion, Szs, lymphoma Lab: Monitor levels NIPE: Reports of ↑ CA risk; topical use for short-term & 2nd line

Tadalafil (Cialis) [Anti-impotence Agent/PDE5] Uses: *Erectile dysfunction* Action: PDE5 inhibitor, increases cGMP and NO levels; relaxes smooth muscles, dilates cavernosal arteries Dose: *Adults.* 10 mg PO before sexual activity w/o regard to meals (range 5–20 mg max) ÷ ↓ 5 mg (10 mg max) w/ renal & hepatic insuff Caution: [B, –] w/ CYP3A4 inhibitor (Table 11) Contra: Nitrates, α-blockers (except tamsulosin), severe hepatic impair Disp: 5-, 10-, 20-mg tabs SE: HA, flushing, dyspepsia, rhinitis, back pain, myalgia hearing loss Interactions: ↑ Effects *W*/ ketoconazole, ritonavir, and other cytochrome P450 CYP3A4 inhibitors; ↑ hypotension *W*/ antihypertensives, nitrates, EtOH; ↓ effects *W*/ P450 CYP3A4 inducers such as rifampin, antacids

NIPE: ↑ Risk of priapism; use barrier contraception to prevent STDs; longest acting of class (36 h)

Talc (Sterile Talc Powder) [Sclerosing Agent]

Uses: *↓ Recurrence of malignant pleural effusions (pleurodesis)* **Action:** Sclerosing agent **Dose:** Mix slurry: 50 mL NS w/ 5-g vial, mix, distribute 25 mL into two 60-mL syringes, volume to 50 mL/syringe w/ NS. Inf each into chest tube, flush w/ 25 mL NS. Keep tube clamped; have pt change positions q15min for 2 h, unclamp tube **Caution:** [X, –] **Contra:** Planned further surgery on site **Disp:** 5 g powder **SE:** Pain, Infxn **NIPE:** May add 10–20 mL 1% lidocaine/syringe; must have chest tube placed, monitor closely while tube clamped (tension pneumothorax), not antineoplastic **NIPE:** Monitor for MI, PE, respiratory distress

Tamoxifen [Antineoplastic/Antiestrogen]

WARNING: CA of the uterus, stroke, and blood clots can occur **Uses:** *Breast CA [postmenopausal, estrogen receptor(+)], ↓ reduction of breast CA in high-risk women, met male breast CA*, ductal carcinoma in situ, mastalgia, pancreatic CA, gynecomastia, ovulation induction **Action:** Nonsteroidal antiestrogen; mixed agonist–antagonist effect **Dose:** 20–40 mg/d (typically 10 mg bid or 20 mg/d) *Prevention:* 10 mg PO bid × 5y **Caution:** [D, –] w/ leukopenia, thrombocytopenia, hyperlipidemia **Contra:** PRG, undiagnosed vag bleeding, h/o thromboembolism **Disp:** Tabs 10, 20 mg, oral soln 10 mg/5 mL **SE:** Uterine malignancy & thrombotic events noted in breast CA prevention trials; menopausal Sxs (hot flashes, N/V) in premenopausal pts; vag bleeding & menstrual irregularities; skin rash, pruritus vulvae, dizziness, HA, peripheral edema; acute flare of bone metastasis pain & ↑ Ca²⁺; retinopathy reported (high dose) **Interactions:** ↑ Effects **W/** bromocriptine, grapefruit juice; ↑ effects *OF* cyclosporine, warfarin; ↓ effects **W/** antacids, aminoglutethimide, estrogens **Labs:** ↑ Ca²⁺, BUN, Cr, LFTs **NIPE:** ⊘ PRG or breast-feeding; use barrier contraception; ↑ risk of photosensitivity—use sunscreen; ↑ risk of PRG in premenopausal women (induces ovulation); brand Nolvadex suspended in US

Tamsulosin (Flomax) [Smooth Muscle Relaxant/Antiadrenergic]

Uses: *BPH* **Action:** Antagonist of prostatic α-receptors **Dose:** 0.4 mg/d, may ↑ to 0.8 mg PO daily; **Caution:** [B, ?] **Contra:** Female gender **Disp:** Caps 0.4 mg **SE:** HA, dizziness, syncope, somnolence, ↓ libido, GI upset, retrograde ejaculation, rhinitis, rash, angioedema, IFIS **Interactions:** ↑ Effects **W/** cimetidine; ↑ hypotension **W/** doxazosin, prazosin, terazosin; **NIPE:** Ensure—test results for prostate CA before drug admin; not for use as antihypertensive; do not open/crush/chew

Tazarotene (Tazorac, Avage) [Keratolytic/Retinoid]

Uses: *Facial acne vulgaris; stable plaque psoriasis up to 20% BSA* **Action:** Keratolytic **Dose:** *Adults & Peds >12 y. Acne:* Cleanse face, dry, & apply thin film daily hs on acne lesions. *Psoriasis:* Apply hs **Caution:** [X, ?/–] **Contra:** Retinoid sensitivity **Disp:** Gel 0.05, 0.1%; cream 0.05%, 0.1% **SE:** Burning, erythema, irritation, rash, photosens, desquamation, bleeding, skin discoloration **Interactions:** ↑ Risk o photosensitivity W/ quinolones, phenothiazine, sulfonamides, tetracyclines, thiazide diuretics **NIPE:** ⊘ PRG or breast-feeding; use contraception; use sunscreen for ↑ photosensitivity risk; D/C w/ excessive pruritus, burning, skin redness or peeling occur until Sxs resolve

Telbivudine (Tyzeka) [Antiretroviral, NRTI] **WARNING:** May cause lactic acidosis and severe hepatomegaly w/ steatosis when used alone or w/ antiretrovirals; D/C may lead to exacerbations of Hep B; monitor LFTs **Uses:** *Rx chronic Hep B* **Action:** Nucleoside RT inhibitor **Dose:** CrCl >50 mL/min: 600 mg PO daily; CrCl 30–49 mL/min: 600 mg q48 h; CrCl <30 mL/min: 600 mg q72h; ESRD: 600 mg q 96h **Caution:** [B; ?/–]; may cause myopathy; follow closely w/ other myopathy causing drugs **Disp:** Tabs 600 mg **SE:** Fatigue, abd pain, N/V/D, HA, URI, nasopharyngitis, ↑ LFTs/CPK, myalgia, flulike Sxs, dizziness, insomnia, dyspepsia **Interactions:** ↑ Risk of myopathy W/ azole antifungals, chloroquine, corticosteroids, cyclosporine, erythromycin, fibrates, hydroxychloroquine, niacin, penicillamine, statins, zidovudine; ↑ risk of renal impair W/ cyclosporine, tacrolimus **Labs:** ↑ LFTs, CPK **NIPE:** Not a cure for Hep B, does not reduce transmission of Hep B by sexual contact or blood contamination

Telithromycin (Ketek) [Antibiotic/Macrolide Derivative] **WARNING:** May be associated with pseudomembranous colitis and hepatic failure **Uses:** *Acute bacterial exacerbations of chronic bronchitis, acute bacterial sinusitis; mild–moderate community-acquired pneumonia* **Action:** Unique macrolide, blocks ↓ protein synth; bactericidal. *Spectrum:* S. aureus, S. pneumoniae, H. influenzae, M. catarrhalis, C. pneumoniae, M. pneumoniae **Dose:** *Chronic bronchitis/sinusitis:* 800 mg (2 tabs) PO daily × 5; *Pneumonia:* 800 mg (2 tabs) PO daily × 7–10 d **Caution:** [C, M] Pseudomembranous colitis, ↑ QTc interval, MyG exacerbations, visual disturbances, hepatic dysfunction; dosing in renal impair unknown **Contra:** Macrolide allergy, use w/ pimozide, w/ MyG **Disp:** Tabs 300, 400 mg **SE:** N/V/D, dizziness, blurred vision **Interactions:** ↑ QTc interval & arrhythmias W/ antiarrhythmics, mesoridazine, quinolone antibiotics, thioridazine; ↑ effects **OF** alprazolam, atorvastatin, benzodiazepines, CCBs, carbamazepine, cisapride, colchicine, cyclosporine, digoxin, ergot alkaloids, felodipine, lovastatin, mirtazapine, midazolam, nateglinide, nefazodone, pimozide, sildenafil, simvastatin, sirolimus, tacrolimus, tadalafil, triazolam, vardenafil, venlafaxine, verapamil; ↓ effects W/ azole antifungals, ciprofloxin, clarithromycin, diclofenac, doxycycline, erythromycin, imatinib, INH, nefazodone, nicardipine, propofol, protease inhibitors, quinidine, verapamil; ↑ effect W/ aminoglutethimide, carbamazepine, nafcillin, nevirapine, phenobarbital, phenytoin, rifampin, rifamycins **Labs:** ↑ LFTs **NIPE:** Take w/o regard to food; ⊘ chew/crush tabs; A CYP450 inhibitor

Telmisartan (Micardis) [Antihypertensive/ARB] **Uses:** *HTN, CHF*, DN **Action:** Angiotensin II receptor antagonist **Dose:** 40–80 mg/d **Caution:** [C (1st tri; D 2nd & 3rd tri), ?/–] **Contra:** Angiotensin II receptor antagonist sensitivity **Disp:** Tabs 20, 40, 80 mg **SE:** Edema, GI upset, HA, angioedema, renal impair, orthostatic ↓ BP **Interactions:** ↑ Effects **W/** EtOH; ↑ effects **OF** digoxin; ↓ effects **OF** warfarin **Labs:** ↑ Cr, ↓ HMG **NIPE:** Take w/o regard to food; ⊘ PRG; use barrier contraception

Temazepam (Restoril) [C-IV] [Sedative/Hypnotic/Benzodi-azepine] Uses: *Insomnia*, anxiety, depression, panic attacks **Action:** Benzodiazepine **Dose:** 15–30 mg PO hs PRN; ↓ in elderly **Caution:** [X, ?/–] Potentiates CNS depressive effects of opioids, barbs, EtOH, antihistamines, MAOIs, TCAs **Contra:** NAG **Disp:** Caps 7.5, 15, 22.5, 30 mg **SE:** Confusion, dizziness, drowsiness, hangover **Interactions:** ↑ Effects **W/** cimetidine, disulfiram, kava kava, valerian; ↑ CNS depression **W/** anticonvulsants, CNS depressants, EtOH; ↑ effects **OF** haloperidol, phenytoin; ↓ effects **W/** aminophylline, dyphylline, OCPs, oxtriphylline, rifampin, theophylline, tobacco; ↓ effects **OF** levodopa **NIPE:** Abrupt D/C after >10 d use may cause withdrawal; ⊘ use in PRG or breast-feeding

Temsirolimus (Torisel Kit) [mTOR Inhibitor] Uses: *Advanced RCC* **Action:** mTOR inhibitor **Dose:** 25 mg IV over 30–60 min × 1 week; continue until tox or progression; pre med w/ 25–50 mg Benadryl 30 min before **Caution:** [D, –] w/ CYP3A4 inhib/inducers (Table 11), avoid grapefruit juice, vaccines, immed postop **Contra:** None **Disp:** 25 mg/mL w/ diluent **SE:** Hypersensitivity Rxn, rash, asthenia, mucositis, N, edema, anorexia, poor wound healing bowel perf **Labs:** ↑ Glucose/lipids/ALP/AST/Cr; ↓ Hct, WBC, plt; monitor Cr, CBC; hold w/ ANC <1000mm^3 or plt <75,000/mm^3 **NIPE:** Combine only w/ provided diluent for IV admin

Tenecteplase (TNKase) [Thrombolytic/Recombinant Tissue Plasminogen Activator] Uses: *Restore perfusion & ↓ mortality w. AMI* **Action:** Thrombolytic; TPA **Dose:** 30–50 mg; see table below

Tenecteplase Dosing

Weight (kg)	TNKase (mg)	TNKase^a Volume (mL)
<60	30	6
≥60–70	35	7
≥70–80	40	8
≥80–90	45	9
≥90	50	10

^{a}From one vial of reconstituted TNKase.

Caution: [C, ?], ↑ Bleeding w/ NSAIDs, ticlopidine, clopidogrel, GPIIb/IIIa antagonists **Contra:** Bleeding, CVA, major surgery (intracranial, intraspinal) or trauma w/in 2 mo **Disp:** Inj 50 mg, reconstitute w/ 10 mL sterile H$_2$O **SE:** Bleeding, allergy **Interactions:** ↑ Risk of bleeding W/ anticoagulants, ASA, clopidogrel, dipyridamole, indomethacin, vitamin K antagonists; ↓ effects W/ aminocaproic acid **Labs:** ↑ PT, PTT, INR **NIPE:** Eval for S/Sxs bleeding; do not shake w/ recons; do *not* use w/ D$_5$W

Tenofovir (Viread) [Antiretroviral/NRTI] WARNING: Lactic acidosis & severe hepatomegaly with steatosis, including fatal cases, have been reported with the use of nucleoside analogs alone or in combo w/ other antiretrovirals. Not OK w/ chronic hepatitis; effects in patients co-infected with Hep B & HIV unknown **Uses:** *HIV Infxn* **Action:** Nucleoside RT inhibitor **Dose:** 300 mg PO daily ? to w/ or w/o meal; CrCl ? = 50 mL/min ? q24h, CrCl 30–49 mL/min q48h, CrCl 10–29 mL/min 2 × week **Caution:** [B, ?/–] Didanosine (separate admin times), lopinavir, ritonavir w/ known risk factors for liver Dz **Contra:** Hypersensitivity **Disp:** Tabs 300 mg **SE:** GI upset, metabolic synd, hepatotox; separate didanosine doses by 2 h **Interactions:** ↑ Effects W/ acyclovir, cidofovir, ganciclovir, indinavir, lopinavir, ritonavir, valacyclovir, food **Labs:** ↑ LFTs, triglycerides **NIPE:** Take w/ food, take 2 h before or 1 h after didanosine, lopinavir/ritonavir; combo product w/ emtricitabine is Truvada

Tenofovir/Emtricitabine (Truvada) [Antiretroviral, Dual NRTI] WARNING: Lactic acidosis & severe hepatomegaly with steatosis, including fatal cases, have been reported with the use of nucleoside analogs alone or in combo w/ other antiretrovirals. Not OK w/ chronic hepatitis; effects in patients co-infected with Hep B & HIV unknown **Uses:** *HIV Infxn* **Action:** Dual nucleotide RT inhibitor **Dose:** 300 mg PO daily w/ or w/o a meal adjust w/ renal impairment **Caution:** w/ known risk factors for liver Dz [B, ?/–] **Contra:** CrCl <30 mL/min; **Disp:** Tabs: 200 mg emtricitabine/300 mg tenofovir **SE:** GI upset, rash, metabolic synd, hepatotox **Interactions:** ↑ Effects W/ acyclovir, cidofovir, ganciclovir, indinavir, lopinavir, ritonavir, valacyclovir, food; ↓ effects OF didanosine, lamivudine, ritonavir **Labs:** ↑ LFTs, triglycerides **NIPE:** Take w/ food, take 2 h before or 1 h after didanosine, lopinavir/ritonavir; causes redistribution and accumulation of body fat; take w/ other antiretrovirals; not a cure for HIV or prevention of opportunistic Infxns

Terazosin (Hytrin) [Antihypertensive/Peripherally Acting Antiadrenergic] Uses: *BPH & HTN* **Action:** α$_1$-Blocker (blood vessel & bladder neck/prostate) **Dose:** Initial, 1 mg PO hs; ↑ 20 mg/d max **Caution:** [C, ?] w/ BB, CCB, ACEI **Contra:** α-Antagonist sensitivity **Disp:** Tabs 1, 2, 5, 10 mg; caps 1, 2, 5, 10 mg **SE:** ↓ BP, & syncope following 1st dose; dizziness, weakness, nasal congestion, peripheral edema, palpitations, GI upset **Interactions:** ↑ Effects W/ antihypertensives, diuretics; ↑ effects OF finasteride; ↓ effects W/ NSAIDs, α-blockers, ephedra, garlic, ginseng, saw palmetto, yohimbe; ↓ effects

OF clonidine **Labs:** ↓ Albumin, HMG, Hct, WBCs **NIPE:** Take w/o regard to food, ⊘ D/C abruptly; caution w/ 1st dose syncope; if for HTN, combine w/ thiazide diuretic

Terbinafine (Lamisil) [Antifungal] **Uses:** *Onychomycosis, athlete's foot, jock itch, ringworm*, cutaneous candidiasis, pityriasis versicolor **Action:** ↓ squalene epoxidase resulting in fungal death **Dose:** *PO:* 250 mg/d PO for 6–12 wk. *Topical:* Apply to area; ↓ in renal/hepatic impair **Caution:** [B, –] ↑ Effects of drug metab by CYP2D6, liver Dz, renal impairment (CrCl <60) **Disp:** Tabs 250 mg; cream, gel, soln 1% **SE:** HA, dizziness, rash, pruritus, alopecia, GI upset, taste perversion, neutropenia, retinal damage, Stevens–Johnson synd **Interactions:** ↑ Effects *W/* cimetidine; ↑ effects *OF* dextromethorphan, theophylline, caffeine; ↓ effects *W/* rifampin; ↓ effects *OF* cyclosporine **Labs:** LFT abnormalities **NIPE:** Effect may take months due to need for new nail growth; do not use occlusive dressings

Terbutaline (Brethine) [Bronchodilator/Sympathomimetic] **Uses:** *Reversible bronchospasm (asthma, COPD); inhibit labor* **Action:** Sympathomimetic; tocolytic **Dose:** *Adults.* Bronchodilator: 2.5–5 mg PO qid or 0.25 mg SQ; repeat in 15 min PRN ;max 0.5 mg in 4 h; *Met-dose inhaler:* 2 inhal q4–6h. *Premature labor:* Acutely 2.5–10 mg/min/IV, gradually ↑ as tolerated q10–20 min; maint 2.5–5 mg PO q4–6h until term *Peds. PO:* 0.05–0.15 mg/kg/dose PO tid; max 5 mg/24h; ↓ in renal failure **Caution:** [B, +] ↑ tox w/ MAOIs, TCAs; DM, HTN, hyperthyroidism, CV disease, convulsive disorders, ↓ K⁺ **Contra:** Component allergy **Disp:** Tabs 2.5, 5 mg; inj 1 mg/mL; met-dose inhaler **SE:** HTN, hyperthyroidism, β₁-adrenergic effects w/ high dose, nervousness, trembling, tachycardia, HTN, dizziness **Interactions:** ↑ Effects *W/* MAOIs, TCAs; ↓ effects *W/* BBs **Labs:** ↑ LFTs, serum glucose **NIPE:** Take oral dose w/ food

Terconazole (Terazol 7) [Antifungal] **Uses:** *Vaginal fungal Infxns* **Action:** Topical triazole antifungal **Dose:** 1 applicatorful or 1 supp intravag hs × 3–7 d **Caution:** [C, ?] **Contra:** Component allergy **Disp:** Vag cream 0.4, 0.8%, vag supp 80 mg **SE:** Vulvar/vag burning **NIPE:** Insert cream or supp high into vag, complete full course of Rx, ⊘ intercourse during drug Rx, ↑ risk of breakdown of latex condoms & diaphragms w/drug

Teriparatide (Forteo) [Antiosteoporotic/Parathyroid Hormone] **WARNING:** ↑ Osteosarcoma risk in animals, therefore only use in pts for whom the potential benefits outweigh risks **Uses:** *Severe/refractory osteoporosis* **Action:** PTH (recombinant) **Dose:** 20 μg SQ daily in thigh or abdomen **Caution:** [C, ?/–] **Contra:** w/ Paget Dz, prior radiation, bone metastases, ↑ Ca²⁺; caution in urolithiasis **Disp:** 3-mL prefilled device (discard after 28 d) **SE:** Orthostatic ↓ BP on administration; N/D, ↑ Ca, leg cramps **Labs:** ↑ Serum Ca²⁺, uric acid, urine Ca²⁺ **NIPE:** ⊘ Take if h/o Paget Dz, bone mets or malignancy, or h/o radiation therapy; take w/o regard to food; not used to prevent osteoporosis; 2 y max use; osteosarcoma in animals

Testosterone (AndroGel, Androderm, Striant, Testim) [CIII] [Androgen Replacement] Uses: *Male hypogonadism* Action: Testosterone replacement; ↑ lean body mass, libido Dose: All daily *AndroGel:* 5 g gel. *Androderm:* Two 2.5- or one 5-mg patch daily. *Striant:* 30-mg buccal tabs bid. *Testim:* One 5-g gel tube. Caution: [N/A, N/A] Contra: PCa, male breast CA Disp: *AndroGel, Testim:* 5-g gel (50-mg test); *Androderm:* 2.5-, 5-mg patches; *Striant:* 30-mg buccal tabs SE: Site Rxns, acne, edema, wt gain, gynecomastia, HTN, ↑ sleep apnea, prostate enlargement Interactions: ↑ Effects *OF* anticoagulants, cyclosporine, insulin, hypoglycemics, oxyphenbutazone; ↑ effects *W/* grapefruit juice; ↓ effects *W/* St. John's Wort Labs: ↑ AST, Cr, Hgb, Hct, LDL, serum alkaline phosphatase, bilirubin, Ca, K, & Na; ↓ thyroid hormones NIPE: Wear gloves if handling transdermal patches; topical drug may cause virilization in female partners. Apply Testoderm to dry shaved scrotal skin (⊘ use chemical depilatories), Androderm to nonscrotal skin, AndroGel to shoulder and upper arms, buccal system, on gum above incisors NIPE: Injectable testosterone enanthate (Delatestryl; Testro-L.A.) & cypionate (Depo-Testosterone) require inj every 14–28 d with highly variable serum levels; PO agents (methyltestosterone & oxandrolone) associated w/ hepatitis/hepatic tumors; transdermal/mucosal forms preferred

Tetanus Immune Globulin [Tetanus Prophylaxis/Immune Serum] Uses: *Passive tetanus immunization* (suspected contaminated wound w/ unknown immunization status, see also Table 8) Action: Passive immunization Dose: *Adults & Peds.* 250–500 units IM (higher dose w/ delayed Rx) Caution: [C, ?] Contra: Thimerosal sensitivity Disp: Inj 250-unit vial/syringe SE: Pain, tenderness, erythema at site; fever, angioedema, muscle stiffness, anaphylaxis Interactions: ↓ Immune response when admin *W/* Td NIPE: Drug does not cause AIDS or hepatitis; may begin active immunization series at different inj site if required

Tetanus Toxoid [Tetanus Prophylaxis/Vaccine] Uses: *Tetanus prophylaxis* Action: Active immunization Dose: Based on previous immunization, Table 8 Caution: [C, ?] Contra: Chloramphenicol use, neurologic Sxs w/ previous use, active Infxn w/ routine primary immunization Disp: Inj tetanus toxoid, fluid, 4–5 Lf units/0.5 mL; tetanus toxoid, adsorbed, 5, 10 Lf units/0.5 mL SE: Local erythema, induration, sterile abscess, chills, fever, neurologic disturbances Interactions: Delay of active immunity if given *W/* tetanus immune globulin; ↓ immune response if given to pts taking corticosteroids or immunosuppressive drugs NIPE: Stress the need of timely completion of immunization series

Tetracycline (Achromycin V, Sumycin) [Antibiotic/Tetracycline] Uses: *Broad-spectrum antibiotic* Action: Bacteriostatic; ↓ protein synth. Spectrum: Gram(+): *Staphylococcus* sp; *Streptococcus* sp; Gram(−): *H. pylori;* Atypicals: *Chlamydia* sp, *Rickettsia* sp, & *Mycoplasma* sp Dose: *Adults.* 250–500 mg PO bid-qid. *Peds > 8 y.* 25–50 mg/kg/24 h PO q6–12h; ↓ w/

renal/hepatic impair, w/o food preferred **Caution:** [D, +] **Contra:** PRG, antacids, w/ dairy products, children =8 y **Disp:** Caps 100, 250, 500 mg; tabs 250, 500 mg; PO susp 250 mg/5 mL **SE:** Photosens, GI upset, renal failure, pseudotumor cerebri, hepatic impair **Interactions:** ↑ Effects *OF* anticoagulants, digoxin; ↓ effects *W/* antacids, cimetidine, laxatives, penicillin, Fe supl, dairy products; ↓ effects *OF* OCPs **Labs:** False - of urinary glucose, serum folate; false ↑ serum glucose **NIPE:** ⊘ Take w/ dairy products; take w/o food; use barrier contraception; can stain tooth enamel & depress bone formation in children

Thalidomide (Thalomid) [Immunomodulatory Agent]

WARNING: Restricted use; use associated w/ severe birth defects and ↑ risk of venous thromboembolism **Uses:** *Erythema nodosum leprosum (ENL)*, GVHD, aphthous ulceration in HIV(+) **Action:** ↓ Neutrophil chemotaxis, ↓ monocyte phagocytosis **Dose:** *GVHD:* 100–1600 mg PO daily. *Stomatitis:* 200 mg bid for 5 d, then 200 mg daily up to 8 wk. *ENL:* 100–300 mg PO qhs **Cautions:** [X, –] May ↑ HIV viral load; h/o Szs **Contra:** PRG; sexually active males not using latex condoms, or females not using 2 forms of contraception **Disp:** 50, 100, 200 mg caps **SE:** Dizziness, drowsiness, rash, fever, orthostasis, Stevens–Johnson synd, peripheral neuropathy, Szs **Interactions:** ↑ Effects *OF* barbiturates, CNS depressants, chlorpromazine, reserpine, EtOH; ↑ peripheral neuropathy *W/* INH, Li, metronidazole, phenytoin **Labs:** Monitor LFTs, WBC, differential, PRG test before start of therapy & monthly during therapy **NIPE:** If also taking drugs that ↓ hormonal contraceptives (carbamazepine, griseofulvin, phenytoin, rifabutin, rifampin) use two other contraceptive methods; take 1 h pc—food will affect absorption; photosensitivity—use sunscreen; ⊘ PRG & breast-feeding; health care provider must register w/ STEPS risk management program; informed consent necessary; immediately D/C if rash develops

Theophylline (Theo24, TheoChron) [Bronchodilator/Xanthine Derivative]

Uses: *Asthma, bronchospasm* **Action:** Relaxes smooth muscle of the bronchi & pulm blood vessels **Dose:** *Adults.* 900 mg PO ÷ q6h; SR products may be ÷ q8–12h (maint). *Peds.* 16–22 mg/kg/24 h PO ÷ q6h; SR products may be ÷ q8–12h (maint); ↓ in hepatic failure **Caution:** [C, +] Multiple interactions (eg, caffeine, smoking, carbamazepine, barbiturates, β-blockers, ciprofloxacin, E-mycin, INH, loop diuretics) **Contra:** Arrhythmia, hyperthyroidism, uncontrolled Szs **Disp:** Elixir 80, 15 mL; soln 80 mg/15 mL; syrup 80, 150 mg/15 mL; caps 100, 200, 250 mg; tabs 100, 125, 200, 250, 300 mg; SR caps 100, 125, 200, 250, 260, 300 mg; SR tabs 100, 200, 300, 400, 450, 600 mg **SE:** N/V, tachycardia, Szs, nervousness, arrhythmias **Notes:** *Levels IV:* Sample 12–24 h after inf started; *Therapeutic:* 5–15 μg/mL; *Toxic:* >20 μg/mL; *1/2 life:* Non-smoking adults 8 h/children and smoking adults 4 h; *Levels PO:* Trough just before next dose; *Therapeutic:* 5–15 μg/mL **Interactions:** ↑ Effects *W/* allopurinol, BBs, CCBs, cimetidine, corticosteroids, macrolide antibiotics, OCPs, quinolones, rifampin, tacrine, tetracyclines, verapamil, zileuton; ↑ effects *OF* digitalis; ↓ effects *W/* barbiturates, loop diuretics, thyroid hormones, tobacco, St John's Wort; ↓ effects *OF* benzodiazepines, Li, phenytoin **Labs:** ↑ Glucose **NIPE:** Use barrier contraception; take w/ food if GI upset; caffeine foods ↑ drug effects; smoking ↓ drug effects

Thiamine [Vitamin B₁] [Vitamin] Uses: *Thiamine deficiency (beriberi), alcoholic neuritis, Wernicke encephalopathy* **Action:** Dietary suppl **Dose: *Adults.*** Deficiency: 100 mg/d IM for 2 wk, then 5–10 mg/d PO for 1 mo. *Wernicke encephalopathy:* 100 mg IV single dose, then 100 mg/d IM for 2 wk. ***Peds.*** 10–25 mg/d IM for 2 wk, then 5–10 mg/24 h PO for 1 mo **Caution:** [A (C if doses exceed RDA), +] **Contra:** Component allergy **Disp:** Tabs 5, 10, 25, 50, 100, 250, 500 mg; inj 100, 200 mg/mL **SE:** Angioedema, paresthesias, rash, anaphylaxis w/ rapid IV **Interactions:** ↑ Effects *OF* neuromuscular blocking drugs **Labs:** Interference w/ theophylline levels **NIPE:** Give IV slowly; IV use associated w/ anaphylactic Rxn

Thiethylperazine (Torecan) [Antiemetic] Uses: *N/V* **Action:** Antidopaminergic antiemetic **Dose:** 10 mg PO, PR, or IM daily–tid; ↓ in hepatic failure **Caution:** [X, ?] **Contra:** Phenothiazine & sulfite sensitivity, PRG **Disp:** Tabs 10 mg; supp 10 mg; inj 5 mg/mL **SE:** EPS, xerostomia, drowsiness, orthostatic ↓ BP, tachycardia, confusion **Interactions:** ↑ Effects *W/* atropine, CNS depressants, epinephrine, Li, MAOIs, TCAs, EtOH; ↑ effects *OF* antihypertensives, phenytoin; ↓ effects *OF* bromocriptine, cabergoline, levodopa **Labs:** ↑ Serum prolactin level, interferes w/ PRG test **NIPE:** May cause tardive dyskinesia; ↑ risk of photosensitivity—use sunscreen

6-Thioguanine [6-TG] (Tabloid) [Purine Antimetabolite] Uses: *AML, ALL, CML* **Action:** Purine-based antimetabolite (substitutes for natural purines interfering w/ nucleotide synth) **Dose:** 2–3 mg/kg/d; ↓ in severe renal/hepatic impair **Caution:** [D, –] **Contra:** Resistance to mercaptopurine **Disp:** Tabs 40 mg **SE:** BM (leucopenia/thrombocytopenia), N/V/D, anorexia, stomatitis, rash, hyperuricemia, rare hepatotox **Interactions:** ↑ Bleeding *W/* anticoagulants, NSAIDs, salicylates, thrombolytics **Labs:** ↑ Serum and urine uric acid **NIPE:** Take w/o food; ↑ fluids to 2–3 L/d; ⊘ exposure to Infxn

Thioridazine   (Mellaril)   [Antipsychotic/Phenothiazine] **WARNING:** Dose-related QT prolongation Uses: *Schizophrenia*, psychosis **Action:** Phenothiazine antipsychotic **Dose: *Adults.*** Initial, 50–100 mg PO tid; maint 200–800 mg/24 h PO in 2–4 ÷ doses. ***Peds >2 y.*** 0.5–3 mg/kg/24 h PO in 2–3 ÷ doses **Caution:** [C, ?] Phenothiazine, QTc-prolonging agents, aluminum **Contra:** Phenothiazine sensitivity **Disp:** Tabs 10, 15, 25, 50, 100, 150, 200 mg; PO conc 30, 100 mg/mL; **SE:** Low incidence of EPS; ventricular arrhythmias; ↓ BP, dizziness, drowsiness, neuroleptic malignant synd, Szs, skin discoloration, photosens, constipation, sexual dysfunction, blood dyscrasias, pigmentary retinopathy, hepatic impair **Interactions:** ↑ Effects *W/* BBs; ↑ effects *OF* anticholinergics, antihypertensives, antihistamines, CNS depressants, nitrates, EtOH; ↓ effects *W/*

barbiturates, Li, tobacco; ↓ effects *OF* levodopa **Labs:** ↑ Serum LFTs; ↓ HMG, Hct, plts, WBC **NIPE:** ↑ Risk of photosensitivity—use sunscreen, take w/ food; ⊘ D/C abruptly; ↓ temp regulation; urine color change to reddish brown; avoid EtOH, dilute PO conc in 2–4 oz Liq

Thiothixene (Navane) [Antipsychotic/Thioxanthene] Uses: *Psychotic disorders* **Action:** Antipsychotic **Dose:** *Adults & Peds > 12 y. Mild–moderate psychosis:* 2 mg PO tid, up to 20–30 mg/d. *Severe psychosis:* 5 mg PO bid; ↑ to max of 60 mg/24 h PRN. *IM use:* 16–20 mg/24 h ÷ bid–qid; max 30 mg/d. *Peds < 12 y.* 0.25 mg/kg/24 h PO ÷ q6–12h **Caution:** [C, ?] **Contra:** Phenothiazine sensitivity **Disp:** Caps 1, 2, 5, 10, 20 mg; PO conc 5 mg/mL; inj 10 mg/mL **SE:** Drowsiness, EPS most common; ↓ BP, dizziness, drowsiness, neuroleptic malignant synd, Szs, skin discoloration, photosens, constipation, sexual dysfunction, blood dyscrasias, pigmentary retinopathy, hepatic impair **Interactions:** ↑ Effects *W/* BBs; ↑ effects *OF* anticholinergics, antihistamines, antihypertensives, CNS depressants, nitrates, EtOH; ↓ effects *W/* barbiturates, Li, tobacco, caffeine; ↓ effects *OF* levodopa **Labs:** ↑ LFTs **NIPE:** ↑ Risk *OF* photosensitivity—use sunscreen; take w/ food; ⊘ D/C abruptly; ↓ temp regulation; darkens urine color; dilute PO conc immediately before use

Tiagabine (Gabitril) [Anticonvulsant] Uses: *Adjunct in partial Szs*, bipolar disorder **Action:** Inhibition of GABA **Dose:** *Adults & Peds = 12 y.* Initial 4 mg/d PO, ↑ by 4 mg during 2nd wk; ↑ PRN by 4–8 mg/d based on response, 56 mg/d max; w/food **Caution:** [C, M] **Contra:** Component allergy **Disp:** Tabs 2, 4, 12, 16 , 20 mg **SE:** Dizziness, HA, somnolence, memory impair, tremors **Interactions:** ↑ Effects *W/* valproate; ↑ effects *OF* CNS depressants, EtOH; ↓ effects *W/* barbiturates, carbamazepine, phenobarbital, phenytoin, primidone, rifampin, ginkgo biloba **NIPE:** Take w/ food; ⊘ D/C abruptly; used in combo w/ other anticonvulsants

Ticarcillin (Ticar) [Antibiotic/Penicillin] Uses: *Infxns due to gram(–) bacteria* (*Klebsiella* sp, *Proteus* sp, *E. coli, Enterobacter* sp, *P. aeruginosa, & Serratia* sp) involving the skin, bone, resp & urinary tract, abdomen, sepsis **Action:** 4th-gen PCN, bactericidal; ↓ cell wall synth. **Spectrum:** Some gram(+) (*Streptococcus* sp, fair *Enterococcus* sp, not MRSA), gram(–) enhanced w/ aminoglycoside use; good anaerobes (*Bacteroides* sp) **Dose:** *Adults.* 3 g IV q4–6h. *Peds.* 200–300 mg/kg/d IV ÷ q4–6h; ↓ w/in renal insuff failure **Caution:** [B, +] PCN sensitivity, renal impair, Sz h/o, Na restriction **Contra:** Allergy to class **Disp:** Inj 1, 3, 6, 20, 30 g **SE:** Interstitial nephritis, anaphylaxis, bleeding, rash, hemolytic anemia **Interactions:** ↑ Effects *W/* probenecid; ↑ effects *OF* anticoagulants, MTX; ↓ effects *W/* tetracyclines, ↓ effects *OF* aminoglycosides **Labs:** ↑ LFTs **NIPE:** Monitor for S/Sxs super Infxn; frequent loose stools may be due to pseudomembranous colitis; used in combo w/ aminoglycosides

Ticarcillin/Potassium Clavulanate (Timentin) [Antibiotic/Penicillin, Beta-Lactamase Inhibitor] Uses: *Infxns of the skin, bone, resp & urinary tract, abdomen, sepsis * **Action:** 4th-gen PCN; bactericidal; ↓ cell wall synth; clavulanic acid blocks β-lactamase. *Spectrum:* Good gram(+), not MRSA; good gram(–) & anaerobes **Dose:** *Adults.* 3.1 g IV q4–6h. *Peds.* 200–300 mg/kg/d IV ÷ q4–6h; ↓ in renal failure **Caution:** [B, +/–] PCN sensitivity **Disp:** Inj 3g/1g IM **SE:** Hemolytic anemia, false + proteinuria; **Interactions:** ↑ Effects *W/* probenecid; ↑ effects *OF* anticoagulants, MRX; ↓ effects *W/* tetracyclines, ↓ effects *OF* aminoglycosides, OCPs **Labs:** False ↑ urine glucose, false + urine proteins **NIPE:** Monitor for S/Sxs super Infxn; frequent loose stools may be due to pseudomembranous colitis; use barrier contraception; often used in combo w/ aminoglycosides; penetrates CNS with meningeal irritation; see also ticarcillin

Ticlopidine (Ticlid) [Antiplatelet/Platelet Aggregation Inhibitor] WARNING: Neutropenia/agranulocytosis, TTP, aplastic anemia reported Uses: *↓ Risk of thrombotic stroke*, protect grafts status post CABG, diabetic microangiopathy, ischemic heart Dz, DVT prophylaxis, graft prophylaxis after renal transplant **Action:** Plt aggregation inhibitor **Dose:** 250 mg PO bid w/ food **Caution:** [B, ?/–], ↑ tox of ASA, anticoagulation, NSAIDs, theophylline **Contra:** Bleeding, hepatic impair, neutropenia, thrombocytopenia **Disp:** Tabs 250 mg **SE:** Bleeding, GI upset, rash **Interactions:** ↑ Effects *W/* anticoagulants, cimetidine, dong quai, evening primrose oil, feverfew, garlic, ginkgo biloba, ginseng, red clover; ↑ effects *OF* ASA, phenytoin, theophylline; ↓ effects *W/* antacids; ↓ effects *OF* cyclosporine, digoxin **Labs:** ↑ LFTs; ↓ plts, RBCs, WBCs; monitor CBC for 1st 3 mo **NIPE:** Take w/food

Tigecycline (Tygacil) [Antibiotic/Related to Tetracycline] Uses: *Rx complicated skin & soft tissue Infxns, & complicated intra-abd Infxns* **Action:** New class: related to tetracycline; *Spectrum:* Broad gram(+), gram(–), anaerobic, some mycobacterial; *E. coli, E. faecalis* (vanco-susceptible isolates), *S. aureus* (meth-susceptible/resistant), *Streptococcus* (*agalactiae, anginosus* grp, *pyogenes*), *C. freundii, E. cloacae, B. fragilis* group, *C. perfringens, Peptostreptococcus* sp **Dose:** *Adults.* 100 mg, then 50 mg q12h IV over 30–60 min every 12 h **Caution:** [D, ?] hepatic impair, monotherapy w/ intestinal perf, not OK in peds **Contra:** Component sensitivity **Disp:** Inj 50 mg vial **SE:** N/V, inj site Rxn **Interactions:** ↑ Risk of bleeding *W/* warfarin; ↓ effectiveness *OF* hormonal contraceptives **Labs:** ↑ LFTs, BUN, Cr, PT, PTT, INR; ↓ K⁺, HMG, Hct, WBCs **NIPE:** ⊘ with children

Timolol (Blocadren) [Antihypertensive/BB] WARNING: Exacerbation of ischemic heart Dz w/ abrupt D/C **Uses:** *HTN & MI* **Action:** β-Adrenergic receptor blocker, β₁, β₂ **Dose:** *HTN:* 10–20 mg bid, up to 60 mg/d. *MI:* 10 mg bid **Caution:** [C (1st tri; D if 2nd or 3rd tri), +] **Contra:** CHF, cardiogenic shock, bradycardia, heart block, COPD, asthma **Disp:** Tabs 5, 10, 20 mg **SE:** Sexual dysfunction, arrhythmia, dizziness, fatigue, CHF **Interactions:** ↑ Effects *W/* antihypertensives, ciprofloxacin, fentanyl, nitrates, quinidine, reserpine; ↑ bradycardia and myocardial depression *W/* cardiac glycosides, diltiazem, reserpine, tacrine,

verapamil; ↑ effects *OF* epinephrine, ergots, flecainide, lidocaine, nifedipine, phenothiazine, prazosin, verapamil; ↓ effects *W/* barbiturates, cholestyramine, colestipol, NSAIDs, penicillin, rifampin, salicylates, sulfinpyrazone, theophylline; ↓ effect *OF* hypoglycemics, sulfonylureas, theophylline **Labs:** ↑ BUN, K⁺, LFTs, uric acid **NIPE:** ⊘ D/C abruptly; ↑ cold sensitivity

Timolol, Ophthalmic (Timoptic) [Antiglaucoma Agent/BB]
Uses: *Glaucoma* **Action:** β-Blocker **Dose:** 0.25% 1 gt bid; ↓ to daily when controlled; use 0.5% if needed; 1 gtt/d gel **Caution:** [C (1st tri; D 2nd or 3rd), ?/+] **Disp:** Soln 0.25/0.5%; Timoptic XR (0.25, 0.5%) gel-forming soln **SE:** Local irritation; see Timolol, above **Additional NIPE:** Depress lacrimal sac 1 min after admin to lessen systemic absorption; admin other drops 10 min before gel

Tinidazole (Tindamax) [Antiprotozoal/Anti-infective]
WARNING: Off-label use discouraged (animal carcinogenicity w/ other drugs in class) **Uses:** *Adults/children >3 y.* *Trichomoniasis & giardiasis; intestinal amebiasis or amebic liver abscess* **Action:** Antiprotozoal nitroimidazole; *Spectrum:* T. vaginalis, G. duodenalis, E. histolytica **Dose:** *Adults.* Trichomoniasis: 2 g PO; Rx partner; *Giardiasis:* 2 g PO; *Amebiasis:* 2 g PO daily × 3; *Amebic liver abscess:* 2 g PO daily × 3–5; *Peds.* Trichomoniasis: 50 mg/kg PO, 2 g/d max; *Giardiasis:* 50 mg/kg PO, 2 g max; *Amebiasis:* 50 mg/kg PO daily × 3, 2 g/d max; *Amebic liver abscess:* 50 mg/kg PO daily × 3–5, 2 g/d max; w/ food **Caution:** [C, D in 1st tri; -] May be cross-resistant with metronidazole; Sz/peripheral neuropathy may require D/C; w/ CNS/hepatic impair **Contra:** Metronidazole allergy, 1st tri PRG, w/ EtOH use **Disp:** Tabs 250, 500 **SE:** CNS disturbances; blood dyscrasias, taste disturbances, N/V, darkens urine **Interactions:** ↑ Effects *OF* anticoagulants, cyclosporine, fluorouracil, lithium, phenytoin, tacrolimus; ↑ effects *W/* cimetidine, ketoconazole; ↑ effects *OF* abd cramping, N/V, HA *W/* disulfiram, EtOH; ↓ effects *W/* cholestyramine, oxytetracycline, phenobarbital, rifampin **Labs:** ↑ LFTs **NIPE:** Crush & disperse in cherry syrup for peds; removed by HD; D/C EtOH during & 3 d after Rx

Tinzaparin (Innohep) [Anticoagulant/LMW Heparin]
WARNING: Risk of spinal/epidural hematomas development w/ spinal anesthesia or lumbar puncture **Uses:** *Rx of DVT w/ or w/o PE* **Action:** LMW heparin **Dose:** 175 units/kg SQ daily at least 6 d until warfarin dose stabilized **Caution:** [B, ?] Pork allergy, active bleeding, mild–moderate renal dysfunction **Contra:** Allergy to sulfites, heparin, benzyl alcohol, HIT **Disp:** Inj 20,000 units/mL **SE:** Bleeding, bruising, thrombocytopenia, inj site pain **Interactions:** ↑ Bleeding *W/* anticoagulants, NSAIDs, salicylates, thrombolytics **Labs:** ↑ LFTs; monitor via anti-Xa levels; *no effect on:* bleeding time, plt Fxn, PT, aPTT **NIPE:** ⊘ Rub inj site, admin deep SQ inj, rotate abd inj sites; causes inj site pain

Tioconazole (Vagistat) [Antifungal]
Uses: *Vaginal fungal Infxns* **Action:** Topical antifungal **Dose:** 1 applicatorful intravag hs (single dose) **Caution:** [C, ?] **Contra:** Component allergy **Disp:** Vag oint 6.5% **SE:** Local burning, itching,

soreness, polyuria **Interactions:** Risk *OF* inactivation of nonoxynol-9 spermacidal **NIPE:** Insert high into vag canal; may cause staining of clothing; refrain from intercourse during drug therapy; risk of latex breakdown of condoms and diaphragm

Tiotropium (Spiriva) [Bronchodilator/Anticholinergic] **Uses:** Bronchospasm w/ COPD, bronchitis, emphysema **Action:** Synthetic anticholinergic-like atropine **Dose:** 1 cap/d inhaled using HandiHaler, *do not* use w/ spacer **Caution:** [C, ?/–] BPH, NAG, MyG, renal impair **Contra:** Acute bronchospasm **Disp:** Inhalation Caps 18 µg **SE:** URI, xerostomia **Interactions:** ↑ Effects *W/* other anticholinergic drugs **Labs:** Monitor FEV$_1$ or peak flow **NIPE:** ⊘ For acute resp episode; take daily at same time

Tipranavir (Aptivus) [Antiretroviral/Protease Inhibitor] **WARNING:** Coadministration w/ ritonavir assoc w/ hepatitis & hepatic decomp w/ fatalities. D/C w/ S/Sxs of hepatitis **Uses:** HIV 1 Infxn w/ highly treatment-experienced pts or HIV 1 strains resistant to multiple protease inhibitors. Must be used w/ ritonavir 200 mg. **Action:** Antiretroviral HIV-1 protease inhibitor **Dose:** 500 mg PO bid w/ food, administer w/ ritonavir 200 mg PO bid **Caution:** [C, –] sulfa allergy, liver Dz **Contra:** Moderate–severe hepatic insuff; concomitant use w/ amiodarone, astemizole, bepridil, cisapride, ergots, flecainide, lovastatin, midazolam, pimozide, propafenone, quinidine, rifampin, simvastatin, terfenadine, triazolam, St. John's Wort **Disp:** Soft gel cap 250 µg; **SE:** HA, GI distress, rash, fatigue, fat redistribution, hyperglycemia, hepatitis, liver Dz, lipid elevations **Interactions:** ↑ Effects *OF* anticoagulants, antiplts, azole antifungals, CCB, clarithromycin, NNRTIs, rifabutin, sildenafil, statins, tadalafil, vardenafil; ↓ effects *W/* antacids, didanosine; ↓ effects OF estrogens, methadone **Labs:** ↑ BS, LFTs, lipids, monitor baseline and periodically **NIPE:** ↑ Bioavailability *W/* high-fat meals; monitor for bleeding in pts w/ hemophilia

Tirofiban (Aggrastat) [Antiplatelet Agent] **Uses:** *Acute coronary synd* **Action:** Glycoprotein IIB/IIIa inhibitor **Dose:** Initial 0.4 µg/kg/min for 30 min, followed by 0.1 µg/kg/min; use in combo w/ heparin; *ACS or PCI:* 0.4 µg/kg/min IV for 30 min, then 0.1 µg/kg/min *(ECC 2005):* ↓ in renal insuff **Caution:** [B, ?/–] **Contra:** Bleeding, intracranial neoplasm, vascular malformation, stroke/surgery/trauma w/in last 30 d, severe HTN **Disp:** Inj 50, 250 µg/mL **SE:** Bleeding, bradycardia, coronary dissection, pelvic pain, rash **Interactions:** ↑ Bleeding risks *W/* anticoagulants, antiplts, NSAIDs, salicylates, dong quai, feverfew, garlic, ginger, ginkgo, horse chestnut; ↓ effects *W/* levothyroxine, omeprazole **Labs:** ↓ HMG, Hct, plts **NIPE:** ⊘ Breast-feeding

Tobramycin (Nebcin) [Antibiotic/Aminoglycoside] **Uses:** *Serious gram(–) Infxns* **Action:** Aminoglycoside; ↓ protein synth. *Spectrum:* Gram(–) bacteria (including *Pseudomonas* sp) **Dose:** *Adults.* 1–2.5 mg/kg/dose IV q8–24h. *Peds.* 2.5 mg/kg/dose IV q8h; ↓ w/ renal insuff **Caution:** [C, M] **Contra:**

Aminoglycoside sensitivity **Disp:** Inj 10, 40 mg/mL **SE:** Nephrotox & ototox **Notes:** Follow CrCl & levels; *Levels: Peak:* 30 min after inf; *Trough:* <0.5 h before next dose; *Therapeutic: Peak:* 5–8 µg/mL, *Trough:* <2 µg/mL; *Toxic peak:* > 12 µg/mL; *1/2 life:* 2 h **Interactions:** ↑ Effects *W/* indomethacin; ↑ nephrotoxic, neurotoxic, and/or ototoxic effects *W/* aminoglycosides, amphotericin B, cephalosporins, cisplatin, IV loop diuretics, methoxyflurane, vancomycin **Labs:** ↑BUN, Cr; ↓ serum K⁺, Na⁺, Ca²⁺, Mg²⁺, plt, WBC; **NIPE:** ↑ Fluids to 2–3 L/d; monitor for super Infxn

Tobramycin Ophthalmic (AKTob, Tobrex) [Antibiotic/ Aminoglycoside] Uses: *Ocular bacterial Infxns* **Action:** Aminoglycoside **Dose:** 1–2 gtt q4h; oint bid–tid; if severe, use oint q3–4h, or 2 gtt q30–60 min, then less frequently **Caution:** [C, M] **Contra:** Aminoglycoside sensitivity **Disp:** Oint & soln tobramycin 0.3% **SE:** Ocular irritation; see Tobramycin **Additional NIPE:** Depress lacrimal sac for 1 min to prevent systemic absorption; ↑ risk of blurred vision & burning

Tobramycin & Dexamethasone Ophthalmic (TobraDex) [Antibiotic/Anti-inflammatory] Uses: *Ocular bacterial Infxns associated w/ significant inflammation* **Action:** Antibiotic w/ anti-inflammatory **Dose:** 0.3% oint apply q3–8h or soln 0.3% apply 1–2 gtt q1–4h **Caution:** [C, M] **Contra:** Aminoglycoside sensitivity **Disp:** Oint & susp 2.5, 5 & 10 mL tobramycin 0.3% & dexamethasone 0.1% **SE:** Local irritation/edema; see Tobramycin **Additional NIPE:** Eval intraocular pressure and lens if prolonged use; use under ophthalmologist's direction

Tolazamide (Tolinase) [Hypoglycemic/Sulfonylurea] Uses: *Type 2 DM* **Action:** Sulfonylurea; ↑ pancreatic insulin release; ↑ peripheral insulin sensitivity; ↓ hepatic glucose output **Dose:** 100–500 mg/d (no benefit >1 g/d) **Caution:** [C, +/–] Elderly, renal or hepatic impair **Disp:** Tabs 100, 250, 500 mg **SE:** HA, dizziness, GI upset, rash, hyperglycemia, photosens, blood dyscrasias **Interactions:** ↑ Effects *W/* chloramphenicol, cimetidine, clofibrate, insulin, MAOIs, phenylbutazone, probenecid, salicylates, sulfonamides, garlic, ginseng; ↓ effects *W/* diuretics **NIPE:** Risk of disulfiram-type Rxn w/ EtOH; take w/ food; use sunscreen

Tolazoline (Priscoline) [Alpha Adrenergic Antagonist] Uses: *Peripheral vasospastic disorders* **Action:** Competitively blocks α-adrenergic receptors **Dose:** *Adults.* 10–50 mg IM/IV/SQ qid. *Neonates.* 1–2 mg/kg IV over 10–15 min, then 1–2 mg/kg/h (adjust w/ ↓ renal Fxn) **Caution:** Avoid alcohol, w/ CAD, renal impairment, CVA, PUD, ↓ BP [C, ?] **Contra:** CAD **Disp:** Inj 25 mg/mL **SE:** ↓ BP, peripheral vasodilation, tachycardia, arrhythmias, GI upset & bleeding, blood dyscrasias, renal failure **Interactions:** ↓ BP *W/* epinephrine, norepinephrine, phenylephrine **NIPE:** Risk of disulfiram-type Rxn w/ EtOH

Tolbutamide (Orinase) [Hypoglycemic/Sulfonylurea] Uses: *Type 2 DM* **Action:** Sulfonylurea; ↑ pancreatic insulin release; ↑ peripheral insulin sensitivity; ↓ hepatic glucose output **Dose:** 500–1000 mg bid; 3 g/d max; ↓ in hepatic failure **Caution:** [C, +] **Contra:** Sulfonylurea sensitivity **Disp:** Tabs 250,

500 mg **SE:** HA, dizziness, GI upset, rash, photosens, blood dyscrasias, hypoglycemia, heartburn **Interactions:** ↑ Effects **W/** anticoagulants, azole antifungals, chloramphenicol, insulin, H_2 antagonists, metformin, phenylbutazone, probenecid, salicylates, sulfonamides, TCAs; ↓ effects **W/** BBs, CCBs, cholestyramine, corticosteroids, hydantoins, INH, OCPs, phenothiazine, phenytoin, rifampin, sympathomimetics, thiazides, thyroid drugs **NIPE:** Risk **OF** disulfiram-type Rxn **W/** EtOH; take w/ food; use barrier contraception; ↑ risk **OF** photosensitivity—use sunscreen

Tolcapone (Tasmar) [Anti-Parkinson Agent/COMT Inhibitor]
WARNING: Cases of fulminant liver failure resulting in death have occurred **Uses:** *Adjunct to carbidopa/levodopa in Parkinson Dz* **Action:** Catechol-O-methyltransferase inhibitor slows levodopa metabolism **Dose:** 100 mg PO tid w/ 1st daily levodopa/carbidopa dose, then dose 6 & 12 h later; ↓ w/ renal impair **Caution:** [C, ?] **Contra:** Hepatic impair; w/ nonselective MAOI **Disp:** Tabs 100 mg, 200 mg **SE:** Constipation, xerostomia, vivid dreams, hallucinations, anorexia, N/D, orthostasis, liver failure, Rhabdomyolysis **Interactions:** ↑ Effects **OF** CNS depressants, SSRIs, TCAs, warfarin, EtOH; ↑ risk **OF** hypertensive crisis with nonselective MAOIs (phenelzine, tranylcypromine) **Labs:** Monitor LFTs **NIPE:** May give w/o regard to food but food ↓ bioavailability of drug, may experience hallucinations; do not abruptly D/C or ↓ dose

Tolmetin (Tolectin) [Analgesic, Anti-inflammatory, Antipyretic/NSAID]
WARNING: May ↑ risk of cardiovascular events & GI bleeding **Uses:** *Arthritis & pain* **Action:** NSAID; ↓ prostaglandins **Dose:** 200–600 mg PO tid; 2000 mg/d max **Caution:** [C (D in 3rd tri or near term), +] **Contra:** NSAID or ASA sensitivity; use for pain post CABG **Disp:** Tabs 200, 600 mg; caps 400 mg **SE:** Dizziness, rash, GI upset, edema, GI bleeding, renal failure **Interactions:** ↑ Effect **OF** aminoglycosides, anticoagulants, cyclosporine, digoxin, insulin, Li, MRX, K-sparing diuretics, sulfonylureas; ↓ effect **W/** ASA, food; ↓ effect **OF** furosemide, thiazides **Labs:** ↑ ALT, AST, serum K^+, BUN, ↓ HMG, Hct **NIPE:** Take w/ food if GI upset; ↑ risk of photosensitivity—use sunscreen

Tolnaftate (Tinactin) [OTC] [Antifungal]
Uses: *Tinea pedis, cruris, corporis, manus, versicolor* **Action:** Topical antifungal **Dose:** Apply to area bid for 2–4 wk **Caution:** [C, ?] **Contra:** Nail & scalp Infxns **Disp:** OTC 1% Liq; gel; powder; topical cream; oint, powder, spray soln **SE:** Local irritation **NIPE:** Avoid ocular contact; Infxn should improve in 7–10 d; ⊘ with children <2 y

Tolterodine (Detrol, Detrol LA) [Anticholinergic/Muscarinic Antagonist]
Uses: *OAB (frequency, urgency, incontinence)* **Action:** Anticholinergic **Dose:** Detrol 1–2 mg PO bid; Detrol LA 2–4 mg/d **Caution:** [C, ?/–] w/ CYP2D6 & 3A3/4 inhibitor (Table 11) **Contra:** Urinary retention, gastric retention, or uncontrolled NAG **Disp:** Tabs 1, 2 mg; Detrol LA tabs 2, 4 mg **SE:** Xerostomia, blurred vision, headache, constipation **Interactions:** ↑ Effects **W/** azole

antifungals, macrolides, grapefruit juice, food; ↑ anticholinergic effects *W/* amantadine, amoxapine, bupropion, clozapine, cyclobenzaprine, disopyramide, olanzapine, phenothiazine, TCAs **NIPE:** May cause blurred vision; LA form may see "intact" pills in stool

Topiramate (Topamax) [Anticonvulsant] Uses: *Adjunctive Rx for complex partial Szs & tonic–clonic Szs*, bipolar disorder, neuropathic pain, migraine prophylaxis **Action:** Anticonvulsant **Dose:** *Adults. Sz:* Total dose 400 mg/d; see insert for 8-wk titration schedule. *Migraine prophylaxis:* Titrate 100 m/d total **Peds 2–16 y:** Initial, 1–3 mg/kg/d PO qhs; titrate per insert to 5–9 mg/kg/d; ↓ w/ renal impair **Caution:** [C, ?/–] **Contra:** Component allergy **Disp:** Tabs 25, 50, 100, 200 mg; caps sprinkles 15, 25, 50 mg **SE:** Wt loss, memory impair, metabolic acidosis, kidney stones, fatigue, dizziness, psychomotor slowing, paresthesias, GI upset, tremor, nystagmus, acute glaucoma requiring D/C **Interactions:** ↑ CNS effects *W/* CNS depressants, EtOH; ↑ effects *OF* phenytoin; ↓ effects *W/* carbamazepine, phenytoin, valproate, ginkgo biloba; ↓ effects *OF* digoxin, OCPs **Labs:** ↑ LFTs **NIPE:** Take w/o regard to food; ⊘ D/C abruptly; use barrier contraception; ↑ fluids to 2–3 L/d; metabolic acidosis responsive to ↓ dose or D/C; D/C requires taper

Topotecan (Hycamtin) [Antineoplastic] **WARNING:** Chemo precautions, for use by health care providers familiar with chemotherapeutic agents, BM suppression possible Uses: *Ovarian CA (cisplatin-refractory), cervical Ca, NSCLC*, sarcoma, breast, ped non-small-cell lung CA **Action:** Topoisomerase I inhibitor; ↓ DNA synth **Dose:** 1.5 mg/m²/d as a 1-h IV inf × 5 d, repeat q3wk; ↓ w/ renal impair **Caution:** [D, –] **Contra:** PRG, breast-feeding **Disp:** Inj 4-mg vials **SE:** ↓ BM, N/V/D, drug fever, skin rash **Interactions:** ↑ Myelosuppression *W/* cisplatin, other neoplastic drugs, radiation therapy; ↑ in duration of neutropenia *W/* filgrastim **Labs:** ↑ AST, ALT, bilirubin; ↓ HMG, Hct, plt, WBCs **NIPE:** Monitor CBC; ⊘ PRG, breast-feeding, immunizations; ⊘ exposure to Infxn; use barrier contraception

Torsemide (Demadex) [Antihypertensive/Loop Diuretic] Uses: *Edema, HTN, CHF, & hepatic cirrhosis* **Action:** Loop diuretic; ↓ reabsorption of Na⁺ & Cl⁻ in ascending loop of Henle & distal tubule **Dose:** 5–20 mg/d PO or IV; 200 mg/d max **Caution:** [B, ?] **Contra:** Sulfonylurea sensitivity **Disp:** Tabs 5, 10, 20, 100 mg; inj 10 mg/mL **SE:** Orthostatic ↓ BP, HA, dizziness, photosens, electrolyte imbalance, blurred vision, renal impair **Notes:** 20 mg torsemide = 40 mg furosemide **Interactions:** ↑ Risk of ototox *W/* aminoglycosides, cisplatin; ↑ effects *W/* thiazides; ↑ effects *OF* anticoagulants, antihypertensives, Li, salicylates; ↓ effects *W/* barbiturates, carbamazepine, cholestyramine, NSAIDs, phenytoin, phenobarbital, probenecid , dandelion **Labs:** Monitor electrolytes, BUN, Cr, glucose, uric acid **NIPE:** Take w/o regard to food; monitor for S/Sxs tinnitus

Tramadol (Ultram, Ultram ER) [Centrally Acting Analgesic/Nonnarcotic] Uses: *Moderate–severe pain* **Action:** Centrally acting analgesic **Dose:** *Adults.* 50–100 mg PO q4–6h PRN, start 25 mg PO qAM, ↑ q3d to 25 mg PO qid; ↑ 50 mg q3d, 400 mg/d max (300 mg if >75 y); XR 100–300 mg PO daily **Peds.** 0.5–1 mg/kg PO q4–6h PRN; ↓ w/ renal insuff **Caution:** [C, ?/–] **Contra:** Opioid dependency; w/ MAOIs; sensitivity to codeine **Disp:** Tabs 50 mg; XR 10, 20, 30 mg **SE:** Dizziness, HA, somnolence, GI upset, resp depression, anaphylaxis **Interactions:** ↑ Effects **W/** antihistamines, CNS depressants, phenothiazine, quinidine, TCAs, EtOH; ↑ risk of serotonin synd **W/** MAOIs, St. John's Wort; ↑ effects **OF** digoxin, warfarin; ↓ effects **W/** carbamazepine **Labs:** ↑ Cr, LFTs, ↓ HMG **NIPE:** Take w/o regard to food; ↓ Sz threshold; tolerance or dependence may develop

Tramadol/Acetaminophen (Ultracet) [Centrally Acting Analgesic/Nonnarcotic] Uses: *Short-term Rx acute pain (<5 d)* Action:
Centrally acting analgesic; nonnarcotic analgesic **Dose:** 2 tabs PO q4–6h PRN; 8 tabs/d max. **Elderly/renal impair:** Lowest possible dose; 2 tabs q12h max if CrCl <30 **Caution:** [C, –] Szs, hepatic/renal impair, or h/o addictive tendencies **Contra:** Acute intox **Disp:** Tab 37.5 mg tramadol/325 mg APAP **SE:** SSRIs, TCAs, opioids, MAOIs ↑ risk of Szs; dizziness, somnolence, tremor, HA, N/V/D, constipation, xerostomia, liver tox, rash, pruritus, ↑ sweating, physical dependence **Interactions:** ↑ Effects **W/** CNS depressants, MAOIs, phenothiazines, quinidine, TCAs, EtOH; ↑ risk of serotonin synd **W/** MAOIs, St. John's Wort; ↑ effects **OF** digoxin, warfarin; ↓ effects **W/** carbamazepine **Labs:** ↑ Cr, LFTs, ↓ HMG **NIPE:** Take w/o regard to food; ⊘ take other acetaminophen-containing drugs; avoid EtOH

Trandolapril (Mavik) [Antihypertensive/ACEI] WARNING:
Use in PRG in 2nd/3rd tri can result in fetal death **Uses:** *HTN*, CHF, LVD, post-AMI **Action:** ACE inhibitor **Dose:** HTN: 2–4 mg/d; CHF/LVD: 4 mg/d; ↓ w/ severe renal/hepatic impair **Caution:** [D, +] ACE inhibitor sensitivity, angioedema w/ ACE inhibitors **Disp:** Tabs 1, 2, 4 mg **SE:** ↓ BP, bradycardia, dizziness, ↑ K+, GI upset, renal impair, cough, angioedema **Notes:** Afro-Americans, minimum dose is 2 mg vs 1 mg in Caucasians **Interactions:** ↑ Effects **W/** diuretics; ↑ effects **OF** insulin, Li; ↓ effects **W/** ASA, NSAIDs **NIPE:** ⊘ Take if PRG or breast-feeding; ⊘ K-containing salt substitutes

Trastuzumab (Herceptin) [Antineoplastic/Monoclonal Antibody] WARNING: Can cause cardiomyopathy and ventricular dysfunction;
infusion Rxns and pulm tox reported **Uses:** *Met breast CA that over express the HER2/neu protein* breast CA adjuvant, w/ doxorubicin, cyclophosphamide, and paclitaxel if pt HER2/neu(+) **Action:** MoAb; binds human EGF receptor 2 protein (HER2); mediates cellular cytotox **Dose:** Per protocol, vary 2 mg/kg/IV/wk **Caution:** [B, ?] CV dysfunction, allergy/inf Rxns **Contra:** Live vaccines **Disp:** Inj form 21 mg/mL **SE:** Anemia, cardiomyopathy, nephrotic synd, pneumonitis **Interactions:** ↑ Risk of cardiac dysfunction **W/** anthracyclines, cyclophosphamide, doxorubicin, epirubicin **Labs:** Monitor cardiac function; ↓ HMG, Hct, WBCs **NIPE:** ⊘ Use dextrose inf soln; ⊘ breast-feed for 6 mo following drug therapy; inf related Rxns minimized w/ acetaminophen, diphenhydramine & meperidine

Trazodone (Desyrel) [Antidepressant]   WARNING: Closely monitor for worsening depression or emergence of suicidality, particularly in pts <24 y **Uses:** *Depression*, hypnotic, augment other antidepressants **Action:** Antidepressant; ↓ reuptake of serotonin & norepinephrine **Dose:** *Adults & Adolescents.* 50–150 mg PO daily–qid; max 600 mg/d. *Sleep:* 50 mg PO, qhs, PRN **Caution:** [C, ?/–] **Contra:** Component allergy **Disp:** Tabs 50, 100, 150, 300 mg **SE:** Dizziness, HA, sedation, N, xerostomia, syncope, confusion, tremor, hepatitis, EPS **Interactions:** ↑ Effects *W/* fluoxetine, phenothiazines; ↑ risk of serotonin syndrome *W/* MAOIs, SSRIs, venlafaxine, St. John's Wort; ↑ CNS depression *W/* barbiturates, CNS depressants, opioids, sedatives, EtOH; ↑ hypotension *W/* antihypertensive, neuroleptics; nitrates, EtOH; ↑ effects *OF* clonidine, digoxin, phenytoin; ↓ effects *W/* carbamazepine **NIPE:** Take w/ food; ↑ fluids to 2–3 L/d; ⊘ D/C abruptly; ↑ risk of priapism; takes 1–2 wk for symptom improvement

Treprostinil Sodium (Remodulin) [Antihypertensive/Vasodilator]   **Uses:** *NYHA class II–IV pulm arterial HTN* **Action:** Vasodilation, inhibits plt aggregation **Dose:** 0.625–1.25 ng/kg/min inj cont inf **Caution:** [B, ?/–] **Contra:** Component allergy **Disp:** 1, 2.5, 5, 10 mg/mL inj **SE:** Additive effects w/ anticoagulants, antihypertensives; inf site Rxns; D (25%), N (22%), HA (27%) **Interactions:** ↑ Effects *W/* antihypertensives; ↑ effects *OF* anticoagulants **NIPE:** Teach care of inf site and pump; use barrier contraception; once med vial used discard after 14 d; initiate in monitored setting; do not D/C or ↓ dose abruptly

Tretinoin, Topical [Retinoic Acid] (Retin-A, Avita, Renova, Retin- A Micro) [Retinoid/Antineoplastic]   **Uses:** *Acne vulgaris, sun-damaged skin, wrinkles* (photo aging), some skin CAs **Action:** Exfoliant retinoic acid derivative **Dose:** *Adults & Peds >12 y.* Apply daily hs (w/ irritation, ↓ frequency). *Photoaging:* Start w/ 0.025%, ↑ to 0.1% over several mo (apply only q3d if on neck area; dark skin may require bid use) **Caution:** [C, ?] **Contra:** Retinoid sensitivity **Disp:** Cream 0.02, 0.025, 0.05, 0.1%; gel 0.01, 0.025, microformulation gel 0.1, 0.04%; Liq 0.05% **SE:** Avoid sunlight; edema; skin dryness, erythema, scaling, changes in pigmentation, stinging, photosens **Interactions:** ↑ photosensitivity *W/* quinolones, phenothiazines, sulfonamides, tetracyclines, thiazides, dong quai, St. John's Wort; ↑ skin irritation *W/* topical sulfur, resorcinol, benzoyl peroxide, salicylic acid; ↑ effects *W/* vitamin A supl and foods *W/* excess vitamin A such as fish oils **NIPE:** ⊘ Apply to mucous membranes, wash skin and apply med after 30 min, wash hands after application; ⊘ breast-feeding, PRG use contraception; use sunscreen

Triamcinolone (Azmacort) [Anti-inflammatory/Corticosteroid]   **Uses:** *Chronic asthma* **Actions:** Topical steroid **Dose:** Two inhalations tid–qid or 4 inhal bid **Caution:** [C, ?] **Contra:** Component allergy **Disp:** Aerosol, metered inhaler 100 µg spray **SE:** Cough, oral candidiasis **Interactions:** ↑ Risk of GI bleed *W/* ASA, NSAIDs; ↑ effects *W/* salmeterol, troleandomycin; ↓ effects *W/* barbiturates, hydantoins, phenytoin, rifampin; ↓ effects *OF* diuretics, insulin, oral hypoglycemics, K supl, salicylates, somatrem, live virus vaccines **Labs:** ↑ Glucose, cholesterol; ↓ serum Ca, K⁺ **NIPE:** Use bronchodilator several minutes before triamcinolone; allow 1 min between repeat inhalations; instruct pts to rinse mouth after use; not for acute asthma

Triamcinolone & Nystatin (Mycolog-II) [Anti-inflammatory, Antifungal/Corticosteroid] Uses: *Cutaneous candidiasis* Action: Antifungal & anti-inflammatory Dose: Apply lightly to area bid; max 25 mg/d Caution: [C, ?] Contra: Varicella; systemic fungal Infxns Disp: Cream & oint 15, 30, 60, 120 mg SE: Local irritation, hypertrichosis, pigmentation changes Interactions: ↓ Effects W/ barbiturates, phenytoin, rifampin; ↓ effects OF salicylates, vaccines NIPE: ⊘ Eyes; ⊘ apply to open skin/wounds, mucous membranes; for short-term use (<7 d)

Triamterene (Dyrenium) [Diuretic/Potassium-Sparing Agent] Uses: *Edema associated w/ CHF, cirrhosis* Action: K⁺-sparing diuretic Dose: Adults. 100–300 mg/24 h PO ÷ daily–bid. Peds. HTN 2–4 mg/kg/d in 1–2 ÷ doses; ↓ w/ renal/hepatic impair Caution: [B (manufacturer; D ed. opinion), ?/–] Contra: ↑ K⁺, renal impair; caution w/ other K⁺-sparing diuretics Disp: Caps 50, 100 mg SE: ↓ K⁺, blood dyscrasias, liver damage, other Rxns Interactions: ↑ Risk of hyperkalemia W/ ACEIs, K supls, K⁺-sparing drugs, K-containing drugs, K salt substitutes; ↑ effects W/ cimetidine, indomethacin; ↑ effects OF amantadine, antihypertensives, Li; ↓ effects OF digitalis Labs: ↑ LFTs, BUN, Cr, glucose, uric acid; ↓ HMG, Hct, plt NIPE: Take w/ food, blue discoloration of urine, ↑ risk of photosensitivity—use sunscreen

Triazolam (Halcion) [C-IV] [Sedative/Hypnotic/Benzodiazepine] Uses: *Short-term management of insomnia* Action: Benzodiazepine Dose: 0.125–0.25 mg/d PO hs PRN; ↓ in elderly Caution: [X, ?/–] Contra: NAG; cirrhosis; concurrent amprenavir, ritonavir, nelfinavir, itraconazole, ketoconazole, nefazodone Disp: Tabs 0.125, 0.25 mg SE: Tachycardia, CP, drowsiness, fatigue, memory impair, GI upset Interactions: ↑ Effects W/ azole antifungals, cimetidine, clarithromycin, ciprofloxin, CNS depressants, disulfiram, digoxin, erythromycin, fluvoxamine, INH, protease inhibitors, troleandomycin, verapamil, EtOH, grapefruit juice, kava kava, valerian; ↓ effects OF levodopa; ↓ effects W/ carbamazepine, phenytoin, rifampin, theophylline NIPE: ⊘ PRG or breast-feeding; ⊘ D/C abruptly after long-term use; Do not prescribe >1 mo supply

Triethanolamine (Cerumenex) [OTC] [Ceruminolytic Agent] Uses: *Cerumen (ear wax) removal* Action: Ceruminolytic agent Dose: Fill ear canal & insert cotton plug; irrigate w/ H₂O after 15 min; repeat PRN Caution: [C, ?] Contra: Perforated tympanic membrane, otitis media Disp: Soln 10, 16, 12 mL SE: Local dermatitis, pain, erythema, pruritus NIPE: Warm soln to body temp before use for better effect

Triethylenethiophosphoramide (Thio-Tepa, Tespa, TSPA) [Alkylating Agent] Uses: *Hodgkin Dz & NHLs; leukemia; breast, ovarian CAs,

preparative regimens for allogeneic & ABMT w/ high doses, intravesical for bladder CA* **Action:** Polyfunctional alkylating agent **Dose:** 0.5 mg/kg q1–4wk, 6 mg/m^2 IM or IV × 4 d q2–4wk, 15–35 mg/m^2 by cont IV inf over 48 h; 60 mg into the bladder & retained 2 h q1–4wk; 900–125 mg/m^2 in ABMT regimens (highest dose w/o ABMT is 180 mg/m^2); 1–10 mg/m^2 (typically 15 mg) IT 1 or 2 ×/wk; 0.8 mg/kg in 1–2 L of soln may be instilled intraperitoneally; ↓ in renal failure **Caution:** [D, –] **Contra:** Component allergy **Disp:** Inj 15, 30 mg **SE:** ↓ BM, N/V, dizziness, HA, allergy, paresthesias, alopecia **Interactions:** ↑ Risk of bleeding w/ anticoagulants, ASA, NSAIDs; ↑ effects *OF* myelosuppressives; ↑ risk of muscular paralysis w/ neuromuscular blockers; ↑ risk of apnea *W/* pancuronium **Labs:** ↑ Uric acid; ↓ HMG, lymphocytes, neutrophils, plts, RBCs, WBCs **NIPE:** ⊘ PRG, lactation, BM suppression, hepatic dysfunction, renal dysfunction; ⊘ ASA or NSAIDs; report s/s of Infxn; intravesical use in bladder CA infrequent today

Trifluoperazine (Stelazine) [Antipsychotic/Phenothiazine]

Uses: *Psychotic disorders* **Action:** Phenothiazine; blocks postsynaptic CNS dopaminergic receptors **Dose:** *Adults.* 2–10 mg PO bid. *Peds 6–12 y.* 1 mg PO daily–bid initial, gradually ↑ to 15 mg/d; ↓ in elderly/debilitated pts **Caution:** [C, ?/–] **Contra:** h/o blood dyscrasias; phenothiazine sensitivity **Disp:** Tabs 1, 2, 5, 10 mg; PO conc 10 mg/mL; inj 2 mg/mL **SE:** Orthostatic ↓ BP, EPS, dizziness, neuroleptic malignant synd, skin discoloration, lowered Sz threshold, photosens, blood dyscrasia **Interactions:** ↑ CNS depression *W/* barbiturates, benzodiazepines, TCAs, EtOH; ↑ effects *OF* antihypertensives, propranolol, ↓ effects *OF* anticoagulants ↓ effects *W/* antacids **Labs:** ↑ LFTs; ↓ WBCs **NIPE:** ↑ Risk of photosensitivity—use sunscreen; urine color may change to pink to reddish-brown; PO conc must be diluted to 60 mL or more prior to administration; requires several wk for onset of effects

Trifluridine Ophthalmic (Viroptic) [Antiviral]

Uses: *Herpes simplex keratitis & conjunctivitis* **Action:** Antiviral **Dose:** 1 gtt q2h (max 9 gtt/d); ↓ to 1 gtt q4h after healing begins; Rx up to 21 d **Caution:** [C, M] **Contra:** Component allergy **Disp:** Soln 1% **SE:** Local burning, stinging **NIPE:** ⊘ <6 y of age; reeval if no improvement in 7 d

Trihexyphenidyl (Artane) [Anti-Parkinson Agent/Anticholinergic]

Uses: *Parkinson Dz* **Action:** Blocks excess acetylcholine at cerebral synapses **Dose:** 2–5 mg PO daily–qid **Caution:** [C, +] **Contra:** NAG, GI obst, MyG, bladder obst **Disp:** Tabs 2, 5 mg; SR caps 5 mg; elixir 2 mg/5 mL **SE:** Dry skin, constipation, xerostomia, photosens, tachycardia, arrhythmia **Interactions:** ↑ Effects *W/* MAOIs, phenothiazine, quinidine, TCAs; ↑ effects *OF* amantadine, anticholinergics, digoxin; ↓ effects *W/* antacids, tacrine; ↓ effects *OF* chlorpromazine, haloperidol, tacrine **NIPE:** Take w/ food; monitor for urinary hesitancy or retention; ⊘ D/C abruptly; ↑ risk of heat stroke

Trimethobenzamide (Tigan) [Antiemetic/Anticholinergic]

Uses: *N/V* **Action:** ↓ Medullary chemoreceptor trigger zone **Dose:** *Adults.* 250 mg

PO or 200 mg PR or IM tid–qid PRN. **Peds.** 20 mg/kg/24 h PO or 15 mg/kg/24 h PR or IM in 3–4 ÷ doses **Caution:** [C, ?] **Contra:** Benzocaine sensitivity **Disp:** Caps 100, 250 mg; supp 100, 200, 300 mg; inj 100 mg/mL **SE:** Drowsiness, ↓ BP, dizziness; hepatic impair, blood dyscrasias, Szs, parkinsonian-like synd **Interactions:** ↑ CNS depression *W/* antidepressants, antihistamines, opioids, sedatives, EtOH; ↑ risk *OF* extrapyramidal effects **NIPE:** In the presence of viral Infxns, may mask emesis *or* mimic CNS effects of Reye synd

Trimethoprim (Trimpex, Proloprim) [Antibiotic/Folate Antagonist]

Uses: *UTI due to susceptible gram(+) & gram(–) organisms*; suppression of UTI **Action:** ↓ Dihydrofolate reductase. **Spectrum:** Many gram(+) & (–) except *Bacteroides* sp, *Branhamella* sp, *Brucella* sp, *Chlamydia* sp, *Clostridium* sp, *Mycobacterium* sp, *Mycoplasma* sp, *Nocardia* sp, *Neisseria* sp, *Pseudomonas* sp, & *Treponema* sp **Dose: Adults.** 100 mg/d PO bid or 200 mg/d PO. **Peds.** 4 mg/kg/d in 2 ÷ doses; ↓ w/ renal failure **Caution:** [C, +] **Contra:** Megaloblastic anemia due to folate deficiency **Disp:** Tabs 100, 200 mg; PO soln 50 mg/5 mL **SE:** Rash, pruritus, megaloblastic anemia, hepatic impair, blood dyscrasias **Interactions:** ↑ Effects *W/* dapsone; ↓ effects *OF* dapsone, phenytoin, procainamide; ↓ efficacy *W/* rifampin **Labs:** ↑ BUN, Cr, bilirubin **NIPE:** ↑ Fluids to 2–3 L/d; ↑ risk of folic acid deficiency

Trimethoprim (TMP)–Sulfamethoxazole (SMX) [Co-Trimoxazole] (Bactrim, Septra) [Antibiotic/Folate Antagonist]

Uses: *UTI Rx & prophylaxis, otitis media, sinusitis, bronchitis* **Action:** SMX ↓ synth of dihydrofolic acid; TMP ↓ dihydrofolate reductase to impair protein synth. **Spectrum:** Includes *Shigella* sp, *P. jiroveci* (formerly *carinii*), & *Nocardia* Infxns, *Mycoplasma* sp, *Enterobacter* sp, *Staphylococcus* sp, *Streptococcus* sp, & more **Dose: Adults.** 1 DS tab PO bid or 5–20 mg/kg/24 h (based on TMP) IV in 3–4 ÷ doses. *P. jiroveci:* 15–20 mg/kg/d IV or PO (TMP) in 4 ÷ doses. *Nocardia:* 10–15 mg/kg/d IV or PO (TMP) in 4 ÷ doses. *UTI prophylaxis:* 1 PO daily. **Peds.** 8–10 mg/kg/24 h (TMP) PO ÷ into 2 doses or 3–4 doses IV; do not use in newborns; ↓ in renal failure; maintain hydration **Caution:** [B (D if near term), +] **Contra:** Sulfonamide sensitivity, porphyria, megaloblastic anemia w/ folate deficiency, significant hepatic impair **Disp:** Regular tabs 80 mg TMP/400 mg SMX; DS tabs 160 mg TMP/800 mg SMX; PO susp 40 mg TMP/200 mg SMX/5 mL; inj 80 mg TMP/400 mg SMX/5 mL **SE:** Allergic skin Rxns, photosens, GI upset, Stevens–Johnson synd, blood dyscrasias, hepatitis **Interactions:** ↑ Effect *OF* dapsone, MTX, phenytoin, sulfonylureas, warfarin, zidovudine; ↑ effects *W/* rifampin; ↓ effect *OF* cyclosporine **Labs:** ↑ Serum bilirubin, alkaline phosphatase, BUN, Cr **NIPE:** ↑ Risk of photosensitivity—use sunscreen; ↑ fluids to 2–3 L/d; synergistic combo

Trimetrexate (Neutrexin) [Anti-infective, Antiprotozoal/ Folic Acid Antimetabolite]

WARNING: Must be used w/ leucovorin to avoid tox **Uses:** *Moderate–severe PCP* **Action:** ↓ dihydrofolate reductase **Dose:** 45 mg/m² IV q24h for 21 d; administer w/ leucovorin 20 mg/m² IV q6h for 24 d; ↓ in hepatic impair **Caution:** [D, ?/–] **Contra:** MTX sensitivity **Disp:** Inj 25, 200 mg/ 25 mg/vial **SE:** Sz, fever, rash, GI upset, anemias, ↑ LFTs, peripheral neuropathy, renal impair **Interactions:** ↑ Effects W/ azole antifungals, cimetidine, erythromycin; ↓ effects W/ rifabutin, rifampin; ↓ effects OF pneumococcal immunization **Labs:** ↑ LFTs, SCr **NIPE:** ⊘ PRG, breast-feeding use contraception; ⊘ exposure to Infxn; use cytotoxic cautions; inf over 60 min

Triptorelin (Trelstar Depot, Trelstar LA) [Antineoplastic/Gonadotropin-Releasing Hormone] Uses: *Palliation of advanced PCa* **Action:** LHRH analog; ↓ GNRH w/ continuous dosing; transient ↑ in LH, FSH, testosterone, & estradiol 7–10 d after 1st dose; w/ chronic/continuous use (usually 2–4 wk), sustained ↓ LH & FSH w/ ↓ testicular or ovarian steroidogenesis similar to surgical castration **Dose:** 3.75 mg IM monthly or 11.25 mg IM q3mo **Caution:** [X, N/A] **Contra:** Not indicated in females **Disp:** Inj depot 3.75 mg; LA 11.25 mg **SE:** Dizziness, emotional lability, fatigue, HA, insomnia, HTN, D, V, ED, retention, UTI, pruritus, anemia, inj site pain, musculoskeletal pain, osteoporosis, allergic Rxns **Interactions:** ↑ Risk of severe hyperprolactinemia W/ antipsychotics, metoclopramide **Labs:** Suppression of pituitary-gonadal Fxn **NIPE:** ⊘ PRG or breast-feeding; may cause hot flashes; initial ↑ bone pain

Trospium Chloride (Sanctura) [Antispasmodic/Anticholinergic] Uses: *OAB* **Action:** Antimuscarinic, antispasmodic **Dose:** 20 mg PO bid; w/ renal impair or >75 y; on empty stomach or 1 h ac **Caution:** [C, ?/–] BOO, GI obst, ulcerative colitis, MyG, renal/hepatic impair **Contra:** NAG, urinary/gastric retention **Disp:** Tabs 20 mg **SE:** Constipation, xerostomia **Interactions:** ↑ Effects W/ amiloride, digoxin, morphine, metformin, procainamide, tenofovir, vancomycin; ↑ effects OF anticholinergics, amiloride, digoxin, morphine, metformin, procainamide, tenofovir, vancomycin **NIPE:** Take w/o food 1 h ac

Urokinase (Abbokinase) [Thrombolytic Enzyme] Uses: *PE, DVT, restore patency to IV catheters* **Action:** Converts plasminogen to plasmin, causes clot lysis **Dose:** *Adults & Peds. Systemic effect:* 4400 units/kg IV over 10 min, then 4400–6000 units/kg/h for 12 h. *Restore catheter patency:* Inject 5000 units into catheter & aspirate up to 2 doses **Caution:** [B, +] **Contra:** Do not use w/in 10 d of surgery, delivery, or organ biopsy; bleeding, CVA, vascular malformation **Disp:** Powder for inj, 250,000-unit vial **SE:** Bleeding, ↓ BP, dyspnea, bronchospasm, anaphylaxis, cholesterol embolism **Interactions:** ↑ Risk of bleeding W/ anticoagulants, ASA, heparin, indomethacin, NSAIDs, phenylbutazone, feverfew, garlic, ginger, ginkgo biloba; ↓ effects W/ aminocaproic acid **Labs:** ↑ PT, PTT; ↓ PT, PTT, INR **NIPE:** Monitor for bleeding q15min for 1st h & q30min for next 7 h

Valacyclovir (Valtrex) [Antiviral/Synthetic Purine Nucleoside] Uses: *Herpes zoster; genital herpes* **Action:** Prodrug of acyclovir ↓ viral DNA replication. *Spectrum:* Herpes simplex I & II **Dose:** 1 g PO tid. *Genital herpes:* 500 mg bid × 7–10 d. *Herpes prophylaxis:* 500–1000 mg/d; ↓ w/ rena failure **Caution:** [B, +] **Disp:** Caplets 500, 1000 mg **SE:** HA, GI upset, dizziness, pruritus, photophobia **Interactions:** ↑ Effects *W/* cimetidine, probenecid **Labs:** ↑ LFTs, Cr ↓ HMG, Hct, plt, WBCs **NIPE:** Take w/regard to food; ↑ fluids to 2–3 L/d; begin drug at 1st sign of S/Sxs

Valganciclovir (Valcyte) [Antiviral/Synthetic Nucleoside]

Uses: *CMV* **Action:** Ganciclovir prodrug; ↓ viral DNA synth **Dose:** Induction, 900 mg PO bid w/ food × 21 d, then 900 mg PO daily; ↓ in renal dysfunction **Caution:** [C, ?/–] Use w/ imipenem/cilastatin, nephrotoxic drugs **Contra:** Allergy to acyclovir, ganciclovir, valganciclovir; ANC HD <500/mm²; plt <25000; Hgb <8 g/dL **Disp:** Tabs 450 mg **SE:** BM suppression, headache, GI upset **Interactions:** ↑ Effects *W/* cytotoxic drugs, immunosuppressive drugs, probenecid; ↑ risks of nephrotox *W/* amphotericin B, cyclosporine; ↑ effects *W/* didanosine **Labs:** ↑ Cr; monitor CBC & Cr **NIPE:** Take w/ food; ⊘ PRG, breast-feeding, EtOH, NSAIDs; use contraception for at least 3 mo after drug Rx

Valproic Acid (Depakene, Depakote) [Anticonvulsant/Carboxylic Acid Derivative]

Uses: *Rx epilepsy, mania; prophylaxis of migraines*, Alzheimer Dz, behavior disorder **Action:** Anticonvulsant; ↑ availability of GABA **Dose:** *Adults & Peds. Szs:* 30–60 mg/kg/24 h PO ÷ tid (after initiation of 10–15 mg/kg/24 h). *Mania:* 750 mg in 3 ÷ doses, ↑ 60 mg/kg/d max. *Migraines:* 250 mg bid, ↑ 1000 mg/d max; ↓ w/ hepatic impair **Caution:** [D, +] **Contra:** Severe hepatic impair **Disp:** Caps 250 mg; syrup 250 mg/5 mL **SE:** Somnolence, dizziness, GI upset, diplopia, ataxia, rash, thrombocytopenia, hepatitis, pancreatitis, prolonged bleeding times, alopecia, wt gain, hyperammonemic encephalopathy reported in pts w/ urea cycle disorders **Notes:** Monitor *Levels: Trough:* just before next dose; *Therapeutic peak:* 50–100 μg/mL; *Toxic trough:* >100 μg/mL; *1/2 life:* 5–20 h; phenobarbital & phenytoin may alter levels **Interactions:** ↑ Effects *W/* clarithromycin, erythromycin, felbamate, INH, phenytoin, salicylates, troleandomycin; ↑ effects *OF* anticoagulants, lamotrigine, nimodipine, phenobarbital, phenytoin, primidone, zidovudine; ↑ CNS depression *W/* CNS depressants, haloperidol, loxapine, maprotiline, MAOIs, phenothiazine, thioxanthenes, TCAs, EtOH; ↓ effects *W/* cholestyramine, colestipol; ↓ effects *OF* clozapine, rifampin **Labs:** ↑ LFTs; altered TFTs; monitor LFTs and serum levels **NIPE:** Take w/ food for GI upset; ⊘ PRG, breast-feeding; D/C abruptly

Valsartan (Diovan) [Antihypertensive/ARB]

WARNING: Use during 2nd/3rd tri of PRG can cause fetal harm **Uses:** HTN, CHF, DN **Action:** Angiotensin II receptor antagonist **Dose:** 80–160 mg/d, max 320 mg/d **Caution:** [C (1st tri; D 2nd & 3rd tri), ?/–] w/ K⁺-sparing diuretics or K⁺ supls **Contra:** Severe hepatic impair, biliary cirrhosis/obst, primary hyperaldosteronism, bilateral RAS **Disp:** Tabs 40, 80, 160, 320 mg, caps: 80, 160 mg **SE:** ↓ BP, dizziness **Interactions:** ↑ Effects *W/* diuretics, Li; ↑ risk of hyperkalemia *W/* K⁺-sparing diuretics, K supls, trimethoprim **Labs:** ↑ K⁺ **NIPE:** Take w/o regard to food; ⊘ PRG, breast-feeding; use contraception

Vancomycin (Vancocin, Vancoled) [Antibiotic/Glycopeptide]
Uses: *Serious MRSA Infxns; enterococcal Infxns; PO Rx of *C. difficile*
pseudomembranous colitis* **Action:** ↓ Cell wall synth. *Spectrum:* Gram(+) bacteria & some anaerobes (includes MRSA, *Staphylococcus* sp, *Enterococcus* sp, *Streptococcus* sp, *C. difficile*) **Dose:** *Adults.* 1 g IV q12h; or 15 mg/kg/dose for colitis 125–500 mg PO q6h. *Peds.* 40–60 mg/kg/24 h IV in ÷ doses q6–12 h. *Neonates.* 10–15 mg/kg/dose q12h; ↓ in renal insuff **Caution:** [C, M] **Contra:** Component allergy; w/ avoid in h/o hearing loss **Disp:** Caps 125, 250 mg; powder 250 mg/5 mL, 500 mg/6 mL for PO soln; powder for inj 500 mg, 1000 mg, 10 g/vial **SE:** Ototoxic & nephrotox, GI upset (PO), neutropenia **Notes:** *Levels: Peak:* 1 h after inf; *Trough:* <0.5 h before next dose; *Therapeutic peak:* 30–40 μg/mL; *Trough:* <2 μg/mL; *Toxic peak:* >50 μg/mL; *Trough:* >15 μg/mL; *1/2 life:* 6–8 h **Interactions:** ↑ Ototox and nephrotox *W/* ASA, aminoglycosides, cyclosporine, cisplatin, loop diuretics; ↓ effects *OF* MRX **Labs:** ↑ BUN, Cr **NIPE:** Take w/ food, ↑ fluid to 2–3 L/d; not absorbed PO, local effect in gut only; give IV dose slowly (over 1–3 h) to prevent "red-man synd" (flushing of head/neck/upper torso); IV product PO for colitis

Vardenafil (Levitra) [Anti-impotence Agent/PDE5]   **WARNING:** May prolong QTc interval **Uses:** *ED* **Action:** PDE5 inhibitor, increases cGMP and NO levels; relaxes smooth muscles, dilates cavernosal arteries **Dose:** 10 mg PO 60 min before sexual activity; 2.5 mg if administered w/ CYP3A4 inhibitors (Table 11); max × 1 =20 mg **Caution:** [B, –] w/ CV, hepatic, or renal Dz **Contra:** Nitrates, ↑ Qtc interval **Disp:** Tabs 2.5, 5, 10, 20 mg tabs **SE:** ∅ BP, HA, dyspepsia, priapism hearing loss **Interactions:** ↑ Effects *W/* erythromycin, ketoconazole indinavir, ritonavir; ↑ risk of hypotension W/α-blockers, nitrates **NIPE:** Take w/o regard to food; ↑ risk of priapism

Varenicline (Chantix) [Nicotinic Acetylcholine Receptor Partial Agonist]   **Uses:** *Smoking cessation* **Action:** Nicotine receptor antagonist **Dose:** *Adults.* 0.5 mg PO daily × 3 d, 0.5 mg bid × 4 d, then 1 mg PO bid for 12 wk total; after meal w/ glass of water **Caution:** [C,?/–] ↓ dose w/ renal impair **Disp:** Tabs 0.5, 1 mg **SE:** N, V, insomnia, flatulence, unusual dreams **Interactions:** May effect metabolism of warfarin, theophylline, insulin; ↑ effects with nicotine replacement drugs **NIPE:** Slowly ↑ dose to ↓ N; initiate 1 wk before desired smoking cessation date

Varicella Virus Vaccine (Varivax) [Vaccine]   **Uses:** *Prevent varicella (chickenpox)* **Action:** Active immunization; live attenuated virus **Dose:** *Adults & Peds.* 0.5 mL SQ, repeat 4–8 wk **Caution:** [C, M] **Contra:** Immunocompromised; neomycin-anaphylactoid Rxn, blood dyscrasias; immunosuppressive drugs; avoid PRG for 3 mo after **Disp:** Powder for inj **SE:** Mild varicella Infxn; fever, local Rxns, irritability, GI upset **Interactions:** ↓ Effects *W/* acyclovir, immunosuppressant drugs **NIPE:** ⊘ Salicylates for 6 wk after immunization; ⊘ PRG for 3 mo after immunization; OK for all children & adults who have not had chickenpox

Vasopressin [Antidiuretic Hormone, ADH] (Pitressin) [Antidiuretic Hormone/ Posterior Pituitary Hormone] Uses: *DI; Rx postop abd distension*; adjunct Rx of GI bleeding & esophageal varices; asystole and PEA pulseless VT & VF, adjunct systemic vasopressor (IV drip) **Action:** Posterior pituitary hormone, potent GI and peripheral vasoconstrictor **Dose:** *Adults & Peds. DI:* 2.5–10 units SQ or IM tid–qid. *GI hemorrhage:* 0.2–0.4 units/min; ↓ in cirrhosis; caution in vascular Dz. *VT/VF:* 40 units IVP X1. *Vasopressor:* 0.01–0.04 units/min **Caution:** [B, +] **Contra:** Allergy **Disp:** Inj 20 units/mL **SE:** HTN, arrhythmias, fever, vertigo, GI upset, tremor **Interactions:** ↑ Vasopressor effects W/ guanethidine, neostigmine; ↑ antidiuretic effects W/ carbamazepine, chlorpropamide, clofibrate, phenformin urea, TCAs; ↓ antidiuretic effects W/ demeclocycline, epinephrine, heparin, Li, phenytoin, EtOH **Labs:** ↑ cortisol level **NIPE:** Take 1–2 glasses H₂O w/ drug; addition of vasopressor to concurrent norepinephrine or epi inf‑sns

Vecuronium (Norcuron) [Skeletal Muscle Relaxant/Nondepolarizing Neuromuscular Blocker] Uses: *Skeletal muscle relaxation* **Action:** Nondepolarizing neuromuscular blocker; onset 2–3 min **Dose:** *Adults & Peds.* 0.1–0.2 mg/kg IV bolus (also rapid intubation *ECC 2005*); maint 0.010–0.015 mg/kg after 25–40 min; additional doses q12–15min PRN; ↓ in severe renal/hepatic impair **Caution:** [C, ?] Drug interactions cause ↑ effect (eg, aminoglycosides, tetracycline, succinylcholine) **Disp:** Powder for inj 10, 20 mg **SE:** Bradycardia, ↓ BP, itching, rash, tachycardia, CV collapse **Interactions:** ↑ Neuromuscular blockade W/ amikacin, clindamycin, gentamicin, neomycin, streptomycin, tobramycin, general anesthetics, quinidine, tetracyclines; ↑ resp depression W/ opioids; ↓ effects W/ phenytoin **NIPE:** Will not provide pain relief or sedation; fewer cardiac effects than succinylcholine

Venlafaxine (Effexor, Effexor XR) [Antidepressant/Serotonin, Norepinephrine, & Dopamine Reuptake Inhibitor] **WARNING:** Monitor for worsening depression or emergence of suicidality, particularly in ped pts Uses: *Depression, generalized anxiety*, social anxiety disorder; obsessive–compulsive disorder, chronic fatigue synd, ADHD, autism **Action:** Potentiation of CNS neurotransmitter activity **Dose:** 75–375 mg/d ÷ into 2–3 equal doses; ↓ w/ renal/hepatic impair **Caution:** [C, ?/–] **Contra:** MAOIs **Disp:** Tabs 25, 37.5, 50, 75, 100 mg; XR caps 37.5, 75, 150 mg **SE:** HTN, ↑ HR, HA, somnolence, GI upset, sexual dysfunction; actuates mania or Szs **Interactions:** ↑ Effects W/ cimetidine, desipramine, haloperidol, MAOIs; ↑ risk of serotonin synd W/ sumatriptan,trazodone, St. John's wort **NIPE:** XR caps swallow whole—◎ chew; take w/ food; ◎ use EtOH; ◎ D/C abruptly; D/C MAOI 14 d before start of this drug; ↑ fluids to 2–3 L/d; may take 2–3 wk for full effects; frequent edema & wt gain

Verapamil (Calan, Isoptin, Verelan) [Antihypertensive, Antianginal, Antiarrhythmic/CCB] Uses: *Angina, HTN, PSVT, AF, atrial flutter*, migraine prophylaxis, hypertrophic cardiomyopathy, bipolar Dz **Action:**

CCB **Dose:** *Adults. Arrhythmias:* 2nd line for PSVT w/ narrow QRS complex & adequate BP 2.5–5 mg IV over 1–2 min; repeat 5–10 mg in 15–30 min PRN (30 mg max). *Angina:* 80–120 mg PO tid, ↑ 480 mg/24 h max. *HTN:* 80–180 mg PO tid or SR tabs 120–240 mg PO daily to 240 mg bid; 2.5–5.0 mg IV over 1–2 min; repeat 5–10 mg, in 5–30 min PRN; or 5-mg bolus q15min (max 30 mg) *(ECC 2005)* **Peds.** *<1 y:* 0.1–0.2 mg/kg IV over 2 min (may repeat in 30 min). *1–16 y:* 0.1–0.3 mg/kg IV over 2 min (may repeat in 30 min); 5 mg max. *PO: 1–5 y:* 4–8 mg/kg/d in 3 ÷ doses. *>5 y:* 80 mg q6–8h; ↓ in renal/hepatic impair **Caution:** [C, +] Amiodarone/β-blockers/flecainide can cause bradycardia; statins, midazolam, tacrolimus, theophylline levels may be ↑; w/ elderly pts **Contra:** Conduction disorders, cardiogenic shock; β-blocker/thiazide combo, dofetilide, pimozide, ranolazine **Disp:** Tabs 40, 80, 120 mg; XR tabs 120, 180, 240 mg; tablets XR 24 h 180, 240, mg; inj 5 mg/2 mL **SE:** Gingival hyperplasia, constipation, ↓ BP, bronchospasm, HR or conduction disturbances **Interactions:** ↑ Effects W/ antihypertensives, nitrates, quinidine, EtOH, grapefruit juice; ↑ effects OF buspirone, carbamazepine, cyclosporine, digoxin, prazosin, quinidine, theophylline; ↓ effects W/ antineoplastics, barbiturates, NSAIDs; ↓ effects OF Li, rifampin **Labs:** ↑ ALT, AST, alkaline phosphatase **NIPE:** Take w/ food; ↑ fluids and bulk foods to prevent constipation

Vinblastine (Velban, Velbe) [Antineoplastic/Vinca Alkaloid]

WARNING: Chemotherapeutic agent; handle w/ caution **Uses:** *Hodgkin Dz & NHLs, mycosis fungoides, CAs (testis, renal cell, breast, non-small-cell lung), AIDS-related Kaposi sarcoma*, choriocarcinoma, histiocytosis **Action:** ↓ Microtubule assembly **Dose:** 0.1–0.5 mg/kg/wk (4–20 mg/m²); ↓ in hepatic failure **Caution:** [D, ?] **Contra:** Intrathecal use **Disp:** Inj 1 mg/mL in 10 mg vial **SE:** ↓ BM (especially leukopenia), N/V, constipation, neurotox, alopecia, rash, myalgia, tumor pain **Interactions:** ↑ Effects W/ erythromycin, itraconazole; ↓ effects W/ glutamic acid, tryptophan; ↓ effects OF phenytoin **Labs:** ↑ Uric acid **NIPE:** ↑ Fluids to 2–3 L/d; ⊘ PRG or breast-feeding; use contraception for at least 2 mo after drug; photosensitivity—use sunscreen; ⊘ admin immunizations

Vincristine (Oncovin, Vincasar PFS) [Antineoplastic/Vinca Alkaloid]

WARNING: Chemotherapeutic agent; handle w/ caution; fatal if administered intrathecally **Uses:** *ALL, breast & small-cell lung CA, sarcoma (eg, Ewing tumor, rhabdomyosarcoma), Wilms tumor, Hodgkin Dz & NHLs, neuroblastoma, multiple myeloma* **Action:** Promotes disassembly of mitotic spindle, causing metaphase arrest **Dose:** 0.4–1.4 mg/m² (single doses 2 mg/max); ↓ in hepatic failure **Caution:** [D, ?] **Contra:** Intrathecal use **Disp:** Inj 1 mg/mL, 5 mg vial **SE:** Neurotox commonly dose limiting, jaw pain (trigeminal neuralgia), fever, fatigue, anorexia, constipation & paralytic ileus, bladder atony; no significant ↓ BM w/ standard doses; tissue necrosis w/ extrav **Interactions:** ↑ Effects W/ CCBs, azole antifungals; ↑ risk of bronchospasm W/ mitomycin; ↓ effects OF digoxin, phenytoin, quinolone antibiotics **Labs:** ↑ Uric acid; ↓ HMG, Hct, plt, WBC

NIPE: ↑ Fluids to 2–3 L/d; reversible hair loss; ⊘ exposure to Infxn; ⊘ admin immunizations

Vinorelbine (Navelbine) [Antineoplastic/Vinca Alkaloid]
WARNING: Chemotherapeutic agent; handle w/ caution **Uses:** *Breast & non-small-cell lung CA* (alone or w/ cisplatin) **Action:** ↓ Polymerization of microtubules, impairing mitotic spindle formation; semisynthetic vinca alkaloid **Dose:** 30 mg/m²/wk; ↓ in hepatic failure **Caution:** [D, ?] **Contra:** Intrathecal use, rotavirus vaccine line **Disp:** Inj 10 mg **SE:** ↓ BM (leukopenia), mild GI, neurotox (6–29%); constipation/paresthesias (rare); tissue damage from extrav **Interactions:** ↑ Risk of granulocytopenia **W/** cisplatin, ↑ pulmonary effects **W/** mitomycin, paclitaxel **Labs:** ↑ LFTs **NIPE:** ⊘ PRG or breast-feeding; use contraception; ⊘ infectious environment; ↑ fluids to 2–3 L/d

Vitamin B₁ See Thiamine
Vitamin B₆ See Pyridoxine
Vitamin B₁₂ See Cyanocobalamin
Vitamin K See Phytonadione
Vitamin, Multi See Multivitamins (Table 13)

Voriconazole (VFEND) [Antifungal/Triazole]
Uses: *Invasive aspergillosis, serious fungal Infxns* **Action:** ↓ Ergosterol synth. *Spectrum:* Fungus: *Aspergillus* sp, *Scedosporium* sp, *Fusarium* sp **Dose:** *Adults & Peds = 12 y. IV:* 6 mg/kg q12h × 2, then 3 mg/kg bid; may ↓ to 3 mg/kg/dose. *PO:* <40 kg: 100 mg q12h, up to 150 mg; >40 kg: 200 mg q12h, up to 300 mg; ↓ w/ mild–moderate hepatic impair; IV w/ renal impair ×1 dose; PO w/o food **Caution:** [D, ?/–] **Contra:** Severe hepatic impair **Disp:** Tabs 50, 200 mg; susp 200 mg/5 mL; 200 mg inj **SE:** Visual changes, fever, rash, GI upset **Interactions:** ↑ Effects **W/** delavirdine, efavirenz; ↑ effects *OF* benzodiazepines, buspirone, CCBs, cisapride, cyclosporine, ergots, pimozide, quinidine, sirolimus, sulfonylureas, tacrolimus; ↓ effects **W/** carbamazepine, mephobarbital, phenobarbital, rifampin, rifabutin **Labs:** ↑ LFTs **NIPE:** Take w/o food; ↑ risk of photosensitivity—use sunscreen; ⊘ PRG or breast-feeding

Vorinostat (Zolinza) [Histone Deacetylase Inhibitor]
Uses: *Rx cutaneous manifestations in cutaneous T-cell lymphoma* **Action:** Histone deacetylase inhibitor **Dose:** 400 mg PO daily w/ food; if intolerant ↓ 300 mg PO d for × 5 d each wk **Caution:** [D; ?/–] w/ warfarin (↑ INR) **Disp:** Caps 100 mg **SE:** N/V/D, dehydration, fatigue, anorexia, dysgeusia, DVT, PE, ↓plt, anemia, hyperglycemia, QTc prolongation **Interactions:** ↑ Risk of thrombocytopenia & GI bleed **W/** HDAC inhibitors (valproic acid) **Labs:** Monitor CBC, lytes (K, Mg, Ca), glucose, & SCr q2wk × 2 mo then monthly; baseline, periodic ECGs **NIPE:** Drink 2 L fluid/d; ⊘ breastfeeding & <18 y of age

Warfarin (Coumadin) [Anticoagulant/Coumarin Derivative]
Uses: *Prophylaxis & Rx of PE & DVT, AF w/ embolization*, other postop indications **Action:** ↓ Vitamin K-dependent clotting factors in order: VII-IX-X-II

Dose: *Adults.* Titrate, INR 2.0–3.0 for most; mechanical valves INR is 2.5–3.5. *ACCP guidelines:* 5 mg initial (unless rapid therapeutic INR needed), may use 7.5–10 mg; ↓ if pt elderly or w/ other bleeding risk factors. *Alternative:* 10–15 mg PO, or IV daily for 1–3 d; maint 2–10 mg/d PO, IV, or follow daily INR initial to adjust dosage (Table 9). *Peds* 0.05–0.34 mg/kg/24 h PO, or IV; follow PT/INR to adjust dosage; monitor vitamin K intake; ↓ w/ hepatic impair/elderly **Caution:** [X, +] **Contra:** Severe hepatic/renal Dz, bleeding, peptic ulcer, PRG **Disp:** Tabs 1, 2, 2.5, 3, 4, 5, 6, 7.5, 10 mg; inj **SE:** Bleeding due to overanticoagulation (PT >3 × control, INR >5.0–6.0) or injury & therapeutic INR; bleeding, alopecia, skin necrosis, purple toe synd **Interactions:** *Common warfarin interactions:* ↑ action W/ APAP, EtOH (w/ liver Dz), amiodarone, cimetidine, ciprofloxacin, cotrimoxazole, erythromycin, fluconazole, flu vaccine, isoniazid, itraconazole, metronidazole, omeprazole, phenytoin, propranolol, quinidine, tetracycline. ↓ action W/ barbiturates, carbamazepine, chlordiazepoxide, cholestyramine, dicloxacillin, nafcillin, rifampin, sucralfate, high-vitamin K foods **Labs:** ↑ PTT; false ↓ serum theophylline levels **NIPE:** Monitor vitamin K intake (↓ effect); INR preferred test; to rapidly correct overanticoagulation, use vitamin K, FFP or both; reddish discoloration of urine; ⊘ PRG or breast-feeding; use barrier contraception; highly teratogenic; caution pt on taking w/ other meds, especially ASA. monitor for bleeding

Zafirlukast (Accolate) [Bronchodilator/Leukotriene Receptor Antagonist]

Uses: *Adjunctive Rx of asthma* **Action:** Selective & competitive inhibitor of leukotrienes *Dose: Adults & Peds = 12 y.* 20 mg bid. *Peds 5–11 y.* 10 mg PO bid (empty stomach) **Caution:** [B, –] Interacts w/ warfarin, ↑ INR **Contra:** Component allergy **Disp:** Tabs 10, 20 mg **SE:** Hepatic dysfunction, usually reversible on D/C; HA, dizziness, GI upset; Churg–Strauss synd **Interactions:** ↑ Effects W/ ASA; ↑ effects OF CCBs, cyclosporine; ↑ risk of bleeding W/ warfarin; ↓ effects W/ erythromycin, theophylline, food **Labs:** ↑ ALT **NIPE:** Take w/o food; ⊘ use for acute asthma attack

Zaleplon (Sonata) [C-IV] [Sedative/Hypnotic]

Uses: *Insomnia* **Action:** A nonbenzodiazepine sedative/hypnotic, a pyrazolopyrimidine **Dose:** 5–20 mg hs PRN; ↓ w/ renal/hepatic insuff, elderly **Caution:** [C, ?/–] w/ mental/psychological conditions **Contra:** Component allergy **Disp:** Caps 5, 10 mg **SE:** HA, edema, amnesia, somnolence, photosens **Interactions:** ↑ CNS depression W/ CNS depressants, imipramine, thoridazine, EtOH; ↓ effects W/ carbamazepine, phenobarbital, phenytoin, rifampin **NIPE:** Rapid effects of drug-take immediately before desired onset; take w/o food ⊘ D/C abruptly

Zanamivir (Relenza) [Antiviral/Neuramidase Inhibitor]

Uses: *Influenza A & B* **Action:** ↓ viral neuraminidase **Dose:** *Adults & Peds > 7 y.* 2 inhal (10 mg) bid for 5 d; initiate w/in 48 h of Sxs **Caution:** [C, M] **Contra:** Pulm Dz **Disp:** Powder for inhal 5 mg **SE:** Bronchospasm, HA, GI upset **Labs:** ↑ ALT, AST, CPK **NIPE:** Does not reduce risk of transmitting virus; uses a Diskhaler for administration

Ziconotide (Prialt) [Pain Control Agent/Nonnarcotic]
WARNING: Psychiatric, cognitive, neurologic impair may develop over several wk; monitor frequently; may necessitate D/C **Uses:** *IT Rx of severe, refractory, chronic pain* **Action:** N-type CCB in spinal cord **Dose:** 2.6 µg/d IT at 0.1 µg/h; may ↑ 0.8 µg/h to total 19.2 µg/d by day 21 **Caution:** [C, ?/–] Reversible psychiatric/neurologic impair **Contra:** Psychosis **Disp:** Inj 25, 100 mg/mL **SE:** Dizziness, N/V, confusion, abnormal vision; may require dosage adjustment **NIPE:** May D/C abruptly; uses specific pumps; do not ↑ more frequently than 2–3 ×/wk; monitor for S/Sxs psychotic behavior & meningitis

Zidovudine (Retrovir) [Antiretroviral/NRTI] **WARNING:** Neutropenia, anemia, lactic acidosis, & hepatomegaly w/ steatosis **Uses:** *HIV Infxn, prevention of maternal HIV, transmission of HIV* **Action:** ↓ RT **Dose:** *Adults.* 200 mg PO tid or 300 mg PO bid or 1–2 mg/kg/dose IV q4h. *PRG:* 100 mg PO 5 ×/d until labor starts; during labor 2 mg/kg over 1 h followed by 1 mg/kg/h until clamping of the cord. *Peds.* 160 mg/m²/dose q8h; ↓ in renal failure **Caution:** [C, ?/–] **Contra:** Allergy **Disp:** Caps 100 mg; tabs 300 mg; syrup 50 mg/5 mL; inj 10 mg/mL **SE:** Hematologic tox, HA, fever, rash, GI upset, malaise, myopathy; **Interactions:** ↑ Effects W/ fluconazole, phenytoin, probenecid, valproic acid; ↑ hematologic tox W/ adriamycin, dapsone, ganciclovir, interferon-a; ↓ effects W/ rifampin, ribavirin, stavudine **NIPE:** Take w/o food; monitor for S/Sxs opportunistic Infxn; monitor for anemia

Zidovudine & Lamivudine (Combivir) [Antiretroviral/NRTI]
WARNING: Neutropenia, anemia, lactic acidosis, & hepatomegaly w/ steatosis **Uses:** *HIV Infxn* **Action:** Combo of RT inhibitors **Dose:** *Adults & Peds >12 y.* 1 tab PO bid; ↓ in renal failure **Caution:** [C, ?/–] **Contra:** Component allergy **Disp:** Caps zidovudine 300 mg/lamivudine 150 mg **SE:** Hematologic tox, HA, fever, rash, GI upset, malaise, pancreatitis **Interactions:** ↑ Effects W/ fluconazole, phenytoin, probenecid, valproic acid; ↑ hematologic tox W/ adriamycin, dapsone, ganciclovir, interferon-a; ↓ W/ rifampin, ribavirin, stavudine **NIPE:** Take w/o food; monitor for S/Sxs opportunistic Infxn; monitor for anemia; combo product ↓ daily pill burden

Zileuton (Zyflo) [Leukotriene Receptor Antagonist] **Uses:** *Chronic Rx of asthma* **Action:** Inhibitor of 5-lipoxygenase **Dose:** *Adults & Peds = 12 y.* 600 mg PO qid **Caution:** [C, ?/–] **Contra:** Hepatic impair **Disp:** Tabs 600 mg **SE:** Hepatic damage, HA, GI upset, leukopenia **Interactions:** ↑ Effects OF propranolol, terfenadine, theophylline, warfarin **Labs:** ↑ WBCs; ↑ LFTs; monitor LFTs every mo × 3, then q2–3mo; **NIPE:** Take w/o regard to food; take on a regular basis; not for acute asthma

Ziprasidone (Geodon) [Antipsychotic/Piperazine Derivative] **WARNING:** ↑ Mortality in elderly with dementia-related psychosis **Uses:** *Schizophrenia, acute agitation* **Action:** Atypical antipsychotic **Dose:** 20 mg PO bid, may ↑ in 2-d intervals up to 80 mg bid; agitation 10–20 mg IM PRN up to

40 mg/d; separate 10-mg doses by 2 h & 20 mg doses by 4h (w/ food) **Caution:** [C, –] w/ ↓ Mg^{2+}, ↓ K^+ **Contra:** QT prolongation, recent MI, uncompensated HF, meds that ↑ QT interval **Disp:** Caps 20, 40, 60, 80 mg; susp 10 mg/mL; Inj 20 mg/mL; susp 10 mg/mL **SE:** Bradycardia, rash, somnolence, resp disorder, EPS, wt gain, orthostatic ↓ BP **Interactions:** ↑ Effects W/ ketoconazole; ↑ effects OF antihypertensives; ↑ CNS depression W/ anxiolytics, sedatives, opioids, EtOH; TCAs, thioridazine; risk of prolonged QT W/ cisapride, chlorpromazine, clarithromycin, diltiazem, erythromycin, levofloxacin, mefloquine, pentamidine, TCAs, thioridazine; ↓ effects W/ amphetamines, carbamazepine; ↓ effects OF levodopa **Labs:** ↑ Glucose; monitor electrolytes **NIPE:** May take weeks before full effects, take w/ food, ↑ risk of tardive dyskinesia

Zoledronic Acid (Zometa, Reclast) [Antihypercalcemic/Biphosphonate]

Uses: *↑ Ca^{2+} of malignancy (HCM),↓ skeletal-related events in CAP, multiple myeloma, & met bone lesions (*Zometa*) postmenopausal osteoporosis, Paget Dz (*Reclast*)* Action: Bisphosphonate; ↓ osteoclastic bone resorption Dose: *HCM:* 4 mg IV over at least 15 min; may retreat in 7 d if adequate renal Fxn. *Bone lesions/myeloma:* 4 mg IV over at least 15 min, repeat q3–4wk PRN; prolonged w/ Cr ↑; *Reclast:* 5 mg IV annually Caution: [C, ?/–] Loop diuretics, aminoglycosides; ASA-sensitive asthmatics; avoid invasive dental procedures w/ CR Contra: Bisphosphonate allergy; w/ dental procedures Disp: Vial 4 mg, 5 mg SE: all are adverse effects ↑ w/ renal dysfunction; fever, flulike Sxs, GI upset, insomnia, anemia; electrolyte abnormalities, osteonecrosis of jaw Interactions: ↑ Risk of hypocalcemia W/ diuretics; ↑ risk of nephrotox W/ aminoglycosides, thalidomide Labs: Follow Cr; effect prolonged w/ Cr increase NIPE: ↑ Fluids to 2–3 L/d; requires vigorous prehydration; do not exceed recommended doses/inf duration to ↓ dose-related renal dysfunction; avoid oral surgery; dental examination recommended prior to therapy; ↓ dose w/ renal dysfunction

Zolmitriptan (Zomig, Zomig XMT, Zomig Nasal) [Analgesic Migraine Agent / 5-HT₁ Receptor Agonist]

Uses: *Acute Rx migraine* Action: Selective serotonin agonist; causes vasoconstriction Dose: Initial 2.5 mg PO, may repeat after 2 h, 10 mg max in 24 h; nasal 5 mg; if HA returns, repeat after 2 h 10 mg max 24 h Caution: [C, ?/–] Contra: Ischemic heart Dz, Prinzmetal angina, uncontrolled HTN, accessory conduction pathway disorders, ergots, MAOIs Disp: Tabs 2.5, 5 mg; Rapid tabs (ZMT) 2.5, 5 mg; nasal 5 mg, SE: Dizziness, hot flashes, paresthesias, chest tightness, myalgia, diaphoresi Interactions: ↑ Effects W/ cimetidine, MAOIs, oral contraceptives, propranolol; ↑ risk of prolonged vasospasms W/ ergots; ↑ risk of serotonin synd W/ sibutramine, SSRIs NIPE: Admin to relieve migraines; not for prophylaxis

Zolpidem (Ambien, Ambien CR) [C-IV] [Sedative/Hypnotic]

Uses: *Short-term Rx of insomnia* Action: Hypnotic agent Dose: 5–10 mg or 12.5 mg CR PO hs PRN; ↓ in elderly (use 6.25 mg CR), hepatic insuff Caution: [B, –] Contra: Breast-feeding Disp: Tabs 5, 10 mg; CR 6.25, 12.5 mg SE: HA, dizziness, drowsiness, N, myalgia **Interactions:** ↑ CNS depression *W/* CNS depressants, sertraline, EtOH; ↑ effects *OF* ketoconazole; ↓ effects *OF* rifampin **NIPE:** Take w/o food; ⊘ DC abruptly if long-term use; may develop tolerance to drug; may be habit-forming; CR delivers a rapid then a longer lasting dose

Zonisamide (Zonegran) [Anticonvulsant/Sulfonamide]
Uses: *Adjunct Rx complex partial Szs* **Action:** Anticonvulsant **Dose:** Initial 100 mg/d PO; may ↑ to 400 mg/d **Caution:** [C, –] ↑ tox w/ CYP3A4 inhibitor; ↓ levels w/ concurrent carbamazepine, phenytoin, phenobarbital, valproic acid **Contra:** Allergy to sulfonamides; oligohydrosis & hypothermia in peds **Disp:** Caps 25, 50, 100 mg **SE:** Dizziness, drowsiness, confusion, ataxia, memory impair, paresthesias, psychosis, nystagmus, diplopia, tremor, anemia, leukopenia, GI upset, nephrolithiasis, Stevens–Johnson synd **Interactions:** ↑ Tox *W/* CYP3A4 inhibitor; ↓ effects *W/* carbamazepine, phenobarbital, phenytoin, valproic acid **Labs:** ↑ Serum alkaline phosphatase, ALT, AST, creatinine, BUN, ↓ glucose, Na **NIPE:** ⊘ D/C abruptly; swallow capsules whole; monitor for ↓ sweating & ↑ body temperature

Zoster Vaccine, Live (Zostavax) [Vaccine] **Uses:** * Prevent varicella zoster in adults >60 y* **Action:** Active immunization (live vaccine), to Herpes zoster **Dose:** *Adults.* 0.65 mL SQ **Contra:** Gelatin, neomycin anaphylaxis; untreated TB, immunocompromised **Caution:** [C,?/–] Not for peds **Disp:** SDV **SE:** Inj site Rxn, HA **Interactions:** ↑ Risk of extensive rash *W/* corticosteroids **NIPE:** ⊘ PRG for at least 3 mo > vaccination; once reconstituted use immediately

COMMONLY USED MEDICINAL HERBS

The following is a guide to some common herbal products. These may be sold separately or in combination with other products. According to the FDA: "Manufacturers of dietary supplements can make claims about how their products affect the structure or function of the body, but they may not claim to prevent, treat, cure, mitigate, or diagnose a disease without prior FDA approval."

Aloe Vera (*Aloe barbadensis*) Uses: Topically for burns, skin irritation, sunburn, wounds; internally used for constipation, amenorrhea, asthma, colds **Actions:** multiple chemical components; aloinosides inhibit H_2O & electrolyte reabsorption & irritates colon which ↑ peristalsis & propulsion; wound healing d/t ↓ production of thromboxane A2, inhibiting bradykinin & histamine; **Available forms:** Apply gel topically 3–5/d PRN; caps 100–200 mg PO hs **Contra:** ⊘ Internally if PRG, lactating, or in children <12 y **Notes/SE:** Abd cramping, D, edema, hematuria, hypokalemia, muscle weakness, dermatitis **Interactions w/ internal use:** ↑ K^+ loss **W/** BB, corticosteroids, diuretics, licorice; ↑ effects **OF** antiarrhythmics, corticosteroids, digoxin, diuretics, hyperglycemias, jimsonweed **Labs:** ↓ K^+, BS **NIPE:** Assess for dehydration, electrolyte imbalance, abd distress **W/** internal use; stimulates uterine contractions & may cause spontaneous abortion

Arnica (*Arnica montana*) Uses: ↓ Swelling & inflammation from acne, blunt injury, bruises, rashes, sprains **Action:** Sesquiterpenoids have shown antibacterial, anti-inflammatory, & analgesic properties **Available forms:** Topical cream spray, oint, tinc; for poultice dilute tinc 3–10 × w/ water & apply PRN **Contra:** Poisonous, ⊘ take internally; ⊘ if pt allergic to arnica, chrysanthemums, marigold, sunflowers **Notes/SE:** Arrhythmias, abd pain, cardiac arrest, contact dermatitis coma, death, hepatic failure, HTN, nervousness, restlessness **Interactions:** ↑ Risk of bleeding **W/** ASA, heparin, warfarin, angelica, anise, asafetida, bogbean, boldo, capsicum, celery, chamomile, clove, danshen, fenugreek, feverfew, garlic, ginger, ginkgo, ginseng, horse chestnut, horseradish, licorice, meadowsweet, onion, pau pain, passion flower, poplar bark, prickly ash, quassia wood, red clover, turmeric, wild carrot, wild lettuce, willow; ↓ effects **OF** antihypertensives **Labs:** None **NIPE:** Apply to broken skin, ⊘ use in PRG & lactation, serious liver & kidney damage w/ internal use, ingestion of flowers & root can cause death, prolonged topical use ↑ risk of allergic reaction

Astragalus (*Astragalus membranaceus*) Uses: Rx of resp In fxns, enhancement of immune system, & HF **Action:** Root saponins ↑ diuresis, ↓ BP; anti-inflammatory action related to the stimulation of macrophages, ↑ antibody formation & ↑ T-lymphocyte proliferation **Available forms:** Caps/tabs 1–4 g tid, PO; Liq ext 4–8 mL/d (1:2 ratio) %doses; dry ext 250 mg (1:8 ratio) tid, PO **Notes/SE:** Immunosuppression w/ doses >28 g **Interactions:** ↑ Effect OF acyclovir, anticoagulants, antihypertensives, antithrombotics, antiplts, interleukin-2, interferon; ↓ effect OF cyclophosphamide **Labs:** ↑ PT, INR **NIPE:** Use cautiously in immunosuppressed pts or those w/ autoimmune Dz

Bilberry (*Vaccinium myrtillus*) **Uses:** Prevent/treat visual problems such as cataract, retinopathy, myopia, glaucoma, macular degeneration; treat vascular problems such as hemorrhoids, & varicose veins **Actions:** Contain anthocyanidins that ↓ vascular permeability, inhibit plt aggregation & thrombus formation, ↑ antioxidant effects on LDLs & liver, ↑ regeneration of rhodopsin in retina **Available forms:** Products should have 25% anthocyanoside content; capes, extracts, dried, or fresh fruit, leaves; eye/vascular problems 240–480 mg PO bid/tid; night vision 60–120 mg of extract PO OD **Contra:** ⊘ PRG or lactation; caution in patients with DM and bleeding disorders **Notes/SE:** Constipation **Interactions:** ↑ Effects OF anticoagulants, antiplts, insulin, NSAIDs, oral hypoglycemics; ↓ effects OF Fe **Labs:** ↑ PT; ↓ glucose, plt aggregation **NIPE:** Large dose of leaves for long periods of time may be poisonous/fatal; take w/o regard to food

Black Cohosh (*Cimicifuga racemosa*) **Uses:** Antitussive; smooth-muscle relaxant; management of menopausal symptoms esp hot flashes, sleep disturbance & anxiety, premenstrual synd, & dysmenorrhea. Anti-inflammatory, peripheral vasodilation, & sedative effects **Action:** Estrogenic activity w/ some studies showing ↓ in LH; vasodilation activity causing ↑ blood flow & hypotensive effects; antimicrobial activity **Available forms:** Dried root/rhizome caps 40–200 mg once/d; fluid ext (1:1) 2–4 mL or 1 tsp once/d; tinc (1:5) 3–6 mL or 1–2 tsp once/d; powdered ext (4:1) 250–500 mg once/d; Remifemin menopause (standardized ext brand name) 20 mg bid **Notes/SE:** Hypotension, bradycardia, N/V, anorexia, HA, miscarriage, nervous system & visual disturbances **Interactions:** Effects OF antihypertensives, estrogen HRT, OCPs, hypnotics, sedatives; tinc may cause a reaction W/ disulfiram & metronidazole; ↑ antiproliferative effect W/ tamoxifen; ↓ effects OF ferrous fumarate, ferrous gluconate, ferrous sulfate **Labs:** May ↓ LH levels & plt counts **NIPE:** Tinc contains large % of EtOH, ⊘ use in PRG or lactation or give to children

Bogbean (*Menyanthes trifoliate*) **Uses:** ↑ Appetite; treat GI distress; anti-inflammatory for arthritis; **Action:** Several chemical constituents include alkaloids (choline, gentianin, gentianidine), flavonoids (hyperin, kaempferol, quercetin, rutin, trifolioside) that act as an anti-inflammatory, and acids (caffeic, chlorogenic, ferulic, folic, palmitic, salicylic, vanillic) that act as bile stimulants & other elements such as carotene, ceryl alcohol, coumarin, iridoid, scopoletin; two compounds produce considerable inhibition of prostaglandin synthesis **Available Forms:** Extract (1:1 dilution) 1–2 mL PO tid with fluid; dried leaf as tea 1–3 g PO tid **Contra:** ⊘ PRG or lactating **Notes/SE:** N/V, bleeding **Interactions:** ↑ Risk of bleeding *W/* anticoagulants, antiplts, ANA, NSAIDs; ↑ Effects *OF* stimulant laxitives; ↓ effects *OF* antacids, H2 antagonists, proton pump inhibitors, sucralfate **Labs:** None **NIPE:** May ↑ uterine contractions; extracts contain EtOH; monitor for S/Sxs bleeding or ↑ bruising; ⊘ if h/o colitis, anemia

Borage (*Borage officinalis*) **Uses:** Oil used for eczema & dermatitis & as a GLA supplement; treat colds, coughs, & bronchitis; anti-inflammatory action used to treat arthritis **Action:** Oil contains GLA & its metabolites produce anti-inflammatory action; topical oil absorbed in skin ↑ fluid retention in stratum corneum; mucilage & malic acid components have expectorant & diuretic actions; contains alkaloids that are hepatotoxic **Available forms:** Caps with 10–25% GLA; 1.1–1.4 g GLA PO OD for joint inflammation; oil topical application bid for dermatitis & eczema **Contra:** ⊘ PRG, lactation, & pts with h/o liver Dz or Sz disorder **Notes/SE:** ↑ Constipation, flatulence, liver dysfunction, Sz **Interactions:** ↑ Risk of bleeding *W/* anticoagulants, antiplts; ↑ effects *OF* antihypertensives; ↓ effects *OF* anticonvulsants, phenothiazine, TCAs; ↓ effects of herb *W/* NSAIDs **Labs:** Monitor LFTs; may ↑ LFTs, PT & INR **NIPE:** Only use herb without UPA alkaloids

Bugleweed (*Lycopus virginicus*) **Uses:** ↓ Hyperthyroid symptoms, analgesic, astringent **Action:** inhibits gonadotropin, prolactin, TSH & IgG antibody activity **Available forms:** Teas, extracts, dried herb **Contra:** ⊘ PRG or lactation, pts with hypothyroidism, pituitary or thyroid tumors, hypogonadism, & CHF **Notes/SE:** Thyroid gland enlargement **Interactions:** ↑ Effects *OF* insulin, oral hypoglycemics, ↑ thyroid suppressing effects *W/* balm leaf & wild thyme plant; ↓ effect *OF* thyroid hormone **Labs:** ↓ FSH, LH, HCG, TSH; monitor BS **NIPE:** ⊘ Substitute for antithyroid drugs; ⊘ if undergoing treatment or diagnostic procedures with radioisotopes; ⊘ stop abruptly

Butcher's Broom (*Ruscus aculeatus*) **Uses:** Rx of circulatory disorders such as PVD, varicose veins, & leg edema; hemorrhoids; diuretic; laxative; inflammation; arthritis **Action:** Vasoconstriction due to direct activation of the α-receptors of the smooth-muscle cells in vascular walls **Available forms:** Raw ext 7–11 mg once/d, PO; tea 1 tsp in 1 cup water; topical oint apply PRN **Notes/SE:** GI upset, N/V **Interactions:** ↑ Effects *OF* anticoagulants, MAOIs; ↓ effects *OF* antihypertensives **Labs:** None **NIPE:** Hypertensive crisis may occur if admin w/ MAOIs; ⊘ use in PRG & lactation

Capsicum (*Capsicum frutescens*) **Uses:** Topical use includes pain relief from arthritis, diabetic neuropathy, postherpetic neuralgia, postsurgical pain; internal uses include circulatory disorders, GI distress, HTN **Actions:** Stimulates skin pain receptors causing burning sensations; desensitization of pain receptors results in pain relief; ↓ lymphocyte production, antibody production, & plt aggregation **Available forms:** Topical creams 0.025–0.25% up to qid; caps 400–500 mg PO tid **Contra:** ⊘ On open sores, in PRG, children <2 y **Notes/SE:** GI irritation, sweating, bronchospasm, respiratory irritation, topical burning, stinging, erythema

Interactions: ↑ Effects *OF* anticoagulants, antiplts, theophylline; ↑ risk of cough *W*/ ACEIs; ↑ risk of anticoagulant effects *W*/ feverfew, garlic, ginger, ginkgo, ginseng; ↑ risk of hypertensive crisis *W*/ MAOIs; ↓ effects *OF* clonidine, methyldopa **Labs:** None **NIPE:** Pain relief may take several weeks; ∅ apply heat on areas *W*/ topical capsicum cream; avoid contact *W*/ eyes or mucous membranes

Cascara (*Rhamnus purshiana*) **Uses:** Laxative **Action:** Stimulates large intestine, ↑ bowel motility & propulsion, **Available forms:** Liq extract 1–5 mL PO OD; **Contra:** ∅ PRG, lactation & IBD **Notes/SE:** N/V, abd cramps, urine discoloration **Interactions:** ↑ Effects *OF* antiarrhythmics, cardiac glycosides; ↑ K⁺ loss *W*/ diuretics, corticosteroids, cardiac glycosides; ↓ effects *W*/ antacids, milk **Labs:** ↓ serum K⁺ **NIPE:** Short-term use; monitor electrolytes; caution w/diuretics

Chamomile (*Matricaria recutita*) **Uses:** Anti-inflammatory, antipyretic, antimicrobial, antispasmodic, astringent, sedative **Action:** Ingredients include α-bisabolol oil, which ↓ inflammation, antispasmodic activity, ↑ healing times for burns & ulcers, & inhibits ulcer formation; apigenin contributes to the anti-inflammatory effect, antispasmodic & sedative effect; azulene inhibits histamine release; chamazulene reduces inflammation & has antioxidant & antimicrobial effects **Available forms:** Teas 3–5 g (1 tbsp) flower heads steeped in water tid–qid, also use as a gargle or compress; fluid ext 1:1 -45% EtOH 1–3 mL tid **Notes/SE:** Allergic reactions if pt allergic to Compositae family (ragweed, sunflowers, asters) eg, angioedema, eczema, contact dermatitis & anaphylaxis **Interactions:** ↑ Effects *OF* CNS depressants, EtOH, anticoagulants, antiplts; ↑ risk *OF* miscarriage; ↓ effects *OF* drugs metabolized by CY4503A4, eg, alprazolam, atorvastatin, diazepam, ketoconazole, verapamil **Labs:** Monitor anticoagulant levels **NIPE:** ∅ PRG, lactation, children <2 y, pt w/ asthma or hay fever

Chondroitin Sulfate **Uses:** Combine w/ glucosamine to Rx arthritis; use as an anticoagulant **Action:** Attracts fluid & nutrients into the joints; inhibits thrombi **Available forms:** 1200 mg once/d, PO, & usually given w/ glucosamine 1500 mg once/d, PO for nl wt adults **Notes/SE:** D, dyspepsia, HA, N/V, restlessness **Interactions:** ↑ Effects *OF* anticoagulants, ASA, NSAIDs **Labs:** None **NIPE:** ∅ PRG & lactation

Comfrey (*Symphytum officinale*) **Uses:** Topical treatment of wounds, bruises, sprains, inflammation **Action:** Multiple chemical components, allantoin promotes cell division, rosmarinic acid has anti-inflammatory effects, tannin possesses astringent effects, mucilage is a demulcent with anti-inflammatory properties, pyrrolizidine alkaloids cause hepatotox **Available forms:** Topical application w/ 5–20% of herb applied on intact skin for up to 10 d **Contra:** ∅ Internally d/t hepatotox, ∅ PRG or lactation **Notes/SE:** N/V, exfoliative dermatitis w/ topical use **Interactions:** ↑ Risk of hepatotox *W*/ ingestion of borage, golden ragwort, hemp, petasites **Labs:** ↑ LFTs, total bilirubin, urine bilirubin **NIPE:** ∅ Use for more than 6 wk in 1 y; ∅ use on broken skin

Coriander (*Coriandrum sativum*) **Uses:** ↑ Appetite, treat D, dyspepsia, flatulence **Action:** Stimulates gastric secretions, spasmolytic effects **Available forms:** Tinc 10–30 gtts PO OD; **Contra:** ⊘ PRG or lactation **Actions/SE:** N/V, fatty liver tumors, allergic skin Rxns **Interactions:** ↑ Effects *OF* oral hypoglycemics **Labs:** Monitor BS **NIPE:** ↑ Risk of photosensitivity—use sunscreen

Cranberry (*Vaccinium macrocarpon*) **Uses:** Prevention UTI; urinary deodorizer in urinary incontinence **Actions:** Interferes with bacterial adherence to epithelial cells of the bladder **Available forms:** Caps 300–500 mg PO bid–qid; unsweetened juice 8–16 oz daily; tinc 3–5 mL **SE:** D, irritation, nephrolithiasis if ↑ urinary Ca oxalate **Interactions:** ↑ Excretion of alkaline drugs such as antidepressants & methotrexate will cause ↓ effectiveness *OF* drug; ↓ effectiveness *OF* Uva-ursi; **Labs:** ↑ Urine pH **NIPE:** Not effective in treating UTI; tinc contains up to 45% EtOH; only unsweetened form effective; regular use may ↓ frequency of bacteriuria with pyria

Dong Quai (*Angelica polymorpha, sinensis*) **Uses:** Dysmenorrhea, PMS, menorrhagia, chronic pelvic Infxn, irregular menstruation. Other reported uses include anemia, HTN, HA, rhinitis, neuralgia, & hepatitis **Action:** Root exts contain at least 6 coumarin derivatives that have anticoagulant, vasodilating, antispasmodic, & CNS-stimulating activity. Studies demonstrate weak estrogen-agonist actions of the ext **Available forms:** Caps 500 mg, 1–2 caps PO, tid; Liq ext 1–2 gtt, tid; tea 1–2 g, tid **Notes/SE:** D, bleeding, photosensitivity, fever **Interactions:** ↑ Effects *OF* anticoagulants, antiplts, estrogens, warfarin; ↑ anticoagulant activity *W/* chamomile, dandelion, horse chestnut, red clover; ↑ risk of disulfiram-like reaction *W/* disulfiram, metronidazole **Labs:** ↑ PT, PTT, INR **NIPE:** Photosensitivity—use sunscreen, ⊘ if breast-feeding or PRG; tincs & exts contain EtOH up to 60%; stop herb 14 d prior to dental or surgical procedures

Echinacea (*Echinacea purpurea*) **Uses:** Immune system stimulant; prevention/Rx of colds, flu; as supportive therapy for colds & chronic Infxns of the resp tract & lower urinary tract **Action:** Stimulates phagocytosis & cytokine production & ↑ resp cellular activity; topically exerts anesthetic, antimicrobial, & antiinflammatory effects **Available forms:** Caps w/ powdered herb equivalent to 300–500 mg, PO, tid; pressed juice 6–9 mL, PO, once/d; tinc 2–4 mL, PO, tid (1:5 dilution); tea 2 tsp (4 g) of powdered herb in 1 cup of boiling water **Notes/SE:** Fever, taste perversion, urticaria, angioedema **Contra:** ⊘ In pts w/ autoimmune Dz, collagen Dz, HIV, leukemia, MS, TB **Interactions:** ↑ Risk of disulfiram-like reaction *W/* disulfiram, metronidazole; ↑risk of exacerbation of HIV or AIDS *W/* echinacea & amprenavir, other protease inhibitors; ↓ effects *OF* azathioprine, basiliximab, corticosteroids, cyclosporine, daclizumab, econazole vag cream, muromonab-CD3, mycophenolate, prednisone, tacrolimus **Labs:** ↑ ALT, AST, lymphocytes, ESR **NIPE:** Large doses of herb interferes w/ sperm activity; ⊘ w/ breast-feeding or PRG; ⊘ continuously for longer than 8 wk w/o a 3-wk break in Rx

Ephedra/Ma Huang **Uses:** Stimulant, aid in wt loss, bronchial dilation **Dose:** Not OK d/t reported deaths (>100 mg/d can be life-threatening). US sales banned by FDA in 2004; bitter orange w/ similar properties has replaced this compound in most wt loss supplements **Caution:** Adverse cardiac events, strokes, death **SE:** Nervousness, HA, insomnia, palpitations, V, hyperglycemia **Interactions:** Digoxin, antihypertensives, antidepressants, DA medications ↑ ALT, AST, total bilirubin, urine bilirubin, serum glucose **NIPE:** Tincs & exts contain EtOH; linked to several deaths; monitor for behavioral mood changes

Evening Primrose Oil (*Oenothera biennis*) **Uses:** PMS, diabetic neuropathy, ADHD, IBS, RA, mastalgia **Action:** Anti-inflammatory, antispasmodic, diuretic, sedative effects related to a high concentration of essential fatty acids especially GLA & CLA & their conversion into prostaglandins **Available forms:** Caps, gel-caps, Liq. dose depends on GLA content. DM neuropathy: 4000 mg–6000 mg PO OD; Eczema 4000 mg PO OD; Mastalgia 3000 mg–4000 mg PO ÷ doses; PMS: 2000 mg–4000 mg PO OD; RA: Up to 5000 mg PO OD **Notes/SE:** Indigestion, N soft stools, flatulence, HA, anorexia, rash **Contra:** ⊘ PRG or lactation; ⊘ persons w/ Sz disorders **Interactions:** ↑ Phenobarbital metabolism, ↓ Sz threshold, ↑ effects *OF* diuretics, sedatives **Labs:** None **NIPE:** May take up to 4 mo for effectiveness, take w/ food

Feverfew (*Tanacetum parthenium*) **Uses:** Anti-inflammatory for arthritis, asthma, digestion problems, fever, migraines, menstrual complaints, threatened abortion **Action:** Active ingredient, parthenolide, inhibits serotonin release, prostaglandin synthesis, plt aggregation, & histamine release from mast cells; several ingredients inhibit activation of polymorphonuclear leukocytes & leukotriene synthesis **Available forms:** Freeze-dried leaf ext 25 mg once/d; caps 300 mg–400 mg tid PO; tinc 15–30 gtt once/d to 0.2–0.7 mg of parthenolide **Notes/SE:** Mouth ulcers, muscle stiffness, joint pain, GI upset, rash **Contra:** ⊘ PRG & lactation or w/ ragweed allergy **Interactions:** ↑ Effects *OF* anticoagulants, antiplts, ↓ effects *OF* Fe absorption **Labs:** ↑ PT, INR, PTT **NIPE:** ⊘ D/C herb abruptly or may experience joint stiffness & pain, headaches, insomnia

Fish Oil Supplements (Omega-3 Polyunsaturated Fatty Acid): **Uses:** CAD, hypercholesterolemia, hypertriglyceridemia, type 2 DM, arthritis **Efficacy:** No definitive data on ↓ cardiac risk in general population; may ↓ lipids and help w/ secondary MI prevention **Dose:** One FDA approved; OTC 1500–3000 mg/d; AHA recommends 1 g/d **Caution:** Mercury contamination possible, some studies suggest ↑ cardiac events **SE:** ↑ Bleed risk, dyspepsia, belching, aftertaste **Interactions:** Anticoagulants

Garlic (*Allium sativum*) **Uses:** Antithrombotic, antilipidemic, antitumor, antimicrobial, antiasthmatic, anti-inflammatory **Action:** Inhibits gram(+) & gram(−) organisms, exerts cholesterol-lowering by preventing gastric lipase fat digestion & fecal excretion of sterols & bile acids & it inhibits free radicals **Available forms:** Teas, tabs, caps, ext, oil, dried powder, syrup, fresh bulb **Notes/SE:**

Dizziness, diaphoresis, HA, N/V, hypothyroidism, contact dermatitis, allergic reactions, oral mucosa irritation, systemic garlic odor, ↓ Hgb production, lysis of RBCs **Interactions:** ↑ Effects *OF* anticoagulants, antiplts, insulin, oral hypoglycemics; ↓ effects *W/* acidophilus **Labs:** ↓ Total cholesterol, LDL, triglycerides, plt aggregation, iodine uptake; ↑ PT, serum IgE **NIPE:** ⊘ PRG, lactation, prior to surgery, GI disorders; report bleeding, bruising, petechiae, tarry stools, monitor CBC, PT

Gentian (*Gentiana lutea*) **Uses:** ↑ Appetite, treat digestive disorders such as colitis, IBS, flatulence **Actions:** Chemical components stimulate digestive juices **Available forms:** Liq extract 2–4g PO OD, tinc 1–3 g PO OD, dried root 2–4 g PO OD **Contra:** ⊘ PRG, lactation, & HTN **Notes/SE:** N/V, HA **Interactions:** ↑ CNS sedation *W/* barbiturates, benzodiazepines, EtOH if extract/tinc contains alcohol; ↓ absorption *OF* Fe salts **Labs:** None **NIPE:** Caution—many herb preps contain up to 60% EtOH

Ginger (*Zingiber officinale*) **Uses:** Antiemetic ↓ N/V; anti-inflammatory relieves pain & swelling of muscle injury, osteoarthritis & RA; antispasmodic action relieves colic, flatulence & indigestion; antiplt; antipyretic; antioxidant; anti-infective against gram(+) & gram(−) bacteria **Action:** Anti-inflammatory effect inhibits prostaglandin, thromboxane, & leukotriene biosynthesis; antiemetic effects due to action on the GI tract; antiplt effect due to the inhibition of thromboxane formation; + inotropic effect on CV system **Available forms:** Dosage form & strength depends on Dz process **General use:** Dried ginger caps 1 g once/d, PO; fluid ext 0.7–2 mL once/d, PO, (2:1 ratio); tabs 500 mg bid–qid, PO; tinc 1.7–5 mL once/d, PO, (1:5 ratio) **Interactions:** ↑ Risk of bleeding *W/* anticoagulants, antiplts; ↑ risk of disulfiram-like reaction *W/* disulfiram, metronidazole **Labs:** ↑ PT **NIPE:** Store herb in cool, dry area; ⊘ PRG, lactation; lack of standardization for herb dosing

Ginkgo Biloba **Uses:** Effective *W/* circulatory disorders, cerebrovascular Dz, & dementia; used to improve alertness & attention span **Action:** Ext flavonoids release neurotransmitters & inhibit monoamine oxidase, which enhances cognitive function; vascular protective action results from relaxation of blood vessels, ↑ tissue perfusion, inhibition of plt aggregation; eradicates free radicals & ↓ polymorphonuclear neutrophils **Available forms:** Dosage depends on diagnosis **General use:** Tabs & caps 40–80 mg tid, PO; tinc 0.5 mL tid, PO; ext 40–80 mg tid, PO **Notes/SE:** Anxiety, D, flatulence, HA, heart palpitations, N/V, restlessness **Interactions:** ↑ Effect *OF* MAOIs; ↑ risk of bleeding *W/* anisindione, dalteparin, dicumarol garlic, heparin, salicylates, warfarin; ↑ risk of coma *W/* trazodone; ↑ effect *OF* carbamazepine, gabapentin, insulin, oral hypoglycemics, phenobarbital, phenytoin; ↓ seizure threshold *W/* bupropion, TCAs **Labs:** ↑ PT **NIPE:** ⊘ PRG & lactation; tincs contain up to 60% EtOH; ⊘ 2 wk prior to surgery

Ginseng (*Panax quinquefolius*) **Uses:** ↑ Physical endurance, quinconcentration, appetite, sleep & stress resistance; ↓ fatigue; antioxidant; aids in glucose control **Action:** Dried root contains ginsenosides, which ↑ natural killer cell activity, & nuclear RNA synthesis, & motor activity **Available forms:** No standard dosage *General use:* Caps 200 mg–500 mg once/d, PO; tea 3 g steeped in boiling water tid PO, tinc 1–2 mg once/d, PO (1:1 dilution) **Notes/SE:** Anxiety, anorexia, chest pain, D, HTN, N/V, palpitations **Interactions:** ↑ Effects *OF* estrogen, hypoglycemics, CNS stimulants, caffeine, ephedra; ↑ risk of bleeding *W/* ibuprofen; ↑ risk *OF* HA, irritability & visual hallucinations *W/* MAOIs; ↓ effects *OF* anisindione, dicumarol, furosemide, heparin, warfarin **Labs:** ↑ Digoxin level falsely; ↓ glucose, PT, INR **NIPE:** ⊘ Use continuously for >3 mo; ⊘ during PRG or lactation; eval for ginseng abuse syndrome w/ symptoms of D, depression, edema, HTN, insomnia, rash & restlessness

Glucosamine Sulfate (chitosamine) **Uses:** Used w/ chondroitin for the Rx of arthritis **Action:** Stimulate the production of cartilage components **Available forms:** Caps/tabs 1500 mg once/d, PO & chondroitin sulfate 1200 mg once/d, PO for adults of nl wt **Notes/SE:** Abd pain, anorexia, constipation or D, drowsiness, HA, heartburn, N/V, rash **Interactions:** ↑ Effects *OF* hypoglycemics **Labs:** Monitor serum glucose levels in diabetics **NIPE:** Take w/ food to reduce GI effects; no uniform standardization of herb

Green Tea (*Camellia sinensis*) **Uses:** Antioxidant, antibacterial, diuretic; prevention of CA, hyperlipidemia, atherosclerosis, dental caries **Actions:** Chemical components include anti-inflammatory, anti-CA, polyphenol, epigallocatechin, & epigallocatechin-3-gallate which inhibit tumor growth; fluoride & tannins demonstrate antimicrobial action against oral bacteria; antioxidant activity delays lipid peroxidation; antimicrobial action due to inhibition of growth of various bacteria including *S. aureus* **Available forms:** Recommend 300–400 mg polyphenol PO OD (3 cups tea = 240–320 mg polyphenol) **Contra:** Caution ↑ intake may cause tannin-induced asthma **Notes/SE:** Tachycardia, insomnia, anxiety, N/V, ↑ BP **Interactions:** ↑ Effects *OF* doxorubicin, ephedrine, stimulant drugs, theophylline; ↑ risk of hypertensive crisis *W/* MAOIs; ↑ bleeding risk *W/* anticoagulants, antiplts; ↓ effects *W/* antacids, dairy products **Labs:** ↑ PT, PTT **NIPE:** Contains caffeine—caution in PRG, infants, and small children & pts *W/* CAD, hyperthyroidism & anxiety disorders; GI distress d/t tannins ↓ *W/* the addition of milk; ↑ tannin content *W/* ↑ brewing times

Guarana (*Paullinia cupana*) **Uses:** Appetite suppressant, CNS stimulant, ↑ sexual performance, ↑ fatigue **Actions:** ↑ Caffine content stiulates cardiac, CNS, & smooth muscle; ↑ diuresis; ↓ plt aggregation **Available forms:** Daily divided doses w/ max 3 g PO daily **Contra:** Avoid in PRG & lactation, CAD, hyperthyroidism, anxiety disorders d/t high caffine content **Notes/SE:** Insomnia, tachycardia, anxiety, N/V, HA, HTN, Sz **Interactions:** ↑ Effects *OF* anticoagulants, antiplts, β-blockers, bronchodilators; ↑ risk of hypertensive crisis *W/* MAOIs; ↑ effects *W/* cimetidine, ciprofloxacin, ephedrine, hormonal contraceptives, theophylline, cola, coffee; ↓ effects *W/* adenosine, antihypertensives, benzodiazepines, Fe, ↓ effects *W/* smoking **Labs:** ↑ PT, PTT **NIPE:** Tincs contain EtOH; may exacerbate GI disorders & HTN

Hawthorn (*Crataegus laevigata*) Uses: Rx of HTN, arrhythmias, HF, stable angina pectoris, insomnia **Action:** ↑ Myocardial contraction by ↓ oxygen consumption, ↓ peripheral resistance, dilating coronary blood vessels, ACE inhibition **Available forms:** Tinc 1–2 mL (1:5 ratio) tid, PO; Liq ext 0.5–1 mL, (1:1 ration) tid, PO **Notes/SE:** Arrhythmias, fatigue, hypotension, N/V, sedation **Interactions:** ↑ Effects *OF* antihypertensives, cardiac glycosides, CNS depressants, & herbs such as adonis, lily of the valley, squill ↓; effects *OF* Fe **Labs:** False ↑ of digoxin **NIPE:** ⊘ PRG & lactation; many tincs contain EtOH

Horsetail (*Equisetum arvense*) Uses: ↑ Strength of bones, hair, nails, & teeth; diuretic, treat dyspepsia, gout; topically used to treat wounds **Actions:** Multiple chemical components; flavonoids ↑ diuretic activity; contains silica which strengthens bones, hair, & nails **Available forms:** Extract 20–40 gtts in H₂O PO tid–qid; topically 10 g herb/L H₂O as compress PRN **Contra:** ⊘ PRG, lactation, w/ children, CAD; contains nicotine & large amts may cause nicotine tox **Notes/SE:** Nicotine tox (N/V, weakness, fever, dizziness, abnormal heart rate, wt loss) **Interactions:** ↑ Effects *OF* digoxin, diuretics, lithium, adonis, lily of the valley; ↑ CNS stimulation *W/* CNS stimulants, theophylline, coffee, tea, cola, nicotine; ↑ K⁺ depletion *W/* corticosteroids, diuretics, stimulant laxatives, licorice; ↑ risk of thiamine deficiency *W/* EtOH use **Labs:** Monitor digoxin, electrolyte, thiamine levels **NIPE:** Tinc contains EtOH which may cause disulfiram-like reaction if taken with benzodiazepines or metronidazole; short-term use only; active components of herb absorbed thru skin

Kava Kava (*Piper methysticum*) Uses: ↓ Anxiety, stress, & restlessness; sedative effect **Action:** Appears to act directly on the limbic system **Available forms:** Standardized ext (70% kavalactones) 100 mg bid–tid, PO **Notes/SE:** ↑ Reflexes, HA, dizziness, visual changes, hematuria, SOB **Interactions:** ↑ Effects *OF* antiplts, benzodiazepines, CNS depressants, MAOIs, phenobarbital; ↑ absorption when taken *W/* food; ↑ in parkinsonian symptoms *W/* kava kava & antiparkinsonian drugs **Labs:** ↑ ALT, AST, urinary RBCs; ↓ albumin, total protein, bilirubin, urea, plts, lymphocytes **NIPE:** ⊘ Take for >3 mo; ⊘ during PRG & lactation

Licorice (*Glycyrrhiza glabra*) Uses: Expectorant, shampoo, GI complaints **Action:** ↑ Mucus secretions, ↓ peptic activity, ↓ scalp sebum secretion **Available forms:** Liq ext, bulk dried root, tea; 15 g once/d PO of licorice root; intake >50 g once/d may cause tox **Notes/SE:** HTN, arrhythmias, edema, hypokalemia, HA, lethargy, rhabdomyolysis **Interactions:** ↑ Drug effects *OF* diuretics, corticosteroids, may prolong QT interval *W/* loratadine, procainamide, quinidine, terfenadine **Labs:** None **NIPE:** Monitor for electrolyte & ECG changes, HTN, mineralocorticoid-like effects; tox more likely w/ prolonged intake of small doses than one large dose

Melatonin (MEL) Uses: Insomnia, jet lag, antioxidant, immunostimulant **Action:** Hormone produce by the pineal gland in response to darkness; declines w/ age **Available forms:** XR caps 1–3 mg once/d 2 h before hs PO **Notes/SE:** HA, confusion, sedation, HTN, tachycardia, hyperglycemia **Interactions:** ↑ Anxiolytic effects *OF* benzodiazepines; ↑ risk of insomnia *W/* cerebral stimulants, methamphetamine, succinylcholine **Labs:** None **NIPE:** ⊘ During PRG & lactation

Milk Thistle (*Silybum marianum*)
Uses: Rx of hepatotox, dyspepsia, liver protectorant **Action:** stimulates protein synthesis, which leads to liver regeneration **Available forms:** Tinc 70–120 mg (70% silymarin) tid, PO **Notes/SE:** D, menstrual stimulation, N/V **Interactions:** ↑ Effects *OF* drugs metabolized by the cytochrome P-450, CYP3A4, CYP2C9 enzymes **Labs:** ↑ PT; ↓ LFTs, serum glucose **NIPE:** ⊘ PRG & lactation; ⊘ pts allergic to ragweed, chrysanthemums, marigolds, daisies

Nettle (*Urtica dioica*)
Uses: Allergic rhinitis, asthma, cough, TB, BPH, bladder inflammation, diuretic, antispasmodic, expectorant, astringent and topically for oily skin, dandruff, & hair stimulant **Actions:** Multiple chemical components have different actions; scopoletin has anti-inflammatory action, root extract ↓ BPH, lectins display immunostimulant action **Available forms:** Caps 150–300 mg PO OD; Liq extract 2–8 mL PO tid **Contra:** ⊘ PRG or lactating or in children <2 y **Notes/SE:** N/V, edema, abd distress, diarrhea, oliguria, edema, local skin irritation **Interactions:** ↑ Effects *OF* diclofenac, diuretics, barbiturates, antipsychotics, opiates; ↓ effects *OF* anticoagulants **Labs:** Monitor electrolytes **NIPE:** Skin contact w/ plant will result in stinging & burning; ↑ intake of foods high in K^+

Rue (*Ruta graveolens*)
Uses: Sedative, spasmolytic for muscle cramps, GI & menstrual disorders, promote lactation, promote abortion via uterine stimulation, anti-inflammatory effect for sports injuries, bruising, arthritis, joint pain **Action:** Contains essential oils, flavonoids, & alkaloids; shown mutagenic & cytotoxic action on cells; produced CV effects due to + chronotropic & inotropic effects on atria; vasodilatory effects reduce BP; shown strengthening effect on capillaries; alkaloids produce antispasmodic & abortifacient activity **Available forms:** Caps, extracts, teas, topical creams, topical oils; topical oil for earache; topical creams to affected areas PRN; teas use 1 tsp/1/4 L H_2O; extract 1/4–1 tsp PO tid with food; caps 1 PO tid with food **Notes/SE:** Dizziness, tremors, hypotension, bradycardia, allergic skin reactions, spontaneous abortion **Contra:** ⊘ During PRG or lactation or give to children; caution in pts with CHF, arrhythmias, or receiving antihypertensive medication **Interactions:** ↑ Inotropic effects *OF* cardiac glycosides; ↑ effects *OF* antihypertensives & warfarin; ↓ effects *OF* fertility drugs **Labs:** ↑ BUN, Cr, LFT **NIPE:** Large doses can be toxic or fatal; research does not establish a safe dose; tincs & extracts contain EtOH; no data with use in children; ⊘ if h/o EtOH abuse or liver disease

Saw Palmetto (*Serenoa repens*)
Uses: Rx of benign prostatic hypertrophy (BPH) stages 1 & 2 (inhibits testosterone-5-α-reductase), ↑ sperm production, ↑ breast size (estrogenic), ↑ sexual vigor, mild diuretic, treat chronic cystitis **Action:** Theorized that sitosterols inhibit conversion of testosterone to dihydrotestosterone

(DHT), which reduces the prostate gland, also competes w/ DHT on receptor sites resulting in antiestrogenic effects **Available forms:** Caps/tabs 160 mg bid, PO; tinc 20–30 gtt qid (1:2 ration); fluid ext, standardized 160 mg bid PO or 320 mg once/d PO **Notes/SE:** Abd pain, back pain, D, dysuria, HA, HTN, N/V, impotence **Contra:** ⊘ PRG, lactation **Interactions:** ↑ Effects *OF* adrenergics, anticoagulants, antiplts, hormones, Fe **Labs:** May affect semen analysis, may cause false ‑ PSA **NIPE:** Take w/ meals to ↓ GI upset, do baseline PSA prior to taking herb, no standardization of herb content

Spirulina (*Spirulina* spp)

Uses: Rx of obesity & as a nutritional supplement **Action:** Contains 65% protein, all amino acids, carotenoids, B-complex vitamins, essential fatty acids & Fe; has been shown to inhibit replicating viral cells **Available forms:** Caps/tabs or powder admin 3–5 g ac, PO **Notes/SE:** Anorexia, N/V **Interactions:** ↑ Effects *OF* anticoagulants; ↓ effects *OF* thyroid hormones due to high iodine content; ↓ absorption *OF* vitamin B$_{12}$ **Labs:** ↑ Serum Ca, alkaline phosphatase; monitor PT, INR **NIPE:** May contain ↑ levels of Hg & radioactive ion content

Stevia (*Stevia rebaudiana*)

Uses: Natural sweetener, hypoglycemic and hypotensive properties **Actions:** Multiple chemical components; sweetness d/t glycoside stevioside; hypotensive effect may be d/t diuretic action or vasodilation action **Available forms:** Liq extract, powder, caps **Notes/SE:** HA, dizziness, bloating **Interactions:** ↑ Hypotensive effects *W/* antihypertensives esp CCB, diuretics **Labs:** Monitor BS **NIPE:** Monitor BP; does not encourage dental caries

St. John's Wort (*Hypericum perforatum*)

Uses: Depression, anxiety, anti-inflammatory, antiviral **Actions:** MAOI in vitro, not in vivo; bacteriostatic & bactericidal, ↑ capillary blood flow, uterotonic activity in animals **Available forms:** Teas, tabs, caps, tinc, oil ext for topical use **Notes/SE:** Photosensitivity (use sunscreen) rash, dizziness, dry mouth, GI distress **Interactions:** Enhance MAOI activity, EtOH, narcotics, sympathomimetics ↑ GH; ↓ digoxin, serum iron, serum prolactin, theophylline **NIPE:** ⊘ PRG, breast-feeding, in or children, ⊘ w/ SSRIs, MAOIs, EtOH, ⊘ sun exposure

Tea Tree (*Melaleuca alternifolia*)

Uses: Rx of superficial wounds (bacterial, viral,& fungal), insect bites, minor burns, cold sores, acne **Action:** Broad-spectrum antibiotic activity against *E. coli, S. aureus, C. albicans* **Available forms:** Topical creams, lotions, oint, oil apply topically PRN **Notes/SE:** Ataxia, contact dermatitis, D, drowsiness, GI mucosal irritation **Interactions:** ↓ Effects *OF* drugs that affect histamine release **Labs:** ↑ Neutrophil count **NIPE:** Caution pt to use externally only; ⊘ apply to broken skin

Valerian (*Valeriana officinalis*)

Uses: Antianxiety, antispasmodic, dysmenorrheal, restlessness, sedative **Action:** Inhibits uptake & stimulates release of GABA, which ↑ GABA concentration extracellularly & causes sedation **Available forms:** Ext 400–900 mg PO 30 min < HS, tea 2–3 g (1 tsp of crude herb) qid,

PRN, tinc 3–5 mL (1/2–1 tsp) (1:5 ratio) PO qid, PRN **Notes/SE:** GI upset, HA, insomnia, N/V, palpitations, restlessness, vision changes **Interactions:** ↑ Effects *OF* barbiturates, benzodiazepines, opiates, EtOH, catnip, hops, kava kava, passion flower, skullcap; ↓ effects *OF* MAOIs, phenytoin, warfarin **Labs:** ↑ ALT, AST, total bilirubin, urine bilirubin **NIPE:** Periodic check of LFTs, unknown effects in PRG & lactation, full effect may take 2–4 wk, taper herb to avoid withdrawal symptoms after long-term use

Unsafe Herbs with Known Toxicity

Agent	Toxicities
Aconite	Salivation, N/V, blurred vision, cardiac arrhythmias
Aristolochic acid	Nephrotox
Calamus	Possible carcinogenicity
Chaparral	Hepatotox, possible carcinogenicity, nephrotox
"Chinese herbal mixtures"	May contain MaHuang or other dangerous herbs
Coltsfoot	Hepatotox, possibly carcinogenic
Comfrey	Hepatotox, carcinogenic
Ephedra/MaHuang	Adverse cardiac events, stroke, Sz
Juniper	High allergy potential, D, Sz, nephrotox
Kava kava	Hepatotox
Licorice	Chronic daily amounts (>30 g/mo) can result in ↓ K+, Na/fluid retention w/HTN, myoglobinuria, hyporeflexia
Life root	Hepatotox, liver cancer
MaHuang/Ephedra	Adverse cardiac events, stroke, Sz
Pokeweed	GI cramping, N/D/V, labored breathing, ↓ BP, Sz
Sassafras	V, stupor, hallucinations, dermatitis, abortion, hypothermia, liver cancer
Usnic acid	Hepatotox
Yohimbine	Hypotension, abdominal distress, CNS stimulation (mania/& psychosis in predisposed individuals)

Yohimbine (*Pausinystalia yohimbe*) Uses: Rx for impotence, aphrodisiac **Action:** Peripherally affects autonomic nervous system by ↓ adrenergic activity & ↑ cholinergic activity; ↑ blood flow **Available forms:** Tabs 5.4 mg tid, PO; doses at 20–30 mg/d may ↑ BP & heart rate **Notes/SE:** Anxiety, dizziness, dysuria, genital pain, HTN, tachycardia, tremors **Interactions:** ↑ Effects *OF* CNS stimulants, MAOIs, SSRIs, caffeine, EtOH; ↑ risk of tox *W/* α-adrenergic blockers, phenothiazines; ↑ yohimbe tox *W/* sympathomimetics; ↑ BP *W/* foods containing tyramine **Labs:** ↑ BUN, Cr **NIPE:** ⊘ w/ caffeine-containing foods w/ herb, may exacerbate mania in patients w/ psychiatric disorders

Tables

TABLE 1
Quick Guide to Dosing of Acetaminophen Based on the Tylenol Product Line

	Suspension[a] Drops and Original Drops 80 mg/0.8 mL Dropperful	Chewable[a] Tablets 80-mg tabs	Suspension[a] Liquid and Original Elixir 160 mg/5 mL	Junior[a] Strength 160-mg Caplets/Chewables	Regular[b] Strength 325-mg Caplets/Tablets	Extra Strength[b] 500-mg Caplets/Gelcaps
Birth–3 mo/ 6–11 lb/ 2.5–5.4 kg	½ dppr[c] (0.4 mL)					
4–11 mo/ 12–17 lb/ 5.5–7.9 kg	1 dppr[c] (0.8 mL)		½ tsp			
12–23 mo/ 18–23 lb/ 8.0–10.9 kg	1½ dppr[c] (1.2 mL)		¾ tsp			
2–3 y/24–35 lb/ 11.0–15.9 kg	2 dppr[c] (1.6 mL)	2 tab	1 tsp			
4–5 y/36–47 lb/ 16.0–21.9 kg		3 tab	1½ tsp			

6–8 y/48–59 lb/ 22.0–26.9 kg	4 tab	2 tsp	2 cap/tab
9–10 y/60–71 lb/ 27.0–31.9 kg	5 tab	2½ tsp	2½ cap/tab
11 y/72–95 lb/ 32.0–43.9 kg	6 tab	4 tsp	3 cap/tab
Adults & children = 12 y = 96 lb = 44.0 kg	4 cap/tab	1 or 2 caps/ tabs	2 caps/ gel

^{a}Doses should be administered 4 or 5 times daily. Do not exceed 5 doses in 24 h.

^{b}No more than 8 dosage units in any 24h period. Not to be taken for pain for more than 10 days or for fever for more than 3 days unless directed by a physician.

^{c}Dropperful.

TABLE 2
Local Anesthetic Comparison Chart for Commonly Used Injectable Agents

Agent	Proprietary Names	Onset	Duration	Maximum Dose mg/kg	Maximum Dose Volume in 70-kg Adult[a]
Bupivacaine	Marcaine	7–30 min	5–7 h	3	70 mL of 0.25% solution
Lidocaine	Xylocaine, Anestacon	5–30 min	2 h	4	28 mL of 1% solution
Lidocaine with epinephrine (1:200,000)		5–30 min	2–3 h	7	50 mL of 1% solution
Mepivacaine	Carbocaine	5–30 min	2–3 h	7	50 mL of 1% solution
Procaine	Novocaine	Rapid	30 min–1 h	10–15	70–105 mL of 1% solution

[a]To calculate the maximum dose if not a 70-kg adult, use the fact that a 1% solution has 10 mg of drug per milliliter.

TABLE 3
Comparison of Systemic Steroids

Drug	Relative Equivalent Dose (mg)	Mineralo-corticoid Activity	Duration (h)	Route
Betamethasone	0.75	0	36–72	PO, IM
Cortisone (Cortone)	25	2	8–12	PO, IM
Dexamethasone (Decadron)	0.75	0	36–72	PO, IV
Hydrocortisone (Solu-Cortef, Hydrocortone)	20	2	8–12	PO, IM, IV
Methylprednisolone acetate (Depo-Medrol)	4	0	36–72	PO, IM, IV
Methylprednisolone succinate (Solu-Medrol)	4	0	8–12	PO, IM, IV
Prednisone (Deltasone)	5	1	12–36	PO
Prednisolone (Delta-Cortef)	5	1	12–36	PO, IM, IV

TABLE 4
Topical Steroid Preparations

Agent	Common Trade Names	Potency	Apply
Aclometasone dipropionate	Aclovate, cream, oint 0.05%	Low	bid/tid
Amcinonide	Cyclocort, cream, lotion, oint 0.1%	High	bid/tid
Betamethasone			
Betamethasone valerate	Valisone cream, lotion 0.01%	Low	qd/bid
Betamethasone valerate	Valisone cream 0.01, 0.1%, oint, lotion 0.1%	Intermediate	qd/bid
Betamethasone dipropionate	Diprosone cream 0.05%	High	qd/bid
Betamethasone dipropionate aerosol 0.1%	Diprosone aerosol 0.1%	Ultrahigh	qd/bid
Betamethasone dipropionate, augmented	Diprolene oint, gel 0.05%	Ultrahigh	bid (2 wk max)
Clobetasol propionate	Temovate cream, gel, oint, scalp, soln 0.05%	Ultrahigh	qd-qid
Clocortolone pivalate	Cloderm cream 0.1%	Intermediate	bid-qid
Desonide	DesOwen, cream, oint, lotion 0.05%	Low	
Desoximetasone			
Desoximetasone 0.05%	Topicort LP cream, gel 0.05%	Intermediate	
Desoximetasone 0.25%	Topicort cream, oint	High	bid-qid
Dexamethasone base	Aeroseb-Dex aerosol 0.01%	Low	
	Decadron cream 0.1%		bid/qid
Diflorasone diacetate	Psorcon cream, oint 0.05%	Ultrahigh	
Fluocinolone			
Fluocinolone acetonide 0.01%	Synalar cream, soln 0.01%	Low	bid/tid
Fluocinolone acetonide 0.025%	Synalar oint, cream 0.025%	Intermediate	bid/tid

314

Fluocinolone acetonide 0.2%	Synalar-HP cream 0.2%	High	bid/tid
Fluocinonide 0.05%	Lidex, anhydrous cream, gel, soln 0.05%	High	bid/tid oint
	Lidex-E aqueous cream 0.05%		
Flurandrenolide	Cordran cream, oint 0.025%	Intermediate	bid/tid
	cream, lotion, oint 0.05%	Intermediate	bid/tid
	tape, 4 mcg/cm²	Intermediate	qd
Fluticasone propionate	Cutivate cream 0.05%, oint 0.005%	Intermediate	bid
Halobetasol	Ultravate cream, oint 0.05%	Very high	bid
Halcinonide	Halog cream 0.025%, emollient base 0.1% cream, oint, sol 0.1%	High	qd/tid
Hydrocortisone			
Hydrocortisone	Cortizone, Caldecort, Hycort, Hytone, etc.	Low	tid/qid
	aerosol 1%, cream 0.5, 1, 2.5%, gel 0.5%, oint 0.5, 1, 2.5%, lotion 0.5, 1, 2.5%, paste 0.5% soln 1%		
Hydrocortisone acetate	Corticaine cream, oint 0.5, 1%	Low	tid/qid
Hydrocortisone butyrate	Locoid oint, soln 0.1%	Intermediate	bid/tid
Hydrocortisone valerate	Westcort cream, oint 0.2%	Intermediate	bid/tid

(Continued)

TABLE 4 (Continued)
Topical Steroid Preparations

Agent	Common Trade Names	Potency	Apply
Mometasone furoate	Elocon 0.1% cream, oint, lotion	Intermediate	qd
Prednicarbate	Dermatop 0.1% cream	Intermediate	bid
Triamcinolone			
Triamcinolone acetonide 0.025%	Aristocort, Kenalog cream, oint, lotion 0.025%	Low	tid/qid
Triamcinolone acetonide 0.1%	Aristocort, Kenalog cream, oint, lotion 0.1%	Intermediate	tid/qid
	Aerosol 0.2-mg/2-sec spray		
Triamcinolone acetonide 0.5%	Aristocort, Kenalog cream, oint 0.5%	High	tid/qid

TABLE 5
Comparison of Insulins

Type of Insulin	Onset (h)	Peak (h)	Duration (h)
Ultra Rapid			
Apidra (glulisine)	Immediate	0.5–1.5	3–5
Humalog (lispro)	Immediate	0.5–1.5	3–5
NovoLog (insulin aspart)	Immediate	0.5–1.5	3–5
Rapid			
Regular Iletin II	0.25–0.5	2–4	5–7
Humulin R	0.5	2–4	6–8
Novolin R	0.5	2.5–5	5–8
Velosulin	0.5	2–5	6–8
Intermediate			
NPH Iletin II	1–2	6–12	18–24
Lente Iletin II	1–2	6–12	18–24
Humulin N	1–2	6–12	14–24
Novolin L	2.5–5	7–15	18–24
Novolin 70/30	0.5	7–12	24
Prolonged			
Ultralente	4–6	14–24	28–36
Humulin U	4–6	8–20	24–28
Lantus (insulin glargine)	4–6	No peak	24
Combination Insulins			
Humalog Mix (lispro protamine/ lispro)	0.25–0.5	1–4	24

TABLE 6
Commonly Used Oral Contraceptives (21 = 21 Active Pills; 28 = 21 Active Pills + 7 Placebo[a])

Monophasics

Drug (Manufacturer)	Estrogen (mcg)	Progestin (mg)	Iron
Alesse 21, 28 (Wyeth)	Ethinyl estradiol (20)	Levonorgestrel (0.1)	
Apri 28 (Barr)	Ethinyl estradiol (30)	Desogestrel (0.15)	
Aviane 28 (Barr)	Ethinyl estradiol (20)	Levonorgestrel (0.1)	
Brevicon 28 (Watson)	Ethinyl estradiol (35)	Norethindrone (0.5)	
Cryselle 28 (Barr)	Ethinyl estradiol (30)	Norgestrel (0.3)	
Demulen 1/35 21, 28 (Pfizer)	Ethinyl estradiol (35)	Ethynodiol diacetate (1)	
Demulen 1/50 21, 28 (Pfizer)	Ethinyl estradiol (50)	Ethynodiol diacetate (1)	
Desogen 28 (Organon)	Ethinyl estradiol (30)	Desogestrel (0.15)	
Estrostep 28 (Warner-Chilcott)[b]	Ethinyl estradiol (20, 30, 35)	Norethindrone acetate (1)	
FemconFe (Warner-Chilcott)	Ethinyl estradiol (35)	Norethindrone (0.4)	75 mg FE
Junel Fe 1/20, 21, 28 (Barr)	Ethinyl estradiol (20)	Norethindrone acetate (1)	7 in 28 days
Junel Fe 1.5/30 21, 28 (Barr)	Ethinyl estradiol (30)	Norethindrone acetate (1.5)	7 in 28 days
Kariva 28 (Barr)	Ethinyl estradiol (20, 0, 10)	Desogestrel (0.15)	
Lessina 28 (Barr)	Ethinyl estradiol (20)	Levonorgestrel (0.1)	
Levlen 21, 28 (Berlex)	Ethinyl estradiol (30)	Levonorgestrel (0.15)	
Levlite 28 (Berlex)	Ethinyl estradiol (20)	Levonorgestrel (0.1)	
Levora 28 (Watson)	Ethinyl estradiol (30)	Levonorgestrel (0.15)	
Loestrin Fe 1.5/30 21, 28 (Warner-Chilcott)	Ethinyl estradiol (30)	Norethindrone acetate (1.5)	7 in 28 days
Loestrin Fe 1/20 21, 28 (Warner-Chilcott)	Ethinyl estradiol (20)	Norethindrone acetate (1)	7 in 28 days

318

Lo/Ovral 21, 28 (Wyeth)	Ethinyl estradiol (30)	Norgestrel (0.3)
Low-Ogestrel 28 (Watson)	Ethinyl estradiol (30)	Norgestrel (0.3)
Microgestin Fe 1/20 21, 28 (Watson)	Ethinyl estradiol (20)	Norethindrone acetate (1) 7 in 28 days
Microgestin Fe 1.5/30 21, 28 (Watson)	Ethinyl estradiol (30)	Norethindrone acetate (1.5) 7 in 28 days
Mircette 28 (Organon)	Ethinyl estradiol (20, 0, 10)	Desogestrel (0.15)
Modicon 28 (Ortho-McNeil)	Ethinyl estradiol (35)	Norethindrone (0.5)
MonoNessa 28 (Watson)	Ethinyl estradiol (35)	Norgestimate (0.25)
Necon 1/50 28 (Watson)	Mestranol (50)	Norethindrone (1)
Necon 0.5/35, 28 (Watson)	Ethinyl estradiol (35)	Norethindrone (0.5)
Necon 1/35 28 (Watson)	Ethinyl estradiol (35)	Norethindrone (1)
Nordette 21, 28 (King)	Ethinyl estradiol (30)	Levonorgestrel (0.15)
Nortrel 0.5/35 28 (Barr)	Ethinyl estradiol (35)	Norethindrone (0.5)
Nortrel 1/35 21, 28 (Barr)	Ethinyl estradiol (35)	Norethindrone (1)
Norinyl 1/35 28 (Watson)	Ethinyl estradiol (35)	Norethindrone (1)
Norinyl 1/50 28 (Watson)	Mestranol (50)	Norethindrone (1)
Ogestrel 28 (Watson)	Ethinyl estradiol (50)	Norgestrel (0.5)
Ortho-Cept 28 (Ortho-McNeil)	Ethinyl estradiol (30)	Desogestrel (0.15)
Ortho-Cyclen 28 (Ortho-McNeil)	Ethinyl estradiol (35)	Norgestimate (0.25)
Ortho-Novum 1/35 28 (Ortho-McNeil)	Ethinyl estradiol (35)	Norethindrone (1)
Ortho-Novum 1/50 28 (Ortho-McNeil)	Mestranol (50)	Norethindrone (1)

(Continued)

TABLE 6 (Continued)
Commonly Used Oral Contraceptives (21 = 21 Active Pills; 28 = 21 Active Pills + 7 Placebo[a])

Monophasics

Drug (Manufacturer)	Estrogen (mcg)	Progestin (mg)	Iron
Ovcon 35 21, 28 (Warner-Chilcott)	Ethinyl estradiol (35)	Norethindrone (0.4)	
Ovcon 50 28 (Warner-Chilcott)	Ethinyl estradiol (50)	Norethindrone (1)	
Ovral 21, 28 (Wyeth-Ayerst)	Ethinyl estradiol (50)	Norgestrel (0.5)	
Portia 28 (Barr)	Ethinyl estradiol (30)	Levonorgestrel (0.15)	
Sprintec 28 (Barr)	Ethinyl estradiol (35)	Norgestimate (0.25)	
Yasmin 28 (Berlex)	Ethinyl estradiol (30)	Drospirenone (3)	
Zovia 1/50E 28 (Watson)	Ethinyl estradiol (50)	Ethynodiol diacetate (1.0)	
Zovia 1/35E 28 (Watson)	Ethinyl estradiol (35)	Ethynodiol diacetate (1.0)	

Multiphasics

Drug	Estrogen (mcg)	Progestin (mg)
Cyclessa 28 (Organon)	Ethinyl estradiol (25)	Desogestrel (0.1, 0.125, 0.15)
Enpresse 28 (Barr)	Ethinyl estradiol (30, 40, 30)	Levonorgestrel (0.05, 0.075, 0.125)
Necon 10/11 21, 28 (Watson)	Ethinyl estradiol (35)	Norethindrone (0.5, 1.0)
Necon 7/7/7 (Watson)	Ethinyl estradiol (35)	Norethindrone (0.5, 0.75, 1.0)
Nortrel 7/7/7 28 (Barr)	Ethinyl estradiol (35)	Norethindrone (0.5, 0.75, 1.0)
Ortho Tri-Cyclen 21, 28 (Ortho-McNeill)	Ethinyl estradiol (25)	Norgestimate (0.18, 0.215, 0.25)

Ortho Tri-Cyclen lo 21, 28 (Ortho-McNeil)	Ethinyl estradiol (35, 35, 35)	Norgestimate (0.18, 0.215, 0.25)
Ortho-Novum 10/11 21 (Ortho-McNeil)	Ethinyl estradiol (35, 35)	Norethindrone (0.5, 1.0)
Ortho-Novum 7/7/7 21 (Ortho-McNeil)	Ethinyl estradiol (35, 35, 35)	Norethindrone (0.5, 0.75, 1.0)

Progestin Only

Drug	Estrogen (mcg)	Progestin (mg)
Tri-Levlen 28 (Berlex)	Ethinyl estradiol (30, 40, 30)	Levonorgestrel (0.05, 0.075, 0.125)
Tri-Nessa 28 (Watson)	Ethinyl estradiol (35)	Norgestimate (0.18, 0.215, 0.25)
Tri-Norinyl 21, 28 (Watson)	Ethinyl estradiol (35, 35, 35)	Norethindrone (0.5, 1.0, 0.5)
Triphasil 21, 28 (Wyeth)	Ethinyl estradiol (30, 40, 30)	Levonorgestrel (0.05, 0.075, 0.125)
Tri-Sprintec (Barr)	Ethinyl estradiol (35)	Norgestimate (0.18, 0.215, 0.25)
Trivora-28 (Watson)	Ethinyl estradiol (30, 40, 30)	Levonorgestrel (0.05, 0.075, 0.125)
Velivet (Barr)	Ethinyl estradiol (25)	Desogestrel (0.1, 0.125, 0.15)
Camila (Barr)	None	Norethindrone (0.35)
Errin (Barr)	None	Norethindrone (0.35)
Jolivette 28 (Watson)	None	Norethindrone (0.35)
Micronor (Ortho-McNeil)	None	Norethindrone (0.35)
Nor-QD (Watson)	None	Norethindrone (0.35)
Nora-BE 28 (Ortho-McNeil)	None	Norethindrone (0.35)
Ovrette (Wyeth-Ayerst)	None	Norgestrel (0.075)

TABLE 6 (Continued)
Commonly Used Oral Contraceptives (21 = 21 Active Pills; 28 = 21 Active Pills + 7 Placebo[a])

Extended-Cycle Combination

Drug	Estrogen (mg)	Progestin (mcg)	Additional Pills
Lybrel (Wyeth) 28 day pack	Ethinyl estradiol (20)	Levonorgestrel (0.09)	None
Yaz (Berlex) 28 day pack[b]	Ethinyl estradiol (20)	Drospirenone 4 (3)	Inert
Loestrin 24 Fe (Warner Chilcott) 28 day pack	Ethinyl estradiol (20)	Norethindrone 4 (1)	Inert
Seasonique 7 (Duramed) 91-day pack	Ethinyl estradiol (30)	Levonorgestrel (0.15)	10 mcg ethinyl estradiol
Seasonale 7 (Duramed) 91-day pack	Ethinyl estradiol (30)	Levonorgestrel (0.15)	Inert

Based in part on data published in the *Medical Letter* Volume 2 (Issue 24) August 2004, Volume 29 (Issue 1266) 2007.

[a]The designations 21 and 28 refer to number of days in regimen available.

[b]Also approved for acne.

TABLE 7
Some Common Oral Potassium Supplements

Brand Name	Salt	Form	mEq Potassium/ Dosing Unit
Glu-K	Gluconate	Tablet	2 mEq/tablet
Kaochlor 10%	KCl	Liquid	20 mEq/15 mL
Kaochlor S-F 10% (sugar-free)	KCl	Liquid	20 mEq/15 mL
Kaochlor Eff	Bicarbonate/ KCl/citrate	Effervescent tablet	20 mEq/tablet
Kaon elixir	Gluconate	Liquid	20 mEq/15 mL
Kaon	Gluconate	Tablet	5 mEq/tablet
Kaon-Cl	KCl	Tablet, SR	6.67 mEq/tablet
Kaon-Cl 20%	KCl	Liquid	40 mEq/15 mL
KayCiel	KCl	Liquid	20 mEq/15 mL
K-Lor	KCl	Powder	15 or 20 mEq/packet
Klorvess	Bicarbonate/ KCl	Liquid	20 mEq/15 mL
Klotrix	KCl	Tablet, SR	10 mEq/tablet
K-Lyte	Bicarbonate/ citrate	Effervescent tablet	25 mEq/tablet
K-Tab	KCl	Tablet, SR	10 mEq/tablet
Micro-K	KCl	Capsule, SR	8 mEq/capsule
Slow-K	KCl	Tablet, SR	8 mEq/tablet
Tri-K	Acetate/bicarbonate and citrate	Liquid	45 mEq/15 mL
Twin-K	Citrate/gluconate	Liquid	20 mEq/5 mL

SR = sustained release.

TABLE 8
Tetanus Prophylaxis

History of Absorbed Tetanus Toxoid Immunization	Clean, Minor Wounds		All Other Wounds[a]	
	Td[b]	TIG[c]	Td[d]	TIG[c]
Unknown or <3 doses	Yes	No	Yes	Yes
=3 doses	No[e]	No	No[f]	No

[a]Such as, but not limited to, wounds contaminated with dirt, feces, soil, saliva, etc; puncture wounds; avulsions; and wounds resulting from missiles, crushing, burns, and frostbite.

[b]Td = tetanus-diphtheria toxoid (adult type), 0.5 mL IM.
- For children <7 y, DPT (DT, if pertussis vaccine is contraindicated) is preferred to tetanus toxoid alone.
- For persons >7 y, Td is preferred to tetanus toxoid alone.
- DT = diphtheria-tetanus toxoid (pediatric), used for those who cannot receive pertussis.

[c]TIG = tetanus immune globulin, 250 U IM.

[d]If only 3 doses of fluid toxoid have been received, then a fourth dose of toxoid, preferably an adsorbed toxoid, should be given.

[e]Yes, if >10 y since last dose.

[f]Yes, if >5 y since last dose.

Source: Based on guidelines from the Centers for Disease Control and Prevention and reported in *MMWR.*

TABLE 9
Oral Anticoagulant Standards of Practice

Thromboembolic Disorder	INR	Duration
Deep Venous Thrombosis & Pulmonary Embolism		
Treatment single episode		
Transient risk factor	2–3	3 mo
Idiopathic	2–3	6–12 mo
Recurrent systemic embolism	2–3	Indefinite
Prevention of Systemic Embolism		
Atrial fibrillation (AF)[a]	2–3	Indefinite
AF: cardioversion	2–3	3 wk prior; 4 wk post sinus rhythm
Valvular heart disease	2–3	Indefinite
Cardiomyopathy	2–3	Indefinite
Acute Myocardial Infarction		
High-risk patients[c]	2–3 + low dose aspirin	
Prosthetic Valves		
Tissue heart valves	2–3	3 mo
Bileaflet mechanical valves in aortic position	2–3	Indefinite
Other mechanical prosthetic valves[b]	2.5–3.5	Indefinite

[a]With high-risk factors or multiple moderate risk factors.

[b]May add aspirin 81 mg to warfarin in patients with caged ball or caged disks valves with additional risk factors.

[c]Large anterior MI, significant heart failure, intracardiac thrombus, and/or history of thromboembolic event.

INR = international normalized ratio.

Source: Based on data published in *Chest* 2004 Sep; 126 (Suppl): 16.

TABLE 10
Antiarrhythmics: Vaughn Williams Classification

Class I: Sodium Channel Blockade

A. **Class Ia:** Lengthens duration of action potential (↑ the refractory period in atrial and ventricular muscle, in SA and AV conduction systems, and Purkinje fibers)
   1. Amiodarone (also class II, III, IV)
   2. Disopyramide (Norpace)
   3. Imipramine (MAO inhibitor)
   4. Procainamide (Pronestyl)
   5. Quinidine
B. **Class Ib:** No effect on action potential
   1. Lidocaine (Xylocaine)
   2. Mexiletine (Mexitil)
   3. Phenytoin (Dilantin)
   4. Tocainide (Tonocard)
C. **Class Ic:** Greater sodium current depression (blocks the fast inward Na^+ current in heart muscle and Purkinje fibers, and slows the rate of ↑ of phase 0 of the action potential)
   1. Flecainide (Tambocor)
   2. Propafenone

Class II: Beta Blocker

D. Amiodarone (also class Ia, III, IV)
E. Esmolol (Brevibloc)
F. Sotalol (also class III)

Class III: Prolong Refractory Period via Action Potential

G. Amiodarone (also class Ia, II, IV)
H. Sotalol

Class IV: Calcium Channel Blocker

I. Amiodarone (also class Ia, II, III)
J. Diltiazem (Cardizem)
K. Verapamil (Calan)

TABLE 11
Cytochrome P-450 Isoenzymes and the Drugs They Metabolize, Inhibit, and Induce[a]

	CYP1A2
Substrates:	Acetaminophen, caffeine, clozapine, imipramine, theophylline, propranolol
Inhibitors:	Most fluoroquinolone antibiotics, fluvoxamine, cimetidine
Inducer:	Tobacco smoking, charcoal-broiled foods, cruciferous vegetables, omeprazole

	CYP2C9
Substrates:	Most NSAIDs (including COX-2), warfarin, phenytoin
Inhibitors:	Fluconazole
Inducer:	Barbiturates, rifampin

	CYP2C19
Substrates:	Diazepam, lansoprazole, omeprazole, phenytoin, pantoprazole
Inhibitors:	Omeprazole, isoniazid, ketoconazole
Inducer:	Barbiturates, rifampin

	CYP2D6
Substrates:	Most β-blockers, codeine, clomipramine, clozapine, codeine, encainide, flecainide, fluoxetine, haloperidol, hydrocodone, 4-methoxy-amphetamine, metoprolol, mexiletine, oxycodone, paroxetine, propafenone, propoxyphene, risperidone, selegiline (deprenyl), thioridazine, most tricyclic antidepressants, timolol
Inhibitors:	Fluoxetine, haloperidol, paroxetine, quinidine
Inducer:	Unknown

	CYP3A
Substrates:	**Anticholinergics:** Darifenacin, oxybutynin, solifenacin, tolterodine **Benzodiazepines:** Alprazolam, midazolam, triazolam **Ca channel blockers:** Diltiazem, felodipine, nimodipine, nifedipine, nisoldipine, verapamil

(Continued)

TABLE 11 (Continued)
Cytochrome P-450 Isoenzymes and the Drugs They Metabolize, Inhibit, and Induce[a]

	Chemotherapy: Cyclophosphamide, erlotinib, ifosfamide, paclitaxel, tamoxifen, vinblastine, vincristine **HIV protease inhibitors:** Amprenavir, atazanavir, indinavir, nelfinavir, ritonavir, saquinavir **HMG-CoA reductase inhibitors:** Atorvastatin, lovastatin, simvastatin **Immunosuppressive agents:** Cyclosporine, tacrolimus **Macrolide-type antibiotics:** Clarithromycin, erythromycin, telithromycin, troleandomycin **Opioids:** Alfentanyl, cocaine, fentanyl, sufentanil **Steroids:** Budesonide, cortisol, 17-β-estradiol, progesterone **Others:** Acetaminophen, amiodarone, carbamazepine, delavirdine, efavirenz, nevirapine, quinidine, repaglinide, sildenafil, tadalafil, trazodone, vardenafil
Inhibitors:	Amiodarone, amprenavir, atazanavir, ciprofloxacin, cisapride, clarithromycin, diltiazem, erythromycin, fluconazole, fluvoxamine, grapefruit juice (in high ingestion), indinavir, itraconazole, ketoconazole, nefazodone, nelfinavir, norfloxacin, ritonavir, telithromycin, troleandomycin, verapamil, voriconazole
Inducer:	Carbamazepine, efavirenz, glucocorticoids, macrolide antibiotics, nevirapine, phenytoin, phenobarbital, rifabutin, rifapentine, rifampin, St. John's wort

[a]Increased or decreased (primarily hepatic cytochrome P-450) metabolism of medications may influence the effectiveness of drugs or result in significant drug–drug interactions. Understanding the common cytochrome P-450 isoforms (eg, CYP2C9, CYP2D6, CYP2C19, CYP3A4) and common drugs that are metabolized by (aka "substrates"), inhibit, or induce activity of the isoform helps minimize significant drug interactions. CYP3A is involved in the metabolism of >50% of drugs metabolized by the liver.

Based on data from Katzug B (ed). *Basic and Clinical Pharmacology,* 9th ed. McGraw-Hill, New York, 2004. *The Medical Letter,* Volume 47, July 4, 2004; http://www.fda.gov/cder/drug/drugreactions (accessed September 16, 2005).

TABLE 12
SSRIs/SNRI/Triptan and Serotonin Syndrome

A life-threatening condition, when selective serotonin reuptake inhibitors (SSRIs) and 5-hydroxytryptamine receptor agonists (triptans) are used together. However, many other drugs have been implicated (see below). Signs and symptoms of serotonin syndrome include the following:
Restlessness, coma, N/V/D, hallucinations, loss of coordination, overactive reflexes, ↑ heart rate/temperature, rapid changes in BP, increased body temperature

Class	Drugs
Antidepressants	MAOIs, TCAs, SSRIs, SNRIs, mirtazapine, venlafaxine
CNS stimulants	Amphetamines, phentermine, methylphenidate, sibutramine
5-HT$_1$ agonists	Triptans
Illicit drugs	Cocaine, methylenedioxymethamphetamine (ecstasy), lysergic acid diethylamide (LSD)
Opioids	Tramadol, pethidine, oxycodone, morphine, meperidine
Others	Buspirone, chlorpheniramine, dextromethorphan, linezolid, lithium, selegiline, tryptophan, St John's wort

Management includes removal of the precipitating drugs, and supportive care. To control agitation serotonin antagonists (cyproheptadine or methysergide) can be used. When symptoms are mild, discontinuation of the medication or medications, and the control of agitation with benzodiazepines may be needed. Critically ill patients may require sedation and mechanical ventilation as well as control of hyperthermia.

Boyer EW, Shannon M. The serotonin syndrome. *N Engl J Med.* 2005;352(11):1112–1120.

TABLE 13
Composition of Selected Multivitamins and Multivitamins with Mineral and Trace Element Supplements

| | Vitamins | | | | | | | | | | | | |
| | Fat Soluble | | | | Water Soluble | | | | | | | | |
	A	D	E	K	C	B₁	B₂	B₃	B₆	Folate	B₁₂	Biotin	B₅
Centrum	70	100	100	31	100	100	100	100	100	100	100	10	100
Centrum Performance	70	100	200	31	200	300	300	200	300	100	300	13	100
Centrum Silver	70	100	150	13	100	100	100	100	150	100	417	10	100
NatureMade Multi Complete	60	100	167	31	200	100	100	100	100	100	100	10	100
NatureMade Multi Daily	60	100	100	NA	100	100	100	100	100	100	100	NA	100
NatureMade Multi Max	60	100	500	50	500	3333	2941	250	2500	100	833	17	500
NatureMade Multi-50+	100	100	200	13	200	200	200	100	200	100	417	10	100
One-A-Day 50+	50	100	110	25	200	300	200	100	300	100	417	10	150
One-A-Day Essential	100	100	100	NA	100	100	100	100	100	100	100	NA	100

One-A-Day Maximum	50	100	100	31	100	100	100	100	100	100	100	10	100
Therapeutic Vitamin	100	100	100	NA	150	200	200	100	150	100	150	10	100
Theragran-M Advanced Formula High Potency	100	100	200	35	150	200	200	100	300	100	200	10	100
Theragran-M Premier High Potency	70	100	200	31	200	267	235	125	200	100	150	10	100
Theragran-M Premier 50 Plus High Potency	70	100	200	13	125	200	176	125	300	100	500	12	150
Therapeutic Vitamin + Minerals Enhanced	100	100	200	NA	150	200	200	100	300	100	200	10	100
Unicap M	100	100	100	NA	100	100	100	100	100	100	100	NA	100
Unicap Senior	100	50	50	NA	100	80	82	80	110	100	50	NA	100
Unicap T	100	100	100	NA	833	667	588	500	300	100	300	NA	250

(Continued)

TABLE 13 (Continued)
Composition of Selected Multivitamins and Multivitamins with Mineral and Trace Element Supplements

	Minerals						Trace Elements						
	Ca	P	Mg	Fe	Zn	I	Se	K	Mn	Cu	Cr	Mo	Other
Centrum	16	11	25	100	100	100	29	2	100	100	100	100	
Centrum Performance	10	5	10	100	100	100	100	2	200	100	100	100	
Centrum Silver	20	5	25	NA	100	100	29	2	100	100	125	100	Lycopene
NatureMade Multi Complete	10	8	25	50	100	100	35	1	100	100	100	33	Ginseng Ginkgo
NatureMade Multi Daily	45	NA	NA	100	100	NA	NA	NA	NA	NA	NA	NA	Lycopene
NatureMade Multi Max	10	4	6	50	100	100	100	1	100	100	100	NA	Lutein
NatureMade Multi 50+	20	5	25	NA	100	100	71	2	100	100	100	33	
NatureMade Multi Complete	10	8	25	50	100	100	35	1	100	100	100	33	Ginseng Ginkgo
NatureMade Multi Daily	45	NA	NA	100	100	NA	NA	NA	NA	NA	NA	NA	Lycopene
NatureMade	10	4	6	50	100	100	100	1	100	100	100	NA	Lutein

NatureMade Multi 50+	20	5	25		100	100	71	2	100	100	100	33	Lutein
One-A-Day 50 Plus	12	NA	25	NA	150	100	150	1	200	NA	150	120	
One-A-Day Essential	NA	NA	NA	NA	NA	NA	NA	NA	NA	NA	NA	NA	
One-A-Day Maximum	16	11	25	100	100	100	29	2	175	100	54	213	
Therapeutic 7 Vitamin	NA	NA	NA	NA	100	100	NA	NA	100	NA	NA	NA	
Theragran-M Advanced Formula High Potency	4	3	26	50	100	100	100	1	100	100	42	100	
Theragran-M Premier High Potency	17	11	25	100	100	100	286	2	100	175	100	107	Lutein
Theragran-M Premier 50 Plus High Potency	20	5	25	0	113	100	286	2	175	100	125	100	Lutein
Therapeutic Vitamin + Minerals Enhanced	4	3	25	50	100	100	100	<1	100	100	42	100	

(Continued)

333

TABLE 13 (Continued)
Composition of Selected Multivitamins and Multivitamins with Mineral and Trace Element Supplements

| | Minerals | | | | | | | Trace Elements | | | | | |
	Ca	P	Mg	Fe	Zn	I	Se	K	Mn	Cu	Cr	Mo	Other
Unicap M	6	5	NA	100	100	100	NA	<1	50	100	NA	NA	
Unicap Senior	10	8	8	56	100	100	NA	<1	50	100	NA	NA	
Unicap T	NA	NA	NA	100	100	100	14	<1	50	100	NA	NA	

Common multivitamins available without a prescription are listed. Most chain stores have generic versions of many of the multivitamin supplements listed above; thus, specific generic brands are not listed. (Many specialty vitamin combinations are available, but not included in this list. (Examples are vitamins B plus C, supplements for a specific condition or organ, pediatric and infant formulations, and prenatal vitamins.)

Values are listed as percentages of the Daily Value based on Recommended Dietary Allowances of vitamins and minerals based on Dietary Reference Intakes (Food and Nutrition Board, Institute of Medicine, National Academy of Science).

¹Common generic brands (when other than the store name itself) are: Osco Drug Central-Vite (Albertson's); Spectravite (CVS); Kirkland Signature Daily Multivitamin (Costco); Whole Source, PharmAssure (Rite Aid); Central-Vite (Safeway); Member's Mark (Sam's Club); Vitasmart (Kmart); Century (Target); A thru Z Select, Super Aytinal, Ultra Choice (Walgreens) Equate Complete or Spring Valley Sentury-Vite (Wal-Mart).

Vitamins: B₁ = Thiamine; B₂ = Riboflavin; B₃ = Niacin; B₅ = Pantothenic Acid; B₆ = Pyridoxine; B₁₂ = Cyanocobalamin. **Elements:** Ca = calcium; Cr = chromium; Cu = copper; Fe = iron; Fl = fluoride; I = iodine; K = potassium; Mg = magnesium; Mo = molybdenum; Mn = manganese; P = phosphorus; Se = selenium; Zn = zinc; NA = not applicable or not available.

Index